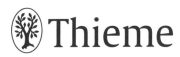

Differential Diagnosis in Neuroimaging

Head and Neck

Steven P. Meyers, MD, PhD, FACR
Professor of Radiology/Imaging Sciences, Neurosurgery, and Otolaryngology
Director, Radiology Residency Program
University of Rochester School of Medicine and Dentistry
Rochester, New York

1538 illustrations

Thieme
New York • Stuttgart • Delhi • Rio de Janeiro

Executive Editor: William Lamsback
Managing Editor: J. Owen Zurhellen IV
Director, Editorial Services: Mary Jo Casey
Editorial Consultant: Judith Tomat
Production Editor: Kenneth L. Chumbley
International Production Director: Andreas Schabert
Vice President, Editorial and E-Product Development: Vera Spillner
International Marketing Director: Fiona Henderson
International Sales Director: Louisa Turrell
Director of Sales, North America: Mike Roseman
Senior Vice President and Chief Operating Officer: Sarah Vanderbilt
President: Brian D. Scanlan

Library of Congress Cataloging-in-Publication Data

Names: Meyers, Steven P., author.
Title: Differential diagnosis in neuroimaging : head and neck /
    Steven P. Meyers.
Description: New York : Thieme, [2017] | Includes bibliographical
    references.
Identifiers: LCCN 2016024610| ISBN 9781626234758 (alk. paper) |
    ISBN 9781626234765 (eISBN)
Subjects: | MESH: Neuroimaging | Central Nervous System
    Diseases—diagnosis | Head—pathology | Neck—pathology
Classification: LCC RC349.D52 | NLM WL 141.5.N47 |
    DDC 616.8/04754—dc23
LC record available at https://lccn.loc.gov/2016024610

© 2017 Thieme Medical Publishers, Inc.
Thieme Publishers New York
333 Seventh Avenue, New York, NY 10001 USA
+1 800 782 3488, customerservice@thieme.com

Thieme Publishers Stuttgart
Rüdigerstrasse 14, 70469 Stuttgart, Germany
+49 [0]711 8931 421, customerservice@thieme.de

Thieme Publishers Delhi
A-12, Second Floor, Sector-2, Noida-201301
Uttar Pradesh, India
+91 120 45 566 00, customerservice@thieme.in

Thieme Publishers Rio de Janeiro, Thieme Publicações Ltda.
Edifício Rodolpho de Paoli, 25º andar
Av. Nilo Peçanha, 50 – Sala 2508
Rio de Janeiro 20020-906, Brasil
+55 21 3172 2297

Cover design: Thieme Publishing Group
Typesetting by Prairie Papers

Printed in China by Asia Pacific Offset   5 4 3 2 1

ISBN 978-1-62623-475-8

Also available as an e-book:
eISBN 978-1-62623-476-5

Important note: Medicine is an ever-changing science undergoing continual development. Research and clinical experience are continually expanding our knowledge, in particular our knowledge of proper treatment and drug therapy. Insofar as this book mentions any dosage or application, readers may rest assured that the authors, editors, and publishers have made every effort to ensure that such references are in accordance with **the state of knowledge at the time of production of the book.**

Nevertheless, this does not involve, imply, or express any guarantee or responsibility on the part of the publishers in respect to any dosage instructions and forms of applications stated in the book. **Every user is requested to examine carefully** the manufacturers' leaflets accompanying each drug and to check, if necessary in consultation with a physician or specialist, whether the dosage schedules mentioned therein or the contraindications stated by the manufacturers differ from the statements made in the present book. Such examination is particularly important with drugs that are either rarely used or have been newly released on the market. Every dosage schedule or every form of application used is entirely at the user's own risk and responsibility. The authors and publishers request every user to report to the publishers any discrepancies or inaccuracies noticed. If errors in this work are found after publication, errata will be posted at www.thieme.com on the product description page.

Some of the product names, patents, and registered designs referred to in this book are in fact registered trademarks or proprietary names even though specific reference to this fact is not always made in the text. Therefore, the appearance of a name without designation as proprietary is not to be construed as a representation by the publisher that it is in the public domain.

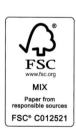

To my parents, for their unwavering encouragement and support along my long journey through formal education.

And to my wife, Barbara, and son, Noah, for their continuous love, support, and patience during this project.

Contents

Preface

As an academic neuroradiologist who has had the privilege of working at a university medical center for the past twenty-five years, I have had many opportunities to continuously learn and be involved in the education of medical students, as well as residents and fellows in radiology, neurosurgery, neurology, otolaryngology, and orthopedics. During my training, I had the opportunity of working with outstanding professors who served as role models for teaching and research. I learned from them that excellent teaching cases are invaluable in the education of our specialty. For the past three decades, I have been collecting and organizing a large teaching file for lectures, as well as an educational resource that can be utilized at the workstation. It is from this large data base that I began writing this three-volume series in my specialty of neuroradiology ten years ago.

The goal of these books is to present the imaging features of neuroradiological abnormalities in an easy-to-use format with extensive utilization of figures for illustration.

This volume of the series, *Differential Diagnosis in Neuroimaging: Head and Neck*, contains chapters describing lesions located in the skull and temporal bone; orbits; paranasal sinuses and nasal cavity; suprahyoid neck; infrahyoid neck; and brachial plexus.

The organization of this and the other books focuses on lists of differential diagnoses of lesions based on anatomic locations in a tabular format. Brief introductory summaries with illustrations are provided at the beginning of most chapters to succinctly provide relevant information, after which tables are presented. Each of the lesions listed in the tables has a column summarizing the pertinent *imaging findings* associated with images for illustration, and a *comments* column summarizing key

clinical data. References are provided in alphabetical order at the end of each chapter. For the reader's convenience, some of the diagnoses are listed in two or more tables. The purpose of this is to minimize or eliminate the need to page back to the same entries in other tables in order to find the desired information.

These books' unique organization helps the reader obtain information efficiently and quickly. Because of the heavy emphasis on providing illustrative images over text, this book format can be an effective guide in narrowing the differential diagnoses of lesions based on their locations and imaging findings.

The other volumes in the series include: *Differential Diagnosis in Neuroimaging: Brain and Meninges*, which covers lesions involving the brain, ventricles, meninges, and neurovascular system in both children and adults; and *Differential Diagnosis in Neuroimaging: Spine*, which includes differential diagnosis tables for congenital and developmental abnormalities, intradural intramedullary lesions (spinal cord lesions), dural and intradural extramedullary lesions, extradural lesions, solitary osseous lesions involving the spine, multifocal lesions and/or poorly-defined signal abnormalities involving the spine, traumatic lesions, and lesions involving the sacrum

I hope these texts will be a valuable resource for practicing radiologists, neurosurgeons, neurologists, otolaryngologists, and orthopedic spine surgeons. These books are intended to become a "well-thumbed text" at the PACS station and clinics. They should also serve as a useful review and teaching guide for trainees in radiology, neurosurgery, neurology, orthopedics, otolaryngology, and other medical specialties, who are preparing for board examinations.

Steven P. Meyers, MD, PhD, FACR

Acknowledgments

I wish to acknowledge the Thieme staff, in particular J. Owen Zurhellen IV, Judith Tomat, William Lamsback, and Kenny Chumbley for their dedication, hard work, and attention to detail. I thank Ms. Colleen Cottrell for her outstanding secretarial work with this project. I also thank Gwendolyn Mack, MFA, Nadezhda D. Kiriyak, BFA, and Katie Tower, BFA, for their creative talents in making illustrations for this book. I thank Sarah Klingenberger and Margaret Kowaluk for helping me optimize the MRI and CT images of this book.

In addition, I wish to acknowledge the following for their contribution of interesting cases: Jeevak Almast, MBBS, Allan Bernstein, MD, Daniel Ginat, MD, Gary M. Hollenberg, MD, Edward Lin, MD, BBA, Peter Rosella, MD, David Shrier, MD, Eric P. Weinberg, MD, Brian Webber, DO, and Andrea Zynda-Weiss, MD.

I extend my appreciation and thanks to my coworkers and physician colleagues (Drs. Bernstein, Hollenberg, Rosella, Shrier, Weinberg, and Zynda-Weiss) at University Medical Imaging, the Outpatient Diagnostic Imaging Facility of the University of Rochester, for making an ideal collaborative environment for teaching and clinical service.

Lastly, I would like to give thanks to my former teachers and mentors for their guidance, encouragement, and friendship.

Illustrations by:

Nadezhda D. Kiriyak: 1.89, 1.90, 1.129, 1.130, 1.131, 3.1, 3.2, 3.4, 5.1, 5.21, 5.52, 5.83, 5.103, 5.110, 6.17

Katie Tower: 6.128

Gwendolyn Mack: 1.1, 1.2, 2.8, 4.1, 4.2, 4.24, 4.25, 4.40, 4.64, 4.82, 4.113, 5.19, 5.53, 7.2

Abbreviations

ABC   Aneurysmal Bone Cyst

ADC   Apparent diffusion coefficient

AML   Acute myelogenous leukemia

ANA   Antinuclear antibodies

ANCA   Anti-neutrophil cytoplasmic antibody

AP   Anteroposterior

AS   Ankylosing spondylitis

ATC   Anaplastic undifferentiated thyroid carcinoma

AVF   Arteriovenous fistula

AVM   Arteriovenous malformation

Ca   Calcium/calcification

CCD   Cleidocranial dysplasia/dysostosis

CHARGE   Syndrome including: Coloboma, Heart anomaly, Atresia choanae, Retardation, Genital hypoplasia, and Ear abnormalities

CIDP   Chronic acquired immune-mediated multifocal demyelinating neuropathy

CISS   Constructive interference steady state

CLL   Chronic lymphocytic leukemia

CML   Chronic myelogenous leukemia

CMT   Charcot-Marie-Tooth disease

CMV   Human cytomegalovirus

CN   Cranial nerve

CNS   Central nervous system

CPA   Cerebellopontine angle

CPPD   Calcium pyrophosphate dihydrate deposition

CSF   Cerebrospinal fluid

CT   Computed tomography

DISH   Diffuse idiopathic skeletal hyperostosis

DTI   Diffusion tensor imaging

DWI   Diffusion weighted imaging

EA   Esophageal atresia

EAC   External auditory canal

EBV   Epstein Barr virus

ECA   External carotid artery

EG   Eosinophilic granuloma

EMA   Epithelial membrane antigen

EMG   Electromyography

FGFR   Fibroblast growth factor receptor

FIESTA   Fast imaging employing steady state acquisition

FLAIR   Fluid attenuation inversion recovery

FS   Frequency selective fat signal suppression

FSE   Fast spin echo

FS-PDWI   Fat-suppressed proton density weighted imaging

FSPGR   Fast spoiled gradient echo imaging

FS-T1WI   Fat-suppressed T1-weighted imaging

FS-T2WI   Fat-suppressed T2-weighted imaging

Gd-contrast   Gadolinium-chelate contrast

GRE   Gradient echo imaging

HD   Hodgkin disease

HIV   Human immunodeficiency virus

HMB-45   Human melanoma black monoclonal antibody

HPF   High power field

HPV   Human papilloma virus

HSV   Herpes simplex virus

HU   Hounsfield unit

IAC   Internal auditory canal

ICA   Internal carotid artery

IP-1   Incomplete partition type 1 of the cochlea

IP-2   Incomplete partition type 2 of the cochlea

IVJ   Internal jugular vein

JIA   Juvenile idiopathic arthritis

LCH   Langerhans cell histiocytosis

MCA   Middle cerebral artery

MEN   Multiple endocrine neoplasia

MIP   Maximum intensity projection

MMN   Multifocal motor neuropathy

MPNST   Malignant peripheral nerve sheath tumor

MPS   Mucopolysaccharidosis

MRA   MR angiography

MRV   MR venography

MS   Multiple sclerosis

NF1   Neurofibromatosis type 1

NF2   Neurofibromatosis type 2

NHL   Non-Hodgkin lymphoma

NSE   Neuron specific enloase

OI   Osteogenesis imperfecta

PC   Phase contrast

PCA   Posterior cerebral artery

PCOM   Posterior communicating artery

PDTC   Poorly differentiated thyroid carcinoma

PDWI   Proton density weighted imaging

PHPV   Persistent hyperplastic primary vitreous

PNET   Primitive neuroectodermal tumor

PSA   Persistent stapedial artery

PVNS   Pigmented villondular synovitis

RF   Radiofrequency

RPS   Retropharyngeal space

PPS   Parapharyngeal space

PPPS   Pre-styloid parapharyngeal space

RPPS   Retro-styloid parapharyngeal space

SCC   Squamous cell carcinoma

SLE   Systemic lupus erythematosus

SMA   Smooth muscle actin antibodies

SNUC   Sinonasal undifferentiated carcinoma

STIR   Short TI inversion recovery imaging

SWI   Susceptibility weighted imaging

S-100   Cellular calcium binding protein in cytoplasm and/or nucleus

T1   Spin-lattice or longitudinal relaxation time (coefficient)

T2   Spin-spin or transverse relaxation time (coefficient)

T2*   Effective spin-spin relaxation time using GRE pulse sequence

T1WI   T1-weighted imaging

T2WI   T2-weighted imaging

TE   Time to echo

TEF   Tracheoesophageal fistula

TR   Pulse repetition time interval

TOF   Time of flight

2D   2 dimensional

3D   3 dimensional

WHO   World Health Organization

Chapter 1
Skull and Temporal Bone

1 Skull and Temporal Bone

Introduction

Skull

The skull is derived from mesenchymal tissue (desmocranium) that surrounds the rostral end of the closed neural tube. The skull and cranial bones are divided into two major portions, the *neurocranium* and *viscerocranium*. The neurocranium is composed of the bones that surround the brain and special sense organs. The viscerocranium refers to the bones of the lower face and jaws.

The neurocranium is divided into two subcategories based on whether the bones develop directly from the embryonic connective tissue/mesenchyme in portions of the desmocranium that surround the brain to form the cranial vault or calvarium (membranous neurocranium) versus those portions that arise via cartilaginous precursors within the desmocranium to form the chondrocranium from which the bones at the skull base develop. These two major pathways of bone development are also referred to as *intramembranous* and *endochondral bone formation* (**Fig. 1.1**).

The desmocranium is derived from paraxial mesoderm and neural crest cells adjacent to the notochord that progressively surround the rostral end of the closed neural tube at the end of the first month of gestation. Primary ossification centers in the membranous neurocranium occur at 9 to 10 weeks of gestation, resulting in formation of the frontal and temporal squamosa and parietal and occipital bones. Other cranial bones that derive from intramembranous bone formation include: the nasal bone, lacrimal bone, zygoma, tympanic bone, and portions of the sphenoid bone (lateral pterygoid bone, some of the greater wing—alisphenoid). The growth of the calvarium is directly related to the relatively rapid progressive growth of the developing brain. Bones of the viscerocranium that also develop via membranous bone formation include the vomer, palatine bone, maxilla, and mandible.

The chondrocranium or chondrobasicranium develops when chondrification centers develop within the desmocranium at 6 to 7 weeks of gestation. These chondrification centers occur between the base of the developing brain and foregut, extending from the nasal region to the foramen magnum. Ossification centers occur in the chondrocranium at 6 to 8 weeks of gestation. At 6 to 7 weeks of gestation, an ossification center can be identified in the basiocciput ventral to the notochord. At 7 weeks, paired ossification centers can be seen in the parietal bones and supraoccipital portions of the occipital bone. At 8 weeks, ossification occurs at the exoccipital bones. Growth and fusion of these and multiple other ossification centers occur during gestation. At birth, 13 ossification centers can be seen in the sphenoid bone and six in the occipital bone. Nonfused ossification centers can be seen at the spheno-occipital and sphenopetrous junctions, petrous apices, sphenoid and occipital bones, and nasal alae and septum.

Most of the clivus portion of the skull base is derived from the four occipital somites at 4 weeks of gestation. Each somite differentiates into an outer dermatome, inner myotome, and medial sclerotome. The mesenchymal tissue of these somites converts into cartilage. The four occipital sclerotomes (also referred to as primary cranial vertebrae) fuse to form the occipital bone and posterior portion of the foramen magnum. The upper two sclerotomes form the basiocciput. The third occipital sclerotome forms the exoccipital bone and jugular tubercles, and the lowermost occipital sclerotome (proatlas) forms the anterior tubercle of the clivus and anterior arch of the foramen magnum, as

Development of the skull

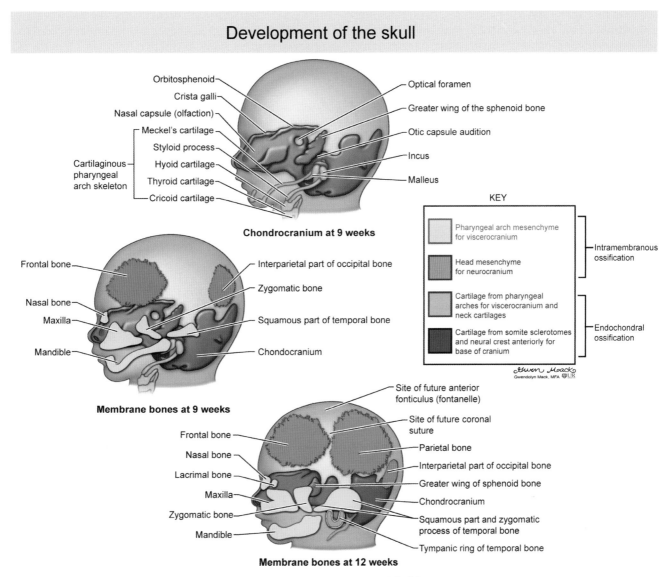

Chondrocranium at 9 weeks

- Orbitosphenoid
- Crista galli
- Nasal capsule (olfaction)
- Meckel's cartilage
- Styloid process
- Hyoid cartilage
- Thyroid cartilage
- Cricoid cartilage
- Cartilaginous pharyngeal arch skeleton
- Optical foramen
- Greater wing of the sphenoid bone
- Otic capsule audition
- Incus
- Malleus

Membrane bones at 9 weeks

- Frontal bone
- Nasal bone
- Maxilla
- Mandible
- Interparietal part of occipital bone
- Zygomatic bone
- Squamous part of temporal bone
- Chondocranium

KEY

Pharyngeal arch mesenchyme for viscerocranium	Intramembranous ossification
Head mesenchyme for neurocranium	
Cartilage from pharyngeal arches for viscerocranium and neck cartilages	Endochondral ossification
Cartilage from somite sclerotomes and neural crest anteriorly for base of cranium	

Gwendolyn Mack, MFA

Membrane bones at 12 weeks

- Frontal bone
- Nasal bone
- Lacrimal bone
- Maxilla
- Zygomatic bone
- Mandible
- Site of future anterior fonticulus (fontanelle)
- Site of future coronal suture
- Parietal bone
- Interparietal part of occipital bone
- Greater wing of sphenoid bone
- Chondrocranium
- Squamous part and zygomatic process of temporal bone
- Tympanic ring of temporal bone

Fig. 1.1 Diagram of developmental chondrification and ossification patterns of skull formation.

well as the lateral atlantal masses of the C1 vertebra and superoposterior portion of the arch of the C1 vertebra. The skull base develops and surrounds the already formed cranial nerves and major arteries, resulting in the formation of the skull-base foramina. The occipital sclerotomes and parachordal cartilages form the condylar and basilar portions of the occipital bone. The polar cartilage and trabecular cartilages of the sphenoid form the sella turcica and sphenoid body, respectively. The nasal capsule and presphenoid cartilage form the ethmoid bone.

Most of the bones of the skull base, except the orbital plate of the frontal bone and lateral portions of the greater wings of the sphenoid bone, are derived by endochondral bone formation and include the sphenoid bone (basisphenoid, orbitosphenoid-lesser wing, presphenoid, postsphenoid portions, some of the greater wing) and occipital bone (bassiocciput and supraoccipital and exoccipital portions). At birth, six components of the occipital bone are observed.

In the first 3 years of life, the anterior and posterior intra-occipital synchondroses begin to fuse. The occipital-mastoid, petro-occipital, and spheno-occipital synchondroses typically remain partially open into the second decade. At birth the sphenoid bone can have 13 ossification centers, most of which usually fuse or assimilate into the sphenoid bone by age 2 years. Pneumatization of the sphenoid sinus begins after the first year, and it progressively enlarges for the next 5 years.

Growth of the membranous calvarial bones is induced by expansion of brain volume and size. Sutures develop when the cranial bones are in close approximation. Sutures contain vascularized, dense, fibrous connective tissue that is oriented into layers related to active growth. At the sutures, there is dynamic mechanical union between adjacent skull bones where bone resorption and progressive appositional bone deposition occur, leading to calvarial bone growth and expansion. Most of the calvarial growth occurs at the sagittal and coronal sutures. The sutures typically widen where they intersect to form the fontanelles. The larger anterior fontanelle occurs at the intersection of the metopic, sagittal, and coronal sutures and closes by the end of the second year. The smaller posterior fontanelle, which occurs at the junction of the sagittal and lambdoid sutures, closes before 3 months.

The fibrous desmocranium develops an outer periosteum at the outer table of the skull and an inner layer adjacent to the inner table (inner periosteum) that fuses with the dura propria derived from mesoderm (also referred to as the periosteal layer of the dura mater). The inner and outer periosteal layers are connected via intrasutural ligaments and skull foramina.

The chondrocranium begins development at 40 days, with the conversion of mesenchyme surrounding the notochord into cartilage next to the base of the brain. During the fifth week of gestation, the notochord is enclosed by the bodies of the upper cervical vertebrae and enters into the basiocciput, where it terminates in the body of the sphenoid bone just below the pituitary fossa and is in contact with the endoderm of the embryonic pharynx. The basiocciput forms the lower two-thirds to three-fourths of the clivus and is derived from the fusion of four occipital sclerotomes. Portions of the chondrocranium persist at birth and are located at the spheno-occipital junction and sphenopetrous junction, within the sphenoid and occipital bones, petrous apices/foramen lacerum, and nasal septum and alae. Synchondroses occur between bones and contain cartilage. The skull base enlarges from appositional growth at endochondral remnants or synchondroses and is related to forces applied by bone expansion and growth at the calvarial sutures. Most of the growth and elongation of the skull base in the postnatal period occurs at the spheno-occipital and sphenopetrous synchondroses. Fusion of the spheno-occipital synchondrosis has been reported to occur in males at 16 to 18.5 years and in females between 14 and 16 years. Fusion of the anterosuperior portions of the petro-occipital synchondrosis occurs at 16 to 18 years, whereas the inferoposterior portions remain as a fissure containing fibrocartilage.

The bones of the skull typically consist of inner and outer tables of compact bone with intervening cancellous bone of the diploic space, which also contains bone marrow. At birth, the bone marrow is typically hematopoietically active, containing red marrow. Red marrow contains 40% water, 40% fat, and 20% protein. A progressive conversion from red to yellow marrow occurs with age, generally from the appendicular skeleton to the axial skeleton. Yellow marrow is hematopoietically inactive and contains 15% water, 80% fat, and 5% protein. These changes can be monitored by observable MRI signal changes. The hematopoietic marrow has low-intermediate signal equal to or slightly lower than muscle on T1-weighted images. Marrow that contains mixed hematopoietic and fat components typically has intermediate signal on T1-weighted images that is slightly higher than muscle but less than fat.

Fatty marrow conversion occurs when the marrow signal is high on T1-weighted images and is similar to fat signal elsewhere in the body. In children less than 3 months old, the MRI signal of marrow in the skull and spine is that of red marrow on T1-weighted imaging. The rate of conversion from red to yellow marrow varies among bones as well as within bones. As the conversion progresses, the marrow signal increases on T1-weighted images. The skull contains 25% of the active hematopoietic marrow at birth. Fatty conversion of skull marrow occurs first in the skull base and facial bones and can be seen with MRI at 2 years of age. Fatty conversion of the calvarium begins in the frontal bones, followed by the parietal bones at ~ 2 years, and can be progressively observed with MRI over the next 13 years. In the clivus, mixed low-intermediate and high signal can be seen at 3 years, with complete fatty conversion seen at 15 years.

The inner portions of the skull can be subdivided into three major compartments: anterior, middle, and posterior cranial fossae (**Fig. 1.2**). The anterior cranial fossa includes the anterior portion of the skull base to the posterior margin of the lesser sphenoid wings. The floor of the anterior cranial fossa is located above the orbits (orbital roof), nasal

Interior base of skull, superior view

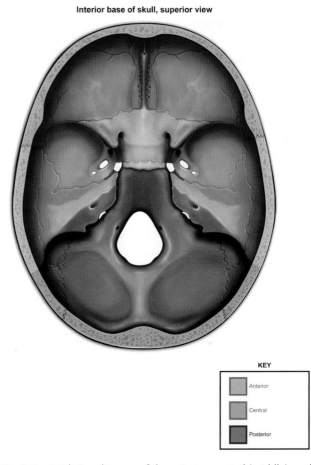

KEY

Anterior

Central

Posterior

Fig. 1.2 Axial view diagram of the anterior, central (middle), and posterior portions of the skull base.

cavity, and ethmoid labyrinths (cribriform plate and crista galli). Within the anterior cranial fossa are the frontal lobes.

The middle cranial fossa is located posterior to the anterior cranial fossa. The anterior border of the middle cranial fossa extends posteriorly from the greater sphenoid wings laterally and upper surface of the sella turcica medially to the superior margins of the petrous ridges of the temporal bones. The floor of the middle cranial fossa is the central skull base, within which are openings for neurovascular foramina, such as the superior orbital fissure, foramen rotundum, vidian canal, foramen ovale, foramen spinosum, carotid artery canal, and jugular foramen.

The posterior cranial fossa is located behind the bassiocciput and basisphenoid, and posterior to the mastoid and petrous portions of the temporal bones. The floor of the posterior cranial fossa is the occipital bone, within which is located the foramen magnum.

References

1. Belden CJ. The skull base and calvaria. Adult and pediatric. Neuroimaging Clin N Am 1998;8(1):1–20
2. Madeline LA, Elster AD. Suture closure in the human chondrocranium: CT assessment. Radiology 1995;196(3):747–756
3. Menezes AH. Craniocervical developmental anatomy and its implications. Childs Nerv Syst 2008;24(10):1109–1122
4. Smoker WRK. Craniovertebral junction: normal anatomy, craniometry, and congenital anomalies. Radiographics 1994;14(2):255–277
5. Smoker WRK, Khanna G. Imaging the craniocervical junction. Childs Nerv Syst 2008;24(10):1123–1145
6. Kanev PM. Congenital malformations of the skull and meninges. Otolaryngol Clin North Am 2007;40(1):9–26, v
7. Laine FJ, Nadel L, Braun IFCT. CT and MR imaging of the central skull base. Part 1: Techniques, embryologic development, and anatomy. Radiographics 1990;10(4):591–602
8. Taccone A, Oddone M, Occhi M, Dell'Acqua AD, Ciccone MA. MRI "road-map" of normal age-related bone marrow. I. Cranial bone and spine. Pediatr Radiol 1995;25(8):588–595
9. Foster K, Chapman S, Johnson K. MRI of the marrow in the paediatric skeleton. Clin Radiol 2004;59(8):651–673

Table 1.1 Congenital and developmental abnormalities involving the skull

- Cephaloceles (frontal, parietal, occipital, sphenoid)
- Atretic parietal cephalocele
- Frontonasal cephalocele
- Frontal-ethmoidal cephalocele, nasal glioma, nasal dermoid
- Sinus pericranii
- Chiari II malformation/Luckenschadel skull
- Achondroplasia
- Basiocciput hypoplasia
- Condylus tertius
- Atlanto-occipital assimilation/nonsegmentation
- Craniosynostosis
- Multiple synostosis syndromes
- Apert syndrome
- Crouzon syndrome
- Other syndromes with premature sutural closure: Disorders related to mutations involving fibroblast growth factor receptors (*FGFR1, FGFR2, FGFR3*)
- Parietal foramina
- Positional plagiocephaly
- Cleidocranial dysplasia/dysostosis
- Wormian bones
- Neurofibromatosis type 1
- Venous lake
- Arachnoid granulation
- Unilateral hemimegalencephaly
- Congenital hydrocephalus
- Macrocephaly from inherited metabolic disorders (Alexander disease, Canavan disease, megalencephalic leukodystrophy with subcortical cysts)
- Microcephaly
- Dyke-Davidoff-Masson syndrome
- Hematopoietic disorders
- Osteopetrosis
- Oxalosis
- Osteogenesis imperfecta
- Epidermoid

Table 1.1 Congenital and developmental abnormalities involving the skull

Lesions or Disorder	Imaging Findings	Comments
Cephaloceles (frontal, parietal, occipital, sphenoid) (**Fig. 1.3, Fig. 1.4,** and **Fig. 1.5**)	Defect in skull through which there is herniation of either meninges and CSF (meningocele) or meninges, CSF/ventricles, and brain tissue (meningoencephaloceles).	Congenital malformation involving lack of separation of neuroectoderm from surface ectoderm, with resultant localized failure of bone formation. Occipital location most common in patients in Western hemisphere, frontoethmoidal location most common site in Southeast Asians. Other sites include parietal and sphenoid bones. Cephaloceles can also result from trauma or surgery.

(continued on page 8)

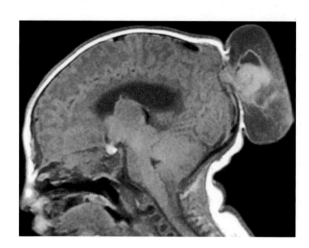

Fig. 1.3 Parietal meningoencephalocele. Sagittal T1-weighted imaging shows a localized skull defect through which damaged brain and meninges extend.

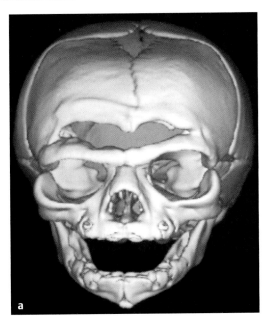 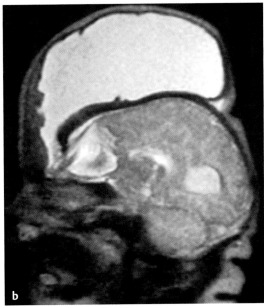

Fig. 1.4 Frontal gliocele. **(a)** Coronal surface-rendered CT shows a defect in the frontal bone. **(b)** Sagittal T2-weighted imaging shows damaged brain tissue and meninges extending through the skull defect. A large gliocele (glial-lined cyst) is seen overlying the upper calvarium.

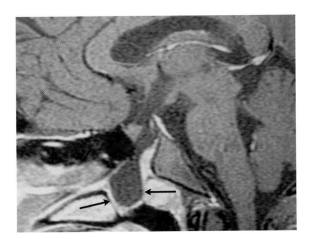

Fig. 1.5 A 17-year-old female with a meningocele (*arrows*) extending inferiorly into the nasopharynx through an osseous defect in the sphenoid bone located posterior to the pituitary gland, as seen on postcontrast fat-suppressed sagittal T1-weighted imaging .

Table 1.1 *(cont.)*   Congenital and developmental abnormalities involving the skull

Lesions or Disorder	Imaging Findings	Comments
Atretic parietal cephalocele (**Fig. 1.6**)	Subcutaneous scalp nodule that often contains high signal on T2-weighted imaging, with thin, low-signal, fibrous bands that are adjacent to a skull defect and may involve intracranial dural venous sinuses. Can result in elevation of the torcular herophili and fenestration of the superior sagittal sinus.	Small defect in the skull (usually parietal bone) through which a small (5–15) cephalocele results in an elevated, hairless, skin-covered scalp lesion. The atretic cephalocele connects to the intracranial space via fibrous bands. May be associated with other anomalies (Dandy-Walker malformation, callosal dysgenesis, others).
Frontonasal cephalocele (**Fig. 1.7**)	Cephalocele occurs between the frontal and nasal bones.	Congenital midline masses that result from lack of normal developmental regression of the embryologic fonticulus frontalis between the frontal bone and nasal bone, with herniation of meninges ± brain tissue through the skull defect.
Frontal-ethmoidal cephalocele, nasal glioma, nasal dermoid (**Fig. 1.8**)	Nasoethmoidal cephaloceles are the most common type and occur between the nasal bones and nasal cartilage. A persistent enlarged foramen cecum is usually present. The sinus tract can contain epidermal inclusion cysts. Gadolinium contrast enhancement of the sinus tract can be seen, with superimposed infection and with or without intracranial extension.	Congenital midline masses that result from lack of normal developmental regression of an embryologic dural projection through the foramen cecum (between the nasal bone and nasal cartilage). Lack of normal separation of the dural projection from the skin can result in a sinus tract, which may eventually contain an epidermal inclusion cyst (dermoid, epidermoid) or extracranial dysplastic brain tissue (nasal glioma) in the nasal cavity or subcutaneous tissue. A nasal dimple is usually present on clinical exam. Sinus tracts can become infected and extend intracranially to cause meningitis, cerebritis, subdural empyema, and/or brain abscess.
Sinus pericranii (**Fig. 1.9**)	Communication between dilated extracranial veins and the intracranial veins or dural venous sinuses through a skull defect or emissary veins.	Lesions are nonpulsatile, asymptomatic, soft tissue masses in the scalp near the midline calvarial sutures and often measure 15 mm. Can increase in size with Valsalva maneuver. Lesions are associated with intracranial anomalies, such as solitary developmental venous anomalies, vein of Galen hypoplasia, vein of Galen aneurysm, dural sinus malformation, and intraosseous arteriovenous malformation. Can be the cutaneous sign of an underlying venous anomaly.

(continued on page 10)

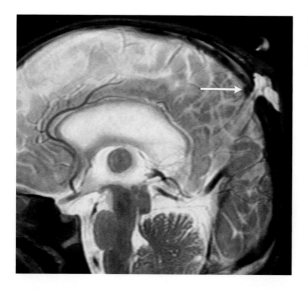

Fig. 1.6   Atretic cephalocele. Sagittal T2-weighted imaging shows a subcutaneous scalp nodule with high signal (*arrow*), which extends intracranially through a small skull defect along an obliquely oriented straight venous sinus.

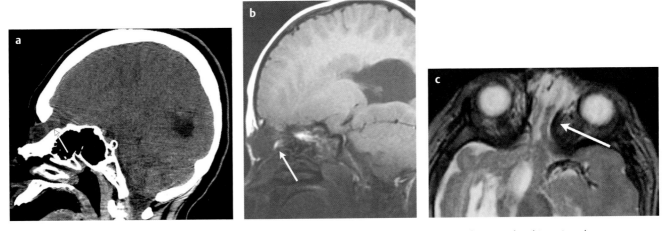

Fig. 1.7 Frontonasal cephalocele. **(a)** Sagittal CT, **(b)** sagittal T1-weighted imaging, and **(c)** axial T2-weighted imaging show an osseous defect between the lower frontal bone and nasal bones traversed by a meningoencephalocele (*arrows* in **a,b,c**).

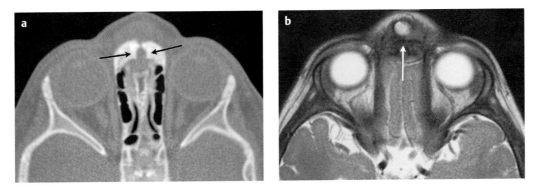

Fig. 1.8 Nasal dermoid. **(a)** An enlarged foramen cecum (*arrows*) is seen on axial CT. **(b)** Within the foramen cecum is a dermoid, seen as a localized zone with high signal (*arrow*) on axial T2-weighted imaging.

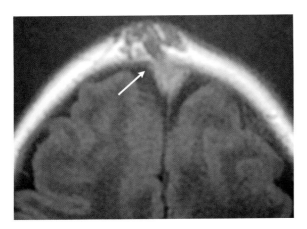

Fig. 1.9 Axial T1-weighted imaging of a 4-week-old female with sinus pericranii that is seen as communication between extracranial veins and the anterior portion of the superior sagittal sinus (*arrow*) through a skull defect.

Table 1.1 *(cont.)*   Congenital and developmental abnormalities involving the skull

Lesions or Disorder	Imaging Findings	Comments
Chiari II malformation/ Luckenschadel skull **(Fig. 1.10)**	Large foramen magnum through which there is an inferiorly positioned vermis associated with a cervicomedullary kink. Myelomeningoceles in nearly all patients, usually in the lumbosacral region. Hydrocephalus and syringomyelia common. Dilated lateral ventricles posteriorly (colpocephaly). Multifocal scalloping at the inner table of the skull (Luckenschadel) can be seen, which often regresses after 6 months.	Complex anomaly involving the cerebrum, cerebellum, brainstem, spinal cord, ventricles, skull, and dura. Failure of fetal neural folds to develop properly results in altered development affecting multiple sites of the CNS. Dysplasia of membranous skull/calvarium in Chiari II (referred to as Luckenschadel skull, lacunar skull, or craniolacunae) can occur, with multifocal thinning of the inner table from nonossified fibrous bone from abnormal collagen development and ossification.
Achondroplasia **(Fig. 1.11)**	The calvarium/skull vault is enlarged in association with a small skull base and narrow foramen magnum. Cervicomedullary myelopathy and/or hydrocephalus can result from a narrowed foramen magnum. The posterior cranial fossa is shallow, and the basal foramina are hypoplastic. Small jugular foramina can restrict venous outflow from the head. Other findings include short, wide ribs, square iliac bones, champagne glass–shaped pelvic inlet, and short pedicles involving multiple vertebrae/congenital spinal canal stenosis.	Autosomal dominant rhizomelic dwarfism that results in abnormal reduced endochondral bone formation. Most common nonlethal bone dysplasia and short-limbed dwarfism, with an incidence of 1/15,000 live births. More than 80–90% are spontaneous mutations involving the gene that encodes the fibroblast growth factor receptor 3 (*FGFR3*) on chromosome 4p16.3. The mutations typically occur on the paternal chromosome and are associated with increased paternal age. The mutated gene impairs endochondral bone formation and longitudinal lengthening of long bones.
Basiocciput hypoplasia **(Fig. 1.12)**	Hypoplasia of the lower clivus results in primary basilar invagination, with the dens extending intracranially by more than 5 mm above Chamberlain's line. Can result in decreased clival-canal angle below the normal range of 150 to 180 degrees, ± syrinx formation in spinal cord.	The lower clivus is a portion of the occipital bone (basiocciput), which is composed of four fused sclerotomes. Failure of formation of one or more of the sclerotomes results in a shortened clivus and primary basilar invagination (dens extending > 5 mm above Chamberlain's line).
Condylus tertius **(Fig. 1.13)**	Ossicle seen between the lower portion of a shortened basiocciput and dens/atlas.	Condylus tertius, or third occipital condyle, results from lack of fusion of the lowermost fourth sclerotome (proatlas) with the adjacent portions of the clivus. This third occipital condyle can form a pseudojoint with the anterior arch of C1 and/or dens, and it can be associated with decreased range of movement.

(continued on page 12)

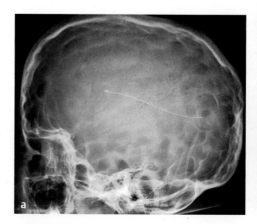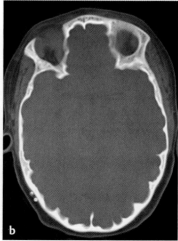

Fig. 1.10   Chiari II malformation/Luckensch-adel skull. **(a)** Lateral radiograph and **(b)** axial CT show multifocal scalloping at the inner table of the skull.

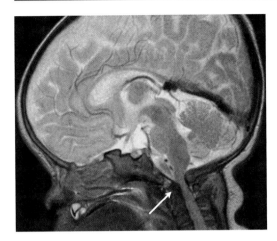

Fig. 1.11 An 8-week-old female with achondroplasia. Sagittal T2-weighted imaging shows a severely narrowed foramen magnum indenting the upper cervical spinal cord (*arrow*). The posterior cranial fossa is shallow.

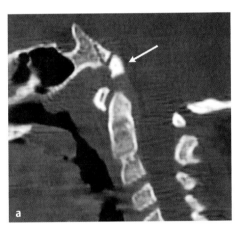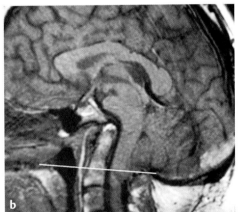

Fig. 1.12 Basiocciput hypoplasia. **(a)** Sagittal CT in an 8-year-old boy shows only minimal formation of the occipital portion of the clivus (*arrow*). **(b)** Sagittal T1-weighted imaging in a 36-year-old man shows hypoplasia of the occipital clivus causing the dens to extend intracranially abnormally above Chamberlain's line (horizontal line in **b**), resulting in an indentation on the pons (basilar invagination).

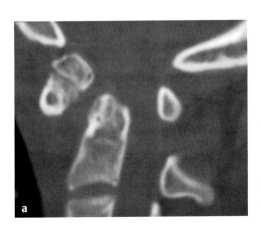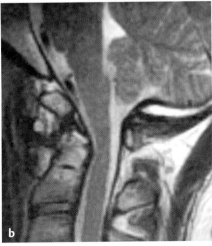

Fig. 1.13 (a) Sagittal CT and **(b)** sagittal T2-weighted imaging in a 16-year-old male show an ossicle (condylus tertius) between the lower portion of a shortened basiocciput and dens/atlas.

Table 1.1 *(cont.)* Congenital and developmental abnormalities involving the skull

Lesions or Disorder	Imaging Findings	Comments
Atlanto-occipital assimilation/ nonsegmentation (**Fig. 1.14**)	Often seen as fusion of the occipital condyle with one or both lateral masses of C1.	Occurs from failure of segmentation of the occipital condyle and the C1 vertebra.
Craniosynostosis (**Fig. 1.15**, **Fig. 1.16**, **Fig. 1.17**, and **Fig. 1.18**)	*Sagittal suture:* Premature closure, most common type (~ 60%), results in an elongated skull (dolichocephaly or scaphocephaly; **Fig. 1.15**). *Coronal or lambdoid suture:* Premature closure, ~ 10%, results in a vertically elongated skull that is asymmetric from the anterior to posterior portions of the skull (brachycephaly), or turricephaly, with narrowed AP dimension and increased height of skull. *Unilateral coronal or lambdoid suture:* Premature closure, with cranial asymmetry from left to right sides (plagiocephaly). *Metopic suture:* Premature closure, results in a wedge-shaped skull with apex anteriorly (trigonocephaly).	Premature closure of cranial suture due to developmental anomaly (primary synostosis), from extraneous causes, such as intrauterine or postnatal trauma, toxins, drugs (aminopterin, dilantin, retinoic acid, valproic acid), metabolic disorders (hyperthyroidism, hypercalcemia, hypophosphatasia, rickets, mucopolysaccharidoses, hydrocephalus, etc.), or lack of brain growth/microcephaly. Sagittal suture closure is the most common (60%), followed by unilateral or bilateral closure of the coronal suture (25%). Premature closure of the metopic suture, resulting in trigonocephaly, occurs in 15%. Only 2–3% have premature closure of the lambdoid suture. Most cases are sporadic, but 8% of coronal craniosynostosis and 2% of sagittal craniosynostosis are related to X-linked hypophosphatemic rickets. Premature sutural closure can result from chromosomal abnormalities (Apert syndrome—mutation on chromosome 10; Saethre-Chotzen syndrome—mutation at chromosome 7p21.2; Pfeiffer syndrome—mutation of chromosome 10; Crouzon syndrome—mutation of chromosome 10).
Multiple synostosis syndromes (**Fig. 1.19**)	Premature synostosis involving more than one suture, with various deformities of skull shape. Associations with underlying anomalies of brain and ventriculomegaly.	Can be sporadic or associated with various genetic disorders, such as Apert syndrome, Crouzon syndrome, etc.
Apert syndrome (**Fig. 1.20**)	Irregular craniosynostosis (bilateral premature closure of coronal sutures is most common), hypertelorism, midface hypoplasia/ underdevelopment, and symmetric complex syndactyly involving hands and feet.	Apert syndrome is the most common syndromic craniosynostosis. It is an autosomal dominant disorder resulting from mutation of the gene for fibroblast growth factor receptor 2 *(FGFR2)* at 10q26.13, with an incidence of 1/55,000 live births. Features include irregular craniosynostosis, midface hypoplasia, syndactyly of fingers and toes. Mental function impairment, often severe, occurs in 70% of cases. High association with brain anomalies (abnormal olfactory bulbs/tracts, malformations of the hippocampi/amygdala-limbic system, septum pellucidum, corpus callosum, gray matter heterotopia, ventriculomegaly). Patients present with headaches, seizures, and conductive hearing loss.

(continued on page 15)

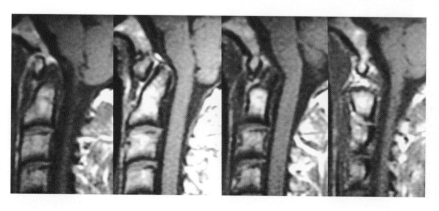

Fig. 1.14 Sagittal T1-weighted imaging shows congenital fusion of the lower clivus with the anterior arch of C1, representing atlanto-occipital assimilation.

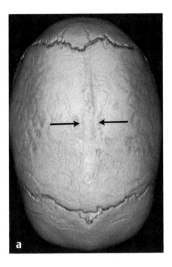
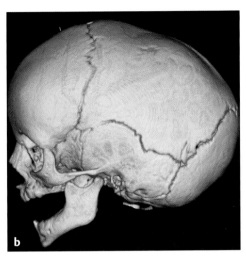

Fig. 1.15 Craniosynostosis. A 9-month-old male with premature fusion of the sagittal suture resulting in scaphocephaly as seen on (a) axial (*arrows*) and (b) sagittal volume-rendered CT.

Fig. 1.16 Craniosynostosis. (a) Angled coronal and (b) sagittal volume-rendered CT of an 11-month-old female shows premature fusion of the coronal suture (*arrows*), resulting in brachycephaly and turricephaly (towerhead appearance).

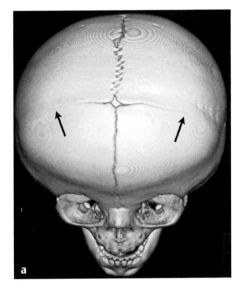
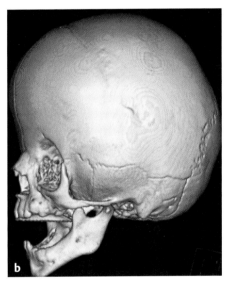

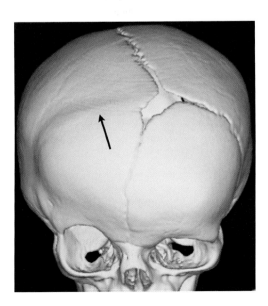

Fig. 1.17 Craniosynostosis. Coronal volume-rendered CT shows premature fusion of the coronal suture on only one side (*arrow*), resulting in plagiocephaly.

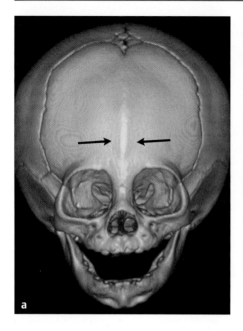

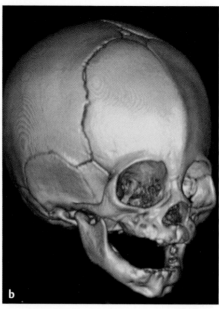

Fig. 1.18 Craniosynostosis. **(a,b)** Volume-rendered CT of a 4-month-old female with premature fusion of the metopic suture (*arrows*), resulting in trigonocephaly.

Fig. 1.19 Multiple synostosis syndrome. **(a)** Lateral and **(b)** axial volume-rendered CT show narrowed AP dimension and increased height of the skull in a 10-month-old male from premature partial closure of the sagittal suture and coronal suture (*arrows*).

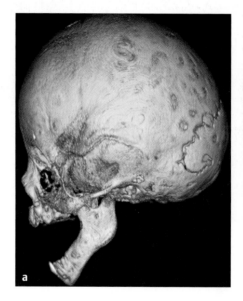

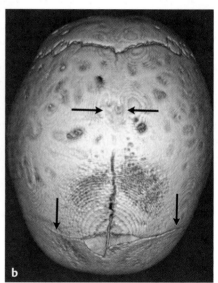

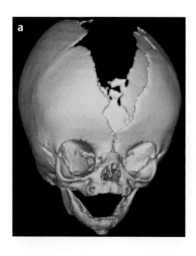

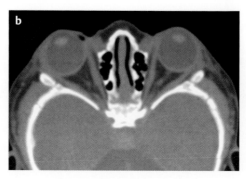

Fig. 1.20 Apert syndrome. **(a)** Coronal volume-rendered CT shows craniosynostosis consisting of premature closure of the coronal suture, resulting in a widened sagittal suture as well as midface hypoplasia/underdevelopment. **(b)** Axial CT shows hypertelorism.

Table 1.1 *(cont.)* Congenital and developmental abnormalities involving the skull

Lesions or Disorder	Imaging Findings	Comments
Crouzon syndrome **(Fig. 1.21)**	Premature ossification and closure of the coronal and lambdoid sutures, causing brachycephaly, followed by early closure of the other sutures. Other findings are shallow orbits, hypertelorism, maxillary hypoplasia, enlarged jaw ± acanthosis nigrans (*FGFR3*), and Chiari I malformation.	Crouzon syndrome is also known as craniofacial dysotosis. It is an autosomal dominant syndrome with mutation of the *FGFR2* gene at 10q26.13 or *FGFR3* at 4p16.3. At birth, findings include craniosynostosis and often fusion of the synchondroses at the skull base. Other clinical findings include maxillary hypoplasia, shallow orbits with proptosis, bifid uvula, ± cleft palate. Up to 70% of patients have Chiari I malformation. Progressive hydrocephalus occurs in 50%.

(continued on page 16)

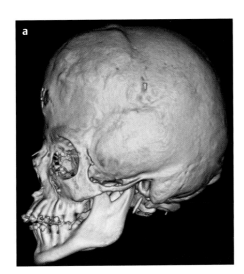 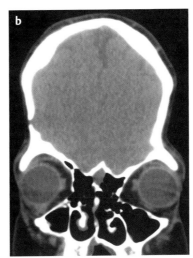 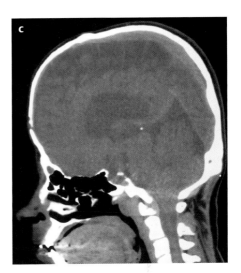

Fig. 1.21 Crouzon syndrome. **(a)** Lateral volume-rendered CT, **(b)** coronal CT, and **(c)** sagittal CT show turricephaly related to prior premature ossification and closure of the coronal and lambdoid sutures. Also seen are shallow orbits, hypertelorism **(a,b)**, and Chiari I malformation **(c)**.

Table 1.1 *(cont.)* Congenital and developmental abnormalities involving the skull

Lesions or Disorder	Imaging Findings	Comments
Other syndromes with premature sutural closure: Disorders related to mutations involving fibroblast growth factor receptors (*FGFR1, FGFR2, FGFR3*)	*Pfeiffer syndrome*: Craniosynostosis (coronal suture with or without sagittal suture—turribrachycephaly; or combined coronal and lambdoid sutures—lobulated "cloverleaf" skull with expansion of calvarial bone between sutures), hypertelorism, Chiari I malformation, hydrocephalus, broad thumbs and toes, and partial syndactyly (**Fig. 1.22**). *Saethre-Chotzen syndrome*: Craniosynostosis (coronal, lambdoid, and/or metopic sutures), brachycephaly, parietal foramina, maxillary hypoplasia, mild syndactyly, and duplicated halluces (**Fig. 1.23**). *Muenke syndrome*: Craniosynostosis (unicoronal, bicoronal, unilateral or bilateral), midfacial hypoplasia, ± thimblelike middle phalanges, ± coned epiphyses, ± tarsal or carpal coalitions.	Autosomal dominant mutations involving fibroblast growth factor receptors (FGFR) 1, 2, or 3 result in hyperplasia of precursor cells involved in osteogenesis. Mutations of the FGFR genes result in different clinical phenotypes, including syndromes with craniosynostosis. Associated with increased paternal age. *Pfeiffer syndrome*: Autosomal dominant syndrome—mutations of *FGFR2* at 10q26.13 or *FGFR1* at 8p11.23-p11.22. *Saethre-Chotzen syndrome*: Autosomal dominant syndrome—mutation of *FGFR2* gene at 10q26.13, or *TWIST1* gene on 7p21.1. *Muenke syndrome*: Autosomal dominant syndrome—mutation involving *FGFR3* at 4p16.3.
Parietal foramina (**Fig. 1.23**)	Bilateral ovoid defects in the posterior parasagittal parietal bones near the vertex. Can involve both inner and outer tables of calvarium, ± traversing blood vessels.	Small or large oval osseous defects secondary to delayed or incomplete ossification of the parietal bone. Often occur adjacent to the sagittal suture. Often autosomal dominant inheritance secondary to mutations of the *MSX2* gene or the *ALX4* gene on chromosome 11p. Usually asymptomatic, can be associated with malformations at the posterior cranial fossa.

(continued on page 18)

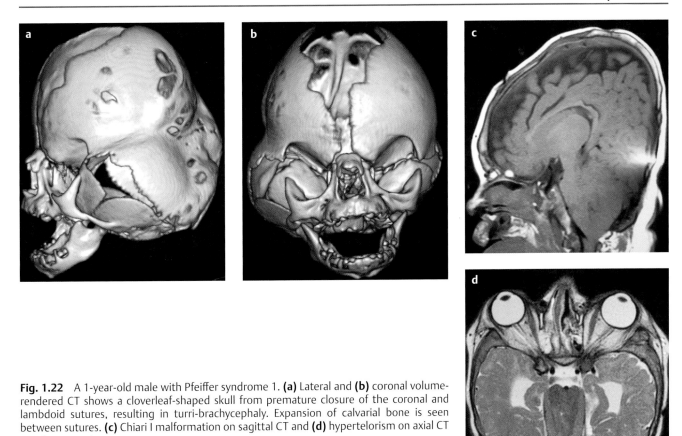

Fig. 1.22 A 1-year-old male with Pfeiffer syndrome 1. **(a)** Lateral and **(b)** coronal volume-rendered CT shows a cloverleaf-shaped skull from premature closure of the coronal and lambdoid sutures, resulting in turri-brachycephaly. Expansion of calvarial bone is seen between sutures. **(c)** Chiari I malformation on sagittal CT and **(d)** hypertelorism on axial CT are also present.

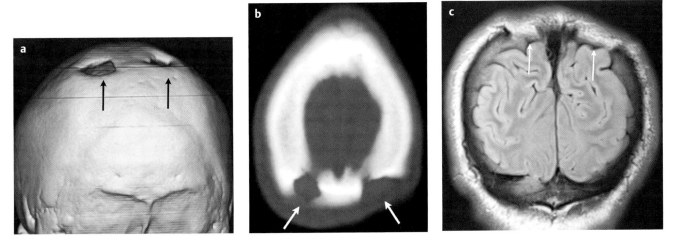

Fig. 1.23 A 20-year-old man with Saethre-Chotzen syndrome. **(a)** Volume-rendered CT, **(b)** axial CT, and **(c)** coronal FLAIR show bilateral parietal foramina (*arrows*).

Table 1.1 *(cont.)*   Congenital and developmental abnormalities involving the skull

Lesions or Disorder	Imaging Findings	Comments
Positional plagiocephaly **(Fig. 1.24)**	Neonates routinely positioned on their side can develop scaphocephaly or, if they sleep on their back, occipital flattening. Can be symmetric or asymmetric.	Deformity of skull by consistent prolonged placement of infant in the same position during rest and sleep. Common in premature neonates on ventilator support. No evidence of premature closure of synostoses is seen.
Cleidocranial dysplasia/ dysostosis **(Fig. 1.25)**	*CT:* Small skull base, brachycephaly, frontal bossing, elongated foramen magnum, hypertelorism, hypoplastic zygoma, stenosis of the external auditory canals, underdeveloped mastoid air cells, choanal stenosis, arched V-shaped palate, and hypoplastic midface and paranasal sinuses. Also observed are hypoplastic or aplastic clavicles.	Autosomal dominant syndrome involving the *RUNX2* gene on chromosome 6p21. Mutations result in haploinsufficiency that affects osteoblast precursor cell differentiation. Loss of one functional gene results in cleidocranial dysplasia/dysostosis; when both genes are abnormal, there is lack of osteoblast differentiation. Involves both membranous and endochondral bone formation. Findings include widening of the fontanelles, *late* sutural closure, broad lateral cranial dimensions, wormian bones in the lambdoid suture, hearing loss (38%), hypoplastic or absent clavicles, multiple spinal anomalies, widened symphysis pubis, short stature, hypoplastic middle and distal phalanges, and supernumerary teeth.
Wormian bones **(Fig. 1.26)**	Small bones within sutures or fontanelles, most common in lambdoid (right side greater than the left) > coronal > sagittal > metopic sutures. Within the fontanelles, wormian bones occur in the asterion > posterior > anterior > orbital fontanelle.	Accessory small bones that occur within sutures and fontanelles of the skull. Can be sporadic (8–15% of general population), or in association with craniosynostosis, osteogenesis imperfecta, Down syndrome, cleidocranial dysostosis/dysplasia, pycnodysostosis, congenital hypothyroidism, or rickets.

(continued on page 20)

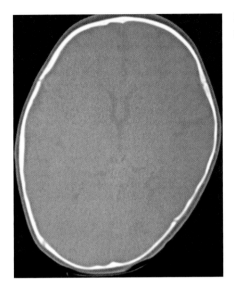

Fig. 1.24 Axial CT of a 7-month-old male shows positional plagiocephaly with a flattened appearance of the left occipital bone. Note that both lambdoid sutures are patent.

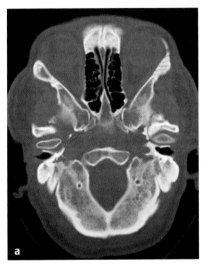

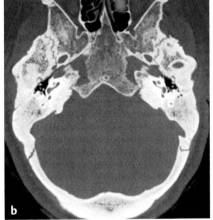

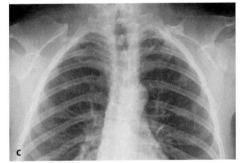

Fig. 1.25 A 35-year-old woman with cleidocranial dysplasia/dysostosis. **(a,b)** Axial CT shows a small skull base, elongated foramen magnum, hypertelorism, hypoplastic zygoma, and underdeveloped mastoid air cells. **(c)** Frontal chest radiograph shows absence of clavicles.

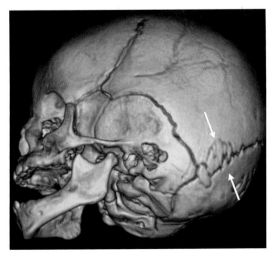

Fig. 1.26 An 8-month-old male with wormian bones (*arrows*) in the right lambdoid suture on volume-rendered CT.

Table 1.1 *(cont.)* Congenital and developmental abnormalities involving the skull

Lesions or Disorder	Imaging Findings	Comments
Neurofibromatosis type 1 **(Fig. 1.27)**	Neurofibromatosis type 1 (NF1) is associated with focal ectasia of intracranial dura, widening of internal auditory canals from dural ectasia, dural and temporal lobe protrusion into orbit through bony defect, bony hypoplasia of greater sphenoid wing, and bone malformation or erosion from plexiform neurofibromas.	Autosomal dominant disorder (1/3,000 births) from mutations involving the neurofibromin gene on chromosome 17q11.2. Represents the most common type of neurocutaneous syndrome. Neurofibronin is a GTPase-activating protein (Ras-GTP) that negatively activates the intracellular signaling protein p21-ras (Ras). Haploinsufficiency or complete deficiency in NF1 results in elevation of Ras activity, which alters cellular proliferation and differentiation of different cell types. Clinical features include café-au-lait spots (skin), axillary freckles, and cutaneous neurofibromas. Patients can have short stature and macrocephaly. Osseous lesions include malformations of sphenoid bone (greater wing hypoplasia/aplasia— usually unilateral), vertebrae, and long bones (tibia/ fibula). More than 50% of osseous malformations of the sphenoid greater wing are associated with NF1. Bone defects can also occur at the lambdoid and sagittal sutures.
Venous lake **(Fig. 1.28)**	*MRI:* Can show gadolinium contrast enhancement and enhancing blood vessels within the diploic space. *CT:* Circumscribed, lobulated, or ovoid radiolucent defect in the calvarium.	Defect in the skull that results from localized dilatation of diploic venous channels.
Arachnoid granulation **(Fig. 1.29)**	Circumscribed ovoid structures within dural venous sinuses, with low signal on T1-weighted imaging and FLAIR, high signal on T2-weighted imaging, and no gadolinium contrast enhancement, ± erosion of adjacent inner table of skull.	Extension of arachnoid membrane into dural venous sinuses. Normal CSF pulsations can result in erosion of adjacent bone.
Unilateral hemimegalencephaly **(Fig. 1.30)**	*MRI:* Nodular or multinodular regions of gray matter heterotopia involving all or part of a cerebral hemisphere, with associated enlargement of the ipsilateral lateral ventricle and hemisphere. Zones with high signal on T2-weighted imaging may occur in the white matter.	Heterogeneous sporadic disorder with hamartomatous overgrowth of one cerebral hemisphere secondary to disturbances in neuronal proliferation and migration and cortical organization. May be associated with unilateral hemihypertrophy and/or cutaneous abnormalities.

(continued on page 22)

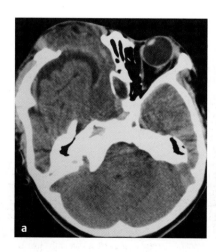

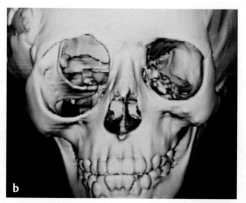

Fig. 1.27 A 10-year-old female with neurofibromatosis type 1. **(a)** Axial CT shows absent greater wing of the right sphenoid bone, with dural and temporal lobe protrusion into the right orbit through the bony defect. **(b)** Coronal volume-rendered CT shows absence of the greater wing of the right sphenoid bone.

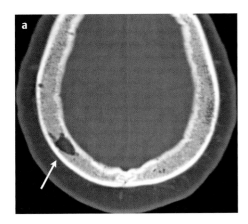 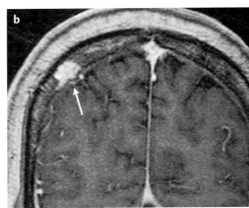

Fig. 1.28 **(a)** A 52-year-old man with a radiolucent venous lake (*arrow*) in the calvarium on axial CT. **(b)** Gadolinium contrast enhancement is seen (*arrow*) on coronal T1-weighted imaging.

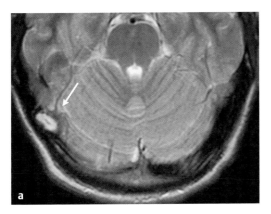 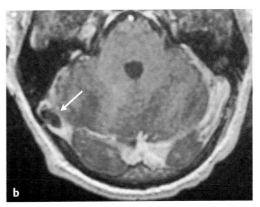

Fig. 1.29 **(a)** A 14-year-old male with an arachnoid granulation within the right transverse venous sinus that has high signal (*arrow*) on axial T2-weighted imaging. **(b)** There is no gadolinium contrast enhancement (*arrow*) on axial T1-weighted imaging. Erosion of the adjacent inner table of skull is seen.

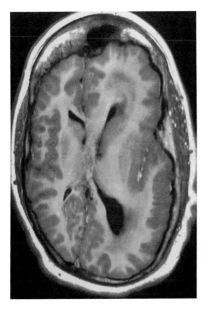

Fig. 1.30 Unilateral hemimegalencephaly. Axial T1-weighted imaging shows asymmetric enlargement of the left side of the skull from enlargement of the left cerebral hemisphere, which has abnormal thickened cerebral cortex and gyri, and slightly enlarged left lateral ventricle.

Table 1.1 *(cont.)* Congenital and developmental abnormalities involving the skull

Lesions or Disorder	Imaging Findings	Comments
Congenital hydrocephalus (**Fig. 1.31**)	*MRI:* With aqueductal stenosis, dilatation of lateral and third ventricles with normal-size fourth ventricle, ± dilatation of only the upper portion of cerebral aqueduct and not the lower portion, ± discrete or poorly defined lesion in midbrain. Subependymal edema can be seen on FLAIR. Macrocephaly is often present.	Incidence is 2 per 1,000 live births. Most common causes are aqueductal stenosis secondary to a small lesion/or neoplasm in the midbrain or debris or adhesions from hemorrhage or inflammatory diseases. May also result from extrinsic compression of the tectal plate and aqueduct from massively enlarged ventricles or ventricular diverticulum. MRI can exclude other lesions causing obstruction of CSF flow through the aqueduct, such as lesions in the posterior third ventricle or posterior cranial fossa. Congenital hydrocephalus also occurs in association with Chiari I, Chiari II, and Dandy-Walker malformations.
Macrocephaly from inherited metabolic disorders (Alexander disease, Canavan disease, megalencephalic leukodystrophy with subcortical cysts)	*Alexander disease* *MRI:* Bilateral symmetric zones of increased signal on T2-weighted imaging (T2WI) and FLAIR in the frontal lobes extending into the temporal and parietal lobes, including the external and extreme capsules, anterior limbs of the internal capsules, subcortical arcuate fibers, midbrain and medulla, and dentate nuclei of the cerebellum. Signal abnormalities in the cerebral white matter can have mass effect early in the disease, with swelling of gyri and narrowing of the lateral ventricles. Increased signal on T2WI and swelling can be seen in the caudate nuclei, basal ganglia, and thalami. Contrast enhancement can be seen in the frontal white matter, periventricular regions, basal ganglia, thalami and brainstem, as well as the optic chiasm. *Canavan disease* *MRI:* Diffuse, abnormal, increased signal on T2-weighted imaging and FLAIR in subcortical cerebral and cerebellar white matter, progressing centripetally to eventually involve the central cerebral white matter and internal capsules, thalami and globus pallidi, cerebellum, and brainstem, with sparing of the caudate nuclei and putamina. Eventual progressive cerebral, cerebellar, and brainstem atrophy. Magnetic resonance spectroscopy shows elevated *N*-acetylaspartate (NAA) peak levels. *Megalencephalic leukodystrophy with subcortical cysts (MLC)* *MRI:* Large brain, with diffuse abnormal high signal on T2-weighted imaging and FLAIR in the cerebral white matter, sparing the cerebral cortex, basal ganglia, and thalami, ± signal changes involving the corpus callosum and internal capsules. Limited involvement of the cerebellum initially. Findings secondary to vacuolation and loss of myelin and degenerative cystic changes. Eventual progressive disappearance of the white matter, which is replaced by fluid. Subcortical cysts typically develop in the anterior temporal lobes, as well as in the frontal and parietal lobes.	Macrocephaly is defined as a head circumference that is more than 2 standard deviations above the mean, or exceeds the 97th percentile by 0.5 cm. *Alexander disease* is a rare, usually sporadic, disease, occasionally autosomal dominant, with three subtypes (infantile, juvenile, and adult). It is caused by mutations of the *GFAP* gene on chromosome 17q21, which encodes glial fibrillary acidic protein. *Canavan disease* is a rare, autosomal recessive neurologic disorder in infants and children that results from mutation of the aspartoacylase gene (*ASPA*) on the short arm of chromosome 17 (17p13-ter). Pathophysiology includes increases in water content and NAA in cerebral white matter, myelin vacuolization and loss, and decreased myelin lipids and proteins. Clinical signs and symptoms begin in the first 6 months after a relatively normal neonatal period. Progressive neurologic decline leads to death, usually at or before 4 years. *Megalencephalic leukodystrophy with subcortical cysts (MLC)* is also referred to as leukoencephalopathy with macrocephaly. MLC is a rare autosomal recessive disease with slow, progressive, clinical deterioration in the first 2 decades. Seventy-five percent of cases are caused by mutations of the *MLC1* gene on chromosome 22qtel, which normally encodes a membrane protein at astrocyte-astrocyte junctions. Another mutation associated with MLC involves the *HEPCAM* gene, which encodes for a glial adhesion (GLIALCAM) protein. Mutated genes result in intramyelinic vacuolation and fibrillary astrogliosis.
Microcephaly (**Fig. 1.32**)	Small brain associated with simplified gyral pattern (usually less than five per hemisphere), shallow sulci, and thin cerebral cortex. Corpus callosum may be thin, deformed, or absent. Zones of gliosis and encephalomalacia are often present.	Head circumference more than 2–3 standard deviations below normal secondary to reduced proliferation of neurons and glial cells. The severity of microcephaly is related to the degree of gyral simplification and severity of corpus callosal anomalies. Can result from a neonatal destructive process, such as hypoxic-ischemic encephalopathy or infection (TORCH). Children are usually severely impaired and often die in their first year of life.

(continued on page 24)

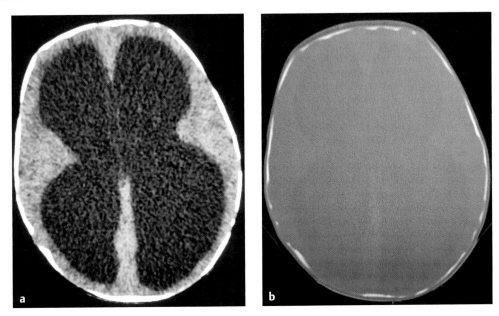

Fig. 1.31 A 3-month-old female with congenital hydrocephalus. **(a,b)** Axial CT shows macrocephaly, markedly dilated lateral ventricles, widened sutures, and multifocal scalloping of the inner tables of the skull.

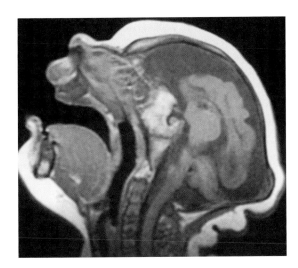

Fig. 1.32 An 8-month-old male with microcephaly with simplified gyral pattern, as seen on sagittal T1-weighted imaging, resulting in a small skull.

Table 1.1 *(cont.)* Congenital and developmental abnormalities involving the skull

Lesions or Disorder	Imaging Findings	Comments
Dyke-Davidoff-Masson syndrome (**Fig. 1.33**)	Atrophy/encephalomalacia of one cerebral hemisphere with compensatory dilatation of ipsilateral lateral ventricle, midline shift, unilateral ipsilateral decrease in size of cranial fossa associated with thickened calvarium, ± enlargement of ipsilateral pneumatized paranasal sinuses and mastoid air cells.	Rare disorder in adolescents presenting with seizures, mental retardation, hemiparesis, or hemiplegia. Can result from congenital injury, such as cerebral infarction from occlusion of the middle cerebral artery, or from postnatal trauma, hemorrhage, ischemia, or infection.
Hematopoietic disorders (See **Fig. 1.85** and **Fig. 1.86**)	Enlargement of the diploic space with red marrow hyperplasia and thinning of the inner and outer tables. Involved marrow has slightly to moderately decreased signal relative to fat on T1- and T2-weighted imaging, isointense to slightly hyperintense signal relative to muscle and increased signal relative to fat on fat-suppressed T2-weighted imaging.	Thickening of diploic space related to erythroid hyperplasia from sickle-cell disease, thalassemia major, or hereditary spherocytosis.
Osteopetrosis (**Fig. 1.34**)	*CT:* Findings include generalized bone sclerosis and hyperostosis, resulting in thickening of the skull, as well as narrowing of the foramina and optic canals. *MRI:* Low signal on T1- and T2-weighted imaging in marrow of endochondral bone (skull base and vertebrae). Expansion of calvarial diploic space, and marrow has low-intermediate to intermediate signal on T1- and T2-weighted imaging.	Osteopetrosis is group of disorders with defective resorption of primary spongiosa and mineralized cartilage secondary to osteoclast dysfunction. Results in failure of conversion of immature woven bone into strong lamellar bone. Consists of four types: the precocious type, an autosomal recessive form (which is usually lethal from medullary crowding secondary to thickened, immature, sclerotic bone, resulting in anemia, thrombocytopenia, and immune dysfunction); the delayed type, an autosomal dominant form described by Albers-Schonberg that can be asymptomatic until there is a pathologic fracture or anemia; the intermediate recessive type, in which patients have short stature, hepatomegaly, and anemia; and tubular acidosis, an autosomal recessive form in which cerebral calcifications occur as well as renal tubular acidosis, mental retardation, muscle weakness, and hypotonia.

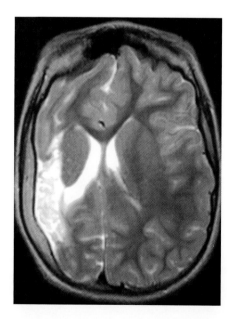

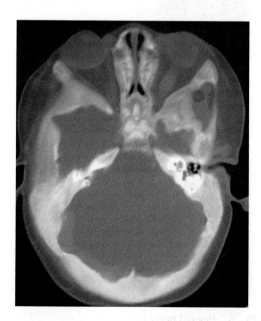

Fig. 1.33 A 7-year-old female with Dyke-Davidoff-Masson syndrome. Axial T2-weighted imaging shows encephalomalacia of the right cerebral hemisphere, with compensatory dilatation of right lateral ventricle, midline shift, and unilateral ipsilateral decrease in size of cranial fossa associated with thickened calvarium.

Fig. 1.34 A 3-month-old male with the precocious type of osteopetrosis. Axial CT shows generalized bone sclerosis and thickening of the skull.

Table 1.1 *(cont.)*   Congenital and developmental abnormalities involving the skull

Lesions or Disorder	Imaging Findings	Comments
Oxalosis (See **Fig. 1.81**)	Global medullary and cortical nephrocalcinosis with resultant renal failure. Early radiographic/CT findings include osteosclerosis and osteopenia, as well as thin transverse sclerotic bands in long bones and skull. Late findings include osteosclerosis and dense intraossoeus sclerotic bands. *MRI:* Decreased signal on T1- and T2-weighted imaging.	Type 1 primary hyperoxaluria is a rare autosomal recessive disorder (1 in 120,000 live births) involving mutations of the *AGXT* gene, which results in a deficiency of the peroxisomal enzyme alanine glyoxylate aminotransferase. Systemic oxalate accumulates and precipitates in bone and multiple organs (kidneys, liver, eye, and heart), resulting in organ failure. Fifty percent of patients have end-stage renal failure at age 15 years. Treatment is combined liver-kidney transplantation.
Osteogenesis imperfecta (**Fig. 1.35**)	Diffuse osteopenia and decreased ossification of skull base, with fractures, infolding of the occipital condyles, elevation of the posterior cranial fossa, and upward migration of the dens into the foramen magnum, resulting in basilar impression (secondary basilar invagination).	Also known as brittle bone disease, osteogenesis imperfecta (OI) has four to seven types. It is a hereditary disorder with abnormal type I fibrillar collagen production and osteoporosis, resulting from mutations involving the *COL1A1* gene on chromosome 17q21.31-q22.05 and the *COL1A2* gene on chromosome 7q22.1. Results in fragile bone prone to repetitive microfractures and remodeling. Type II is the most severe, secondary to the insufficient quantity and quality of collagen. Most Type II OI patients die within the first year from intracerebral hemorrhage or respiratory failure. The other types are associated with bone fractures and deformities, discoloration of sclera, hearing loss, scoliosis, and short stature, ± respiratory problems.

(continued on page 26)

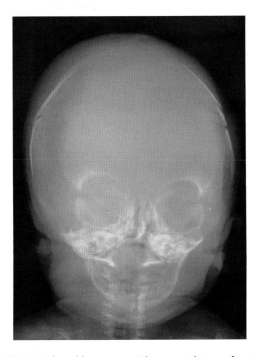

Fig. 1.35   A 1-day-old neonate with neonatal type of osteogenesis imperfecta (type II, which presents in the perinatal period and is usually lethal). AP radiograph shows prominent diffuse osteopenia.

Table 1.1 *(cont.)*   Congenital and developmental abnormalities involving the skull

Lesions or Disorder	Imaging Findings	Comments
Epidermoid (See **Fig. 1.57**)	*MRI:* Well-circumscribed spheroid or multilobulated extra-axial ectodermal-inclusion cystic lesions with low-intermediate signal on T1-weighted imaging and high signal on T2-weighted imaging and diffusion-weighted imaging. Mixed low, intermediate, or high signal on FLAIR images, with no gadolinium contrast enhancement. Often insinuate along CSF pathways, with resulting chronic deformation of adjacent neural tissue (brainstem, brain parenchyma). Commonly located in posterior cranial fossa (cerebellopontine angle cistern) > parasellar/middle cranial fossa. Can occur within or erode the adjacent skull. *CT:* Well-circumscribed spheroid or multilobulated extra-axial ectodermal-inclusion cystic lesions with low-intermediate attenuation ± bone erosion.	Nonneoplastic congenital or acquired extra-axial off-midline lesions filled with desquamated cells and keratinaceous debris, usually with a mild mass effect on adjacent brain, and infratentorial > supratentorial locations. Occur in adults, in males and females equally often, ± related clinical symptoms. Commonly located in posterior cranial fossa (cerebellopontine angle cistern) > parasellar/middle cranial fossa.

Table 1.2   Solitary lesions involving the skull

- Malignant Tumors
  - Metastatic disease
  - Myeloma/plasmacytoma
  - Lymphoma
  - Chordoma
  - Chondrosarcoma
  - Osteosarcoma
  - Ewing's sarcoma
  - Invasive pituitary tumor
  - Squamous cell carcinoma
  - Nasopharyngeal carcinoma
  - Adenoid cystic carcinoma
  - Esthesioneuroblastoma
  - Sinonasal undifferentiated carcinoma (SNUC)
  - Rhabdomyosarcoma
- Benign Tumors
  - Meningioma
  - Hemangiopericytoma
  - Schwannoma
  - Neurofibroma
  - Paraganglioma
  - Giant cell tumor
  - Enchondroma
  - Chondroblastoma
  - Osteoma
  - Osteoblastoma
  - Osteoid osteoma
- Tumorlike Lesions
  - Epidermoid
  - Fibrous dysplasia
  - Aneurysmal bone cysts (ABCs)
  - Aneurysm/pseudoaneurysm
  - Hemangioma
  - Venous lake
  - Paget disease
  - Notochord rest
  - Arachnoid granulation
- Inflammatory Lesions
  - Osteomyelitis
  - Mucocele/pyocele
  - Cholesterol granuloma
  - Langerhans' cell histiocytosis
- Traumatic Lesions
  - Cephalohematoma
  - Fracture

Table 1.2 Solitary lesions involving the skull

Lesions	Imaging Findings	Comments
Malignant Tumors		
Metastatic disease (**Fig. 1.36** and **Fig. 1.37**)	Single well-circumscribed or poorly defined lesion involving the skull. *CT:* Lesions are usually radiolucent and may also be sclerotic, ± extraosseous tumor extension, usually + contrast enhancement, ± compression of neural tissue or vessels. *MRI:* Single well-circumscribed or poorly defined lesion involving the skull, with low-intermediate signal on T1-weighted imaging, intermediate-high signal on T2-weighted imaging, usually showing gadolinium contrast enhancement, ± bone destruction, ± compression of neural tissue or vessels.	Metastatic lesions are proliferating neoplastic cells that are located in sites or organs separated or distant from their origins. Metastatic carcinoma is the most frequent malignant tumor involving bone. In adults, metastatic lesions to bone occur most frequently from carcinomas of the lung, breast, prostate, kidney, and thyroid, as well as from sarcomas. Primary malignancies of the lung, breast, and prostate account for 80% of bone metastases. Metastatic tumor may cause variable destructive or infiltrative changes in single or multiple sites.

(continued on page 28)

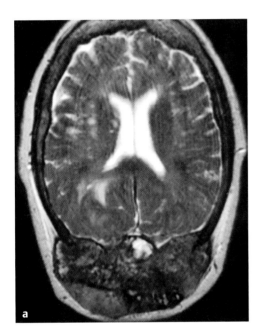
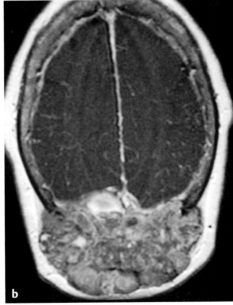

Fig. 1.36 A 75-year-old woman with metastatic tumor from lung carcinoma destroying the posterior portion of the skull. **(a)** The tumor has mixed low and intermediate signal on axial T2-weighted imaging and **(b)** shows heterogeneous gadolinium contrast enhancement on axial T1-weighted imaging.

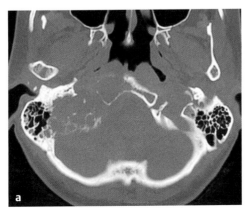
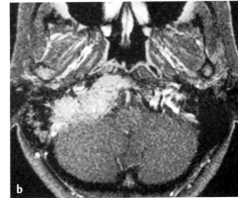

Fig. 1.37 **(a)** Metastatic breast carcinoma destroying the right temporal bone and adjacent occipital bone, as seen on axial CT. **(b)** The metastatic tumor shows gadolinium contrast enhancement on axial fat-suppressed T1-weighted imaging.

Table 1.2 *(cont.)* Solitary lesions involving the skull

Lesions	Imaging Findings	Comments
Myeloma/plasmacytoma (**Fig. 1.38**)	Multiple myeloma or single plasmacytoma are well-circumscribed or poorly defined lesions involving the skull and dura. *CT:* Lesions have low-intermediate attenuation, usually + contrast enhancement, + bone destruction. *MRI:* Well-circumscribed or poorly defined lesions involving the skull and dura, with low-intermediate signal on T1-weighted imaging, intermediate-high signal on T2-weighted imaging, usually showing gadolinium contrast enhancement, + bone destruction.	Multiple myeloma are malignant tumors composed of proliferating antibody-secreting plasma cells derived from single clones. Multiple myeloma primarily involves bone marrow. A solitary myeloma or plasmacytoma is an infrequent variant in which a neoplastic mass of plasma cells occurs at a single site of bone or soft tissues. In the United States, 14,600 new cases occur each year. Multiple myeloma is the most common primary neoplasm of bone in adults. Median age at presentation = 60 years. Most patients are older than 40 years. Tumors occur in the vertebrae > ribs > femur > iliac bone > humerus > craniofacial bones > sacrum > clavicle > sternum > pubic bone > tibia.
Lymphoma	Well-circumscribed or poorly defined lesion involving the skull. *CT:* Lesion has low-intermediate attenuation and may show contrast enhancement, ± bone destruction. *MRI:* Lesion has low-intermediate signal on T1-weighted imaging, intermediate to high signal on T2-weighted imaging, + gadolinium contrast enhancement. It is locally invasive and is associated with bone erosion/destruction and intracranial extension with meningeal involvement.	Lymphomas are a group of lymphoid tumors whose neoplastic cells typically arise within lymphoid tissue (lymph nodes and reticuloendothelial organs). Unlike leukemia, lymphoma usually arises as discrete masses. Lymphomas are subdivided into Hodgkin disease (HD) and non-Hodgkin lymphoma (NHL). Distinction between HD and NHL is useful because of differences in clinical and histopathologic features, as well as treatment strategies. HD typically arises in lymph nodes and often spreads along nodal chains, whereas NHL frequently originates at extranodal sites and spreads in an unpredictable pattern. Almost all primary lymphomas of bone are B-cell NHL.
Chordoma (**Fig. 1.39**)	Chordomas are well-circumscribed lobulated lesions found along the dorsal surface of clivus, vertebral bodies, or sacrum, + localized bone destruction. *CT:* Lesions have low-intermediate attenuation, ± calcifications from destroyed bone carried away by tumor, + contrast enhancement. *MRI:* Lesions have low-intermediate signal on T1-weighted images, high signal on T2-weighted imaging, + gadolinium contrast enhancement (usually heterogeneous). Chordomas are locally invasive and associated with bone erosion/destruction, encasement of vessels (usually without arterial narrowing) and nerves. Skull base-clivus is a common location, usually in the midline for conventional chordomas, which account for 80% of skull base chordomas. Chondroid chordomas tend to be located off midline near skull base synchondroses..	Chordomas are rare, locally aggressive, slow-growing, low to intermediate grade malignant tumors derived from ectopic notochordal remnants along the axial skeleton. Chondroid chondromas (5–15% of all chordomas) have both chordomatous and chondromatous differentiation. Chordomas that contain sarcomatous components are referred to as dedifferentiated or sarcomatoid chordomas (5% of all chordomas). Chordomas account for 2–4% of primary malignant bone tumors, 1–3% of all primary bone tumors, and less than 1% of intracranial tumors. The annual incidence has been reported to be 0.18 to 0.3 per million. Dedifferentiated chordomas or sarcomatoid chordomas account for less than 5% of all chordomas. For cranial chordomas, patients' mean age = 37 to 40 years.
Chondrosarcoma (**Fig. 1.40**)	Lobulated lesions with bone destruction at synchondroses. *CT:* Lesions have low-intermediate attenuation associated with localized bone destruction, ± chondroid matrix calcifications, + contrast enhancement. *MRI:* Lesions have low-intermediate signal on T1-weighted imaging, high signal on T2-weighted imaging (T2WI), ± matrix mineralization-low signal on T2WI, + gadolinium contrast enhancement (usually heterogeneous). Tumors are locally invasive and are associated with bone erosion/destruction and encasement of vessels and nerves. Skull base petro-occipital synchondrosis is a common location, usually off midline.	Chondrosarcomas are malignant tumors containing cartilage formed within sarcomatous stroma. They can contain areas of calcification/mineralization, myxoid material, and/or ossification. Chondrosarcomas rarely arise within synovium. They represent from 12 to 21% of malignant bone lesions, 21–26% of primary sarcomas of bone, 9–14% of all bone tumors, 6% of skull base tumors, and 0.15% of all intracranial tumors.

(continued on page 30)

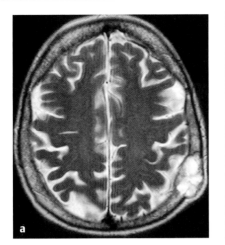
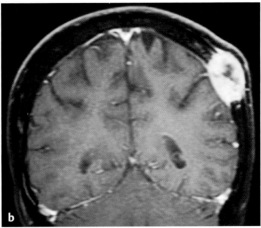

Fig. 1.38 **(a)** A 65-year-old woman with a plasmacytoma involving the left parietal bone that has high signal on axial T2-weighted imaging. **(b)** The tumor shows gadolinium contrast enhancement on coronal fat-suppressed T1-weighted imaging.

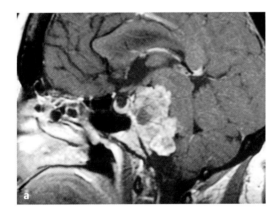
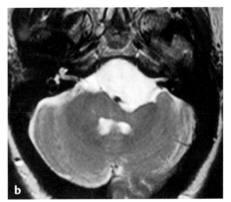

Fig. 1.39 **(a)** A 55-year-old woman with a chordoma along the dorsal surface of the clivus that shows gadolinium contrast enhancement on sagittal T1-weighted imaging and **(b)** high signal on axial T2-weighted imaging.

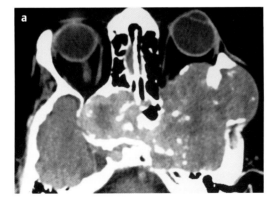
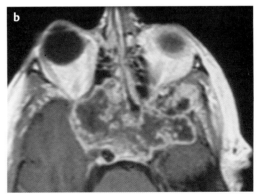

Fig. 1.40 An 81-year-old woman with a large chondrosarcoma involving both middle cranial fossae, the suprasellar cistern, sphenoid and ethmoid sinuses, and left orbit. **(a)** The tumor is associated with bone destruction and has mixed intermediate and low attenuation as well as chondroid calcifications on axial CT. **(b)** The tumor has peripheral lobulated and irregular curvilinear gadolinium contrast enhancement on axial T1-weighted imaging.

Table 1.2 *(cont.)*   Solitary lesions involving the skull

Lesions	Imaging Findings	Comments
Osteosarcoma (**Fig. 1.41**)	Destructive lesions involving the skull base. *CT:* Tumors have low-intermediate attenuation, usually + matrix mineralization/ossification, and often contrast enhancement (usually heterogeneous). *MRI:* Tumors often have poorly defined margins and commonly extend from the marrow through destroyed bone cortex into adjacent soft tissues. Tumors usually have low-intermediate signal on T1-weighted imaging. Zones of low signal often correspond to areas of tumor calcification/mineralization and/or necrosis. Zones of necrosis typically have high signal on T2-weighted imaging (T2WI), whereas mineralized zones usually have low signal on T2WI. Tumors can have variable signal on T2WI and fat-suppressed (FS) T2WI, depending on the relative amounts of calcified/mineralized osteoid, chondroid, fibroid, and hemorrhagic and necrotic components. Tumors may have low, low-intermediate, or intermediate to high signal on T2WI and FS T2WI. After gadolinium contrast administration, osteosarcomas typically show prominent enhancement in nonmineralized/calcified portions.	Osteosarcomas are malignant tumors composed of proliferating neoplastic spindle cells, which produce osteoid and/or immature tumoral bone. Occur in children as primary tumors, and in adults they are associated with Paget disease, irradiated bone, chronic osteomyelitis, osteoblastoma, giant cell tumor, and fibrous dysplasia.
Ewing's sarcoma (**Fig. 1.42**)	*CT:* Destructive lesions involving the skull base, with low-intermediate attenuation, can show contrast enhancement (usually heterogeneous). *MRI:* Destructive lesions involving the skull base, with low-intermediate signal on T1-weighted imaging, mixed low, intermediate, and high signal on T2-weighted imaging, + gadolinium contrast enhancement (usually heterogeneous).	Malignant primitive tumor of bone composed of undifferentiated small cells with round nuclei. Accounts for 6–11% of primary malignant bone tumors, 5–7% of primary bone tumors. Usually occurs between the ages of 5 and 30, and in males more than in females. Ewing's sarcomas commonly have translocations involving chromosomes 11 and 22: t(11;22) (q24:q12), which results in fusion of the FL1-1 gene at 11q24 to the EWS gene at 22q12. Ewing's sarcoma is locally invasive, with high metastatic potential. Rarely involves the skull base.
Invasive pituitary tumor (**Fig. 1.43**)	*CT:* Often have intermediate attenuation, ± necrosis, ± cyst, ± hemorrhage, usually show contrast enhancement, can extend into suprasellar cistern with waist at diaphragma sella, ± extension into cavernous sinus, and can invade the skull base. *MRI:* Often have intermediate signal on T1- and T2-weighted imaging and signal is often similar to gray matter, ± necrosis, ± cyst, ± hemorrhage, usually show prominent gadolinium contrast enhancement, extension into suprasellar cistern with waist at diaphragma sella, ± extension into cavernous sinus, and occasionally invade skull base.	Histologically benign pituitary macroadenomas or pituitary carcinomas can occasionally have an invasive growth pattern with extension into the sphenoid bone, clivus, ethmoid sinus, orbits, and/or interpeduncular cistern.

(continued on page 32)

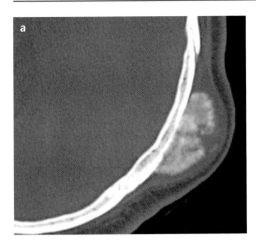

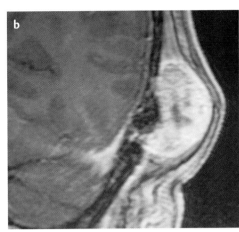

Fig. 1.41 (a) A 57-year-old woman with a primary osteosarcoma at the surface of the outer table of the skull, which contains mineralized osteoid matrix as seen on axial CT. **(b)** The tumor shows gadolinium contrast enhancement on sagittal T1-weighted imaging, with additional findings of localized destruction of the outer table of the skull.

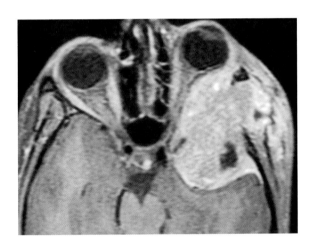

Fig. 1.42 An 11-year-old female with a primary Ewing's sarcoma in the left middle cranial fossa and left orbit associated with bone destruction. The tumor shows gadolinium contrast enhancement on axial T1-weighted imaging.

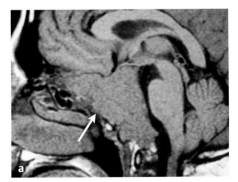

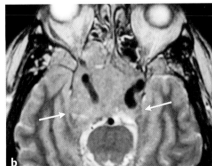

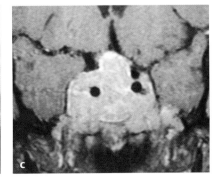

Fig. 1.43 A 44-year-old man with an aggressive pituitary carcinoma invading the sphenoid and occipital portions of the clivus, cavernous sinuses, and sphenoid sinus. **(a)** The tumor has intermediate signal on sagittal T1-weighted imaging (*arrow*), **(b)** intermediate to slightly high signal on axial T2-weighted imaging (*arrows*), and **(c)** gadolinium contrast enhancement on coronal fat-suppressed T1-weighted imaging.

Table 1.2 *(cont.)* Solitary lesions involving the skull

Lesions	Imaging Findings	Comments
Squamous cell carcinoma **(Fig. 1.44)**	*CT:* Tumors have intermediate attenuation and mild contrast enhancement. Can be large lesions (± necrosis and/or hemorrhage). *MRI:* Destructive lesions in the nasal cavity, paranasal sinuses, nasopharynx, ± intracranial extension via bone destruction or perineural spread. Lesions have intermediate signal on T1-weighted imaging, intermediate-slightly high signal on T2-weighted imaging, and mild gadolinium contrast enhancement. Can be large lesions (± necrosis and/or hemorrhage).	Malignant epithelial tumors originating from the mucosal epithelium of the paranasal sinuses (maxillary, 60%; ethmoid, 14%; sphenoid and frontal sinuses, 1%) and nasal cavity (25%). Include both keratinizing and nonkeratinizing types. Account for 3% of malignant tumors of the head and neck. Occur in adults usually > 55 years old, and in males more than in females. Associated with occupational or other exposure to tobacco smoke, nickel, chlorophenols, chromium, mustard gas, radium, and material in the manufacture of wood products.
Nasopharyngeal carcinoma	*CT:* Tumors have intermediate attenuation and mild contrast enhancement. Can be large lesions (± necrosis and/or hemorrhage). *MRI:* Invasive lesions in the nasopharynx (lateral wall/ fossa of Rosenmüller, and posterior upper wall); ± intracranial extension via bone destruction or perineural spread; intermediate signal on T1-weighted imaging, intermediate-slightly high signal on T2-weighted imaging; often shows gadolinium contrast enhancement. Can be large lesions (± necrosis and/or hemorrhage).	Carcinomas arising from the nasopharyngeal mucosa with varying degrees of squamous differentiation. Subtypes include squamous cell carcinoma, nonkeratinizing carcinoma (differentiated and undifferentiated), and basaloid squamous cell carcinoma. Occurs at higher frequency in Southern Asia and Africa than in Europe and the Americas. Peak ages: 40–60 years. Occurs two to three times more frequently in men than in women. Associated with Epstein-Barr virus, diets containing nitrosamines, and chronic exposure to tobacco smoke, formaldehyde, chemical fumes, and dust.
Adenoid cystic carcinoma	*CT:* Tumors have intermediate attenuation and variable mild, moderate, or prominent contrast enhancement. *MRI:* Destructive lesions with intracranial extension via bone destruction or perineural spread, with intermediate signal on T1-weighted imaging, intermediate-high signal on T2-weighted imaging, and variable mild, moderate, or prominent gadolinium contrast enhancement.	Basaloid tumor comprised of neoplastic epithelial and myoepithelial cells. Morphologic tumor patterns include tubular, cribriform, and solid. Accounts for 10% of epithelial salivary neoplasms. Most commonly involves the parotid, submandibular, and minor salivary glands (palate, tongue, buccal mucosa, and floor of the mouth, other locations). Perineural tumor spread common, ± facial nerve paralysis. Usually occurs in adults > 30 years old. Solid type has the worst prognosis. Up to 90% of patients die within 10–15 years of diagnosis.
Esthesioneuroblastoma **(Fig. 1.45)**	*CT:* Tumors have intermediate attenuation and variable mild, moderate, or prominent contrast enhancement. *MRI:* Locally destructive lesions with low-intermediate signal on T1-weighted imaging, intermediate-high signal on T2-weighted imaging, + prominent gadolinium contrast enhancement. Location: superior nasal cavity, ethmoid air cells with occasional extension into the other paranasal sinuses, orbits, anterior cranial fossa, and cavernous sinuses. *PET/CT:* FDG is useful for staging of disease and detection of metastases.	Also referred to as olfactory neuroblastoma, these malignant neoplasms of neuroectodermal origin arise from olfactory epithelium in the upper nasal cavity and cribriform region. Tumors consist of immature neuroblasts with variable nuclear pleomorphism, mitoses, and necrosis. Tumor cells occur in a neurofibrillary intercellular matrix. Esthesioneuroblastoma has a bimodal age of occurrence in adolescents (11–20 years old) and adults (50–60 years old) and occurs in males more than in females.
Sinonasal undifferentiated carcinoma (SNUC) **(Fig. 1.46)**	*CT:* Tumors have intermediate attenuation and variable mild, moderate, or prominent contrast enhancement. *MRI:* Locally destructive lesions, usually larger than 4 cm, with low-intermediate signal on T1-weighted imaging, intermediate-high signal on T2-weighted imaging, + prominent gadolinium contrast enhancement. Location: superior nasal cavity, ethmoid air cells with occasional extension into the other paranasal sinuses, orbits, anterior cranial fossa, and cavernous sinuses.	Malignant tumor composed of pleomorphic neoplastic cells with medium to large nuclei, prominent single nucleoli, and small amounts of eosinophilic cytoplasm. Mitotic activity is typically high and necrosis is common. Immunoreactive to CK7, CK8, CK19, ± to p53, epithelial membrane antigen, and neuron-specific enolase. Poor prognosis, with 5-year survival less than 20%.

(continued on page 34)

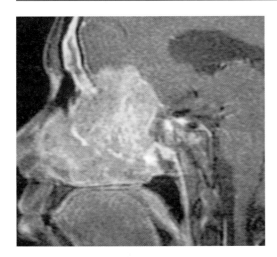

Fig. 1.44 A 37-year-old woman with a poorly differentiated squamous cell carcinoma in the nasal cavity and ethmoid and sphenoid sinuses that extends intracranially through destructive bone changes at the skull base. The tumor shows gadolinium contrast enhancement on sagittal fat-suppressed T1-weighted imaging.

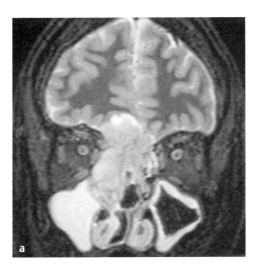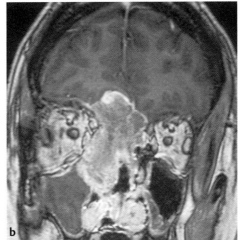

Fig. 1.45 A 30-year-old woman with an esthesioneuroblastoma in the ethmoid sinuses, right nasal cavity, and right maxillary sinus that extends intracranially through destructive bone changes at the skull base. **(a)** The tumor has heterogeneous slightly high signal on coronal STIR and **(b)** shows heterogeneous gadolinium contrast enhancement on coronal T1-weighted imaging.

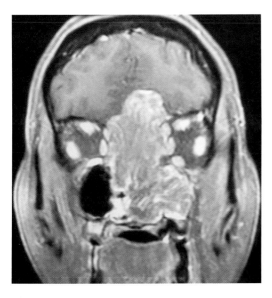

Fig. 1.46 A 41-year-old woman with sinonasal undifferentiated carcinoma in the nasal cavity and ethmoid and sphenoid sinuses that extends intracranially through destructive bone changes at the skull base. The tumor shows gadolinium contrast enhancement on coronal fat-suppresssed T1-weighted imaging.

Table 1.2 *(cont.)* Solitary lesions involving the skull

Lesions	Imaging Findings	Comments
Rhabdomyosarcoma	*CT:* Soft tissue lesions that usually have circumscribed or irregular margins. Calcifications are uncommon. Tumors can have mixed CT attenuation, with solid zones of soft tissue attenuation, cystic appearing and/or necrotic zones, and occasional foci of hemorrhage, ± bone invasion and destruction. *MRI:* Tumors can have circumscribed and/or poorly defined margins, and typically have low-intermediate signal on T1-weighted imaging and heterogeneous signal (various combinations of intermediate, slightly high, and/or high signal) on T2-weighted imaging (T2WI) and fat-suppressed T2WI. Tumors show variable degrees of gadolinium contrast enhancement, ± bone destruction and invasion.	Malignant mesenchymal tumors with rhabdomyoblastic differentiation that occur primarily in soft tissue, and only very rarely in bone. There are three subgroups of rhabdomyosarcoma: embryonal (50–70%), alveolar (18–45%), and pleomorphic (5–10%). Embryonal and alveolar rhabdomyosarcomas occur primarily in children < 10 years old, and pleomorphic rhabdomyosarcomas occur mostly in adults (median age in the sixth decade). Alveolar and pleomorphic rhabdomyosarcomas occur frequently in the extremities. Embryonal rhabdomyosarcomas occur mostly in the head and neck.
Benign Tumors		
Meningioma **(Fig. 1.47, Fig. 1.48**, and **Fig. 1.49)**	Extra-axial well-circumscribed dura-based lesions. Location: supra- > infratentorial, parasagittal > convexity > sphenoid ridge > parasellar > posterior fossa > optic nerve sheath > intraventricular. Some meningiomas can invade bone or occur predominantly within bone. *CT:* Tumors have intermediate attenuation, usually prominent contrast enhancement, ± calcifications, ± hyperostosis of adjacent bone. *MRI:* Tumors often have intermediate signal on T1-weighted imaging, intermediate-slightly high signal on T2-weighted imaging, and typically prominent gadolinium contrast enhancement, ± calcifications, ± hyperostosis and/or invasion of adjacent skull. Some meningiomas have high signal on diffusion-weighted imaging although these findings can be seen with both benign and atypical tumors.	Benign slow-growing tumors involving cranial and/or spinal dura that are composed of neoplastic meningothelial (arachnoidal or arachnoid cap) cells. Usually solitary and sporadic, but can also occur as multiple lesions in patients with neurofibromatosis type 2. Most are benign, although ~ 5% have atypical histologic features. Anaplastic meningiomas are rare (< 3% of meningiomas). Meningiomas account for up to 26% of primary intracranial tumors. Annual incidence is 6 per 100,000. Typically occur in adults (> 40 years old), and in women more than in men. Can result in compression of adjacent brain parenchyma, encasement of arteries, and compression of dural venous sinuses. Rarely, invasive/malignant types occur.

(continued on page 36)

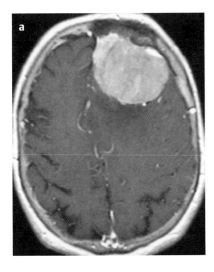

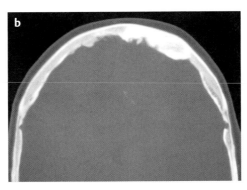

Fig. 1.47 **(a)** A 75-year-old woman with a gadolinium-enhancing meningioma in the left frontal region on axial T1-weighted imaging. **(b)** The tumor has associated hyperostosis in the adjacent skull on axial CT.

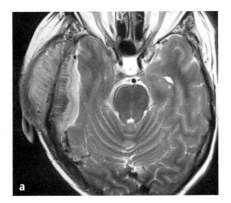

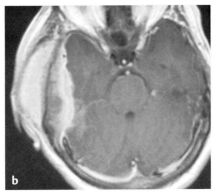

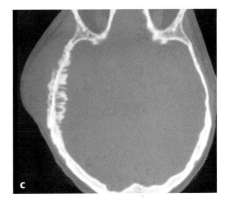

Fig. 1.48 **(a)** A 55-year-old woman with a WHO grade II–III atypical meningioma in the right temporal region that invades and extends through the skull into the adjacent extracranial soft tissues, as seen on axial T2-weighted imaging. **(b)** The tumor shows gadolinium contrast enhancement on axial T1-weighted imaging and **(c)** and is associated with hair-on-end periosteal reaction, as seen on axial CT.

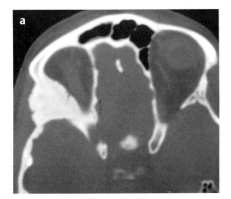

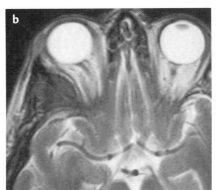

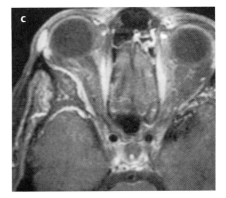

Fig. 1.49 A 52-year-old woman with an intraosseous meningioma. **(a)** Axial CT shows thickening and hyperostosis at the posterolateral wall of the right orbit. **(b)** The intraosseous meningioma has mostly low signal on axial T2-weighted imaging as well as thin zones of slightly high signal at sites of extraosseous extension. **(c)** The small zones of extraosseous tumor at the lateral orbit and anterior middle cranial fossa show gadolinium contrast enhancement on axial fat-suppressed T1-weighted imaging.

Table 1.2 *(cont.)* Solitary lesions involving the skull

Lesions	Imaging Findings	Comments
Hemangiopericytoma **(Fig. 1.50)**	*MRI:* Solitary dura-based and/or intraosseous tumors ranging from 2 to 7 cm in diameter that have low-intermediate signal on T1-weighted imaging, intermediate-slightly high signal on T2-weighted imaging, and usually prominent gadolinium contrast enhancement, often with a dural tail, as well as calcifications. Intratumoral hemorrhage and cystic or necrotic foci can occur in 30%. *Magnetic resonance spectroscopy:* Relative ratios of myo-inositol, glucose, and glutathione with respect to glutamate are higher in hemangiopericytomas than in meningiomas. *CT:* Extra-axial mass lesions that are often well circumscribed. Tumors have intermediate attenuation with or without calcifications and usually show prominent contrast enhancement. Can erode or invade adjacent bone.	Rare (WHO grade II) neoplasms that account for 0.4% of primary intracranial tumors and that are 50 times less frequent than meningiomas. Tumors composed of closely packed cells with scant cytoplasm and round, ovoid, or elongated nuclei with moderately dense chromatin. Numerous slitlike vascular channels are seen that are lined by flattened endothelial cells, ± zones of necrosis. Immunoreactive to vimentin (85%), factor XIIIa (80–100%), and variably to Leu-7 and CD34. Associated with abnormalities involving chromosome 12. Typically occur in young adults (mean age = 43 years), and in males more than in females. Sometimes referred to as angioblastic meningioma or meningeal hemangiopericytoma, tumors arise from vascular cells—pericytes. Frequently recur.
Schwannoma **(Fig. 1.51)**	*MRI:* Circumscribed ovoid or spheroid lesions with low-intermediate signal on T1-weighted imaging, high signal on T2-weighted imaging (T2WI) and fat-suppressed T2WI, and usually prominent gadolinium (Gd) contrast enhancement. High signal on T2WI and Gd contrast enhancement can be heterogeneous in large lesions due to cystic degeneration and/or hemorrhage. Schwannomas involving the skull include those from CN V (trigeminal nerve cistern/Meckel's cave), CN VI (Dorello canal), CN VII and CN VIII (internal auditory canal and cerebellopontine angle cistern), CN IX, CN X, and CN XI (jugular foramen). *CT:* Circumscribed ovoid or spheroid lesions with intermediate attenuation, + contrast enhancement. Large lesions can have cystic degeneration and/or hemorrhage, ± erosion of adjacent bone.	Schwannomas are benign encapsulated tumors that contain differentiated neoplastic Schwann cells. Multiple schwannomas are often associated with neurofibromatosis type 2 (NF2), which is an autosomal dominant disease involving a gene at chromosome 22q12. In addition to schwannomas, patients with NF2 can also have multiple meningiomas and ependymomas. Schwannomas represent 8% of primary intracranial tumors and 29% or primary spinal tumors. The incidence of NF2 is 1/37,000 to 1/50,000 newborns. Age at presentation is 22 to 72 years (mean age = 46 years). Peak incidence is in the fourth to sixth decades. Many patients with NF2 present in the third decade with bilateral vestibular schwannomas.
Neurofibroma **(Fig. 1.52)**	*MRI:* *Solitary neurofibromas:* Circumscribed spheroid, ovoid, or lobulated extra-axial lesions with low-intermediate signal on T1-weighted imaging (T1WI), intermediate-high signal on T2-weighted imaging (T2WI), + prominent gadolinium (Gd) contrast enhancement. High signal on T2WI and Gd contrast enhancement can be heterogeneous in large lesions. *Plexiform neurofibromas* appear as curvilinear and multinodular lesions involving multiple nerve branches and have low to intermediate signal on T1WI and intermediate, slightly high to high signal on T2WI and fat-suppressed T2WI, with or without bands or strands of low signal. Lesions usually show gadolinium contrast enhancement. *CT:* Ovoid or fusiform lesions with low-intermediate attenuation. Lesions can show contrast enhancement. Often erode adjacent bone.	Benign nerve sheath tumors that contain mixtures of Schwann cells, perineural-like cells, and interlacing fascicles of fibroblasts associated with abundant collagen. Unlike schwannomas, neurofibromas lack Antoni A and B regions and cannot be separated pathologically from the underlying nerve. Most frequently occur as sporadic, localized, solitary lesions, less frequently as diffuse or plexiform lesions. Multiple neurofibromas are typically seen with neurofibromatosis type 1 (NF1), which is an autosomal dominant disorder (1/2,500 births) resulting from mutations of the neurofibromin gene on chromosome 17q11.2. NF1 is the most common type of neurocutaneous syndrome and is associated with neoplasms of the central and peripheral nervous systems (optic gliomas, astrocytomas, plexiform and solitary neurofibromas) and skin (café-au-lait spots, axillary and inguinal freckling). Also associated with meningeal and skull dysplasias, as well as hamartomas of the iris (Lisch nodules).

(continued on page 38)

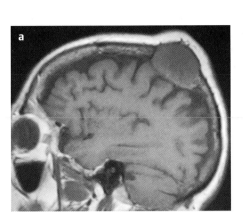
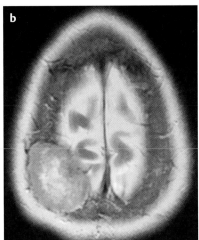
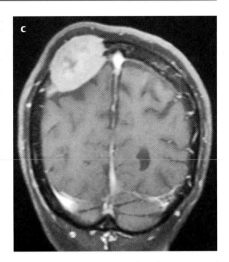

Fig. 1.50 An 81-year-old woman with a hemangiopericytoma in the skull destroying both the inner and outer tables and with intracranial and extracranial tumor extension. **(a)** The tumor has intermediate signal on sagittal T1-weighted imaging and **(b)** mixed intermediate and high signal on axial T2-weighted imaging, as well as **(c)** gadolinium contrast enhancement on coronal fat-suppressed T1-weighted imaging.

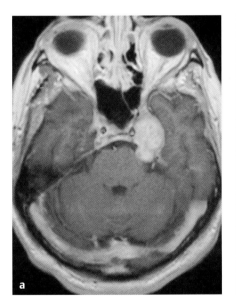
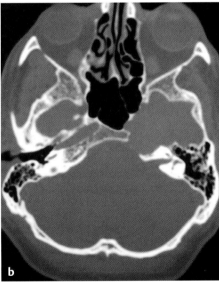

Fig. 1.51 **(a)** A 70-year-old man with a left trigeminal nerve schwannoma that shows gadolinium contrast enhancement on axial T1-weighted imaging. **(b)** The tumor is associated with adjacent chronic erosive osseous changes on axial CT.

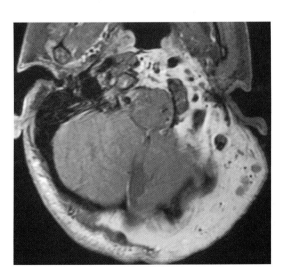

Fig. 1.52 A 19-year-old woman with neurofibromatosis type 1. A gadolinium-enhancing plexiform neurofibroma in the superficial soft tissues is associated with erosion and remodeling of the left occipital and temporal bones and extends into the left carotid, retropharyngeal, and prevertebral spaces on axial fat-suppressed T1-weighted imaging.

Table 1.2 *(cont.)* Solitary lesions involving the skull

Lesions	Imaging Findings	Comments
Paraganglioma **(Fig. 1.53)**	Ovoid or fusiform lesions with low-intermediate attenuation. *MRI:* Spheroid or lobulated lesion with intermediate signal on T1-weighted imaging (T1WI), intermediate-high signal on T2-weighted imaging (T2WI) and fat-suppressed T2WI, ± tubular zones of flow voids, usually prominent gadolinium contrast enhancement, ± foci of high signal on T1WI from mucin or hemorrhage, ± peripheral rim of low signal (hemosiderin) on T2WI. *CT:* Lesions can show contrast enhancement. Often erode adjacent bone.	Benign encapsulated neuroendocrine tumors that arise from neural crest cells associated with autonomic ganglia (paraganglia) throughout the body. Lesions, also referred to as chemodectomas, are named according to location (glomus jugulare, tympanicum, vagale). Paragangliomas represent 0.6% of tumors of the head and neck and 0.03% of all neoplasms.
Giant cell tumor	*MRI:* Often well-defined lesions with thin, low-signal margins on T1-weighted imaging (T1WI) and T2-weighted imaging (T2WI). Solid portions of giant cell tumors often have low to intermediate signal on T1WI, intermediate to high signal on T2WI, and high signal on fat-suppressed T2WI. Signal heterogeneity on T2WI is not uncommon. Zones of low signal on T2WI and T2* imaging may be seen secondary to hemosiderin. Aneurysmal bone cysts can be seen in 14% of giant cell tumors, resulting in cystic zones with variable signal and fluid–fluid levels, ± cortical destruction and extraosseous tumor extension. *CT:* Radiolucent lesions with relatively narrow zones of transition. Zones of cortical thinning are typical. Expansion and zones of cortical destruction are commonly seen. No matrix mineralization.	Aggressive tumors composed of neoplastic, ovoid, mononuclear cells and scattered multinucleated osteoclast-like giant cells (derived from fusion of marrow mononuclear cells). Can occasionally be seen associated with Paget disease in older patients. Up to 10% of all giant cell tumors are malignant. Account for ~ 5 to 9.5% of all bone tumors and up to 23% of benign bone tumors. Median age at presentation = 30 years. Eighty percent occur in patients more than 20 years old. Tumors typically occur in long bones, and rarely in the spine and skull.
Enchondroma **(Fig. 1.54)**	*MRI:* Lobulated intramedullary tumors that usually have low-intermediate signal on T1-weighted imaging and intermediate signal on proton density-weighted imaging. On T2-weighted imaging (T2WI) and fat-suppressed T2WI, lesions usually have predominantly high signal, with foci and/or bands of low signal representing areas of matrix mineralization and fibrous strands. Lesions typically show gadolinium contrast enhancement in various patterns (peripheral curvilinear lobular, central nodular/septal and peripheral lobular, or heterogeneous diffuse). *CT:* Lobulated intramedullary lesion that usually has low-intermediate attenuation and contains areas of chondroid matrix mineralization and fibrous strands.	Benign intramedullary lesions composed of hyaline cartilage, enchondromas represent ~ 10% of benign bone tumors. Enchondromas can be solitary (88%) or multiple (12%). Ollier's disease is a dyschondroplasia involving endochondrally formed bone resulting in multiple enchondromas (enchondromatosis). Metachondromatosis is a combination of enchondromatosis and osteochondromatosis and is rare. Maffucci's disease refers to a syndrome in which there are multiple enchondromas and soft tissue hemangiomas, and is very rare. Age at presentation is 3 to 83 years (median age = 35 years, mean age = 38 to 40 years), with a peak in the third and fourth decades.
Chondroblastoma	*MRI:* Ovoid or fusiform lesions with low-intermediate signal on T1-weighted imaging and intermediate to high signal on T2-weighted imaging (T2WI) and fat-suppressed T2WI. Punctate zones of low signal on T2WI and fat-suppressed T2WI can be seen within tumors secondary to chondroid matrix mineralization. Lesions typically show moderate to prominent gadolinium contrast enhancement. Often erode adjacent bone. Poorly-defined zones with high signal on T2WI and FS T2WI and corresponding Gd-contrast enhancement are typically seen in the marrow adjacent to the lesions representing inflammatory reaction from prostaglandin synthesis by these tumors. *CT:* Tumors often have fine lobular margins and typically have low-intermediate attenuation containing chondroid matrix mineralization (50%). Contrast enhancement may be seen. Cortical destruction is uncommon.	Benign cartilaginous tumors with chondroblast-like cells and areas of chondroid matrix formation that rarely occur in the craniofacial bones. If chondroblastoma involves craniofacial bones, the squamous portion of the temporal bone is the most common location. Usually occur in children and adolescents, median = 17 years, mean = 16 years for lesions in long bones, mean = 28 years in other bones. Most cases are diagnosed between the ages of 5 and 25.

(continued on page 40)

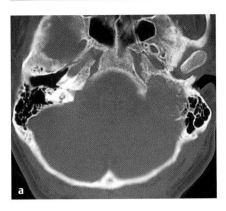
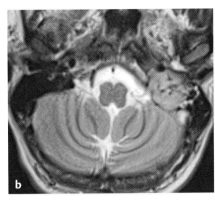
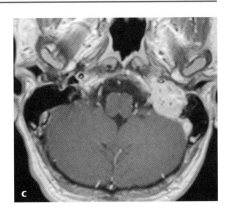

Fig. 1.53 **(a)** Axial CT shows a paraganglioma/glomus jugulare with erosive destructive changes involving the left temporal bone and including the jugular foramen. **(b)** The tumor has slightly high signal on axial fat-suppressed T2-weighted imaging as well as small flow voids. **(c)** The tumor shows prominent gadolinium contrast enhancement on axial T1-weighted imaging.

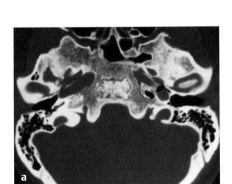
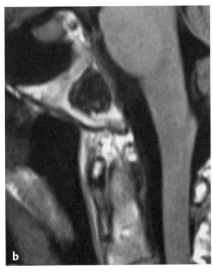
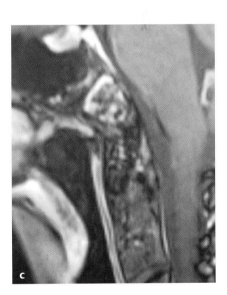

Fig. 1.54 **(a)** A 44-year-old woman with an enchondroma within the clivus, which has dense chondroid mineralization on axial CT and **(b)** low signal on sagittal T1-weighted imaging. **(c)** The lesion shows peripheral and central curvilinear gadolinium contrast enhancement on sagittal fat-suppressed T1-weighted imaging.

Table 1.2 *(cont.)* Solitary lesions involving the skull

Lesions	Imaging Findings	Comments
Osteoma (**Fig. 1.55**)	*MRI:* Well-circumscribed lesions involving the skull, with low-intermediate signal on T1- and T2-weighted imaging and typically no significant gadolinium contrast enhancement. *CT:* Well-circumscribed lesions involving the skull, with high attenuation.	Benign primary bone tumors composed of dense lamellar, woven, and/or compact cortical bone, usually located at the surface of the skull or paranasal sinuses (frontal > ethmoid > maxillary > sphenoid). Account for less than 1% of primary benign bone tumors. Age at presentation ranges from 16 to 74 years, with tumors most frequent in the sixth decade.
Osteoblastoma	*MRI:* Spheroid or ovoid zone measuring greater than 1.5 to 2 cm located within medullary and/or cortical bone. Can have irregular, distinct, or indistinct margins. Tumors have low-intermediate signal on T1-weighted imaging and low-intermediate and/or high signal on T2-weighted imaging (T2WI) and fat-suppressed (FS) T2WI. Calcifications or areas of mineralization can be seen as zones low signal on T2WI. After gadolinium (Gd) contrast administration, osteoblastomas show variable degrees of enhancement. Zones of thickened cortical bone and medullary sclerosis are often seen adjacent to osteoblastomas, ± secondary aneurysmal bone cysts. Poorly defined zones of high signal on T2WI and FS T2WI and corresponding Gd contrast enhancement can be seen in the marrow adjacent to osteoblastomas as well as within the extraosseous soft tissues. *CT:* Expansile radiolucent lesion greater than 1.5 cm surrounded by bony sclerosis. Lesions can show contrast enhancement. The radiolucent lesions typically arise in medullary bone and may or may not contain internal calcifications.	Rare, benign, bone-forming tumors that are histologically related to osteoid osteomas. Osteoblastomas are larger than osteoid osteomas and show progressive enlargement. Osteoblastomas typically produce well-vascularized osteoid, with woven bone spicules surrounded by osteoblasts. Account for 3 to 6% of primary benign bone tumors and < 1 to 2% of all primary bone tumors. Age at presentation ranges from 1 to 30 years (median age = 15 years and mean age = 20 years). Approximately 90% of lesions occur in patients < 30 years old. Osteoblastomas occasionally occur in older adults up to 78 years old. Rarely involve the skull.
Osteoid osteoma (**Fig. 1.56**)	*MRI:* Dense fusiform thickening of bone cortex that has low -intermediate signal on T1-weighted imaging (T1WI), proton density-weighted imaging, T2-weighted imaging (T2WI), and fat-suppressed (FS) T2WI. Within the thickened cortex, a spheroid or ovoid zone (nidus) measuring less than 1.5 cm is seen. The nidus can have irregular, distinct, or indistinct margins relative to the adjacent region of cortical thickening. The nidus can have low-intermediate signal on T1WI and low-intermediate or high signal on T2WI and FS T2WI. Calcifications in the nidus can be seen as low signal on T2WI. After gadolinium contrast administration, variable degrees of enhancement are seen at the nidus. *CT:* Intraosseous, circumscribed, radiolucent lesion less than 1.5 cm in diameter surrounded by bony sclerosis. Lesions often have low-intermediate attenuation centrally, often show contrast enhancement, and are surrounded by a peripheral rim of increased attenuation from associated bony sclerosis.	Benign osteoblastic lesion composed of a circumscribed < 1.5 cm nidus of vascularized osteoid trabeculae surrounded by osteoblastic sclerosis, and usually surrounded by reactive bone formation. The lesions are usually painful and have limited growth potential. Focal pain and tenderness associated with the lesion are often worse at night and are relieved by aspirin. Osteoid osteoma accounts for 11 to 13% of primary benign bone tumors and 3 to 4% of all primary bone tumors. Age at presentation is 6 to 30 years (median age = 17 years). Approximately 75% occur in patients < 25 years old. Rare cases have been reported in older adults up to 72 years old.

(continued on page 42)

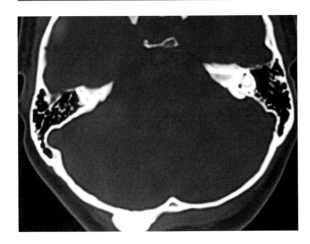

Fig. 1.55 Axial CT shows an osteoma at the outer surface of the right occipital bone.

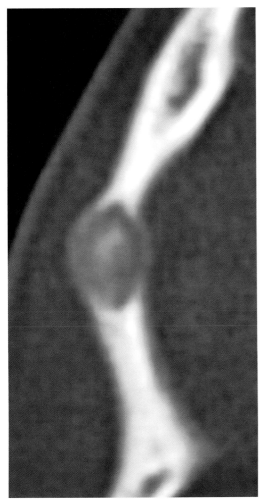

Fig. 1.56 Axial CT shows an osteoid osteoma in the right frontal bone. The slightly expansile lesion has intermediate attenuation and a central calcification.

Table 1.2 *(cont.)* Solitary lesions involving the skull

Lesions	Imaging Findings	Comments
Tumorlike Lesions		
Epidermoid (**Fig. 1.57**)	*MRI:* Well circumscribed lesions with low-intermediate signal on T1-weighted imaging, high signal on T2-weighted imaging and diffusion-weighted imaging, mixed low, intermediate, and/or high signal on FLAIR, and no gadolinium contrast enhancement. *CT:* Circumscribed radiolucent lesion within the skull, ± bone expansion or erosion.	Epidermoid cysts are ectoderm-lined inclusion cysts that contain only squamous epithelium, desquamated skin epithelial cells, and keratin. Result from persistence of ectodermal elements at sites of neural tube closure and suture closure. Can be intraosseous or intracranial extra-axial lesions. Occur in adults, in males and females equally often, ± related clinical symptoms.
Fibrous dysplasia (**Fig. 1.58** and **Fig. 1.59**)	*MRI:* Features depend on the proportions of bony spicules, collagen, fibroblastic spindle cells, and hemorrhagic and/or cystic changes. Lesions are usually well circumscribed and have low or low-intermediate signal on T1-weighted imaging. On T2-weighted imaging, lesions have variable mixtures of low, intermediate, and/or high signal, often surrounded by a low-signal rim of variable thickness. Internal septations and cystic changes are seen in a minority of lesions. Bone expansion is commonly seen. All or portions of the lesions can show gadolinium contrast enhancement in a heterogeneous, diffuse, or peripheral pattern. Can have associated secondary-type aneurysmal bone cysts. *CT:* Lesions involving the skull are often associated with bone expansion. Lesions have variable density and attenuation on radiographs and CT, respectively, depending on the degree of mineralization and number of bony spicules in the lesions. Attenuation coefficients can range from 70 to 400 Hounsfield units. Lesions can have a ground-glass radiographic appearance secondary to the mineralized spicules of immature woven bone in fibrous dysplasia. Sclerotic borders of varying thickness can be seen surrounding parts or all of the lesions.	Benign medullary fibro-osseous lesion of bone, most often sporadic, involving a single site, referred to as monostotic fibrous dysplasia (80–85%), or in multiple locations (polyostotic fibrous dysplasia). Results from developmental failure in the normal process of remodeling primitive bone to mature lamellar bone, with resultant zone or zones of immature trabeculae within dysplastic fibrous tissue. The lesions do not mineralize normally and can result in cranial neuropathies from neuroforaminal narrowing, facial deformities, sinonasal drainage disorders, and sinusitis. McCune-Albright syndrome accounts for 3% of polyostotic fibrous dysplasia and may include the presence of pigmented cutaneous macules (sometimes referred to as café-au-lait spots) with irregular indented borders that are ipsilateral to bone lesions, precocious puberty, and/or other endocrine disorders, such as acromegaly, hyperthyroidism, hyperparathyroidism, and Cushing's syndrome. *Leontiasis ossea* is a rare form of polyostotic fibrous dyplasia that involves the craniofacial bones and results in facial enlargement and deformity. Age at presentation: < 1 year to 76 years; 75% occur before the age of 30 years. Median age for monostotic fibrous dysplasia = 21 years; mean and median ages for polyostotic fibrous dysplasia are between 8 and 17 years. Most cases are diagnosed in patients between the ages of 3 and 20 years.

(continued on page 44)

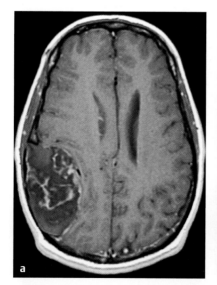 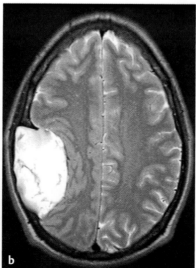 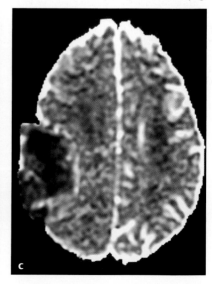

Fig. 1.57 A 39-year-old man with an epidermoid in the right side of the skull associated with both intracranial and extracranial extension though eroded bone. **(a)** The lesion had mostly low signal with small areas of high signal on axial T1-weighted imaging, **(b)** mostly high signal on axial T2-weighted imaging, and **(c)** restricted diffusion on axial ADC.

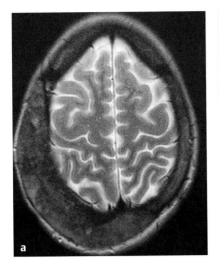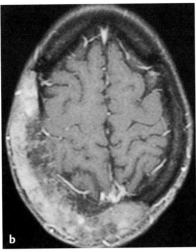

Fig. 1.58 A 29-year-old woman with fibrous dysplasia. **(a)** The expansile abnormality involving the right and posterior skull has mixed low and intermediate signal on axial T2-weighted imaging and **(b)** shows heterogeneous gadolinium contrast enhancement on axial T1-weighted imaging.

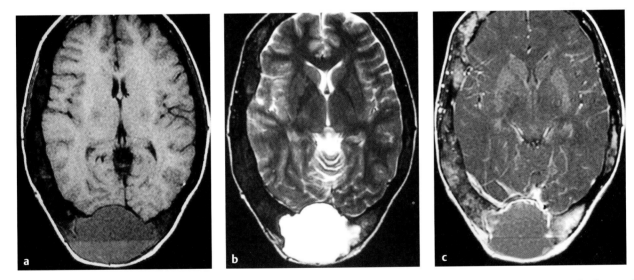

Fig. 1.59 A 28-year-old woman with fibrous dysplasia involving the right and posterior portions of the skull. **(a)** The expansile abnormality involving the right skull has mixed low and intermediate signal on axial T1-weighted imaging and **(b)** T2-weighted imaging and **(c)** shows heterogeneous gadolinium contrast enhancement on axial T1-weighted imaging. An aneurysmal cyst is seen at the dorsal portion of the skull involved with fibrous dysplasia, which has a fluid–fluid level on axial T1-weighted imaging, high signal on axial T2-weighted imaging, and thin peripheral gadolinium contrast enhancement on axial T1-weighted imaging.

Table 1.2 *(cont.)* Solitary lesions involving the skull

Lesions	Imaging Findings	Comments
Aneurysmal bone cysts (ABCs) (**Fig. 1.60**; see **Fig. 1.59**)	*CT:* Circumscribed radiolucent lesion with variable low, intermediate, and high attenuation, ± lobulations, ± one or multiple fluid–fluid levels. *MRI:* Circumscribed lesion with variable low, intermediate, high, and/or mixed signal on T1- and T2-weighted imaging, ± surrounding thin zone of low signal on T2-weighted imaging, ± lobulations, ± one or multiple fluid–fluid levels.	Tumorlike expansile bone lesions containing cavernous spaces filled with blood. ABCs can be primary bone lesions (two-thirds) or secondary to other bone lesions/tumors (such as giant cell tumors, chondroblastomas, osteoblastomas, osteosarcomas. chondromyxoid fibromas, nonossifying fibromas, fibrous dysplasia, fibrosarcomas, malignant fibrous histiocytomas, and metastatic disease). ABCs rarely involve the skull.
Aneurysm/pseudoaneurysm (**Fig. 1.61**)	*CT:* Focal circumscribed lesion with low-intermediate and/or high attenuation. *MRI:* Focal circumscribed lesion with layers of low, intermediate, and/or high signal on T1- and T2-weighted imaging secondary to layers of thrombus, as well as a signal void representing a patent lumen. *CTA and contrast-enhanced MRA* show contrast enhancement of nonthrombosed portions within lumens of aneurysms.	Abnormal dilatation of artery secondary to acquired/degenerative cause, connective tissue disease, atherosclerosis, trauma, infection (mycotic), arteriovenous malformation, drugs, or vasculitis.
Hemangioma (**Fig. 1.62**)	*MRI:* Circumscribed or poorly marginated structures (< 4 cm in diameter) in marrow of skull (often frontal bone) with intermediate-high signal on T1-weighted imaging (often isointense to marrow fat), high signal on T2-weighted imaging (T2WI) and fat-suppressed T2WI, and typically gadolinium contrast enhancement, ± widening of diploic compartment. *CT:* Expansile lesions with a radiating pattern of bony trabeculae oriented toward the center.	Benign lesions of bone composed of capillary, cavernous, and/or malformed venous vessels. Considered to be a hamartomatous disorder. Age at presentation is 1 to 84 years (median age = 33 years).
Venous lake (See **Fig. 1.28**)	*MRI:* Can show gadolinium contrast enhancement and enhancing blood vessels within the diploic space. *CT:* Circumscribed lobulate or ovoid radiolucent defect in the calvarium.	Defect in the skull that results from localized dilatation of diploic venous channels.
Paget disease	*MRI:* Most cases involving the skull are the late or inactive phases. Findings include osseous expansion and cortical thickening with low signal on T1- and T2-weighted imaging. The inner margins of the thickened cortex can be irregular and indistinct. Zones of low signal on T1- and T2-weighted imaging can be seen in the diploic marrow secondary to thickened bony trabeculae. Marrow in late or inactive phases of Paget disease can have signal similar to normal marrow, contain focal areas of fat signal, have low signal on T1- and T2-weighted imaging secondary to regions of sclerosis, and have areas of high signal on fat-suppressed T2-weighted imaging due to edema or persistent fibrovascular tissue. *CT:* Lesions often have mixed intermediate and high attenuation. Irregular/indistinct borders between marrow and inner margins of the outer and inner tables of the skull.	Paget disease is a chronic skeletal disease in which there is disordered bone resorption and woven bone formation, resulting in osseous deformity. A paramyxovirus may be the etiologic agent. Paget disease is polyostotic in up to 66% of patients. Paget disease is associated with a risk of less than 1% for developing secondary sarcomatous changes. Occurs in 2.5 to 5% of Caucasians more than 55 years old, and 10% of those more than 85 years old. Can result in narrowing of neuroforamina, with cranial nerve compression and basilar impression, ± compression of brainstem.

(continued on page 46)

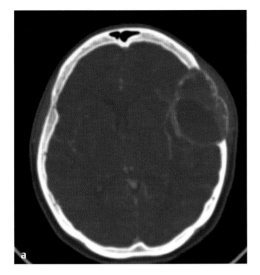

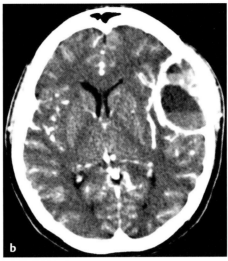

Fig. 1.60 An aneurysmal bone cyst is seen in the left skull. **(a)** Axial CT shows the expansile lesion to have thinned bone margins and **(b)** to contain several fluid–fluid levels.

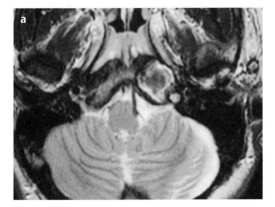

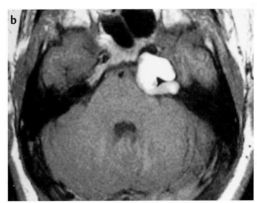

Fig. 1.61 A pseudoaneurysm of the left internal carotid artery is seen in the left carotid canal. **(a)** The expansile lesion has mixed low signal peripherally and low and high signal centrally on axial T2-weighted imaging. **(b)** The lesion has mostly high signal on axial T1-weighted imaging.

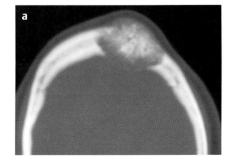

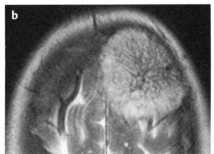

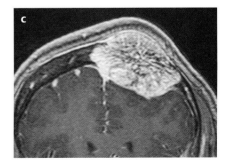

Fig. 1.62 A 33-year-old woman with a hemangioma in the left frontal bone. **(a)** The expansile lesion has a radiating pattern of bony trabeculae oriented toward the center on axial CT. **(b)** The lesion has mostly intermediate-high signal on axial T2-weighted imaging and contains thin bands of low signal, which correspond to bony trabeculae. **(c)** The lesion shows gadolinium contrast enhancement on coronal T1-weighted imaging.

Table 1.2 *(cont.)* Solitary lesions involving the skull

Lesions	Imaging Findings	Comments
Notochord rest (**Fig. 1.63**)	*MRI:* Circumscribed zone within the clivus inferior to the sella, with low-intermediate signal on T1-weighted imaging and high signal on T2-weighted imaging and fat-suppressed T2-weighted imaging, + gadolinium contrast enhancement. *CT:* Usually no findings. Can occasionally appear as a localized radiolucent abnormality.	During the fifth week of gestation, the notochord is enclosed by the bodies of the upper cervical vertebrae and enters into the basiocciput, where it terminates in the body of the sphenoid bone just below the pituitary fossa. Lack of normal involution of the notochord results in benign aggregates of physaliferous cells within bone. Notochord rests usually are stable in size.
Arachnoid granulation (See **Fig. 1.29**)	Circumscribed ovoid structures within dural venous sinuses, with low signal on T1-weighted imaging and FLAIR, high signal on T2-weighted imaging, and no gadolinium contrast enhancement, ± erosion of adjacent inner table of skull.	Extension of arachnoid membrane into dural venous sinuses. Normal CSF pulsations can result in erosion of adjacent bone.
Inflammatory Lesions		
Osteomyelitis (**Fig. 1.64**)	*CT:* Zones of abnormally decreased attenuation, focal sites of bone destruction, ± complications, including subgaleal empyema, epidural empyema, subdural empyema, meningitis, cerebritis, intra-axial abscess, and venous sinus thrombosis. *MRI:* Zones with low-intermediate signal on T1-weighted imaging and high signal on T2-weighted imaging (T2WI) and fat-suppressed T2WI, ± high signal on diffusion-weighted imaging and low signal on ADC. Usually shows heterogeneous gadolinium (Gd) contrast enhancement, ± adjacent intracranial dural and/or leptomeningeal Gd contrast enhancement, ± abnormal high T2 signal and contrast enhancement of brain tissue/abscess formation.	Osteomyelitis (bone infection) of the skull can result from surgery, trauma, hematogenous dissemination from another source of infection, or direct extension of infection from an adjacent site, such as the paranasal sinuses, nasal cavity, petrous apex air cells, and/or mastoid air cells and middle ear.
Mucocele/pyocele (**Fig. 1.65**)	*CT:* Airless expanded sinus filled with mucus (10–18 HU). *MRI:* Lesion with low signal on T1-weighted imaging (T1WI) and high signal on T2-weighted imaging (T2WI), can have high signal on T1WI and low signal on T2WI from inspissated secretions with high protein content or related to superimposed infection-pyocele.	Inflammation/infection of paranasal sinuses can cause obstruction of the sinus ostium, resulting in accumulation of mucus and desquamated epithelium. Progressive remodeling and expansion of sinus bone walls into orbits and cranial compartments. Distribution is frontal sinuses (65%), ethmoid air cells (25%), and maxillary sinuses (10%).

(continued on page 48)

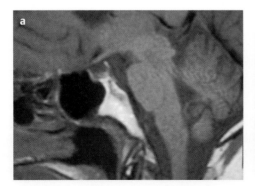
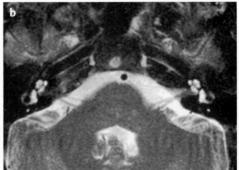

Fig. 1.63 A 53-year-old man with a notochord rest that is seen as a curvilinear zone within the clivus below the sella, which has **(a)** intermediate signal on sagittal T1-weighted imaging and **(b)** high signal on axial fat-suppressed T2-weighted imaging.

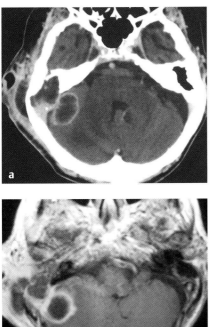

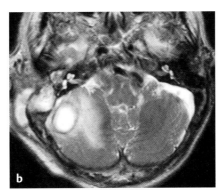

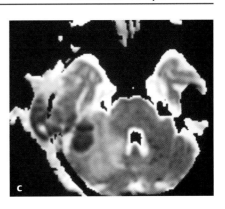

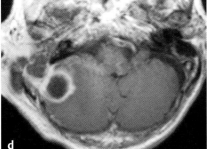

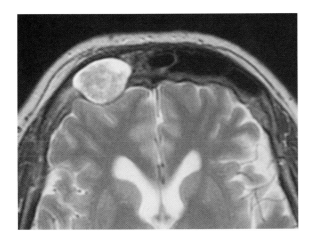

Fig. 1.64 **(a)** Osteomyelitis involving the right mastoid bone associated with osteolysis on axial postcontrast CT as well as intra-axial and extracranial abscesses. The collections of purulent material in the mastoid, extra-cranial and right cerebellar abscesses have **(b)** high signal on axial T2-weighted imaging, **(c)** restricted diffusion on axial ADC, and **(d)** peripheral gadolinium contrast enhancement on axial T1-weighted imaging.

Fig. 1.65 A 56-year-old woman with a mucocele in the right frontal sinus. The expansile lesion has thin bone margins and contains mixed high and intermediate signal on fat-suppressed T2-weighted imaging.

Table 1.2 *(cont.)* Solitary lesions involving the skull

Lesions	Imaging Findings	Comments
Cholesterol granuloma **(Fig. 1.66)**	*MRI:* Circumscribed lesion measuring between 2 and 4 cm in the marrow of the petrous bone, often associated with mild bone expansion. Lesions usually have high signal on T1-weighted imaging (T1WI) and fat-suppressed (FS) T1WI. Lesions may have high, intermediate, and/or low signal on T2-weighted imaging (T2WI) and FS T2WI. A peripheral rim of low signal on T2WI may also be seen due to hemosiderin. *CT:* Circumscribed radiolucent lesion measuring between 2 and 4 cm in the marrow of the petrous bone, often associated with mild bone expansion. Lesions usually have low attenuation.	Lesions occur in young and middle-aged adults and occur when there is obstruction of mucosa-lined air cells in the petrous bone. Multiple cycles of hemorrhage and granulomatous reaction result in an expansile osteolytic lesion containing cholesterol granules, chronic inflammatory cells, red blood cells, hemosiderin, fibrous tissue, and debris.
Langerhans' cell histiocytosis **(Fig. 1.67)**	Single or multiple circumscribed soft-tissue lesions in the marrow of the skull associated with focal bony destruction/erosion with extension extra- or intracranially or both. *CT:* Lesions usually have low-intermediate attenuation, + contrast enhancement, ± enhancement of the adjacent dura. *MRI:* Lesions typically have low-intermediate signal on T1-weighted imaging and heterogeneous slightly high to high signal on T2-weighted imaging (T2WI) and fat-suppressed (FS) T2WI. Poorly defined zones of high signal on T2WI and FS T2WI are usually seen in the marrow and soft tissues peripheral to the lesions secondary to inflammatory changes. Lesions typically show prominent gadolinium contrast enhancement in marrow and extraosseous soft tissue portions.	Disorder of reticuloendothelial system in which bone marrow–derived dendritic Langerhans' cells infiltrate various organs as focal lesions or in diffuse patterns. Langerhans' cells have eccentrically located ovoid or convoluted nuclei within pale to eosinophilic cytoplasm. Lesions often consist of Langerhans' cells, macrophages, plasma cells, and eosinophils. Lesions are immunoreactive to S-100, CD1a, CD-207, HLA-DR, and β_2-microglobulin. Prevalence of 2 per 100,000 children < 15 years old; only a third of lesions occur in adults. Localized lesions (eosinophilic granuloma) can be single or multiple in the skull, usually at the skull base. Single lesions are commonly seen in males more than in females, and in patients < 20 years old. Proliferation of histiocytes in medullary bone results in localized destruction of cortical bone with extension into adjacent soft tissues. Multiple lesions are associated with Letterer-Siwe disease (lymphadenopathy hepatosplenomegaly), in children < 2 years old and Hand-Schüller-Christian disease (lymphadenopathy, exophthalmos, diabetes insipidus) in children 5–10 years old.
Traumatic Lesions		
Cephalohematoma	Hematoma located beneath periosteum of outer table, does not cross suture lines, ± skull fracture, ± subdural hematoma.	Results from birth trauma (complication of forceps delivery), associated with 1% of births.
Fracture **(Fig. 1.68)**	*Nondisplaced/nondepressed skull fractures:* Abnormal low signal on T1-weighted imaging and high signal on T2-weighted imaging in marrow at the site of fracture, ± subgaleal hematoma, ± epidural hematoma, ± subdural hematoma, ± subarachnoid hemorrhage. *Depressed skull fracture:* Angulation and internal displacement of fractured skull, abnormal low signal on T1-weighted imaging and high signal on T2-weighted imaging in marrow at the site of fracture, ± subgaleal hematoma, ± epidural hematoma, ± subdural hematoma, ± subarachnoid hemorrhage.	Traumatic fractures of the skull can involve the calvarium or skull base, with significant complications that can include epidural hematoma, subdural hematoma, subarachnoid hemorrhage, and CSF leakage (rhinorrhea, otorrhea).

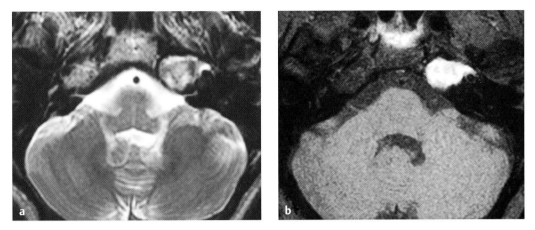

Fig. 1.66 A 40-year-old man with a cholesterol granuloma in the left petrous bone. **(a)** The expansile lesion has mixed high, intermediate, and low signal on axial T2-weighted imaging and **(b)** high signal on axial fat-suppressed T1-weighted imaging.

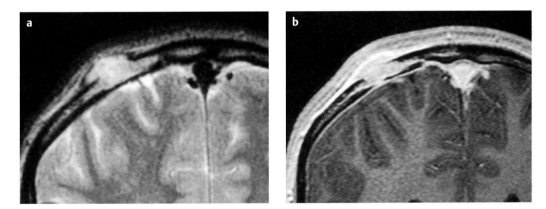

Fig. 1.67 A 14-year-old female with Langerhans' cell histiocytosis and an eosinophilic granuloma in the skull. **(a)** The intramedullary lesion erodes the inner and outer tables of the skull and has high signal on coronal T2-weighted imaging. **(b)** The lesion shows gadolinium contrast enhancement on coronal T1-weighted imaging.

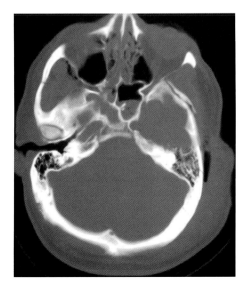

Fig. 1.68 Axial CT shows fractures at the anterior left temporal region, lateral right maxillary wall, and right zygoma.

Table 1.3   Multiple lesions involving the skull

- Malignant Tumors
  - Metastatic malignancies
  - Multiple myeloma
  - Lymphoma
- Benign Tumors
  - Schwannomas
  - Neurofibromas
- Tumorlike Lesions
  - Polyostotic fibrous dysplasia
  - Cystic angiomatosis/lymphangiomatosis
  - Paget disease
  - Hyperostosis frontalis
- Inflammatory Lesions
  - Langerhans' cell histiocytosis
  - Mucoceles

Table 1.3   Multiple lesions involving the skull

Lesions	Imaging Findings	Comments
Malignant Tumors		
Metastatic malignancies (**Fig. 1.69** and **Fig. 1.70**)	Multiple well-circumscribed or poorly defined lesions involving the skull. *CT:* Lesions are usually radiolucent, may also be sclerotic, ± extraosseous tumor extension through sites of bone destruction, usually + contrast enhancement, ± compression of neural tissue or vessels. *MRI:* Multiple well-circumscribed or poorly defined lesions involving the skull, with low-intermediate signal on T1-weighted imaging, intermediate-high signal on T2-weighted imaging, and usually gadolinium contrast enhancement, ± bone destruction, ± compression of neural tissue or vessels.	Metastatic lesions represent proliferating neoplastic cells that are located in sites or organs separated or distant from their origins. Metastatic carcinoma is the most frequent malignant tumor involving bone. In adults, metastatic lesions to bone occur most frequently from carcinomas of the lung, breast, prostate, kidney, and thyroid, as well as from sarcomas. Primary malignancies of the lung, breast, and prostate account for 80% of bone metastases. Metastatic tumor may cause variable destructive or infiltrative changes in single or multiple sites.
Multiple myeloma (**Fig. 1.71**)	Well-circumscribed or poorly defined lesions involving the skull and dura. *CT:* Lesions have low-intermediate attenuation, usually + contrast enhancement, + bone destruction. *MRI:* Well-circumscribed or poorly defined lesions involving the skull and dura, with low-intermediate signal on T1-weighted imaging, intermediate-high signal on T2-weighted imaging, and usually gadolinium contrast enhancement, + bone destruction	Multiple myeloma are malignant tumors comprised of proliferating antibody-secreting plasma cells derived from single clones. Multiple myeloma primarily involves bone marrow. A solitary myeloma or plasmacytoma is an infrequent variant in which a neoplastic mass of plasma cells occurs at a single site of bone or soft tissue. In the United States, 14,600 new cases occur each year. Multiple myeloma is the most common primary neoplasm of bone in adults. Median age at presentation = 60 years. Most patients are > 40 years old. Tumors occur in the vertebrae > ribs > femur > iliac bone > humerus > craniofacial bones > sacrum > clavicle > sternum > pubic bone > tibia.

(continued on page 52)

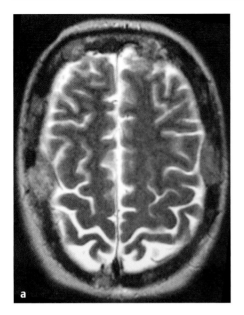

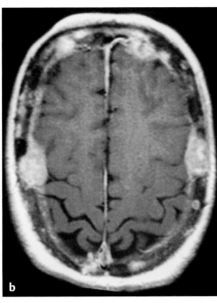

Fig. 1.69 A 68-year-old woman with metastatic breast carcinoma who has multiple lesions in skull marrow associated with bone destruction and extraosseous tumor extension. **(a)** The tumors have intermediate to slightly high signal on axial T2-weighted imaging and **(b)** show gadolinium contrast enhancement on axial T1-weighted imaging. Thickened contrast enhancing dura is also seen from neoplastic invasion.

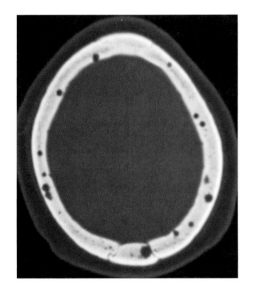

Fig. 1.70 A 65-year-old man with renal cell carcinoma who has multiple osteolytic metastases involving the skull on axial CT.

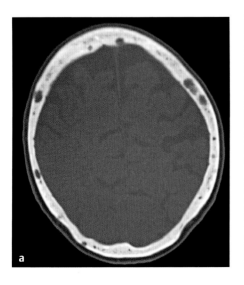

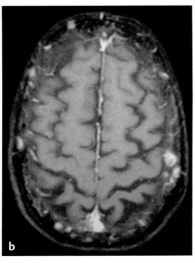

Fig. 1.71 **(a)** Multiple osteolytic lesions from multiple myeloma are seen in the skull on axial CT. **(b)** The lesions show gadolinium contrast enhancement on axial fat-suppressed T1-weighted imaging.

Table 1.3 *(cont.)*   Multiple lesions involving the skull

Lesions	Imaging Findings	Comments
Lymphoma	Single or multiple well-circumscribed or poorly defined lesions involving the skull. *CT:* Lesions have low-intermediate attenuation and may show contrast enhancement, ± bone destruction. *MRI:* Lesions have low-intermediate signal on T1-weighted imaging, intermediate to high signal on T2-weighted imaging, + gadolinium contrast enhancement. Can be locally invasive and associated with bone erosion/destruction, and intracranial extension with meningeal involvement.	Lymphomas are a group of lymphoid tumors whose neoplastic cells typically arise within lymphoid tissue (lymph nodes and reticuloendothelial organs). Unlike leukemia, lymphomas usually arise as discrete masses. Lymphomas are subdivided into Hodgkin disease (HD) and non-Hodgkin lymphoma (NHL). Distinction between HD and NHL is useful because of differences in clinical and histopathologic features, as well as treatment strategies. HD typically arises in lymph nodes and often spreads along nodal chains, whereas NHL frequently originates at extranodal sites and spreads in an unpredictable pattern. Almost all primary lymphomas of bone are B-cell NHL.
Benign Tumors		
Schwannomas **(Fig. 1.72)**	*MRI:* Circumscribed spheroid or ovoid lesions with low-intermediate signal on T1-weighted imaging, high signal on T2-weighted imaging (T2WI) and fat-suppressed T2WI, and usually prominent gadolinium (Gd) contrast enhancement. High signal on T2WI and Gd contrast enhancement can be heterogeneous in large lesions due to cystic degeneration and/or hemorrhage. Schwannomas involving the skull include those from CN V (trigeminal nerve cistern/Meckel's cave), CN VI (Dorello canal), CN VII and CN VIII (internal audittory canal and cerebellopontine angle cistern), CN IX, CN X, and CN XI (jugular foramen). *CT:* Circumscribed spheroid or ovoid lesions with intermediate attenuation, + contrast enhancement. Large lesions can have cystic degeneration and/or hemorrhage, ± erosion of adjacent bone.	Schwannomas are benign encapsulated tumors that contain differentiated neoplastic Schwann cells. Multiple schwannomas are often associated with neurofibromatosis type 2 (NF2), which is an autosomal dominant disease involving a gene at chromosome 22q12. In addition to schwannomas, patients with NF2 can also have multiple meningiomas and ependymomas. Schwannomas represent 8% of primary intracranial tumors and 29% of primary spinal tumors. The incidence of NF2 is 1/37,000 to 1/50,000 newborns. Age at presentation is 22 to 72 years (mean age = 46 years). Peak incidence is in the fourth to sixth decades. Many patients with NF2 present in the third decade with bilateral vestibular schwannomas.
Neurofibromas	*MRI: Solitary neurofibromas* Circumscribed spheroid, ovoid, or lobulated extra-axial lesions with low-intermediate signal on T1-weighted imaging (T1WI), intermediate-high signal on T2-weighted imaging (T2WI), + prominent gadolinium contrast enhancement. High signal on T2WI and gadolinium (Gd) contrast enhancement can be heterogeneous in large lesions. *Plexiform neurofibromas* appear as curvilinear and multinodular lesions involving multiple nerve branches and have low to intermediate signal on T1WI and intermediate, slightly high to high signal on T2WI and fat-suppressed T2WI, with or without bands or strands of low signal. Lesions usually show Gd contrast enhancement. *CT:* Ovoid or fusiform lesions with low-intermediate attenuation. Lesions can show contrast enhancement. Often erode adjacent bone.	Benign nerve sheath tumors that contain mixtures of Schwann cells, perineural-like cells, and interlacing fascicles of fibroblasts associated with abundant collagen. Unlike schwannomas, neurofibromas lack Antoni A and B regions and cannot be separated pathologically from the underlying nerve. Multiple neurofibromas are typically seen with neurofibromatosis type 1 (NF1), which is an autosomal dominant disorder (1/2,500 births) caused by mutations in the neurofibromin gene on chromosome 17q11.2. NF1 is the most common type of neurocutaneous syndrome and is associated with neoplasms of the central and peripheral nervous systems (optic gliomas, astrocytomas, plexiform and solitary neurofibromas) and skin (café-au-lait spots, axillary and inguinal freckling). Also associated with meningeal and skull dysplasias, as well as hamartomas of the iris (Lisch nodules).

(continued on page 54)

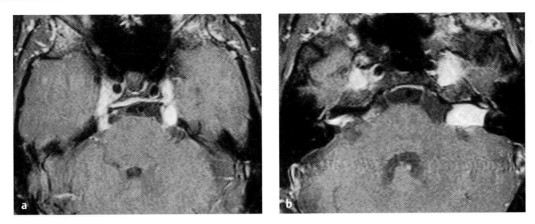

Fig. 1.72   **(a,b)** A 27-year-old man with neurofibromatosis type 2 who has gadolinium-enhancing schwannomas involving CN V, VII, and VIII on axial fat-suppressed T1-weighted imaging. The schwannomas are associated with chronic erosive osseous changes of the adjacent skull.

Table 1.3 *(cont.)* Multiple lesions involving the skull

Lesions	Imaging Findings	Comments
Tumorlike Lesions		
Polyostotic fibrous dysplasia (**Fig. 1.73**)	*CT:* Lesions involving the skull are often associated with bone expansion. Lesions have variable density and attenuation on radiographs and CT, respectively, depending on the degree of mineralization and number of the bony spicules in the lesions. Attenuation coefficients can range from 70 to 400 Hounsfield units. Lesions can have a ground-glass radiographic appearance secondary to the mineralized spicules of immature woven bone in fibrous dysplasia. Sclerotic borders of varying thickness can be seen surrounding parts or all of the lesions.	Benign medullary fibro-osseous lesion of bone, most often sporadic, involving a single site, referred to as *monostotic* fibrous dysplasia (80 to 85%), or in multiple locations (*polyostotic* fibrous dysplasia). Results from developmental failure in the normal process of remodeling primitive bone to mature lamellar bone, with resultant zone or zones of immature trabeculae within dysplastic fibrous tissue. These lesions do not mineralize normally and can result in cranial neuropathies from neuroforaminal narrowing, facial deformities, sinonasal drainage disorders, and sinusitis.
	MRI: Features depend on the proportions of bony spicules, collagen, fibroblastic spindle cells, and hemorrhagic and/or cystic changes. Lesions are usually well circumscribed and have low or low-intermediate signal on T1-weighted imaging. On T2-weighted imaging, lesions have variable mixtures of low, intermediate, and/or high signal, often surrounded by a low-signal rim of variable thickness. Internal septations and cystic changes are seen in a minority of lesions. Bone expansion is commonly seen. All or portions of the lesions can show gadolinium contrast enhancement in a heterogeneous, diffuse, or peripheral pattern.	McCune-Albright syndrome accounts for 3% of polyostotic fibrous dysplasia and may include the presence of pigmented cutaneous macules (sometimes referred to as café-au-lait spots) with irregular indented borders that are ipsilateral to bone lesions, precocious puberty, and/or other endocrine disorders, such as acromegaly, hyperthyroidism, hyperparathyroidism, and Cushing's syndrome. *Leontiasis ossea* is a rare form of polyostotic fibrous dyplasia that involves the craniofacial bones, resulting in facial enlargement and deformity. Age at presentation is < 1 year to 76 years; 75% of cases occur before the age of 30 years. Median age for monostotic fibrous dysplasia = 21 years; mean and median ages for polyostotic fibrous dysplasia are between 8 and 17 years. Most cases are diagnosed in patients between the ages of 3 and 20 years.

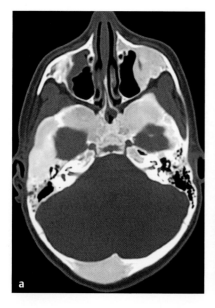
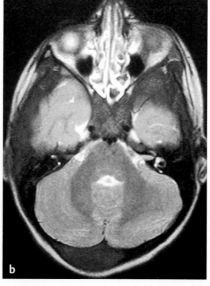

Fig. 1.73 A 5-year-old female with polyostotic fibrous dysplasia who has multiple expansile bone lesions involving the skull. **(a)** The lesions have a ground-glass appearance on axial CT and **(b)** low-intermediate signal on axial T2-weighted imaging.

Lesions	Imaging Findings	Comments
Cystic angiomatosis/ lymphangiomatosis	*MRI:* Circumscribed, poorly defined, or diffuse osseous lesions, typically with mixed low-intermediate and/or high signal on T1-weighted imaging and high signal on T2-weighted imaging (T2WI) and fat-suppressed T2WI, associated with thickened vertical trabeculae, usually with gadolinium contrast enhancement. *CT:* Multiple, ovoid, radiolucent, expansile bone lesions that can have a honeycomb or soap-bubble appearance, ± radiating pattern of bony trabeculae oriented toward the center.	Rare disorder with multiple intraosseous or soft tissue lesions containing endothelium-lined spaces with delicate walls not surrounded by neoplastic or reactive tissue.
Paget disease (See **Fig. 1.84** and **Fig. 1.105**)	*CT:* Lesions often have mixed intermediate and high attenuation. Irregular/indistinct borders between marrow and inner margins of the outer and inner tables of the skull. *MRI:* Most cases involving the skull are the late or inactive phases. Findings include osseous expansion and cortical thickening with low signal on T1- and T2-weighted imaging. The inner margins of the thickened cortex can be irregular and indistinct. Zones of low signal on T1- and T2-weighted imaging can be seen in the diploic marrow secondary to thickened bony trabeculae. Marrow in late or inactive phases of Paget disease can have signal similar to normal marrow, contain focal areas of fat signal, have low signal on T1- and T2-weighted imaging secondary to regions of sclerosis, and have areas of high signal on fat-suppressed T2-weighted imaging due to edema or persistent fibrovascular tissue.	Paget disease is a chronic skeletal disease in which there is disordered bone resorption and woven bone formation, resulting in osseous deformity. A paramyxovirus may be the etiologic agent. Paget disease is polyostotic in up to 66% of patients. Paget disease is associated with a risk of less than 1% for developing secondary sarcomatous changes. Occurs in 2.5 to 5% of Caucasians > 55 years old, and 10% of those > 85 years old. Can result in narrowing of neuroforamina, with cranial nerve compression and basilar impression, ± compression of brainstem.
Hyperostosis frontalis (**Fig. 1.74**)	*CT:* Expansion of the medullary portion of the frontal bone extending intracranially with well-defined cortical margins of the inner table of the skull. *MRI:* Marrow signal is typically within normal limits.	Benign bilateral bone overgrowth involving the inner table of the frontal bone, most often seen in elderly women.

(continued on page 56)

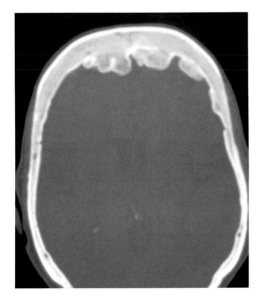

Fig. 1.74   An 83-year-old woman with hyperostosis frontalis, which is seen as inward lobulated expansion of the medullary portion of the frontal bone with well-defined thin cortical margins on axial CT.

Table 1.3 *(cont.)* Multiple lesions involving the skull

Lesions	Imaging Findings	Comments
Inflammatory Lesions		
Langerhans' cell histiocytosis (**Fig. 1.75**)	Single or multiple circumscribed soft tissue lesions in the marrow of the skull associated with focal bony destruction/erosion, with extension extra- or intracranially or both. *CT:* Lesions usually have low-intermediate attenuation, + contrast enhancement, ± enhancement of the adjacent dura. *MRI:* Lesions typically have low-intermediate signal on T1-weighted imaging and heterogeneous slightly high to high signal on T2-weighted imaging (T2WI) and fat-suppressed (FS) T2WI. Poorly defined zones of high signal on T2WI and FS T2WI are usually seen in the marrow and soft tissues peripheral to the lesions secondary to inflammatory changes. Lesions typically show prominent gadolinium contrast enhancement in marrow and extraosseous soft tissue portions.	Disorder of the reticuloendothelial system in which bone marrow–derived dendritic Langerhans' cells infiltrate various organs as focal lesions or in diffuse patterns. Langerhans' cells have eccentrically located ovoid or convoluted nuclei within pale to eosinophilic cytoplasm. Lesions often consist of Langerhans' cells, macrophages, plasma cells, and eosinophils. Lesions are immunoreactive to S-100, CD1a, CD-207, HLA-DR, and β_2-microglobulin. Prevalence of 2 per 100,000 children < 15 years old; only a third of lesions occur in adults. Localized lesions (eosinophilic granuloma) can be single or multiple in the skull, usually at the skull base. Single lesions are commonly seen in males more than in females, and in patients < 20 years old. Proliferation of histiocytes in medullary bone results in localized destruction of cortical bone with extension into adjacent soft tissues. Multiple lesions are associated with Letterer-Siwe disease (lymphadenopathy hepatosplenomegaly) in children < 2 years old, and Hand-Schüller-Christian disease (lymphadenopathy, exophthalmos, diabetes insipidus) in children 5–10 years old.
Mucoceles (**Fig. 1.76**)	*CT:* Airless expanded sinus with mucus (10–18 HU). *MRI:* Lesion with low signal on T1-weighted imaging and high signal on T2-weighted imaging. Lesions can have high signal on T1-weighted imaging and low signal on T2-weighted imaging from inspissated secretions with high protein content and/or infection-pyocele.	Inflammation/infection of paranasal sinuses can cause obstruction of the sinus ostium, resulting in accumulation of mucus and desquamated epithelium. Progressive remodeling and expansion of sinus bone walls into orbits and cranial compartments. Distribution is frontal sinuses (65%), ethmoid air cells (25%), and maxillary sinuses (10%).

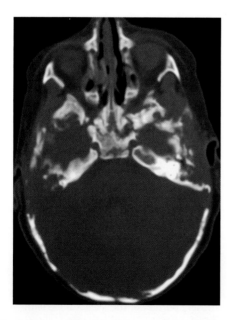

Fig. 1.75 A 2-year-old female with Langerhans' cell histiocytosis who has multiple osteolytic eosinophilic granulomas involving the skull on axial CT.

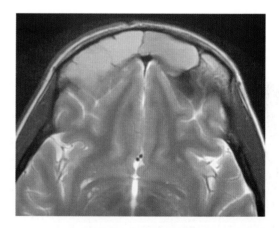

Fig. 1.76 Axial T2-weighted imaging shows bilateral mucoceles involving the frontal sinuses.

Table 1.4   Diffuse abnormalities involving the skull

- Chiari II malformation/Luckenschadel skull
- Achondroplasia
- Cleidocranial dysplasia/dysostosis (CCD)
- Congenital hydrocephalus
- Osteopetrosis
- Oxalosis
- Osteogenesis imperfecta (OI)
- Renal osteodystrophy/secondary hyperparathyroidism
- Paget disease
- Hematopoietic disorders
- Metastatic disease
- Leukemia

Table 1.4   Diffuse abnormalities involving the skull

Lesions	Imaging Findings	Comments
Chiari II malformation/ Luckenschadel skull **(Fig. 1.77)**	Large foramen magnum through which there is an inferiorly positioned vermis associated with a cervicomedullary kink. Myelomeningoceles in nearly all patients, usually in the lumbosacral region. Hydrocephalus and syringomyelia are common. Dilated lateral ventricles posteriorly (colpocephaly). Multifocal scalloping at the inner table of skull (Luckenschadel) can be seen, but it often regresses after 6 months.	Complex anomaly involving the cerebrum, cerebellum, brainstem, spinal cord, ventricles, skull, and dura. Failure of fetal neural folds to develop properly, resulting in altered development affecting multiple sites of the CNS. Dysplasia of membranous skull/ calvarium in Chiari II (referred to as Luckenschadel, lacunar skull, or craniolacunae) can occur with multifocal thinning of the inner table caused by nonossified fibrous bone due to abnormal collagen development and ossification.

(continued on page 58)

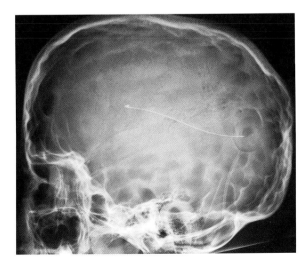

Fig. 1.77   Chiari II malformation/Luckenschadel. Lateral radiograph shows multifocal scalloping at the inner table of the skull.

Table 1.4 *(cont.)* Diffuse abnormalities involving the skull

Lesions	Imaging Findings	Comments
Achondroplasia **(Fig. 1.78)**	The calvarium/skull vault is enlarged in association with a small skull base and narrow foramen magnum. Cervicomedullary myelopathy and/or hydrocephalus can result from a narrowed foramen magnum. The posterior cranial fossa is shallow, and basal foramina are hypoplastic. Small jugular foramina can restrict venous outflow from the head. Other findings include short wide ribs, square iliac bones, champagne-glass-shaped pelvic inlet, and short pedicles involving multiple vertebrae/congenital spinal canal stenosis.	Autosomal dominant rhizomelic dwarfism that results in abnormal reduced endochondral bone formation. Most common nonlethal bone dysplasia and short-limbed dwarfism, with an incidence of 1/15,000 live births. More than 80–90% are spontaneous mutations involving the gene that encodes the fibroblast growth factor receptor 3 (*FGFR3*) on chromosome 4p16.3. The mutations typically occur on the paternal chromosome and are associated with increased paternal age. The mutated gene impairs endochondral bone formation and longitudinal lengthening of long bones.
Cleidocranial dysplasia/ dysostosis (CCD) **(Fig. 1.79)**	*CT:* Small skull base, brachycephaly, frontal bossing, elongated foramen magnum, hypertelorism, hypoplastic zygoma, stenosis of the external auditory canals, underdeveloped mastoid air cells, choanal stenosis, arched V-shaped palate, and hypoplastic midface and paranasal sinuses.	Autosomal dominant syndrome involving the *RUNX2* gene on chromosome 6p21. Mutations result in haploinsufficiency that affects osteoblast precursor cell differentiation. Loss of one functional gene results in CCD; when both genes are abnormal, lack of osteoblast differentiation. CCD involves both membranous and endochondral bone formation. Findings include widening of the fontanelles, *late* sutural closure, broad lateral cranial dimensions, wormian bones in the lambdoid suture, hearing loss (38%), hypoplastic or absent clavicles, multiple spinal anomalies, widened symphysis pubis, short stature, hypoplastic middle and distal phalanges, and supernumerary teeth.
Congenital hydrocephalus (See **Fig. 1.31**)	*MRI:* With aqueductal stenosis, dilatation of lateral and third ventricles with normal-size fourth ventricle, ± dilatation of only the upper portion of cerebral aqueduct and not the lower portion, ± discrete or poorly defined lesion in midbrain. Subependymal edema can be seen on FLAIR	Incidence is 2 per 1,000 live births. Most common cause is aqueductal stenosis secondary to a small lesion or neoplasm in the midbrain, debris or adhesions from hemorrhage, or inflammatory diseases. MRI can exclude other lesions causing obstruction of CSF flow through the aqueduct, such as lesions in the posterior third ventricle or posterior cranial fossa. Congenital hydrocephalus also occurs in association with Chiari I, Chiari II, and Dandy-Walker malformations
Osteopetrosis **(Fig. 1.80)**	*CT:* Findings include generalized bony sclerosis and hyperostosis, resulting in thickening of the skull, as well as narrowing of the foramina and optic canals. *MRI:* Low signal on T1- and T2-weighted imaging in marrow of endochondral bone (skull base and vertebrae). Expansion of calvarial diploic space, and marrow has low-intermediate to intermediate signal on T1- and T2-weighted imaging.	Osteopetrosis is a group of disorders with defective resorption of primary spongiosa and mineralized cartilage secondary to osteoclast dysfunction. Results in failure of conversion of immature woven bone into strong lamellar bone. Consists of four types: the precocious type, an autosomal recessive form (which is usually lethal from medullary crowding secondary to thickened, immature, sclerotic bone, resulting in anemia, thrombocytopenia, and immune dysfunction); the delayed type, an autosomal dominant form described by Albers-Schonberg that can be asymptomatic until there is a pathologic fracture or anemia; the intermediate recessive type, in which patients have short stature, hepatomegaly, and anemia; and tubular acidosis, an autosomal recessive form in which cerebral calcifications occur, as well as renal tubular acidosis, mental retardation, muscle weakness, and hypotonia.

(continued on page 60)

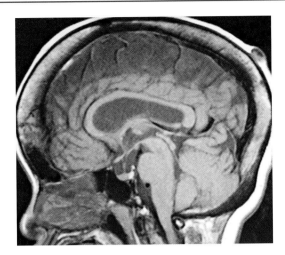

Fig. 1.78 A 48-year-old woman with achondroplasia. Sagittal T1-weighted imaging shows a narrowed foramen magnum, small skull base and posterior cranial fossa, and enlarged and thickened calvarium.

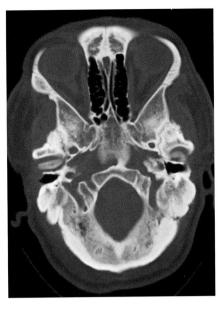

Fig. 1.79 A 35-year-old woman with cleidocranial dysplasia/dysostosis. Axial CT shows a small skull base with thickened bone and elongated foramen magnum, as well as underdeveloped mastoid air cells.

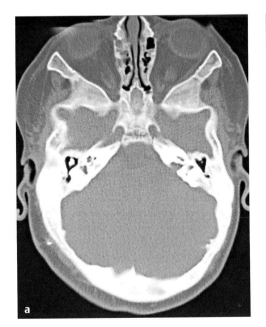

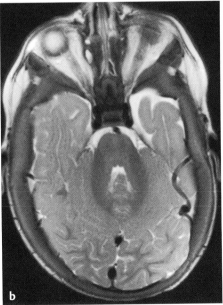

Fig. 1.80 A 3-month-old male with osteopetrosis. **(a)** Axial CT shows generalized bone sclerosis and thickening of the skull. **(b)** The marrow in the expanded diploic space has low-intermediate signal on axial T2-weighted imaging.

Table 1.4 *(cont.)* Diffuse abnormalities involving the skull

Lesions	Imaging Findings	Comments
Oxalosis (**Fig. 1.81**)	Global medullary and cortical nephrocalcinosis with resultant renal failure. *CT:* Early findings include osteosclerosis, osteopenia, and thin, transverse, sclerotic bands in long bones and skull. Late findings include osteosclerosis and dense intraossoeus sclerotic bands. *MRI:* Decreased signal of bone marrow on T1- and T2-weighted imaging.	Type 1 primary hyperoxaluria is a rare autosomal recessive disorder (1 in 120,000 live births) involving mutations of the *AGXT* gene, which results in a deficiency of the peroxisomal enzyme alanine glyoxylate aminotransferase. Systemic oxalate accumulates and precipitates in multiple organs (kidneys, liver, eye, heart, and bone), resulting in organ failure. Fifty percent of patients have end-stage renal failure at 15 years. Treatment is combined liver–kidney transplantation.
Osteogenesis imperfecta (OI) (**Fig. 1.82**)	Diffuse osteopenia, decreased ossification of skull base with fractures, infolding of the occipital condyles, elevation of the posterior cranial fossa, and upward migration of the dens into the foramen magnum, resulting in basilar impression (secondary basilar invagination).	Also known as brittle bone disease, OI has four to seven types. OI is a hereditary disorder with abnormal type I fibrillar collagen production and osteoporosis resulting from mutations involving the *COL1A1* gene on chromosome 17q21.31-q22.05 and the *COL1A2* gene on chromosome 7q22.1. Results in fragile bone prone to repetitive microfractures and remodeling. Type II is the most severe type, secondary to insufficient quantity and quality of collagen. Most patients with Type II die within the first year from intracerebral hemorrhage or respiratory failure. The other types are associated with bone fractures and deformities, discoloration of sclera, hearing loss, scoliosis, and short stature, ± respiratory problems.
Renal osteodystrophy/ secondary hyperparathyroidism (**Fig. 1.83**)	*CT:* Trabecular bone resorption with a salt-and-pepper appearance from mixed osteolysis and osteosclerosis, osteiitis fibrosa cystica, cortical thinning, coarsened trabecular pattern, and osteolytic lesions/brown tumors. Another pattern is ground-glass appearance with indistinct corticomedullary borders. *MRI:* Zones of low signal on T1- and T2-weighted imaging corresponding to regions of bone sclerosis. Circumscribed zones with high signal on T2-weighted imaging can be due to osteolytic lesions or brown tumors.	Osteoblastic and osteoclastic changes that occur in bone as a result of chronic end-stage renal disease, secondary hyperparathyroidism (hyperplasia of parathyroid glands), and osteomalacia (abnormal vitamin D metabolism). Can result in pathologic fracture. Unlike in secondary hyperparathyroidism, diffuse or patchy bone sclerosis infrequently occurs.
Paget disease (**Fig. 1.84;** see **Fig. 1.105**)	Expansile sclerotic/lytic process involving the skull. *CT:* Lesions often have mixed intermediate high attenuation. Irregular/indistinct borders between marrow and inner margins of the outer and inner tables of the skull. *MRI:* The MRI features of Paget disease vary based on the phases of the disease. Most cases involving the skull are the late or inactive phases. Findings include osseous expansion and cortical thickening with low signal on T1- and T2-weighted imaging. The inner margins of the thickened cortex can be irregular and indistinct. Zones of low signal on T1- and T2-weighted imaging can be seen in the diploic marrow secondary to thickened bony trabeculae. Marrow in late or inactive phases of Paget disease can have signal similar to normal marrow, contain focal areas of fat signal, have low signal on T1- and T2-weighted imaging secondary to regions of sclerosis, have areas of high signal on fat-suppressed T2-weighted imaging from edema or persistent fibrovascular tissue, or have various combinations of the aforementioned.	Paget disease is a chronic skeletal disease in which there is disordered bone resorption and woven bone formation, resulting in osseous deformity. A paramyxovirus may be the etiologic agent. Paget disease is polyostotic in up to 66% of patients. Paget disease is associated with a risk of < 1% for developing secondary sarcomatous changes. Occurs in 2.5 to 5% of Caucasians more than 55 years old, and 10% of those more than 85 years old. Can result in narrowing of neuroforamina, with cranial nerve compression and basilar impression, ± compression of brainstem.

(continued on page 62)

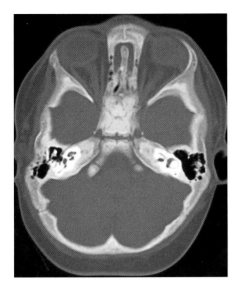

Fig. 1.81 A 2-year-old female with oxalosis. Axial CT shows diffuse increased attenuation of the skull as well as thin intraosseous sclerotic bands.

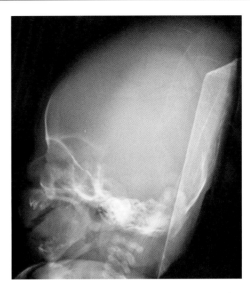

Fig. 1.82 A 1-day-old neonate with neonatal type of osteogenesis imperfecta (type II). Lateral radiograph shows prominent diffuse osteopenia.

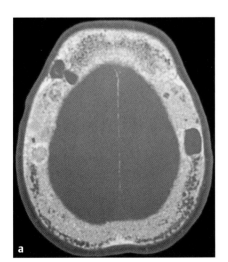

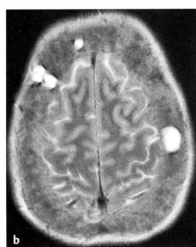

Fig. 1.83 Renal osteodystrophy/secondary hyperparathyroidism. **(a)** Axial CT shows the thickened skull with mixed osteolysis and osteosclerosis, cortical thinning, coarsened trabecular pattern, and osteolytic lesions/brown tumors. Also seen are zones with ground-glass appearance and indistinct corticomedullary borders. **(b)** Axial T2-weighted imaging shows heterogeneous mixed low and intermediate signal in marrow, as well as circumscribed ovoid zones with high signal.

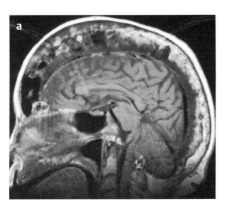

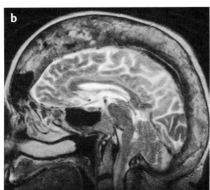

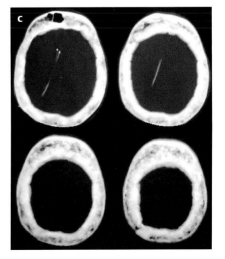

Fig. 1.84 An 81-year-old woman with Paget disease involving the skull and associated basilar impression. The interface between the diploic space and the inner and outer tables is obscured, and there is osseous expansion. The marrow has mixed low, intermediate, and high signal on **(a)** sagittal T1-weighted imaging and **(b)** sagittal T2-weighted imaging. **(c)** Axial CT shows mixed sclerosis within the expanded calvarium.

Table 1.4 *(cont.)* Diffuse abnormalities involving the skull

Lesions	Imaging Findings	Comments
Hematopoietic disorders (**Fig. 1.85** and **Fig. 1.86**)	*MRI:* Enlargement of the diploic space, with red marrow hyperplasia and thinning of inner and outer tables. Involved marrow has low-intermediate signal on T1-weighted imaging (slightly to moderately decreased signal relative to fat), intermediate to slightly high signal on T2-weighted imaging (isointense to slightly hyperintense signal to muscle) and increased signal relative to fat on fat-suppressed T2-weighted imaging. Expansion of marrow space causes reduced pneumatization of paranasal sinuses. Similar imaging findings can result from chronic cyanotic heart disease and long-term treatment with granulocyte colony stimulating factor (GCSF) for severe congenital neutropenia. Bone infarcts and extramedullary hematopoesis can also occur. *β-thalassemia* *Conventional radiography:* Findings are seen after 1 year. Hair-on-end appearance of dense bony trabeculae that are perpendicular to the thinned inner and outer tables of the skull, periosteal elevation, and osteopenia.	Inherited anemias (sickle-cell disease, thalassemia, hereditary spherocytosis) cause ineffective erythropoiesis, which results in elevated levels of erythropoietin and hyperplasia of normal red marrow elements. Expansion of bone marrow by up to 15- to 30-fold can occur. In *sickle-cell disease* (most common type), abnormal hemoglobin S is combined with itself or other hemoglobin types (C, D, E, or thalassemia). Sickling of red blood cells is most severe with hemoglobin SS, SC, and S-thalassemia. *β-thalassemia* is characterized by deficient synthesis of beta chains of hemoglobin, resulting in an excess of alpha chains that causes dysfunctional hematopoiesis and hemolysis. Treatment is iron chelation therapy and transfusions.
Metastatic disease (**Fig. 1.87**)	Multiple well-circumscribed or poorly defined lesions involving the skull, dura, leptomeninges, and/or choroid plexus. *MRI:* Multiple well-circumscribed or poorly defined lesions involving the skull, dura, leptomeninges, and/or choroid plexus, with low-intermediate signal on T1-weighted imaging, intermediate-high signal on T2-weighted imaging, and usually gadolinium contrast enhancement, ± bone destruction, ± compression of neural tissue or vessels. Leptomeningeal tumor often best seen on postcontrast images. *CT:* Lesions are usually radiolucent, may also be sclerotic, ± extraosseous tumor extension, usually + contrast enhancement, ± compression of neural tissue or vessels.	Metastatic lesions represent proliferating neoplastic cells that are located in sites or organs separated or distant from their origins. Metastatic lesions can disseminate hematogenously via arteries or veins, along CSF pathways, along surgical tracts, and along lymphatic structures. Metastatic carcinoma is the most frequent malignant tumor involving bone. In adults, metastatic lesions to bone occur most frequently from carcinomas of the lung, breast, prostate, kidney, and thyroid, as well as from sarcomas. Primary malignancies of the lung, breast, and prostate account for 80% of bone metastases. Metastatic tumor may cause variable destructive or infiltrative changes in single or multiple sites.
Leukemia (**Fig. 1.88**)	*MRI:* Diffuse abnormal signal in the marrow, with low-intermediate signal on T1-weighted imaging, intermediate-high signal on T2-weighted imaging, ± gadolinium contrast enhancement, ± bone destruction. *CT:* ± zones of bone destruction.	Leukemias are neoplastic proliferations of hematopoietic cells. Myeloid sarcomas (also referred to as chloromas, granulocytic sarcomas) are focal tumors composed of myeloblasts and neoplastic granulocyte precursor cells and occur in 2% of patients with acute myelogenous leukemia. These lesions can involve the skull marrow, leptomeninges, and brain. Intracranial lesions can be solitary or multiple.

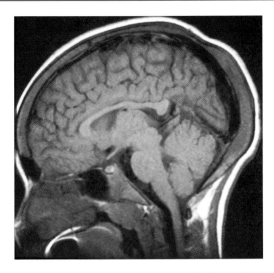

Fig. 1.85 Patient with sickle-cell anemia who has enlargement of the diploic space with red marrow hyperplasia, which has low-intermediate signal on sagittal T1-weighted imaging.

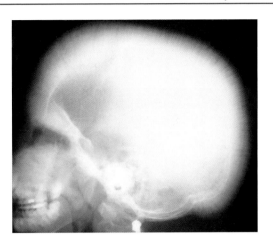

Fig. 1.86 Lateral radiograph of a patient with β-thalassemia shows enlarged calvarium with a hair-on-end appearance of dense bony trabeculae that are perpendicular to the thinned inner and outer tables of the skull. Expanded bone fills the maxillary sinuses.

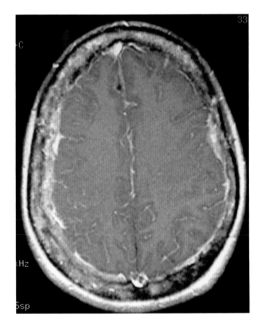

Fig. 1.87 A 33-year-old woman with diffuse metastatic tumor from breast carcinoma involving the calvarial marrow that shows gadolinium contrast enhancement, multiple sites of destruction of the outer and inner tables, and intracranial tumor extension to involve the dura.

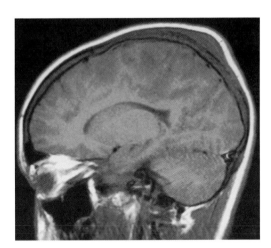

Fig. 1.88 A 12-year-old female with leukemia (ALL) involving the skull that is seen as low-intermediate signal in the marrow as well as sites of destruction of the inner and outer tables with extracranial neoplastic extension on sagittal T1-weighted imaging.

1.5 Abnormalities Involving the Craniovertebral Junction

The craniovertebral junction consists of the occipital bone, C1 and C2 vertebrae, and connecting ligaments. The articulations of the occipital-atlanto (C0–C1) and atlanto-axial (C1–C2) joints are different from the lower cervical levels. With the occipital-atlanto articulation, the occipital condyles rest along the superior facets of the lateral masses of C1. This configuration allows for 20 degrees of flexion and extension while limiting axial rotation and lateral flexion. With the C1–C2 articulation, a small rounded facet (fovea dentis) at the dorsal aspect of the anterior arch of C1 articulates with the anterior margin of the dens. This configuration enables the skull and atlas to rotate laterally as a unit around the vertical axis of the dens. Ligaments at the craniovertebral junction include the alar, transverse, and apical ligaments (**Fig. 1.89** and **Fig. 1.90**). The alar ligaments connect the lateral margins of the odontoid process with the lateral masses of C1 and medial margins of the foramen magnum. The alar ligaments limit atlanto-axial rotation. The transverse ligament extends medially from the tubercles at the inner aspects of the lateral articulating masses of C1 behind the dens, stabilizing the dens to the anterior arch of C1. The transverse ligament is the horizontal portion of the cruciform ligament, which also has fibers that extend from the transverse ligament superiorly to the clivus and inferiorly to the posterior surface of the dens. The apical ligament (middle odontoid ligament) extends from the upper margin of the dens to the anterior clival portion of the foramen magnum. The tectorial membrane is an upward extension from the posterior longitudinal ligament that connects with the body of C2 and the occipital bone (jugular tubercle and cranial base). Above the C2 level, the tectorial membrane merges with dura mater. The anterior and posterior atlanto-occipital membranes are superior extensions of the flaval ligament.

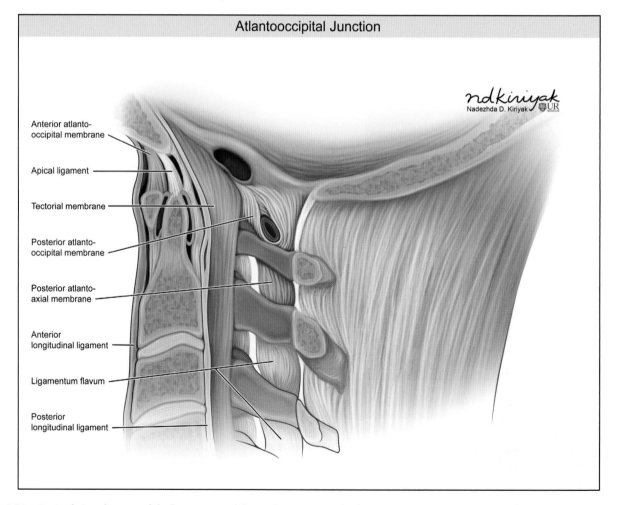

Atlantooccipital Junction

Anterior atlanto-occipital membrane

Apical ligament

Tectorial membrane

Posterior atlanto-occipital membrane

Posterior atlanto-axial membrane

Anterior longitudinal ligament

Ligamentum flavum

Posterior longitudinal ligament

Nadezhda D. Kiriyak

Fig. 1.89 Sagittal view diagram of the ligaments stabilizing the craniovertebral junction.

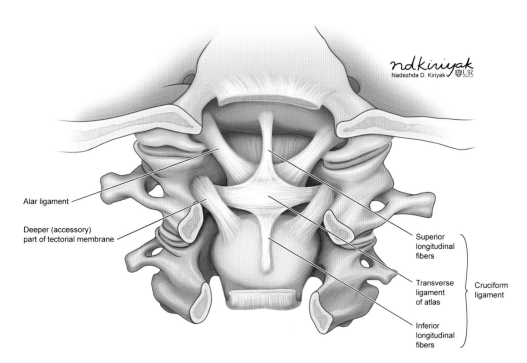

Internal Craniocervical Ligaments

Alar ligament

Deeper (accessory)
part of tectorial membrane

Superior
longitudinal
fibers

Transverse
ligament
of atlas

Cruciform
ligament

Inferior
longitudinal
fibers

Fig. 1.90 Posterior view diagram of the dorsal aspects of the cruciform ligament, alar ligaments, and tectorial membrane.

Table 1.5 Abnormalities involving the craniovertebral junction

- Congenital/Developmental
    - Basiocciput hypoplasia
    - Chiari I malformation
    - Chiari II malformation
    - Chiari III malformation
    - Condylus tertius
    - Atlanto-occipital assimilation/nonsegmentation
    - Atlas anomalies
    - Os odontoideum
    - Achondroplasia
    - Down syndrome (Trisomy 21)
    - Ehlers-Danlos syndrome
    - Mucopolysaccharidosis (MPS)
    - Osteogenesis imperfecta (OI)
    - Neurenteric cyst
    - Ecchordosis physaliphora
- Osteomalacia
    - Renal osteodystrophy/secondary hyperparathyroidism
    - Paget disease
    - Fibrous dysplasia
    - Hematopoietic disorders
- Traumatic Lesions
    - Fracture of skull base

- Atlanto-occipital dislocation
- Jefferson fracture (C1)
- Hangman's fracture (C2)
- Odontoid fracture (C2)
- Inflammation
    - Osteomyelitis/epidural abscess
    - Langerhans' cell histiocytosis
    - Rheumatoid arthritis
    - Calcium pyrophosphate dihydrate (CPPD) deposition
- Malignant Neoplasms
    - Metastatic disease
    - Myeloma
    - Chordoma
    - Chondrosarcoma
    - Squamous cell carcinoma
    - Nasopharyngeal carcinoma
    - Adenoid cystic carcinoma
    - Invasive pituitary tumor
- Benign Neoplasms
    - Meningioma
    - Schwannoma
    - Neurofibroma
- Tumorlike Lesions
    - Epidermoid
    - Arachnoid cyst
    - Mega cisterna magna

Table 1.5 Abnormalities involving the craniovertebral junction

Lesions	Imaging Findings	Comments
Congenital/Developmental		
Basiocciput hypoplasia (**Fig. 1.91**)	Hypoplasia of the lower clivus results in primary basilar invagination. Results in elevation of the dens more than 5 mm above Chamberlain's line (line between the hard palate and opisthion, the posterior margin of the foramen magnum on sagittal MRI). Can also result in abnormally decreased clival-canal angle below the normal range of 150 to 180 degrees, ± syrinx formation in spinal cord.	The lower clivus is a portion of the occipital bone (basiocciput), which is composed of four fused sclerotomes. Failure of formation of one or more of the sclerotomes results in a shortened clivus and primary basilar invagination (dens extending > 5 mm above Chamberlain's line). Can be associated with hypoplasia of the occipital condyles. The occipital condyles develop from the ventral segment of the proatlas derived from the fourth occipital sclerotome.
Chiari I malformation (**Fig. 1.92**)	Cerebellar tonsils extend more than 5 mm below the foramen magnum in adults, 6 mm in children < 10 years old. Syringohydromyelia occurs in 20 to 40% of cases. Hydrocephalus in 25%. Basilar impression in 25%. Less common associations are Klippel-Feil anomaly and atlanto-occipital assimilation.	Cerebellar tonsillar ectopia. Most common anomaly of CNS. Not associated with myelomeningocele.
Chiari II malformation (**Fig. 1.93**)	Large foramen magnum through which there is an inferiorly positioned vermis associated with a cervicomedullary kink. Myelomeningoceles occur in nearly all patients, usually in the lumbosacral region. Hydrocephalus and syringomyelia are common. Dilated lateral ventricles posteriorly (colpocephaly). Multifocal scalloping at the inner table of the skull (Luckenschadel) can be seen, but it often regresses after 6 months.	Complex anomaly involving the cerebrum, cerebellum, brainstem, spinal cord, ventricles, skull, and dura. Failure of fetal neural folds to develop properly results in altered development affecting multiple sites of the CNS. Dysplasia of membranous skull/calvarium in Chiari II (referred to as Luckenschadel, lacunar skull, or craniolacunae) can occur, with multifocal thinning of the inner table due to nonossified fibrous bone caused by abnormal collagen development and ossification.
Chiari III malformation (See **Fig. 1.13**)	Features of Chiari II plus lower occipital or high cervical encephalocele.	Rare anomaly associated with high mortality.
Condylus tertius (**Fig. 1.94**)	Ossicle seen between the lower portion of a shortened basiocciput and the dens/atlas.	Condylus tertius, or third occipital condyle, results from lack of fusion of the lowermost fourth sclerotome (proatlas) with the adjacent portions of the clivus. The third occipital condyle can form a pseudojoint with the anterior arch of C1 and/or dens and can be associated with decreased range of movement.

(continued on page 68)

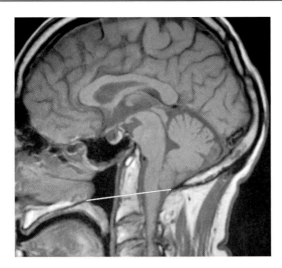

Fig. 1.91   Sagittal T1-weighted imaging shows basiocciput hypoplasia, with the dens extending intracranially above Chamberlain's line by more than 5 mm.

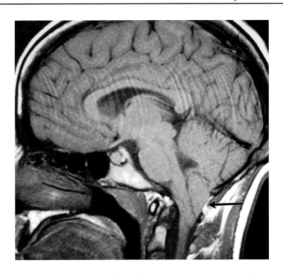

Fig. 1.92   Sagittal T1-weighted imaging in a 19-year-old woman shows a Chiari I malformation, with the cerebellar tonsils (*arrow*) extending below the foramen magnum to the level of the posterior arch of the C1 vertebra. The fourth ventricle has a normal appearance (*arrows*).

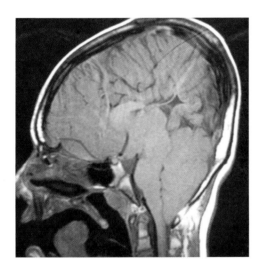

Fig. 1.93   Sagittal T1-weighted imaging of a patient with a Chiari II malformation shows a small posterior cranial fossa and a large foramen magnum through which the cerebellum extends inferiorly. There is absence of the normal shape of the fourth ventricle. Hypoplasia of the posterior portion of the corpus callosum is also seen.

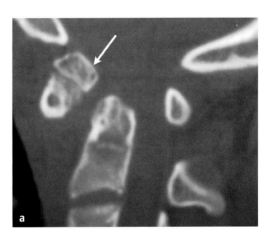

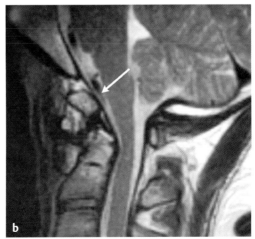

Fig. 1.94   Condylus tertius. **(a)** Sagittal CT and **(b)** sagittal T2-weighted imaging of a 16-year-old male show an ossicle (condylus tertius) between the lower portion of a shortened basiocciput and dens/atlas (*arrows*).

Table 1.5 *(cont.)*   Abnormalities involving the craniovertebral junction

Lesions	Imaging Findings	Comments
Atlanto-occipital assimilation/ nonsegmentation (**Fig. 1.95**; see **Fig. 1.14**)	Often seen as fusion of the occipital condyle with the anterior arch, posterior arch, one or both lateral masses of C1, or combinations of the above, ± associated congenital anomalies, which occur in 20% of cases, such as external ear deformities, cleft palate, C2–C3 nonsegmentation, and/or cervical ribs.	Most common congenital osseous anomaly involving the craniovertebral junction. Failure of segmentation of the occipital condyles (fourth occipital sclerotome) and the C1 vertebra (first cervical sclerotome). Can be associated with C1–C2 instability.
Atlas anomalies (**Fig. 1.96** and **Fig. 1.97**)	Unilateral or bilateral hypoplasia/aplasia of the posterior arch of C1. Clefts can also be seen in C1, most commonly at the posterior arch in the midline.	The first spinal sclerotome forms the atlas, while caudal portions of the proatlas form the lateral masses and upper portions of the posterior arch. Anomalies include aplasia of C1, or partial aplasia/hypoplasia of the posterior arch, ± atlanto-axial subluxation. Another more common anomaly involving C1 is rachischisis, clefts in the altas arches caused by developmentally defective cartilage formation. Clefts most commonly occur in the posterior arch in the midline (> 90%), followed by lateral clefts, and anterior clefts.
Os odontoideum (**Fig. 1.98** and **Fig. 1.99**)	Separate corticated bony structure positioned below the basion and superior to the C2 body at site of normally expected dens, often associated with enlargement of the anterior arch of C1 (which may sometimes be larger than the adjacent os odontoideum). Instability can result when the gap between the os and the body of C2 is above the plane of the superior articular facets and below the transverse ligament.	Independent bony structure positioned superior to the C2 body at site of normally expected dens, often associated with hypertrophy of the anterior arch of C1, ± cruciate ligament incompetence/instability (± zone of high signal on T2-weighted imaging in spinal cord). Os odontoideum can be associated with Klippel-Feil anomaly, spondyloepiphyseal dysplasia, Down syndrome, and Morquio syndrome. Os odontoideum is considered to be a normal variant or arising from a childhood injury (between 1 and 4 years), with fracture/separation of the cartilaginous plate between the dens and body of axis.
Achondroplasia (**Fig. 1.100**)	The calvarium/skull vault is enlarged in association with a small skull base and narrow foramen magnum. Cervicomedullary myelopathy and/or hydrocephalus can result from a narrowed foramen magnum. The posterior cranial fossa is shallow, and basal foramina are hypoplastic. Small jugular foramina can restrict venous outflow from the head. Other findings include short wide ribs, square iliac bones, champagne-glass-shaped pelvic inlet, and short pedicles involving multiple vertebrae/congenital spinal canal stenosis.	Autosomal dominant rhizomelic dwarfism that results in abnormal reduced endochondral bone formation. Most common nonlethal bone dysplasia and short-limbed dwarfism, with an incidence of 1/15,000 live births. More than 80–90% are spontaneous mutations involving the gene that encodes the fibroblast growth factor receptor 3 (*FGFR3*) on chromosome 4p16.3. The mutations typically occur on the paternal chromosome and are associated with increased paternal age. The mutated gene impairs endochondral bone formation and longitudinal lengthening of long bones.

(continued on page 71)

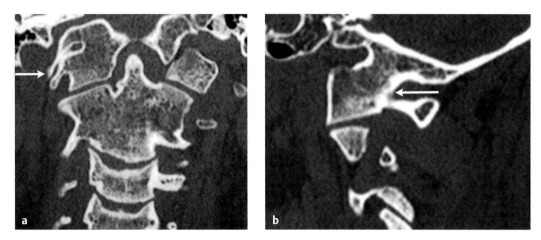

Fig. 1.95 **(a)** Coronal and **(b)** and sagittal CT show unilateral nonsegmentation (assimilation) involving the right occipital condyle and right lateral articulating mass of the C1 vertebra (*arrows*). Also seen is nonsegmentation involving the C2 and C3 vertebrae (Klippel-Feil anomaly).

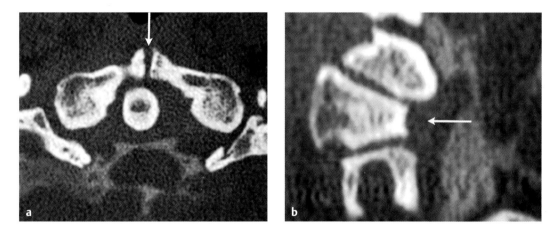

Fig. 1.96 **(a)** Axial and **(b)** sagittal CT images of a 58-year-old woman show absence of the posterior arch of C1 (*arrow* in **b**). Also seen is an anterior cleft in C1 (*arrow* in **a**).

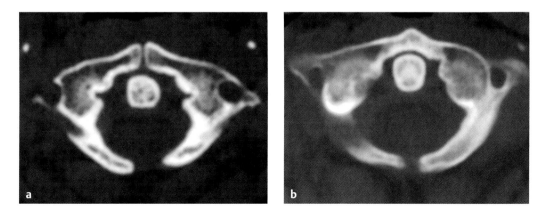

Fig. 1.97 Atlas anomalies. **(a)** Axial CT of a 13-year-old female shows clefts involving both the posterior and anterior arches of C1. **(b)** Axial CT of a 30-year-old woman shows a posterior cleft of C1.

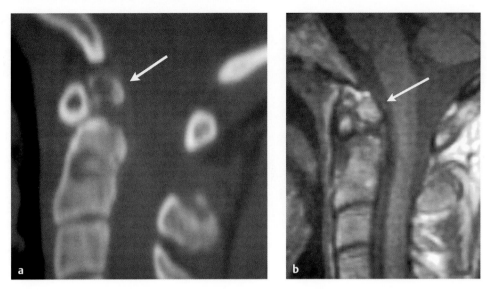

Fig. 1.98 A 38-year-old woman with an os odontoideum. **(a)** Sagittal CT and **(b)** and sagittal T1-weighted imaging show a corticated bony structure (*arrows*) positioned below the basion and superior to the C2 body at the normally expected site of the dens. Os odontoideum is often associated with enlargement of the anterior arch of C1 (which may sometimes be larger than the adjacent os odontoideum).

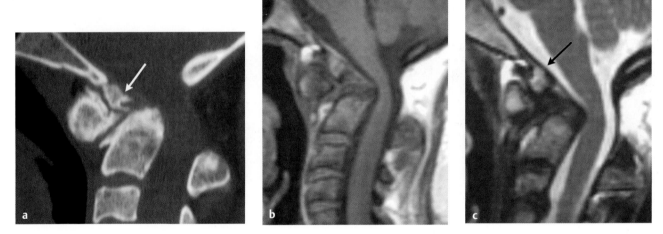

Fig. 1.99 A 16-year-old male with an os odontoideum. **(a)** Sagittal CT, **(b)** sagittal T1-weighted imaging, and **(c)** T2-weighted imaging show a corticated bony structure (*arrow* in **a** and **c**) positioned below the basion and superior to the C2 body. Enlargement of the anterior arch of C1 is seen that is larger than the adjacent os odontoideum. An abnormally decreased clivis canal angle is present.

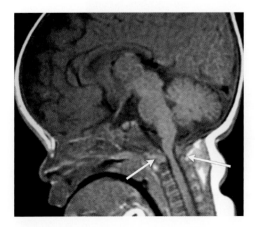

Fig. 1.100 An 8-week-old female with achondroplasia. Sagittal T1-weighted imaging shows a severely narrowed foramen magnum (*arrows*) indenting the upper cervical spinal cord. The posterior cranial fossa is shallow.

Table 1.5 *(cont.)* Abnormalities involving the craniovertebral junction

Lesions	Imaging Findings	Comments
Down syndrome (Trisomy 21) **(Fig. 1.101)**	Separation between the anterior arch of C1 and the anterior margin of the upper dens by more than 5 mm and narrowing of the spinal canal, ± indentation on the spinal cord.	Most common genetic disorder, with an incidence of 1 in 733 live births. Can be associated with atlanto-occipital instability (up to 60%) or atlanto-axial instability (up to 30%). Can result from ligamentous laxity, ± associated persistent synchondroses, posterior C1 rachischisis, and os odontoideum (6%).
Ehlers-Danlos syndrome	Separation between the anterior arch of C1 and the anterior margin of the upper dens by more than 5 mm and narrowing of the spinal canal, ± indentation on the spinal cord.	Mutation involving genes involved with the formation or processing of collagen, which results in ligamentous laxity at the atlanto-axial joint.

(continued on page 72)

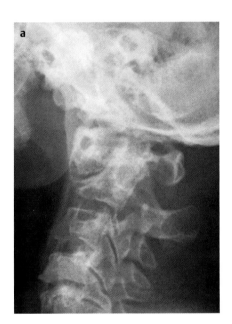 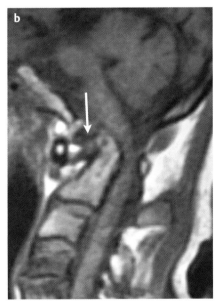

Fig. 1.101 A 46-year-old woman with Down syndrome. **(a)** Lateral radiograph and **(b)** sagittal T1-weighted imaging show separation *(arrow)* between the anterior arch of C1 and the anterior margin of the upper dens by more than 5 mm, resulting in narrowing of the spinal canal and ventral indentation on the spinal cord.

Table 1.5 *(cont.)* Abnormalities involving the craniovertebral junction

Lesions	Imaging Findings	Comments
Mucopolysaccharidosis (MPS) **(Fig. 1.102)**	*MRI:* Hypoplastic/dysplastic dens (deceased height, broad base with flattened tip) and soft tissue thickening adjacent to the dens at the C1–C2 level that has low-intermediate signal on T1- and T2-weighted imaging. Most commonly occurs with Morquio syndrome (type IV) and Hurler syndrome (type I). Can result in spinal canal stenosis. Findings include wedge-shaped vertebral bodies with anterior beaks (central, Morquio; anteroinferiorly, Hurler/Hunter), decreased heights of vertebral bodies, widened discs, spinal canal stenosis, thick clavicles, paddle-shaped ribs, widened symphysis pubis, flared iliac bones, widening of the femoral necks, ± absent femoral heads, coxa valga, shortened metacarpal bones, Madelung's deformity, and diaphyseal widening of long bones. Marrow MRI signal may be within normal limits or slightly decreased on T1-weighted imaging and/or slightly increased on T2-weighted imaging.	Inherited disorders of glycosaminoglycan (GAG) catabolism caused by defects in specific lysosomal enzymes. MPS I (Hurler, Scheie syndromes) is a deficiency of α-L-iduronidase; MPS II (Hunter syndrome) is an X-linked deficiency of iduronate-2-sulfatase; MPS III (Sanfilippo A, B, C, D syndrome) is an autosomal recessive deficiency of enzymes that break down heparin sulfate; MPS IV (Morquio syndrome), is an autosomal recessive deficiency of *N*-acetylgalactosamine-6-sulfatase; MPS VI (Maroteaux-Lamy syndrome) is an autosomal deficiency of *N*-acetylgalatosamine-4-sulfatase; MPS VII (Sly syndrome) is an autosomal recessive deficiency of β-glucuronidase; and MPS IX is a hyaluronidase deficiency. Disorders are characterized by accumulation of GAGs in lysosomes, extracellular matrix, joint fluid, and connective tissue, resulting in axonal loss and demyelination. Treatments include enzyme replacement and bone marrow transplantation.
Osteogenesis imperfecta (OI) **(Fig. 1.103)**	Diffuse osteopenia, decreased ossification of skull base with microfractures, infolding of the occipital condyles, elevation of the posterior cranial fossa and posterior cranial fossa, and upward migration of the dens into the foramen magnum, resulting in basilar impression (secondary basilar invagination).	Also known as brittle bone disease, OI has four to seven types. OI is a hereditary disorder with abnormal type I fibrillar collagen production and osteoporosis resulting from mutations involving the *COL1A1* gene on chromosome 17q21.31-q22.05 and the *COL1A2* gene on chromosome 7q22.1. OI results in fragile bone prone to repetitive microfractures and remodeling. Type IV is most commonly associated with abnormalities at the craniovertebral junction.
Neurenteric cyst **(Fig. 1.104)**	*MRI:* Well-circumscribed, spheroid, intradural, extra-axial lesions, with low, intermediate, or high signal on T1- and T2-weighted imaging and FLAIR and usually no gadolinium contrast enhancement. *CT:* Circumscribed, intradural, extra-axial structures with low-intermediate attenuation. Usually no contrast enhancement.	Neurenteric cysts are malformations in which there is a persistent communication between the ventrally located endoderm and the dorsally located ectoderm secondary to developmental failure of separation of the notochord and foregut. Obliteration of portions of a dorsal enteric sinus can result in cysts lined by endothelium, fibrous cords, or sinuses. Observed in patients < 40 years old. Location: thoracic > cervical > posterior cranial fossa > craniovertebral junction > lumbar. Usually midline in position and often ventral to the spinal cord or brainstem. Associated with anomalies of the adjacent vertebrae and clivus.
Ecchordosis physaliphora	*MRI:* Circumscribed lesion ranging in size from 1 to 3 cm, with low signal on T1-weighted imaging, intermediate signal on FLAIR, and high signal on T2-weighted imaging. Typically shows no gadolinium contrast enhancement. *CT:* Lesions typically have low attenuation, ± remodeling/erosion of adjacent bone, ± small calcified bone stalk.	Congenital benign hamartoma composed of gelatinous tissue with physaliphorous cell nests derived from ectopic vestigial notochord. Incidence at autopsy ranges from 0.5 to 5%. Usually located intradurally, dorsal to the clivus and dorsum sella within the prepontine cistern, and rarely dorsal to the upper cervical spine or sacrum. Rarely occurs as an extradural lesion. Derived from an ectopic notochordal remnant or from extension of extradural notochord at the dorsal wall of the clivus through the adjacent dura into the subarachnoid space. Typically is asymptomatic and is observed as an incidental finding in patients between the ages of 20 and 60 years.

(continued on page 74)

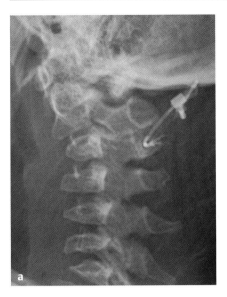
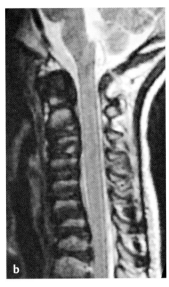

Fig. 1.102 A 9-year-old male with Morquio type of mucopolysaccharidosis. **(a)** Lateral radiograph shows wedge-shaped vertebral bodies with anterior beaks. **(b)** Sagittal T2-weighted imaging shows soft tissue thickening adjacent to the dens at the C1–C2 level that has low-intermediate signal.

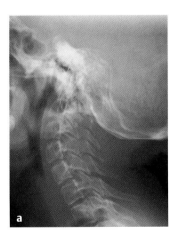
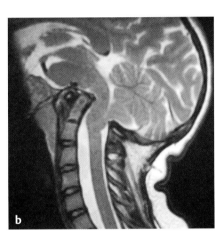

Fig. 1.103 A 15-year-old female with osteogenesis imperfecta. **(a)** Lateral radiograph shows diffuse osteopenia and basilar invagination. **(b)** Sagittal T2-weighted imaging shows upward intracranial extension of the dens, which indents the pontomedullary junction.

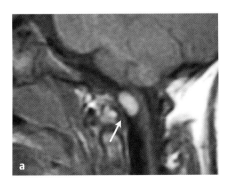
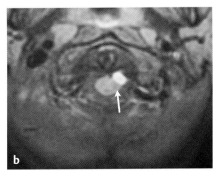
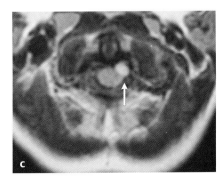

Fig. 1.104 An intradural neurenteric cyst is seen anteriorly within the thecal sac on the left at the C1–C2 level. The cyst has high signal on **(a)** sagittal T1-weighted imaging (*arrow*) and **(b)** fat-suppressed T1-weighted imaging (*arrow*), and high signal on **(c)** axial FLAIR (*arrow*). The high signal of the lesion on fat-suppressed T1-weighted imaging is related to elevated protein content within the fluid of the cystic lesion.

Table 1.5 *(cont.)* Abnormalities involving the craniovertebral junction

Lesions	Imaging Findings	Comments
Osteomalacia		
Renal osteodystrophy/ secondary hyperparathyroidism (See **Fig. 1.83**)	*CT:* Trabecular bone resorption with a salt-and-pepper appearance from mixed osteolysis and osteosclerosis, osteiitis fibrosa cystica, cortical thinning, coarsened trabecular pattern, and osteolytic lesions/brown tumors. Another pattern is ground-glass appearance with indistinct corticomedullary borders. *MRI:* Zones of low signal on T1- and T2-weighted imaging corresponding to regions of bone sclerosis. Circumscribed zones with high signal on T2-weighted imaging can be due to osteolytic lesions or brown tumors.	Secondary hyperparathyroidism related to renal failure/end-stage kidney disease is more common than primary hyperparathyroidism. Osteoblastic and osteoclastic changes occur in bone as a result of secondary hyperparathyroidism (hyperplasia of parathyroid glands secondary to hypocalcemia in end-stage renal disease related to abnormal vitamin D metabolism) and primary hyperparathyroidism (hypersecretion of PTH from parathyroid adenoma or hyperplasia). Can result in pathologic fractures due to osteomalacia. Unlike secondary hyperparathyroidism, primary hyperparathyroidism infrequently has diffuse or patchy bony sclerosis. Brown tumors are more common in primary than in secondary hyperparathyroidism.
Paget disease (**Fig. 1.105**)	Expansile sclerotic/lytic process involving the skull. *CT:* Lesions often have mixed intermediate and high attenuation. Irregular/indistinct borders between marrow and inner margins of the outer and inner tables of the skull. *MRI:* MRI features vary based on the phases of the disease. Most cases involving the skull are the late or inactive phases. Findings include osseous expansion and cortical thickening with low signal on T1- and T2-weighted imaging. The inner margins of the thickened cortex can be irregular and indistinct. Zones of low signal on T1- and T2-weighted imaging can be seen in the diploic marrow secondary to thickened bony trabeculae. Marrow in late or inactive phases of Paget disease can have signal similar to normal marrow, contain focal areas of fat signal, have low signal on T1- and T2-weighted imaging secondary to regions of sclerosis, have areas of high signal on fat-suppressed T2-weighted imaging caused by edema or persistent fibrovascular tissue, or have various combinations of the aforementioned.	Paget disease is a chronic skeletal disease in which there is disordered bone resorption and woven bone formation, resulting in osseous deformity. A paramyxovirus may be the etiologic agent. Paget disease is polyostotic in up to 66% of patients. Paget disease is associated with a risk of < 1% for developing secondary sarcomatous changes. Occurs in 2.5 to 5% of Caucasians more than 55 years old, and in 10% of those more than 85 years old. Can result in narrowing of neuroforamina, with cranial nerve compression and basilar impression, ± compression of brainstem.
Fibrous dysplasia (**Fig. 1.106**)	*CT:* Lesions involving the skull are often associated with bone expansion. Lesions have variable density and attenuation on radiographs and CT, respectively, depending on the degree of mineralization and number of the bony spicules in the lesions. Attenuation coefficients can range from 70 to 400 Hounsfield units. Lesions can have a ground-glass radiographic appearance secondary to the mineralized spicules of immature woven bone in fibrous dysplasia. Sclerotic borders of varying thickness can be seen surrounding parts or all of the lesions. *MRI:* Features depend on the proportions of bony spicules, collagen, fibroblastic spindle cells, and hemorrhagic and/or cystic changes. Lesions are usually well circumscribed and have low or low-intermediate signal on T1-weighted imaging. On T2-weighted imaging, lesions have variable mixtures of low, intermediate, and/or high signal, often surrounded by a low-signal rim of variable thickness. Internal septations and cystic changes are seen in a minority of lesions. Bone expansion is commonly seen. All or portions of the lesions can show gadolinium contrast enhancement in a heterogeneous, diffuse, or peripheral pattern.	Benign medullary fibro-osseous lesion of bone, most often sporadic. Fibrous dysplasia involving a single site is referred to as monostotic (80–85%) and that involving multiple locations is known as polyostotic fibrous dysplasia. Results from developmental failure in the normal process of remodeling primitive bone to mature lamellar bone, with resultant zone or zones of immature trabeculae within dysplastic fibrous tissue. The lesions do not mineralize normally and can result in cranial neuropathies caused by neuroforaminal narrowing, facial deformities, sinonasal drainage disorders, and sinusitis. Age at presentation is < 1 year to 76 years; 75% of cases occur before the age of 30 years. Median age for monostotic fibrous dysplasia = 21 years; mean and median ages for polyostotic fibrous dysplasia are between 8 and 17 years. Most cases are diagnosed in patients between the ages of 3 and 20 years.

(continued on page 76)

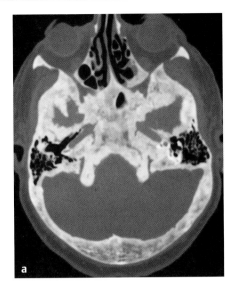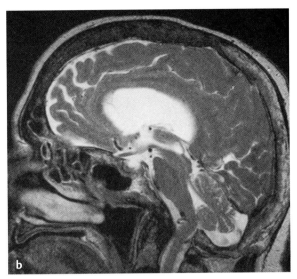

Fig. 1.105 An 84-year-old woman with Paget disease involving the skull. **(a)** Axial CT shows diffuse expansion of bone containing mixed intermediate and high attenuation, with irregular/indistinct borders between marrow and inner margins of the outer and inner tables of the skull. **(b)** Sagittal T2-weighted imaging shows osseous expansion, cortical thickening with low signal, and marrow with heterogeneous low and intermediate signal. There is a flattening deformity of the skull base (platybasia) secondary to the effects of gravity on the softened pagetoid bone.

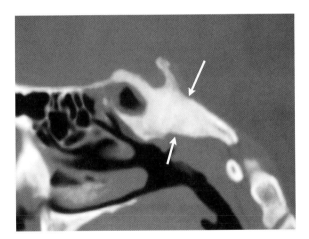

Fig. 1.106 Sagittal CT shows diffuse sclerosis of the clivus caused by fibrous dysplasia (*arrows*).

Table 1.5 *(cont.)*   Abnormalities involving the craniovertebral junction

Lesions	Imaging Findings	Comments
Hematopoietic disorders (See **Fig. 1.85** and **Fig. 1.86**)	Enlargement of the diploic space, with red marrow hyperplasia and thinning of the inner and outer tables. Involved marrow has slightly to moderately decreased signal relative to fat on T1-weighted imaging and T2-weighted imaging, isointense to slightly hyperintense signal relative to muscle and increased signal relative to fat on fat-suppressed T2-weighted imaging.	Thickening of diploic space related to erythroid hyperplasia caused by inherited anemias, such as sickle-cell disease, thalassemia major, and hereditary spherocytosis. Sickle cell disease is the most common hemoglobinopathy, in which abnormal hemoglobin S is combined with itself, or other hemoglobin types such as C, D, E, or thalassemia. Hemoglobin SS, SC, and S-thalassemia have the most sickling of erythrocytes. In addition to marrow hyperplasia seen in sickle-cell disease, bone infarcts and extramedullary hematopoeisis can also occur. Beta-thalassemia is a disorder in which there is deficient synthesis of β chains of hemoglobin, resulting in excess α chains in erythrocytes, causing dysfunctional hematopoiesis and hemolysis. The decrease in β chains can be severe in the major type (homozygous), moderate in the intermediate type (heterozygous), or mild in the minor type (heterozygous).
Traumatic Lesions		
Fracture of skull base (**Fig. 1.107**)	*CT:* Fracture line, ± displaced fragments, epidural or subdural hematoma. *MRI:* Abnormal low signal on T1-weighted imaging and high signal on T2-weighted imaging in marrow at the site of fracture, ± abnormal high signal on T2-weighted imaging involving the brainstem and/or spinal cord, ± subgaleal hematoma, ± epidural hematoma, ± subdural hematoma, ± subarachnoid hemorrhage.	Traumatic fractures of the skull (calvarium and/or skull base), occipital condyles, C1, and/or C2 can be associated with traumatic injury of brainstem and upper spinal cord, epidural hematoma, subdural hematoma, subarachnoid hemorrhage, and CSF leakage (rhinorrhea, otorrhea).
Atlanto-occipital dislocation (**Fig. 1.108**)	*CT:* Abnormal increased distance from the basion of the clivus to the tip of the odontoid, as measured by the basion–axial interval (BAI) and/or basion–dental interval (BDI). The BAI is the distance from the basion to a line drawn along the dorsal surface of the C2 body (normal range of BAI for adults is –4 to 12 mm, for children, 0–12 mm). The BDI is used only in patients more than 13 years old and is the distance from the basion to the tip of the dens (normal range is 2–12 mm). *MRI:* Disruption/tears of alar ligaments and tectorial membrane with associated abnormal high T2 signal and capsular edema.	Unstable traumatic injury with disruption of the alar ligaments and tectorial membrane between the occiput and C1, with or without injury to the brainstem and/or upper spinal cord. Most commonly occurs in children.
Jefferson fracture (C1) (**Fig. 1.109**)	*CT:* Rough-edged fractures of the arch of C1, often with multiple fracture sites.	Compression burst fracture of the arch of C1, often stable, but can be unstable when there is disruption of transverse or posterior ligament or comminution of anterior arch. Often associated with fractures of other cervical vertebrae.
Hangman's fracture (C2) (**Fig. 1.110**)	Disrupted ring of C2 caused by bilateral pedicle fractures separating the C2 body from the posterior arch of C2. Skull, C1, and C2 body are displaced anterior with respect to C3.	Unstable injury due to traumatic bilateral pedicle fractures caused by hyperextension and distraction mechanisms, with separation of the C2 body from the posterior arch of C2. Fractures can extend into the C2 body and/or through the foramen transversarium, with injury/occlusion of the vertebral artery. Often associated with spinal cord injury.

(continued on page 78)

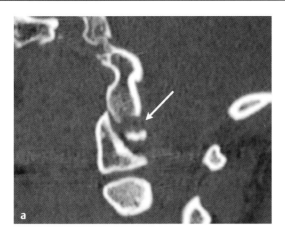
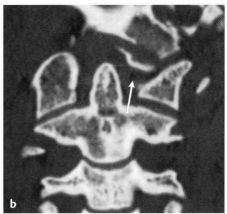

Fig. 1.107 **(a)** Sagittal and **(b)** coronal CT images show a displaced fracture (*arrows*) of the left occipital condyle in a 20-year-old woman.

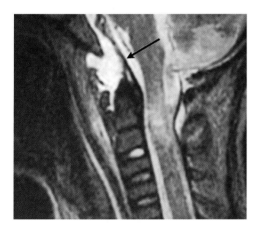

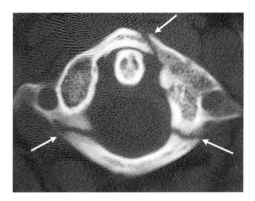

Fig. 1.109 Axial CT of a 45-year-old woman with a Jefferson fracture with three fracture sites (*arrows*) involving C1.

Fig. 1.108 A 5-year-old male with atlanto-occipital dislocation. Sagittal T2-weighted imaging shows disruption of the alar ligaments and tectorial membrane (*arrow*), with adjacent abnormal high-signal fluid and abnormal high signal in the spinal cord and cerebellum representing severe injuries.

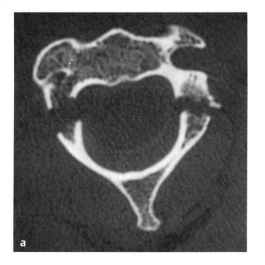
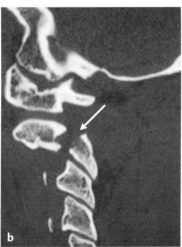

Fig. 1.110 **(a)** Axial and **(b)** sagittal CT show a hangman's fracture with bilateral pedicle fractures separating the C2 body from the posterior arch of C2 (*arrow*).

Table 1.5 *(cont.)* Abnormalities involving the craniovertebral junction

Lesions	Imaging Findings	Comments
Odontoid fracture (C2) (**Fig. 1.111** and **Fig. 1.112**)	*Type I:* Fracture at the upper portion of the dens above the transverse ligament (unstable) due to avulsion at the alar ligament. *Type II:* Transverse fracture through the lower portion of the dens (may be unstable). *Type III:* Oblique fracture involving the dens and body of C2 (usually stable).	Traumatic fracture involving the upper, mid, and/or lower portions of the dens.
Inflammation		
Osteomyelitis/epidural abscess (**Fig. 1.113**)	*CT:* Zones of abnormal decreased attenuation, focal sites of bone destruction, ± complications, including subgaleal empyema, epidural empyema, subdural empyema, meningitis, cerebritis, intra-axial abscess, and venous sinus thrombosis. *MRI:* Zones with low-intermediate signal on T1-weighted imaging and high signal on T2-weighted imaging and fat-suppressed T2-weighted imaging, ± high signal on diffusion-weighted imaging and low signal on ADC. Usually there is heterogeneous gadolinium (Gd) contrast enhancement, ± adjacent intracranial dural and/or leptomeningeal Gd contrast enhancement, ± abnormal high T2 signal and contrast enhancement of brain tissue/abscess formation.	Osteomyelitis (bone infection) of the skull can result from surgery, trauma, hematogenous dissemination from another source of infection, or direct extension of infection from an adjacent site, such as the paranasal sinuses, nasal cavity, petrous apex air cells, and/or mastoid air cells and middle ear.
Langerhans' cell histiocytosis (**Fig. 1.114**)	Single or multiple circumscribed soft tissue lesions in the marrow of the skull associated with focal bony destruction/erosion and with extension extra- or intracranially or both. *CT:* Lesions usually have low-intermediate attenuation, + contrast enhancement, ± enhancement of the adjacent dura. *MRI:* Lesions typically have low-intermediate signal on T1-weighted imaging and heterogeneous slightly high to high signal on T2-weighted imaging (T2WI) and fat-suppressed (FS) T2WI. Poorly defined zones of high signal on T2WI and FS T2WI are usually seen in the marrow and soft tissues peripheral to the lesions secondary to inflammatory changes. Lesions typically show prominent gadolinium contrast enhancement in marrow and extraosseous soft tissue portions.	Disorder of reticuloendothelial system in which bone marrow-derived dendritic Langerhans' cells infiltrate various organs as focal lesions or in diffuse patterns. Langerhans' cells have eccentrically located ovoid or convoluted nuclei within pale to eosinophilic cytoplasm. Lesions often consist of Langerhans' cells, macrophages, plasma cells, and eosinophils. Lesions are immunoreactive to S-100, CD1a, CD-207, HLA-DR, and β$_2$-microglobulin. Prevalence of 2 per 100,000 children < 15 years old; only a third of lesions occur in adults. Localized lesions (eosinophilic granuloma) can be single or multiple in the skull, usually at the skull base. Single lesions are commonly seen in males more than in females, and in patients < 20 years old. Proliferation of histiocytes in medullary bone results in localized destruction of cortical bone with extension into adjacent soft tissues. Multiple lesions are associated with Letterer-Siwe disease (lymphadenopathy hepatosplenomegaly), in children < 2 years old, and Hand-Schüller-Christian disease (lymphadenopathy, exophthalmos, diabetes insipidus) in children 5–10 years old.

(continued on page 80)

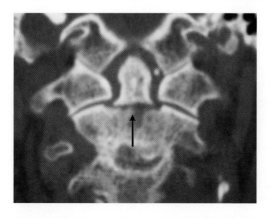

Fig. 1.111 Type II odontoid fracture. Coronal CT shows a transverse fracture through the lower portion of the dens (*arrow*).

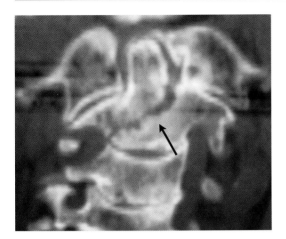

Fig. 1.112 Type III odontoid fracture. Coronal CT shows an oblique fracture (*arrow*) involving the dens and body of C2.

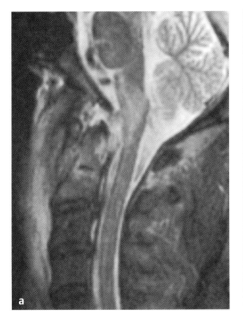

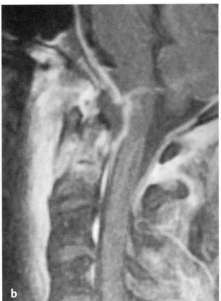

Fig. 1.113 A 59-year-old man with pyogenic osteomyelitis and epidural abscess at the craniovertebral junction. **(a)** Sagittal fat-suppressed T2-weighted imaging shows abnormal high signal in the marrow of the C1 and C2 vertebrae and lower clivus, with **(b)** corresponding abnormal gadolinium contrast enhancement on fat-suppressed T1-weighted imaging. A peripherally enhancing fluid collection (epidural abscess) is seen indenting the ventral margin of the spinal cord at the C1–C2 level. Abnormal gadolinium contrast enhancement is also seen in the prevertebral soft tissues, representing a phlegmon.

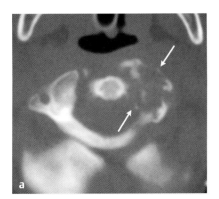

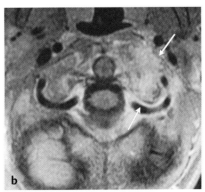

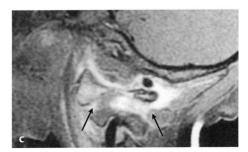

Fig. 1.114 A 23-year-old man with an eosinophilic granuloma involving the left occipital condyle. **(a)** Axial CT shows an osteolytic lesion (*arrows*). **(b)** Axial and **(c)** sagittal fat-suppressed T1-weighted MRI images show the lesion (*arrows*) to have prominent intraosseous gadolinium contrast enhancement, with ill-defined margins that extend into, and involve the adjacent soft tissues.

Table 1.5 *(cont.)* Abnormalities involving the craniovertebral junction

Lesions	Imaging Findings	Comments
Rheumatoid arthritis (**Fig. 1.115** and **Fig. 1.116**)	*MRI:* Hypertrophied synovium (pannus) can be diffuse, nodular, and/or villous, and usually has low to intermediate or intermediate signal on T1-weighted imaging. On T2-weighted imaging, pannus can have low to intermediate, intermediate, and/or slightly high to high signal. Signal heterogeneity of hypertrophied synovium on T2-weighted imaging can result from variable amounts of fibrin, hemosiderin, and fibrosis. Chronic fibrotic nonvascular synovium usually has low signal on T1- and T2-weighted imaging. Hypertrophied synovium can show prominent homogeneous or variable heterogeneous gadolinium contrast enhancement. Erosion of the dens and destruction of the transverse ligament can occur, as well as basilar impression. *CT:* Zones of erosion and/or destruction of the dens and atlas, ± basilar impression/invagination.	Chronic multisystem disease of unknown etiology with persistent inflammatory synovitis involving peripheral joints in a symmetric distribution. Can result in progressive destruction of cartilage and bone, leading to joint dysfunction. Affects ~ 1% of the world's population. Eighty percent of adult patients present between the ages of 35 and 50 years. Patients with juvenile idiopathic arthritis range in age from 5 to 16 years (mean = 10.2 years). Most common type of inflammatory synovitis causing destructive/erosive changes of cartilage, ligaments, and bone. cervical spine involvement two-thirds of patients, juvenile and adult types.
Calcium pyrophosphate dihydrate (CPPD) deposition (**Fig. 1.117**)	*CT:* Thickened synovium at C1–C2 containing multiple calcifications. *MRI:* At the C1–odontoid articulation, hypertophy of synovium can be seen, with low-intermediate signal on T1- and T2-weighted imaging. Small zones of low signal may correspond to calcifications seen with CT. Minimal or no gadolinium contrast enhancement.	CPPD disease is a common disorder, usually in older adults, in which there is deposition of CPPD crystals, resulting in calcifications of hyaline and fibrocartilage, and is associated with cartilage degeneration, subchondral cysts, and osteophyte formation. Symptomatic CPPD disease is referred to as pseudogout because of overlapping clinical features with gout. Usually occurs in the knee, hip, shoulder, elbow, and wrist, and occasionally at the odontoid–C1 articulation.
Malignant Neoplasms		
Metastatic disease (**Fig. 1.118**)	Single or multiple well-circumscribed or poorly defined lesions involving the skull. *CT:* Lesions are usually radiolucent and may also be sclerotic, ± bone destruction with extraosseous tumor extension, usually + contrast enhancement, ± compression of neural tissue or vessels. *MRI:* Single or multiple well-circumscribed or poorly defined lesions involving the skull, with low-intermediate signal on T1-weighted imaging, intermediate-high signal on T2-weighted imaging, and usually gadolinium contrast enhancement, ± bone destruction, ± compression of neural tissue or vessels.	Metastatic lesions represent proliferating neoplastic cells that are located in sites or organs separated or distant from their origins. Metastatic carcinoma is the most frequent malignant tumor involving bone. In adults, metastatic lesions to bone occur most frequently from carcinomas of the lung, breast, prostate, kidney, and thyroid, as well as from sarcomas. Primary malignancies of the lung, breast, and prostate account for 80% of bone metastases. Metastatic tumor may cause variable destructive or infiltrative changes in single or multiple sites.

(continued on page 82)

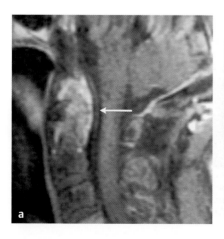 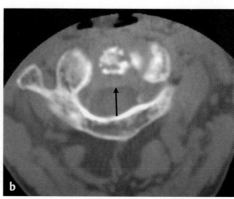

Fig. 1.115 A 72-year-old woman with rheumatoid arthritis. **(a)** Sagittal fat-suppressed T1-weighted imaging shows gadolinium-enhancing pannus (*arrow*) at the C1-dens joint eroding the cortical margins and extending into the marrow. **(b)** Axial CT shows erosive changes involving the dens (*arrow*) caused by the pannus.

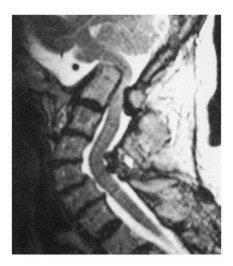

Fig. 1.116   A 60-year-old woman with rheumatoid arthritis that eroded the transverse ligament, resulting in upward intracranial displacement of the dens that compresses the ventral margin of the medulla on sagittal T2-weighted imaging.

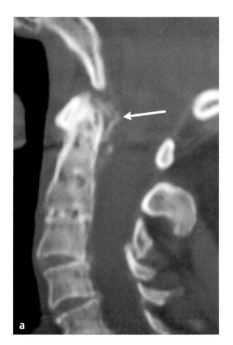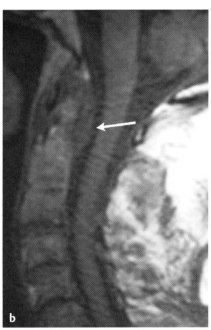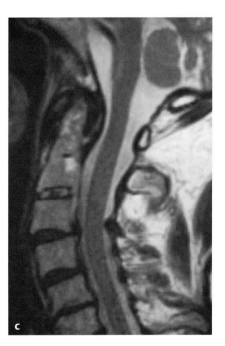

Fig. 1.117   An 80-year-old man with calcium pyrophosphate dihydrate (CPPD) deposition at the C1–odontoid articulation. **(a)** Sagittal CT shows thickened synovium containing multiple calcifications (*arrow*). **(b)** The hypertrophied synovium (*arrow*) has intermediate signal on sagittal T1-weighted imaging and **(c)** low-intermediate signal on sagittal T2-weighted imaging.

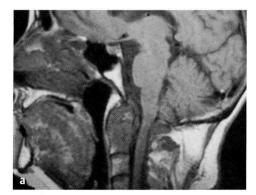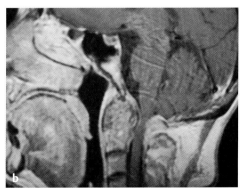

Fig. 1.118 A 76-year-old woman with metastatic breast carcinoma involving the marrow of the dens that has intermediate signal on **(a)** sagittal T1-weighted imaging and shows gadolinium contrast enhancement on **(b)** sagittal T1-weighted imaging. The tumor destroys cortical bone and extends into the prevertebral and epidural spaces causing spinal canal compression.

Table 1.5 (*cont.*)   Abnormalities involving the craniovertebral junction

Lesions	Imaging Findings	Comments
Myeloma	Plasmacytoma (solitary myeloma) or multiple myeloma are well-circumscribed or poorly defined lesions involving the skull and dura. *CT:* Lesions have low-intermediate attenuation, usually + contrast enhancement, + bone destruction. *MRI:* Well-circumscribed or poorly defined lesions involving the skull and dura, with low-intermediate signal on T1-weighted imaging, intermediate-high signal on T2-weighted imaging, and usually gadolinium contrast enhancement, + bone destruction.	Multiple myeloma are malignant tumors comprised of proliferating antibody-secreting plasma cells derived from single clones. Multiple myeloma primarily involves bone marrow. A solitary myeloma or plasmacytoma is an infrequent variant in which a neoplastic mass of plasma cells occurs at a single site of bone or soft tissues. In the United States, 14,600 new cases occur each year. Multiple myeloma is the most common primary neoplasm of bone in adults. Median age at presentation = 60 years. Most patients are more than 40 years old. Tumors occur in the vertebrae > ribs > femur > iliac bone > humerus > craniofacial bones > sacrum > clavicle > sternum > pubic bone > tibia.
Chordoma (**Fig. 1.119**)	Well-circumscribed lobulated lesions along the dorsal surface of the clivus, vertebral bodies, or sacrum, + localized bone destruction. *CT:* Lesions have low-intermediate attenuation, ± calcifications from destroyed bone carried away by tumor, + contrast enhancement. *MRI:* Lesions have low-intermediate signal on T1-weighted imaging, high signal on T2-weighted imaging, + gadolinium contrast enhancement (usually heterogeneous). Chordomas are locally invasive and associated with bone erosion/destruction, encasement of vessels (usually without luminal narrowing) and nerves. Skull base-clivus is a common location, usually in the midline for conventional chordomas, which account for 80% of skull base chordomas. Chondroid chordomas tend to be located off midline near skull base synchondroses..	Chordomas are rare, locally aggressive, slow-growing, low to intermediate grade malignant tumors derived from ectopic notochordal remnants along the axial skeleton. Chondroid chondromas (5–15% of all chordomas) have both chordomatous and chondromatous differentiation. Chordomas that contain sarcomatous components are referred to as dedifferentiated chordomas or sarcomatoid chordoma (5% of all chordomas). Chordomas account for 2–4% of primary malignant bone tumors, 1–3% of all primary bone tumors, and < 1% of intracranial tumors. The annual incidence has been reported to be 0.18 to 0.3 per million. Dedifferentiated chordomas or sarcomatoid chordomas account for less than 5% of all chordomas. For cranial chordomas, patients' mean age= 37 to 40 years.
Chondrosarcoma	Lobulated lesions with bone destruction at synchondroses. *CT:* Lesions have low-intermediate attenuation associated with localized bone destruction, ± chondroid matrix calcifications, + contrast enhancement. *MRI:* Lesions have low-intermediate signal on T1-weighted imaging, high signal on T2-weighted imaging, ± matrix mineralization-low signal on T2-weighted images, + gadolinium contrast enhancement (usually heterogeneous), locally-invasive associated with bone erosion/destruction, encasement of vessels and nerves, skull base petro-occipital synchondrosis common location, usually off midline.	Chondrosarcomas are malignant tumors containing cartilage formed within sarcomatous stroma. Chondrosarcomas can contain areas of calcification/mineralization, myxoid material, and/or ossification. Chondrosarcomas rarely arise within synovium. Chondrosarcomas represent 12–21% of malignant bone lesions, 21–26% of primary sarcomas of bone, 9–14% of all bone tumors, 6% of skull base tumors, and 0.15% of all intracranial tumors.
Squamous cell carcinoma (See **Fig. 1.44**)	*MRI:* Destructive lesions in the nasal cavity, paranasal sinuses, and nasopharynx, ± intracranial extension via bone destruction or perineural spread. Intermediate signal on T1-weighted imaging, intermediate-slightly high signal on T2-weighted imaging, and mild gadolinium contrast enhancement. Can be large lesions (± necrosis and/or hemorrhage). *CT:* Tumors have intermediate attenuation and mild contrast enhancement. Can be large lesions (± necrosis and/or hemorrhage).	Malignant epithelial tumors originating from the mucosal epithelium of the paranasal sinuses (maxillary sinus, 60%; ethmoid sinus, 14%; sphenoid and frontal sinuses, 1%) and nasal cavity (25%). Includes both keratinizing and nonkeratinizing types. Accounts for 3% of malignant tumors of the head and neck. Occurs in adults, usually > 55 years old, and in males more than in females. Associated with occupational or other exposure to tobacco smoke, nickel, chlorophenols, chromium, mustard gas, radium, and material in the manufacture of wood products.

Lesions	Imaging Findings	Comments
Nasopharyngeal carcinoma (See **Fig. 1.45**)	*CT:* Tumors have intermediate attenuation and mild contrast enhancement. Can be large lesions (± necrosis and/or hemorrhage). *MRI:* Invasive lesions in the nasopharynx (lateral wall/fossa of Rosenmüller, and posterior upper wall), ± intracranial extension via bone destruction or perineural spread. Lesions have intermediate signal on T1-weighted imaging, intermediate-slightly high signal on T2-weighted imaging, and often gadolinium contrast enhancement. Can be large lesions (± necrosis and/or hemorrhage).	Carcinomas arising from the nasopharyngeal mucosa with varying degrees of squamous differentiation. Subtypes include squamous cell carcinoma, nonkeratinizing carcinoma (differentiated and undifferentiated), and basaloid squamous cell carcinoma. Occur at higher frequency in Southern Asia and Africa than in Europe and the Americas. Peak ages: 40–60 years. Nasopharyngeal carcinoma occurs two to three times more frequently in men than in women. Associated with Epstein-Barr virus, diets containing nitrosamines, and chronic exposure to tobacco smoke, formaldehyde, chemical fumes, and dust.
Adenoid cystic carcinoma (See **Fig. 1.236**)	*MRI:* Destructive lesions with intracranial extension via bone destruction or perineural spread, with intermediate signal on T1-weighted imaging, intermediate-high signal on T2-weighted imaging, and variable mild, moderate, or prominent gadolinium contrast enhancement. *CT:* Tumors have intermediate attenuation and variable mild, moderate, or prominent contrast enhancement.	Basaloid tumor comprised of neoplastic epithelial and myoepithelial cells. Morphologic tumor patterns include tubular, cribriform, and solid. Accounts for 10% of epithelial salivary neoplasms. Most commonly involves the parotid, submandibular, and minor salivary glands (palate, tongue, buccal mucosa, and floor of the mouth, as well as other locations). Perineural tumor spread is common, ± facial nerve paralysis. Usually occurs in adults > 30 years old. Solid type has the worst prognosis. Up to 90% of patients die within 10–15 years of diagnosis.
Invasive pituitary tumor (See **Fig. 1.43**)	*MRI:* Tumors often have intermediate signal on T1- and T2-weighted imaging, often similar to gray matter, ± necrosis, ± cyst, ± hemorrhage, and usually show prominent gadolinium contrast enhancement. Tumor can extend into the suprasellar cistern with waist at diaphragma sella, ± extension into cavernous sinus, and occasionally invades skull base. *CT:* Tumors often have intermediate attenuation, ± necrosis, ± cyst, ± hemorrhage, and usually show contrast enhancement. Tumor can extend into the suprasellar cistern with waist at diaphragma sella, ± extension into cavernous sinus, and can invade the skull base.	Histologically benign pituitary macroadenomas or pituitary carcinomas can occasionally have an invasive growth pattern, with extension into the sphenoid bone, clivus, ethmoid sinus, orbits, and/or interpeduncular cistern.

(continued on page 84)

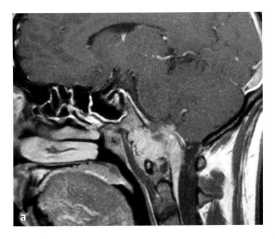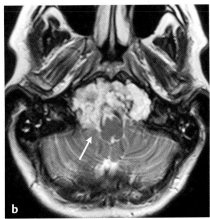

Fig. 1.119   A 44-year-old woman with a chordoma destroying the lower clivus that shows gadolinium contrast enhancement on **(a)** sagittal T1-weighted imaging and has heterogeneous mostly high signal on **(b)** axial T2-weighted imaging (*arrow*). The tumor extends into the ventral portion of the craniovertebral junction and upper ventral portion of the spinal canal.

Table 1.5 *(cont.)*   Abnormalities involving the craniovertebral junction

Lesions	Imaging Findings	Comments
Benign Neoplasms		
Meningioma (**Fig. 1.120**)	Extra-axial dura-based lesions, well circumscribed, supra- > infratentorial. Some meningiomas can invade bone or occur predominantly within bone. *MRI:* Tumors often have intermediate signal on T1-weighted imaging and intermediate-slightly high signal on T2-weighted imaging, and typically show prominent gadolinium contrast enhancement, ± calcifications, ± hyperostosis and/or invasion of adjacent skull. Some meningiomas have high signal on diffusion-weighted imaging. *CT:* Tumors have intermediate attenuation, usually prominent contrast enhancement, ± calcifications, ± hyperostosis of adjacent bone.	Benign slow-growing tumors involving cranial and/or spinal dura that are composed of neoplastic meningothelial (arachnoidal or arachnoid cap) cells. Usually solitary and sporadic but can also occur as multiple lesions in patients with neurofibromatosis type 2. Most are benign, although ~ 5% have atypical histologic features. Anaplastic meningiomas are rare and account for less than 3% of meningiomas. Meningiomas account for up to 26% of primary intracranial tumors. Annual incidence is 6 per 100,000. Typically occur in adults (> 40 years old), and in women more than in men. Can result in compression of adjacent brain parenchyma, encasement of arteries, and compression of dural venous sinuses.
Schwannoma	*MRI:* Circumscribed ovoid or spheroid lesions with low-intermediate signal on T1-weighted imaging, high signal on T2-weighted imaging (T2WI) and fat-suppressed T2WI, and usually prominent gadolinium (Gd) contrast enhancement. High signal on T2WI and Gd contrast enhancement can be heterogeneous in large lesions due to cystic degeneration and/or hemorrhage. *CT:* Circumscribed ovoid or spheroid lesions with intermediate attenuation, + contrast enhancement. Large lesions can have cystic degeneration and/or hemorrhage, ± erosion of adjacent bone.	Schwannomas are benign encapsulated tumors that contain differentiated neoplastic Schwann cells. Multiple schwannomas are often associated with neurofibromatosis type 2 (NF2), which is an autosomal dominant disease involving a gene mutation at chromosome 22q12. In addition to schwannomas, patients with NF2 can also have multiple meningiomas and ependymomas. Schwannomas represent 8% of primary intracranial tumors and 29% or primary spinal tumors. The incidence of NF2 is 1/37,000 to 1/50,000 newborns. Age at presentation is 22 to 72 years (mean age = 46 years). Peak incidence is in the fourth to sixth decades. Many patients with NF2 present in the third decade with bilateral vestibular schwannomas.
Neurofibroma (**Fig. 1.121**)	*MRI:* *Solitary neurofibromas:* Circumscribed spheroid, ovoid, or lobulated extra-axial lesions with low-intermediate signal on T1-weighted imaging (T1WI), intermediate-high signal on T2-weighted imaging (T2WI), + prominent gadolinium (Gd) contrast enhancement. High signal on T2WI and Gd contrast enhancement can be heterogeneous in large lesions. *Plexiform neurofibromas* appear as curvilinear and multinodular lesions involving multiple nerve branches and have low to intermediate signal on T1WI and intermediate, slightly high to high signal on T2WI and fat-suppressed T2WI, with or without bands or strands of low signal. Lesions usually show gadolinium contrast enhancement. *CT:* Ovoid or fusiform lesions with low-intermediate attenuation. Lesions can show contrast enhancement. Often erode adjacent bone.	Benign nerve sheath tumors that contain mixtures of Schwann cells, perineural-like cells, and interlacing fascicles of fibroblasts associated with abundant collagen. Unlike schwannomas, neurofibromas lack Antoni A and B regions and cannot be separated pathologically from the underlying nerve. Most frequently occur as sporadic, localized, solitary lesions, less frequently as diffuse or plexiform lesions. Multiple neurofibromas are typically seen with neurofibromatosis type 1, which is an autosomal dominant disorder (1/2,500 births) caused by mutations of the neurofibromin gene on chromosome 17q11.2.

(continued on page 86)

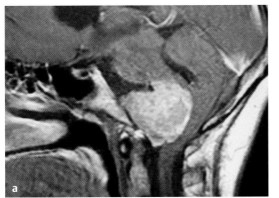
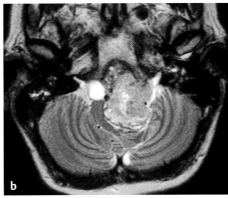

Fig. 1.120 **(a)** Sagittal T1-weighted imaging shows a gadolinium-enhancing meningioma (transitional cell type) along the endocranial surface of the clivus that displaces posteriorly the brainstem and cerebellum. **(b)** The meningioma has mixed intermediate and slightly high on axial T2-weighted imaging.

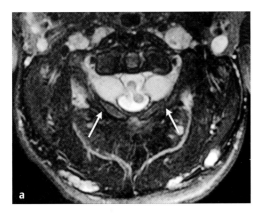
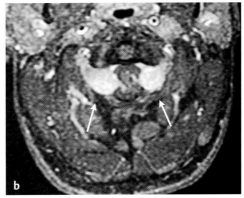

Fig. 1.121 A 22-year-old woman with neurofibromatosis type 1 who has multiple neurofibromas that have high signal on **(a)** axial T2-weighted imaging and show gadolinium contrast enhancement on **(b)** axial fat-suppressed T1-weighted imaging, including two bilateral epidural neurofibromas (*arrows*) that compress and deform the thecal sac and spinal cord.

Table 1.5 *(cont.)* Abnormalities involving the craniovertebral junction

Lesions	Imaging Findings	Comments
Tumorlike Lesions		
Epidermoid (**Fig. 1.122**)	*MRI:* Well-circumscribed lesion with low-intermediate signal on T1-weighted imaging, high signal on T2-weighted imaging and diffusion-weighted imaging, and mixed low, intermediate, and/or high signal on FLAIR. No gadolinium contrast enhancement. *CT:* Circumscribed radiolucent lesion within the skull, ± bone expansion or erosion. Extra-axial lesions often have low attenuation.	Epidermoid cysts are ectoderm-lined inclusion cysts that contain only squamous epithelium, desquamated skin epithelial cells, and keratin. Result from persistence of ectodermal elements at sites of neural tube closure and suture closure. Can occur within bone or as an extra-axial lesion.
Arachnoid cyst (**Fig. 1.123**)	*MRI:* Well-circumscribed extra-axial lesion with low signal on T1-weighted imaging, FLAIR, and diffusion-weighted imaging and high signal on T2-weighted imaging similar to CSF. No gadolinium contrast enhancement. Common locations: anterior middle cranial fossa > suprasellar/quadrigeminal > frontal convexities > posterior cranial fossa. *CT:* Well-circumscribed extra-axial lesions with low attenuation and no contrast enhancement.	Nonneoplastic congenital, developmental, or acquired extra-axial lesions filled with CSF, usually with mild mass effect on adjacent brain, ± related clinical symptoms. Locations: supratentorial > infratentorial. Occur in males more than in females.
Mega cisterna magna (**Fig. 1.124**)	*MR and CT:* Variably enlarged posterior cranial fossa with prominent cisterna magna. The fourth ventricle and vermis are often within normal limits in size and configuration. The cerebellar tonsils are typically normal in position relative to the foramen magnum.	Developmental variant with slightly enlarged posterior cranial fossa associated with a large cisterna magna. Some cases may represent a mild form of the Dandy-Walker spectrum when there is associated mild hypoplasia of the inferior vermis.

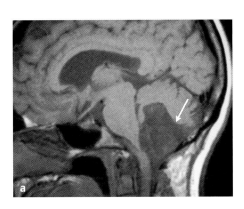 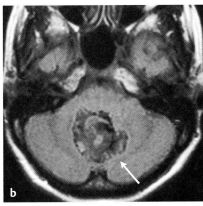 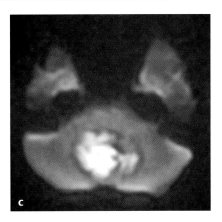

Fig. 1.122   Epidermoid in the inferior portion of the fourth ventricle, foramen of Magendie, and foramen magnum that has heterogeneous mostly low signal on **(a)** sagittal T1-weighted imaging (*arrow*), mixed low, intermediate, and slightly high signal on **(b)** axial FLAIR (*arrow*), and **(c)** restricted diffusion on axial diffusion-weighted imaging.

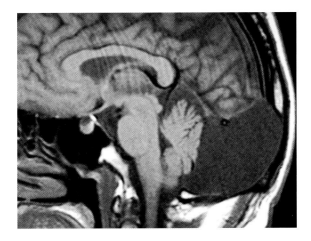 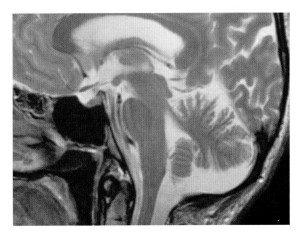

Fig. 1.123   Sagittal T1-weighted imaging shows a large arachnoid cyst with CSF signal in the posterior cranial fossa associated with anterior displacement of the vermis and erosion of the inner table of the occipital bone.

Fig. 1.124   Sagittal T2-weighted imaging shows a slightly enlarged posterior cranial fossa with prominent cisterna magna filled with CSF located below the cerebellum and cerebellar tonsils.

1.6 Temporal Bone

At 3 weeks of gestation, formation of the temporal bone begins from an otic placode on the surface of the primitive hindbrain. Invagination of the otic placode into a pit progresses into the otic cyst. Division of the otic cyst forms the cochlear and vestibular pouches. The cochlear pouch gives rise to the cochlear duct and saccule. The vestibular pouch gives rise to the vestbular duct, utricle, and semicircular ducts. Eventual chondrification and vacuolization of the otic cyst lead to formation of the perilymphatic space in concert with ossification to form the bony labyrinth. The organ of Corti develops in the cochlear duct, and the ampullae form within the semicircular ducts.

Osseous Anatomy

The temporal bone develops from five ossification centers, including the squamous, mastoid, tympanic, petrous, and styloid bones, which fuse after birth (**Fig. 1.125**).

The squamous segment is the outer portion, which forms part of the skull surface where the temporalis muscle and fascia attach. A curved projection from the outer inferior surface extends anteriorly to fuse with a projection from the zygoma to form the zygomatic arch. At the inferior surface are the glenoid fossa of the temporomandibular joint and the upper posterior wall of the outer ear meatus. The anterior border is the sphenoid bone and the

posterior border is the occipital bone. The medial osseous border is along the tympanic segment.

The mastoid segment is the most posterior portion of the temporal bone. The upper margin articulates with the lower portion of the parietal bone, and the lower margin articulates with the occipital bone. The mastoid bone typically has a pneumatized portion containing varying amounts of multiple air cells. Mucous membranes line an irregular mastoid air cell (aditus ad antrum) that is contiguous with the middle ear cavity (typanic antrum). The upper margin of the tympanic antrum is bone of varying thickness, referred to as the tegmen typani, which separates the middle ear from the middle cranial fossa. Along the inner surface of the mastoid bone is a groove (sigmoid sulcus) within which is the transverse dural venous sinus. A thin osseous plate usually separates the sigmoid sulcus from the mastoid air cells. A triangular bone (scutum) at the roof of the attic forms the upper attachment of the tympanic membrane.

The tympanic segment of the temporal bone is located anterior to the mastoid segment and inferior to the squamous segment. The tympanic segment forms most of the wall of the osseous external auditory canal. The medial portion forms the tympanic sulcus, where the other portions of the tympanic membrane attach.

The petrous segment is a wedge-shaped dense bone containing the otic capsule and internal auditory canal (**Fig. 1.126**). The osseous borders are the greater wing of the sphenoid bone anteriorly and the occipital bone inferiorly. Laterally, the petrous segment fuses with the squamous and mastoid segments. The upper anterior surface forms the posterior border of the middle cranial fossa, and

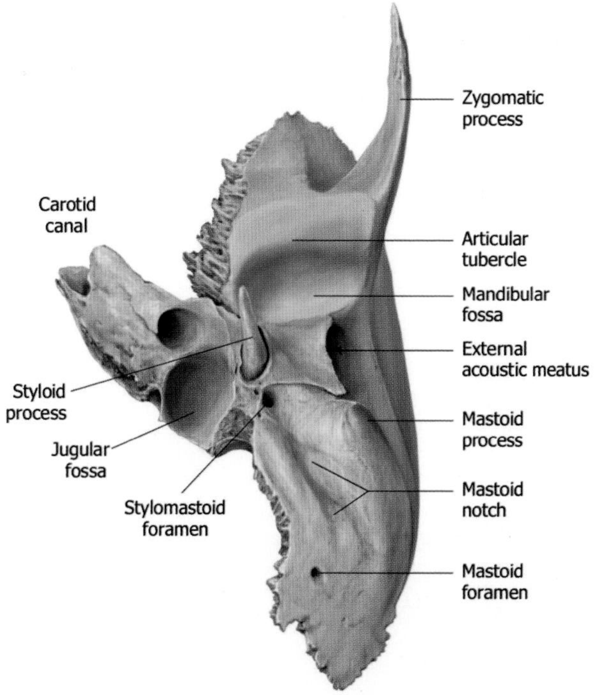

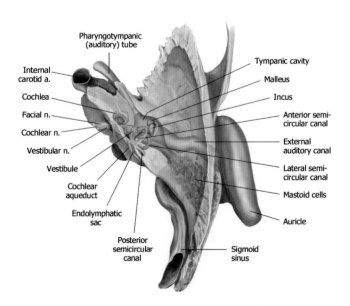

Fig. 1.125 Basal inferior view of the osseous components of the temporal bone. From THIEME Atlas of Anatomy: Head and Neuroanatomy, © Thieme 2007, Illustration by Karl Wesker.

Fig. 1.126 Basal view of the anatomic relationships among the osseous temporal bone and the external, middle, and inner ear structures and sigmoid sinus. From THIEME Atlas of Anatomy: Head and Neuroanatomy, © Thieme 2007, Illustration by Karl Wesker.

the posterior surface forms the anterior margin of the posterior cranial fossa.

The styloid segment is the smallest segment and is a thin osseous projection at the inferior surface of the temporal bone. It is a site of attachment for the stylohyoid and stylomandibular ligaments, as well as the stylohyoid, stylopharyngeal, and styloglossus muscles.

External Auditory Canal

The external auditory is up to 25 mm long and extends from the auricle to the outer surface of the tympanic membrane. The walls of the lateral third portion of the canal are composed of fibrocartilaginous tissue, and the walls of the medial two-thirds are primarily osseous (**Fig. 1.127**).

Middle Ear

The middle ear extends from the inner margin of the tympanic membrane to the otic capsule. The middle ear cavity is separated into three major portions based on their positions relative to the tympanic membrane and annulus. The *epitympanum* is the space above a line drawn horizontally from the upper margin of the tympanic annulus. The epitympanum contains the mallear head and body of the incus. The epitympanum is contiguous with the mastoid antrum via the aditus ad antrum. The superior lateral epitympanic recess (Prussak's space) is located deep to the scutum and pars flaccida and lateral to the mallear head and is a common site of acquired cholesteatomas.

The *mesotympanum* is the space between lines drawn medially from the tympanic membrane and contains the other portions of the ossicular chain.

The *hypotympanum* is the space below the horizontal line drawn from the inferior margin of the tympanic membrane and is filled with air only.

The lateral border of the middle ear is the tympanic membrane. The upper anterior portion of the tympanic membrane is attached to the scutum, and the other portions attach to the tympanic annulus. The upper portion of the tympanic membrane is thin and slightly loose and is referred to as the pars flaccida. The lower portion of the tympanic membrane is more rigid and is referred to as the pars tensa. The ossicular chain is located within the middle ear and consists of the malleus, incus, and stapes (**Fig. 1.128**). The manubrium of the malleus is attached to the tympanic membrane. The neck of the malleus connects the manubrium to its head, where it articulates with the body of the incus. The malleus is stabilized by superior, anterior, and lateral mallear ligaments. The long process of the incus connects to the lenticular process, which articulates with the capitulum (head) of the stapes at the incudostapedial joint. The head of the stapes (capitulum) is contiguous with the anterior and posterior crura (arches), which attach to the stapes footplate at the oval window. The stapedius muscle, innervated by cranial nerve VII, attaches to, and stabilizes, the capitulum of the stapes. The tensor tympani muscle, innervated by cranial nerve V, extends medial to the pharyngotympanic tube to attach to the neck of the malleus. These muscles moderate intense sounds to minimize cochlear injury.

At the posterior lower wall of the middle ear cavity is the pyramidal eminence, which contains the descending portion of the facial nerve. Medial to the pyramidal eminence is the sinus tympani, and the facial nerve recess is located laterally.

The pharyngotympanic (eustachian) tube is a 40 mm pathway containing both an osseous dorsal portion opening at the lower middle ear and a cartilaginous ventral portion opening in the nasopharynx anterior to the torus tubarius. The lining of this pathway includes pseudostratified ciliated columnar epithelium and Schneiderian cells. The walls of the tube are normally collapsed but transiently open during swallowing, mastication, and yawning, when pressures equalize between the middle ear and nasopharynx. Secretions in the middle ear drain via the eustachian tube into the nasopharynx by ciliary action of the epithelium as well as the equalization of pressure between both ends of the tube.

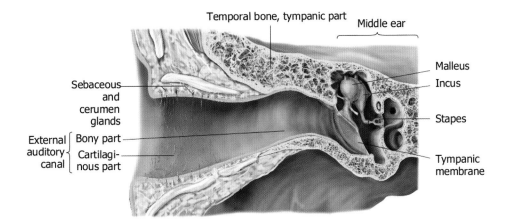

Fig. 1.127 Coronal view diagram of the external auditory canal and relationship to the middle and inner ear structures. From THIEME Atlas of Anatomy: Head and Neuroanatomy, © Thieme 2007, Illustration by Karl Wesker.

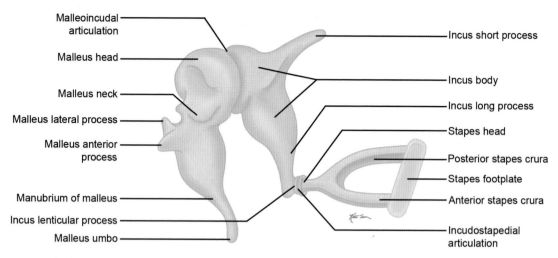

Malleoincudal articulation
Malleus head
Malleus neck
Malleus lateral process
Malleus anterior process
Manubrium of malleus
Incus lenticular process
Malleus umbo

Incus short process
Incus body
Incus long process
Stapes head
Posterior stapes crura
Stapes footplate
Anterior stapes crura
Incudostapedial articulation

Fig. 1.128 Coronal view diagram of the anatomic relationships of the ossicular chain within the middle ear.

Inner Ear

The inner ear is composed of the dense bone of the otic capsule, within which are the cochlea, modiolus, vestibule, semicircular canals, vestibular and cochlear aqueducts, oval and round windows, and internal auditory canal. Transmission of sound waves is funneled from the outer ear though the external auditory canal to cause vibrations of the tympanic membrane, which are transferred to the oval window by the ossicular chain (**Fig. 1.129**). Vibrations at the oval window cause pressure variations in the endolymph of the central cochlear duct (scala media) containing the tectorial membrane whose movement on specialized hair cells of the organ of Corti results in neuro-electric depolarization of cochlear nerve cells (**Fig. 1.130**). The nerve impulses are transmitted to the spiral ganglia at the cochlear base, and then to the cochlear nuclei of the dorsal lower pons via the cochlear nerve (CN VIII), thalamic medial geniculate body, and superior temporal gyrus.

The cochlea is a spiral structure measuring 30 mm in length and consists of two and a half to less than three turns, which are referred to as the basal, middle, and apical turns. High-frequency sounds are detected in the basal turn, middle frequencies in the middle turn, and low frequencies in the apical turn. A centrally located osseous structure (modiolus) within the cochlea contains the spiral ganglion and links to the spiral lamina, which separates the cochlea into the scala vestibuli, scala media, and scala tympani. The scala media spirals through the cochlear turns and communicates with the saccule, and it is separated from the perilymph-filled scala vestibuli by the Reissner vestibular membrane and from the scala tympani by the basal tectorial membrane. The scala vestibuli and tympani are contiguous at the helicotrema. The round window is located posterior to the oval window at the border between the scala tympani and middle ear. The cochlear aqueduct contains the perilymphatic duct, which is a thin channel measuring up to 10 mm in length and 0.1 mm in width and which extends from the scala tympani at the basal cochlear turn to the lateral margin of the jugular foramen. The function of the cochlear duct is to regulate perilymph and CSF pressures.

The vestibular system of the inner ear functions to maintain balance and neurologic orientation with regard to static body position or dynamic motions that have linear and angular accelerations. The functional portion of the vestibular system is the interconnected membranous labyrinth, which consists of the endolymph-containing saccule and utricle within the vestibule, and the semicircular ducts within each of the osseous semicircular canals. The saccule and utricle contain maculae that are involved with assessment of balance and linear acceleration, and the superior, lateral, and posterior semicircular ducts contain ampullae involved in the detection of angular acceleration. The semicircular ducts converge at the crus commune, which connects to the utricle. The utriculosaccular duct connects the anterior saccule with the posterior utricle. The saccule connects to the endolymph of the scala media and cochlear and vestibular aqueducts. The vestibular aqueduct is a bony channel containing an endolymphatic duct that extends posteroinferiorly from the upper posterior vestibule to the endolymphatic sac. The vestibular aqueduct normally measures less than 1.5 mm. Between the outer margins of the membranous labyrinth and osseous semicircular canals is the perilymph fluid. Development of the inner ear structures progresses in a specific pattern. External and/or internal factors can arrest the normal sequence of inner ear development, resulting in various anomalies, as shown in **Fig. 1.131**.

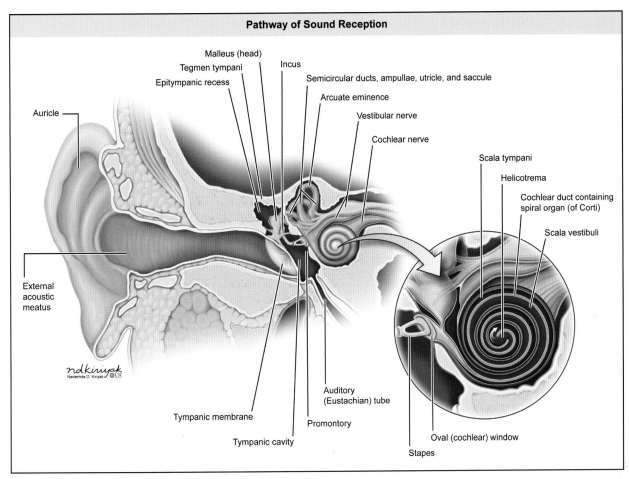

Fig. 1.129 Coronal view diagram of the pathway of sound transmission to the inner ear.

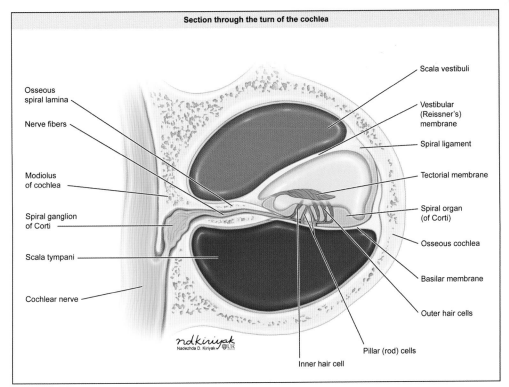

Fig. 1.130 Coronal view diagram through the cochlea shows the scala vestibuli and scala tympani in relationship to the organ of Corti.

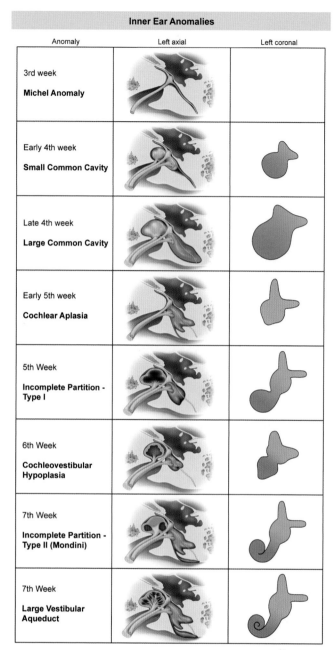

Inner Ear Anomalies

Anomaly	Left axial	Left coronal
3rd week **Michel Anomaly**		
Early 4th week **Small Common Cavity**		
Late 4th week **Large Common Cavity**		
Early 5th week **Cochlear Aplasia**		
5th Week **Incomplete Partition - Type I**		
6th Week **Cochleovestibular Hypoplasia**		
7th Week **Incomplete Partition - Type II (Mondini)**		
7th Week **Large Vestibular Aqueduct**		

Fig. 1.131 Diagram of the relationship of the developmental stages of the inner ear to congenital anomalies. (Adapted from references 3 and 5.)

Internal Auditory Canal

The internal auditory canal is an intraosseous posteromedial to anterolateral channel within the petrous bone, with its endocranial opening oriented 45 degrees with respect to the long axis of the petrous bone. The inner opening (porus acusticus) is wider than the lateral portion (fundus). The facial nerve located at the anterosuperior portion of the canal, the cochlear nerve of CN VIII at the anteroinferior portion, and the superior and inferior vestibular nerves of CN VIII at the posterior portion. The inner auditory branch of the basilar artery is also in the canal. A horizontal osseous plate at the fundus is the falciform crest, which divides the channel into superior and inferior portions. The fundus can also be divided into an anterior and posterior channel by a vertical bone plate referred to as Bill's bar.

The facial nerve (CN VII) extends from the upper anterior portion of the internal auditory canal in an anterolateral direction through a narrow canal in the petrous bone to the geniculate ganglion. At the geniculate ganglion, the superficial petrosal nerve courses medially to supply preganglionic parasympathetic secretomotor fibers to the lacrimal gland from the superior salivatory nucleus in the lower pons. The other larger portion of CN VII extends posterolaterally from the geniculate ganglion under the lateral semicircular canal as the tympanic portion of CN VII, which continues to the pyramidal eminence, where it turns inferiorly as the mastoid portion, exiting caudally at the stylomastoid foramen. This portion of CN VII sends efferent motor fibers from the motor nuclear column in the ventrolateral pontine tegmentum to the muscles of facial expression, to the posterior belly of the digastric, and to the stylohyoid and stapedius muscles. The motor nerve of CN VII extends from its nucleus in the lower pons where it loops dorsally around the abducens nerve (CN VI) nucleus, forming a bulge in the floor of the fourth ventricle (referred to as the facial colliculus) prior to its exit from the anterolateral portion of the pons. The chorda tympani is a branch of the facial nerve carrying sensory and taste fibers from the anterior two-thirds of the tongue. The chorda tympani separates from the mastoid portion of CN VII just above the stylomastoid foramen and extends superiorly within its bony canal into the middle ear passing between the malleus and incus, and exiting the skull through the petrotympanic fissure where it joins the lingual nerve in the masticator space. The chorda tympani supplies parasympathetic secretomotor fibers to the submandibular and sublingual glands from the superior salivatory nucleus in the pons. Taste sensations from the anterior two-thirds of the tongue that are carried in the chorda tympani from the lingual nerve connect to the geniculate ganglion and to the nucleus of the solitary tract (nucleus tractus solitarii) in the upper medulla.

The vestibulocochlear nerve (CN VIII) is involved in the specialized neural sensations of hearing and balance. The cochlear portion of CN VIII carries auditory sensory input from the cochlea to the dorsal and ventral cochlear nuclei in the lateral aspects of the inferior cerebellar peduncle (restiform body). Postsynaptic fibers continue superiorly to the lateral lemniscus in the posterior pons, inferior colliculi in the midbrain, and medial geniculate bodies of the thalami, with eventual termination in the superior temporal gyri.

Sensory input from the vestibular nerves of CN VIII within the posterior portion of the internal auditory canal continues to the central vestibular nuclei in each half of the brainstem, which have commissural fibers that connect to the contralateral nuclei.

Carotid Artery Canal

The internal carotid artery enters the skull at the carotid foramen and ascends anterior to the jugular bulb and courses anteromedially within the petrous carotid canal. At the level of the cochlea, a thin osseous plate covers the canal.

Jugular Foramen

The jugular foramen is located within the sigmoid sulcus along the endocranial surface of the mastoid segment and extends anterolaterally and inferiorly between the petrous segment and the occipital bone. An osseous spur (jugular spine) separates the anteromedial pars nervosa from the posterolateral pars vascularis. The pars vascularis contains the jugular bulb (which drains most of the venous blood from the sigmoid sinus), as well as cranial nerves X and XI. A cutaneous branch from CN X (Arnold's nerve) at the lateral wall of the jugular foramen extends along the mastoid segment of CN VII in the mastoid canaliculus. The pars nervosa contains CN IX and the inferior petrosal sinus (draining venous blood from the cavernous sinus), which extends inferiorly to eventually connect with the jugular vein below the skull base. A tympanic branch from CN IX (Jacobson's nerve) adjacent to the jugular spine extends into the middle ear with the inferior tympanic artery via the inferior tympanic canaliculus. Schwannomas and paragangliomas can involve the Jacobson's and Arnold's nerves.

Table 1.6 Congenital and developmental anomalies involving the temporal bone

- External Auditory Canal (EAC)
  - Congenital dysplasia of the EAC
  - Narrowing of EAC
- Middle Ear
  - Hypoplasia of middle ear
  - Unilateral agenesis, aplasia, and hypoplasia of the internal carotid artery
  - Aberrant position of the internal carotid artery
  - Persistent stapedial artery (PSA)
  - Dehiscence of the jugular vein bulb
  - High position of the jugular bulb
- Ossicles
  - Malformation of ossicles
  - Osseous fusion bar
- Inner Ear
  - Cochlear vestibule and semicircular canals
  - Michel anomaly (labyrinthine aplasia)
  - Cochlear aplasia
  - Small common cavity anomaly
  - Common cavity anomaly
  - Cochlear hypoplasia
  - Cochlea, incomplete partition type I (IP-I)
  - Cochlea, incomplete partition type II (IP-II)– Mondini malformation
  - Large vestibular aqueduct syndrome
  - X-linked stapes gusher
- Vestibule and Semicircular Canals
  - Globular vestibule with dilated semicircular canal
  - Aplasia/hypoplasia of semicircular canals
  - Dehiscence of the superior semicircular canal
  - Atresia/congenital absence of the oval window
- Internal Auditory Canals (IACs)
  - Hypoplasia of IACs
  - Dilatation of IACs
- Syndromes Associated with Abnormal Development of the Temporal Bones
  - Branchiootorenal syndrome
  - CHARGE syndrome
  - Hemifacial microsomia (Goldenhar syndrome, oculoauriculovertebral spectrum)

Table 1.6 Congenital and developmental anomalies involving the temporal bone

Anatomical Entity/ Anomalies	Imaging Findings	Comments
External Auditory Canal (EAC)		
Congenital dysplasia of the EAC (**Fig. 1.132** and **Fig. 1.133**)	Partial or complete atresia of the EAC, with bone present between middle ear and deformed external ear, ± small middle ear, ± malformations (absence or partial atresia) or fusion of ossicles, ± abnormal position of CN VII, ± calcified tympanic membrane, ± oval window atresia.	Failure of first branchial groove to develop into the normal EAC and middle ear. Can be associated with Crouzon syndrome, Goldenhar syndrome, cleidocranial dysplasia, and Pierre Robin syndrome. Inner ear anomalies occur in < 10%.
Narrowing of EAC (**Fig. 1.134**)	Narrowing of membranous and osseous portions of the EAC.	Developmental narrowing of the membranous and osseous portions of the EAC, along with a mild form of congenital dysplasia of the external ear. Can be seen with Crouzon syndrome, Goldenhar syndrome, cleidocranial dysplasia, CHARGE syndrome, and Pierre Robin syndrome.
Middle Ear		
Hypoplasia of middle ear (**Fig. 1.135**)	Small size of middle ear, ± malformations of the ossicles.	May occur as unilateral or bilateral anomaly. Can be associated with Crouzon syndrome, Goldenhar syndrome, cleidocranial dysplasia, CHARGE syndrome, and Pierre Robin syndrome.
Unilateral agenesis, aplasia, and hypoplasia of the internal carotid artery (**Fig. 1.136**)	Absence or near complete absence of the internal carotid artery and petrous carotid canal.	Rare congenital anomalies involving the internal carotid artery, ranging from agenesis (complete absence), aplasia (presence of vestigial remnants), to hypoplasia. Occurs in < 0.1% of the population.

(continued on page 96)

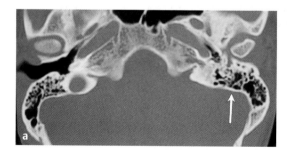 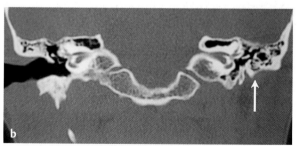

Fig. 1.132 Congenital dysplasia of the external auditory canal in an 8-year-old male. **(a)** Axial and **(b)** coronal CT images show atresia of the left osseous external auditory canal (*arrows*) in comparison to the normal right temporal bone. This is nonsyndromic congenital dysplasia because the ipsilateral mandible and zygomatic arch are normal in size and shape.

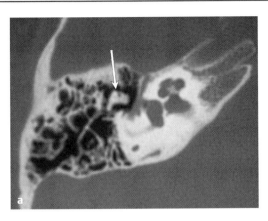
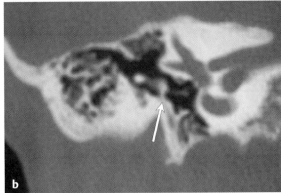

Fig. 1.133 Congenital dysplasia (nonsyndromic type) of the external auditory canal in a 6-year-old female. **(a)** Axial and **(b)** coronal CT images show atresia of the right osseous external auditory canal. The malleus and incus are malformed and fused (*arrows*), including a bony bar to the wall of the middle ear (*arrow* in **b**).

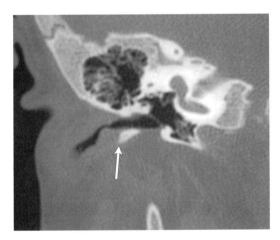

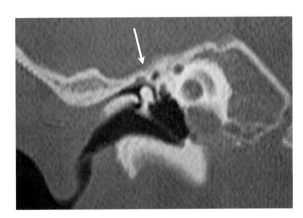

Fig. 1.135 Coronal CT image shows hypoplasia of the epitympanic portion of the middle ear (*arrow*).

Fig. 1.134 Narrowing/hypoplasia of the membranous portions of the right external auditory canals (*arrow*) in a 1-year-old female as seen on coronal CT.

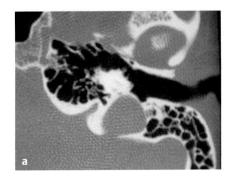
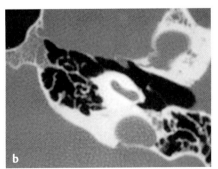
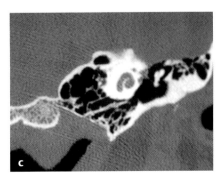

Fig. 1.136 Unilateral agenesis of the left internal carotid artery. The left internal carotid artery is completely absent at the levels of **(a)** the jugular foramen and **(b)** basal turn of the cochlea on axial CT, and **(c)** at the level of the cochlea on coronal CT.

Table 1.6 *(cont.)* Congenital and developmental anomalies involving the temporal bone

Anatomical Entity/ Anomalies	Imaging Findings	Comments
Aberrant position of the internal carotid artery (**Fig. 1.137**)	Abnormal position of the internal carotid artery (ICA), which enters the middle ear posteriorly through an enlarged inferior tympanic canaliculus lateral to the expected site of the petrous carotid canal. The anomalous artery courses anteriorly over the cochlear promontory to connect with the horizontal petrous ICA via a dehiscent carotid bone plate. The aberrant ICA within the middle ear is usually smaller in caliber than the contralateral normal ICA.	Congenital arterial variation related to altered formation of the extracranial ICA resulting from agenesis of the normal first embryonic segment of the ICA. A collateral alternative developmental pathway occurs where the proximal ICA originates from the ascending pharyngeal artery connecting to the inferior tympanic artery, which extends superiorly through the inferior tympanic canal into the middle ear where it anastomoses with the caroticotympanic artery, and the lateral petrous portion of the ICA. As a result, the ICA is positioned laterally within the middle ear cavity. Often an incidental finding with surgical planning implications. Also, a characteristic narrowing of the inferior tympanic artery occurs as it passes through the inferior tympanic canal at the skull base.
Persistent stapedial artery (PSA) (**Fig. 1.138**)	Commonly occurs as an anomalous small artery associated with an aberrant internal carotid artery (ICA) or as an isolated anomaly. Findings include an absent ipsilateral foramen spinosum. The small tubular PSA extends from the ICA along the cochlear promontory through the stapes and then adjacent to the tympanic segment of CN VII to an enlarged tympanic facial nerve canal, where it enters the middle cranial fossa as the middle meningeal artery.	Rare vascular anomaly that is often associated with an aberrant ICA. Results from lack of normal evolution of the embryonic hyoid artery (from the second anterior embryonic aortic arch) into the stapedial artery, with eventual formation of the branches of the external carotid arteries supplying the orbits, meninges, and lower face, as well as the small caroticotympanic and superior tympanic arteries. Lack of normal involution of the stapedial artery results in a persistent stapedial artery, which extends from the ICA into the middle ear, passing through the stapes near the course of the tympanic portion of CN VII and extending intracranially to supply the middle meningeal artery. As a result, the middle meningeal artery is not supplied by the external carotid artery and internal maxillary artery. There is no ipsilateral foramen spinosum.
Dehiscence of the jugular vein bulb (**Fig. 1.139**)	Protrusion of the jugular bulb into the posteroinferior portion of the middle ear related to deficient or absent bone at the jugular plate.	Venous variant anatomy with the jugular bulb extending superiorly and laterally into the middle ear through localized deficiency/dehiscence of the jugular plate. May be associated with pulsatile tinnitus, Ménière disease, and hearing loss. Important to report for surgical planning.
High position of the jugular bulb	The upper portion of the jugular bulb is located above the base of the internal auditory canal/basilar turn of the cochlea. Does not protrude into the middle ear.	Developmental venous variant with positioning of the upper portion of the jugular bulb above the base of the internal auditory canal. Usually an incidental finding.
Ossicles		
Malformation of ossicles (**Fig. 1.140** and **Fig. 1.141**)	Abnormal formation or osseous fusion of one or more ossicles, which can occur as isolated unilateral or bilateral anomalies, or in association with various malformation syndromes.	The most common isolated ossicular malformation is stapes footplate fixation, which is usually bilateral. Anomalies involving the incus and malleus are usually unilateral. Syndromes associated with ossicular malformations include the CHARGE syndrome, branchiootorenal syndrome, hemifacial microsomia (Goldenhar syndrome, oculoauriculovertebral spectrum) branchio-oculo-facial syndrome, and Treacher Collins syndrome.
Osseous fusion bar (**Fig. 1.142**)	Osseous connection of one or more ossicles with the wall of the middle ear.	Congenital or developmental ankylosis with bone connecting the ossicles (malleus > incus > stapes) to the wall of the middle ear. Results in conductive hearing loss. Can be associated with external ear dysplasia or chronic inflammatory disease/tympanosclerosis.

(continued on page 99)

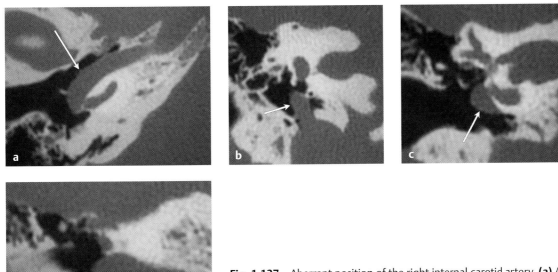

Fig. 1.137 Aberrant position of the right internal carotid artery. **(a)** Axial CT image shows the right internal carotid artery (*arrow*) passing through the middle ear positioned lateral to the basal turn of the cochlea. **(b)** The aberrant right internal carotid (*arrow*) enters the middle ear from below at the level of the round window on coronal CT. **(c)** The artery passes anteromedially (*arrow*) along the cochlear promontory; **(d)** it then enters the petrous carotid canal (*arrow*).

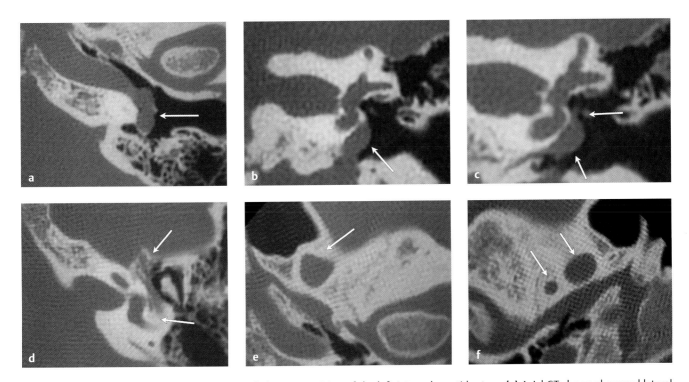

Fig. 1.138 Persistent stapedial artery (PSA) and aberrant position of the left internal carotid artery. **(a)** Axial CT shows abnormal lateral position of the left internal carotid artery (*arrow*) within the middle ear. **(b)** The artery enters the posterior portion of the middle ear (*arrow*), as seen on coronal CT. **(c)** The PSA is seen as a small branch (*upper arrow*) arising from the upper portion of the internal carotid artery (*lower arrow*) on coronal CT. **(d)** The PSA then passes through the stapes and is located parallel to the tympanic portion of the facial nerve (*arrows*), as seen on axial CT, before it extends intracranially to form the middle meningeal artery. **(e)** Because of this alternate pathway of the middle meningeal artery from the PSA, the foramen spinosum is absent posterolateral to the foramen ovale (*arrow*), **(f)** in comparison to the contralateral side, which has a normal foramen spinosum (*arrow on the on the left*), lateral to the foramen ovale (*arrow on the right*).

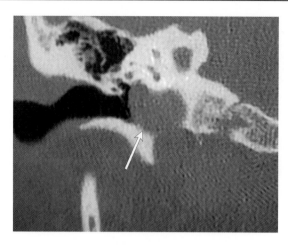

Fig. 1.139 High-riding jugular bulb with extension into the middle ear, as seen on coronal CT. There is bony dehiscence where the jugular vein protrudes into the middle ear (*arrow*).

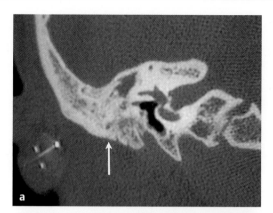

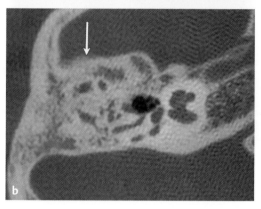

Fig. 1.140 Atresia of the right external auditory canal with a thick bone plate (*arrows*). There is near complete absence of the ossicles except for a portion of the stapes as seen on **(a)** coronal and **(b)** axial CT.

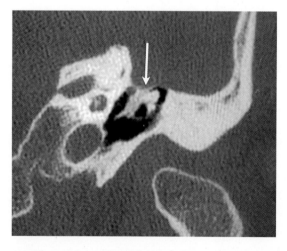

Fig. 1.141 A 41-year-old man with branchiootorenal syndrome, with associated severe malformation and fusion of the malleus and incus, as well as osseous fusion to the roof of the middle ear (*arrow*) on coronal CT.

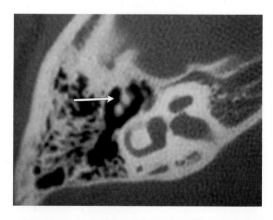

Fig. 1.142 A 7-year-old female with conductive hearing loss from an osseous fusion bar (*arrow*) between the malleus and wall of the middle ear on axial CT.

Table 1.6 *(cont.)* Congenital and developmental anomalies involving the temporal bone

Anatomical Entity/ Anomalies	Imaging Findings	Comments
Inner Ear		
Cochlear vestibule and semicircular canals		Rare anomalies that account for 20% of congenital sensorineural hearing loss and that can be seen on CT. The other 80% of congenital causes of sensorineural hearing loss involve anomalies of the membranous structures of the inner ear, which cannot be seen on CT. Cochlear malformations (in descending order of frequency) are: cochlea, incomplete partition type II/Mondini; cochlea, incomplete partition type I; common cavity; hypoplasia and aplasia; and Michel anomaly. Vestibular malformations (in descending order of frequency) are dilation, common cavity, and aplasia (see **Fig. 1.131**).
Michel anomaly (labyrinthine aplasia) **(Fig. 1.143)**	Bilateral or unilateral absence of the otic capsule, including the cochlea, vestibule, semicircular canals, and vestibular aqueduct. Hypoplasia of the petrous apex, internal auditory canal, and aberrant course of CN VII are often seen.	Rare anomaly (6% of cochlear malformations). Unilateral or bilateral. Complete absence of the inner ear structures results from lack of development of the otic placode, which normally occurs by the third gestational week. Cochlea and vestibular nerves are absent. Can result from mutations, such as *FGF3* and *HOXA1* genes.

(continued on page 100)

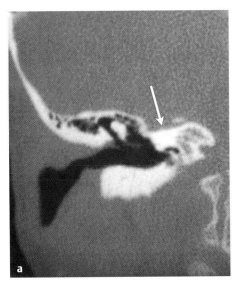 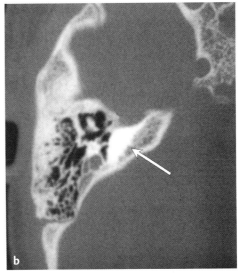

Fig. 1.143   Labyrinthine aplasia (Michel anomaly/aplasia). **(a)** Coronal and **(b)** axial CT images show complete lack of the cochlea, vestibule, and semicircular canals (*arrows*). (From Swartz JD, Loevner LA. Imaging of the Temporal Bone. New York: Thieme; 2008.)

Table 1.6 *(cont.)* Congenital and developmental anomalies involving the temporal bone

Anatomical Entity/ Anomalies	Imaging Findings	Comments
Cochlear aplasia (**Fig. 1.144**)	Unilateral or bilateral complete absence of the cochlea with normal, dilated, or hypoplastic vestibule and semicircular canals. Flattening of cochlear promontory. Absence of cochlear nerve and cochlear nerve canal. Hypoplastic internal auditory canal.	Deafness from rare anomaly (5% of cochlear malformations) with absent development of the cochlea, with or without hypoplastic/malformed vestibule and semicircular canals, caused by arrest of differentiation of the otic capsule at late third week of gestation.
Small common cavity anomaly (**Fig. 1.145**)	Small, ovoid, radiolucent cystic-appearing zone representing the combined cochlea and vestibule, lacking differentiation on CT and with high signal on T2-weighted imaging, ± absent or malformed posterior and/or superior semicircular canals.	Rare anomaly (< 1% of inner ear malformations). Unilateral or bilateral. Caused by arrest of differentiation of the otic capsule at the fourth week of gestation, the time of early formation of the otic placode. Results in a radiolucent zone containing the undifferentaited cochlea and vestibule, with associated deafness or severe sensorineural hearing loss. Idiopathic or related to mutation of the *HOXA1* gene.
Common cavity anomaly (**Fig. 1.146**)	Ovoid, radiolucent, common zone representing undifferentiated combined cochlea and vestibule, ± absent or malformed posterior and/or superior semicircular canals, seen on CT, with high signal on T2-weighted imaging.	Rare anomaly (8% of cochlear malformations). Caused by arrest of differentiation of the otic capsule between the fourth and fifth weeks of gestation after formation of the otic placode. The common cavity is larger than that caused by the earlier arrested development that results in the small common cavity. Idiopathic or related to mutation of *HOXA1* gene.
Cochlear hypoplasia (**Fig. 1.147**)	Cochlea and vestibule are separate structures but the cochlea is smaller than normal, often with only one turn and a "bud-shaped" end. The vestibule and semicircular canals may be normal size or small/ hypoplastic.	Arrest of differentiation of the otic capsule at the sixth week of gestation. Accounts for up to 12% of cochlear malformations.
Cochlea, incomplete partition type I (IP-I) (**Fig. 1.148**)	Dimensions of cochlea and vestibule are grossly within normal limits to slightly enlarged, but lack normal internal architecture, with absent internal septations. The cochlea lacks a modiolus and interscalar septum. There is also thinning of the bone (lamina cribrosa) separating the internal auditory canal from the basal turn of the cochlea. The cochlea and vestibule have a radiolucent "figure 8" shape, ± dilated horizontal semicircular canal and vestibule. Cochlear nerve is absent or hypoplastic. Cochlear nerve canal can be widened. Vestibular aqueduct is not dilated. Internal auditory canal is often enlarged.	Accounts for 20% of cochlear malformations. Unilateral or bilateral cystic cochleovestibular malformation with empty cochlea and vestibule without dilated vestibular aqueduct. Arrest of differentiation of the otic capsule at the fifth week of gestation. Usually profound sensorineural hearing loss.

(continued on page 102)

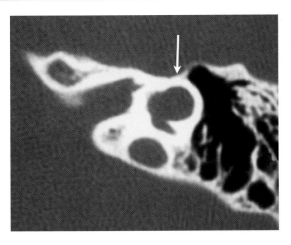

Fig. 1.144 Cochlear aplasia. Axial CT shows dilated vestibule and lateral semicircular canal and absence of the cochlea (*arrow*).

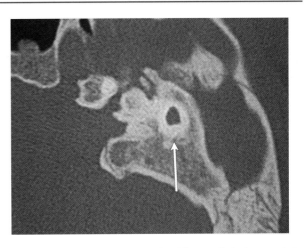

Fig. 1.145 Small common cavity (cochleovestibular) anomaly in a 21-year-old woman. Axial CT shows a small single cavity in the left temporal bone (*arrow*).

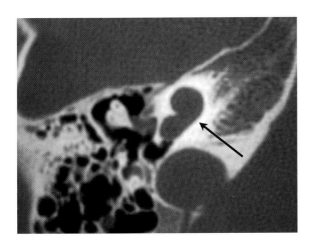

Fig. 1.146 Common cavity anomaly in a 5-year-old female. Axial CT shows a common cavity (*arrow*) representing a combined dilated and malformed cochlea, vestibule, and semicircular canals without partitions.

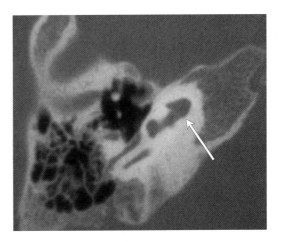

Fig. 1.147 Cochlear hypoplasia in a 3-year-old female. Axial CT shows the basal turn of the cochlea terminating in a bud-shaped end (*arrow*).

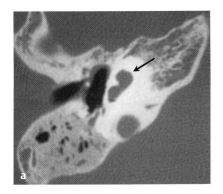
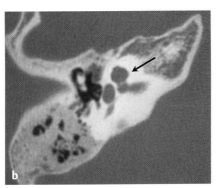
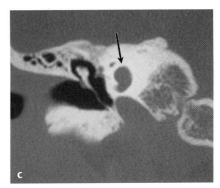

Fig. 1.148 Incomplete partition, type I, in a 9-year-old female. **(a,b)** Axial CT shows a cystic cochlea (*arrows*) with absent modiolus and cystic vestibule. A small bony partition between the cochlea and vestibule is seen **(b),** consistent with a more developed anomaly than the common cavity anomaly. **(c)** Coronal CT shows a cystic cochlear apex (*arrow*). A dilated vestibular aqueduct was not present.

Table 1.6 *(cont.)* Congenital and developmental anomalies involving the temporal bone

Anatomical Entity/ Anomalies	Imaging Findings	Comments
Cochlea, incomplete partition type II (IP-II)— Mondini malformation (**Fig. 1.149** and **Fig. 1.150**)	Dimensions of cochlea and vestibule are grossly within normal limits. Modiolus is partially formed, cochlea consists of only 1.5 turns, with fusion of the middle and apical turns, vestibules are mildly dilated, and vestibular aqueducts are abnormally enlarged.	Unilateral or bilateral. Accounts for up to 19% of cochlear malformations. More differentiated than IP-I. Caused by arrest of differentiation of the otic capsule at the seventh week of gestation. The basal portion of the modiolus is present, with rudimentary formation of the spiral ganglia and nerve endings. Hearing gain from cochlear implants is greater for IP-II than for IP-I.
Large vestibular aqueduct syndrome (**Fig. 1.151**)	Bilateral or unilateral dilatation of the vestibular aqueducts, ± varying degrees of modiolar deficiency. On MRI, dilated endolymphatic sacs with high signal on T2-weighted imaging are seen.	Progressive sensorineural hearing loss beginning in childhood associated with dilatation of the vestibular aqueducts (greater than 1.5 mm in diameter). Lack of other osseous anomalies of the cochlea, vestibules, and semicircular canals on CT. Vestibular aqueducts may progressively enlarge, suggesting an acquired, versus congenital, etiology. Accounts for up to 15% of cochleovestibular malformations.
X-linked stapes gusher (**Fig. 1.152**)	Bilateral dilatation of the fundi of the internal auditory canals, thinning or absence of the bone (lamina cribrosa) separating the internal auditory canals from the basal turn of the cochlea, with widened cochlear nerve canal. The cochlea also has a "corkscrew" appearance resulting from absence of both the modiolus and interscalar septum. The labyrinthine segment of the facial nerve is widened.	Rare, congenital, X-linked mixed and profound sensorineural hearing loss related to abnormality at the Xq13q21.1 region and *POU3F4* gene. Accounts for 2% of cochlear malformations. Consists of bilateral malformation and dilatation of the fundi of the internal auditory canals and absence of bone separating the internal auditory canals from the cochlea (lamina cribrosa), which results in communication of the subarachnoid CSF with the perilymph of the cochlea. Fixation of stapes footplates is usually present. Patients are at high risk for gushing of perilymphatic fluid during attempted stapedectomy, resulting in worsening of sensorineural hearing loss.

(continued on page 104)

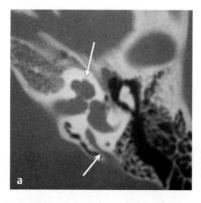 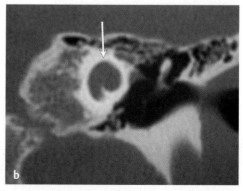

Fig. 1.149 Incomplete partition, type II (Mondini malformation), in a 5-year-old male. **(a)** Axial CT shows a dilated vestibular aqueduct (*posterior arrow*), deficient modiolus (*anterior arrow*), and dilated vestibule. **(b)** Coronal CT shows a bulbous cochlear apex (*arrow*).

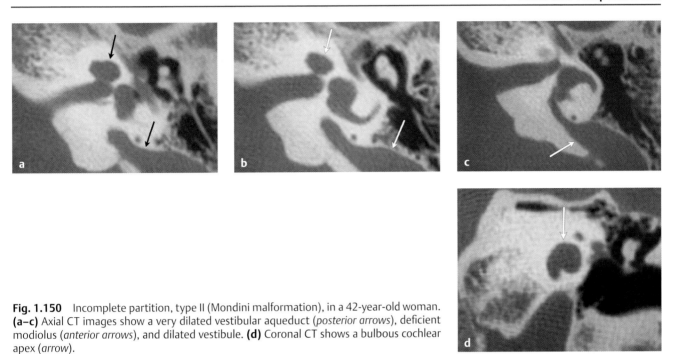

Fig. 1.150   Incomplete partition, type II (Mondini malformation), in a 42-year-old woman. **(a–c)** Axial CT images show a very dilated vestibular aqueduct (*posterior arrows*), deficient modiolus (*anterior arrows*), and dilated vestibule. **(d)** Coronal CT shows a bulbous cochlear apex (*arrow*).

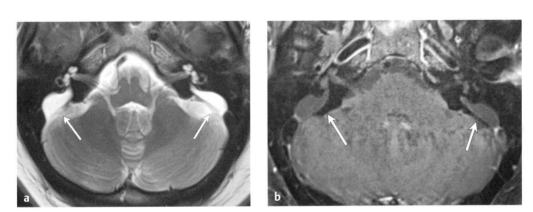

Fig. 1.151   Dilated vestibular aqueducts. **(a)** Axial T2-weighted imaging shows bilateral dilated vestibular aqueducts (*arrows*) and endolymphatic sacs, which show no abnormal contrast enhancement on **(b)** axial fat-suppressed T1-weighted imaging.

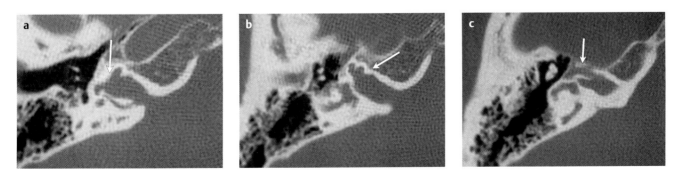

Fig. 1.152   X-linked stapes gusher in a 44-year-old man. **(a,b)** Axial CT images show dilatation of the fundus of the internal auditory canal (*arrows*) and absence of the bone (lamina cribosa) separating the internal auditory canal from the basal turn of the cochlea, with a widened cochlear nerve canal. The cochlea has a corkscrew appearance resulting from absence of both the modiolus and interscalar septum. **(c)** The labyrinthine segment of the facial nerve (*arrow*) is widened, as seen on axial CT.

Table 1.6 *(cont.)* Congenital and developmental anomalies involving the temporal bone

Anatomical Entity/ Anomalies	Imaging Findings	Comments
Vestibule and Semicircular Canals		
Globular vestibule with dilated semicircular canal (**Fig. 1.153**)	Gobular vestibule with adjacent dilated semicircular canal, most often involving the lateral semicircular canal.	Most common malformation involving the vestibule and semicircular canals. Patients may experience vertigo and sensorineural hearing loss.
Aplasia/hypoplasia of semicircular canals (**Fig. 1.154** and **Fig. 1.155**)	Aplasia or hypoplasia of one or more semicircular canals with or without hypoplastic vestibule.	Malformations involving the vestibule and semicircular canals. Can be isolated anomalies or associated with CHARGE syndrome (hypoplastic vestibule and semicircular canal) or branchiootorenal syndrome (hypoplastic semicircular canal, hypoplastic middle and apical turns of cochlea).
Dehiscence of the superior semicircular canal (**Fig. 1.156**)	Lack of bone covering the superior semicircular canal seen on high-resolution CT.	Developmental absence or severe thinning of bone covering the superior semicircular canal that can result in abnormal flow dynamics of endolymph in the semicircular canals. Can result in disequilibrium, oscillopsia, and/or Tulio phenomenon (vertigo with or without nystagmus caused by sound). Osseous dehiscence can also involve the lateral and posterior semicircular canals.
Atresia/congenital absence of the oval window (**Fig. 1.157**)	The oval window is abnormally covered by bone. Associated abnormalities include malformations of the ossicular chain, with dysplastic or absent stapes, and inferomedial positioning of the tympanic portion of CN VII.	Uncommon embryologic defect with maximal conductive hearing loss beginning at birth or in early childhood. Associated with malposition of the tympanic portion of CN VII.

(continued on page 106)

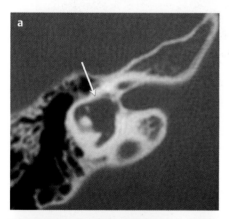

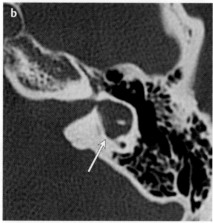

Fig. 1.153 **(a)** Globular vestibule (*arrow*) in a 5-year-old male, as seen on axial CT. **(b)** Axial CT in another patient shows globular vestibule (*arrow*) and dilated lateral semicircular canal (LSCC) in the left inner ear.

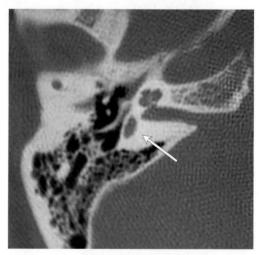

Fig. 1.154 Aplasia of the semicircular canals in a 22-year-old man with CHARGE syndrome. Axial CT shows a normal-shaped cochlea, as well as a vestibule without semicircular canals (*arrow*).

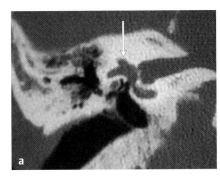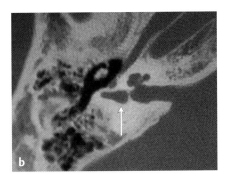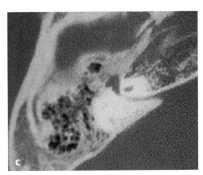

Fig. 1.155 Hypoplasia of the superior semicircular canal (SCC) and aplasia of the posterior SCC in a 20-year-old man as seen on **(a)** coronal (*arrow*) and **(b,c)** axial CT. The cochlea is normal shaped. The superior SCC (*arrow*) is small in height **(a)**, and **(b)** the posterior SCC (*arrow*) is not seen. The superior SCC is not seen at the level of the labyrinthine facial nerve canal on axial CT **(c)**.

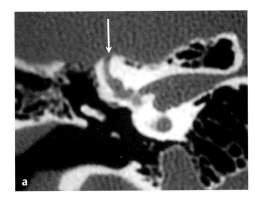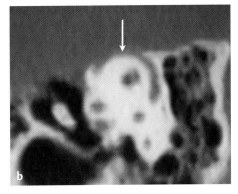

Fig. 1.156 Bony dehiscence of superior semicircular canal (SCC). **(a)** Coronal CT and **(b)** reconstructed CT image parallel to the superior SCC show absence of bony cortex (*arrows*) that would normally cover the roof of the superior SCC.

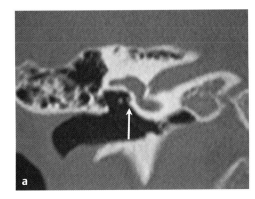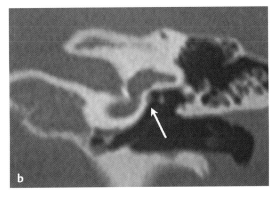

Fig. 1.157 Atresia/congenital absence of the oval window in a 6-year-old female. Coronal CT of **(a)** the right and **(b)** the left temporal bones show both oval windows covered by bone (*arrows*). The tympanic portions of both CN VII are abnormally positioned inferomedially over the atretic, bone-covered oval windows.

Table 1.6 *(cont.)* Congenital and developmental anomalies involving the temporal bone

Anatomical Entity/ Anomalies	Imaging Findings	Comments
Internal Auditory Canals (IACs)		
Hypoplasia of IACs **(Fig. 1.158)**	Unilateral or bilateral small IACs seen with CT and MRI.	Hypoplasia of the IACs can be seen with labyrinthine aplasia, cochlear aplasia/hypoplasia, common cavity anomaly, cleidocranial dysplasia, and hemifacial microsomia/Goldenhar syndrome.
Dilatation of IACs **(Fig. 1.159)**	Unilateral or bilateral enlarged/dilated IACs seen with CT and MRI.	Abnormally enlarged IACs can be idiopathic or associated with branchiootorenal syndrome and X-linked stapes gusher.
Syndromes Associated with Abnormal Development of the Temporal Bones		
Branchiootorenal syndrome **(Fig. 1.160)**	*CT:* Findings include dilated eustachian tubes, stenosis/ narrowing of the external auditory canals, hypoplastic middle ears, malformed and/or fused ossicles, hypoplasia of cochlea and/or one or more semicircular canals, dilated vestibular aqueducts, and widened and flared internal auditory canals.	Autosomal dominant disorder with sensorineural and/ or conductive hearing loss secondary to mutations of the *EYA1* gene on chromosome 8q13.3 or the *SIX* gene on chromosome 19q13.3. Incidence: 1/40,000. Other abnormalities include preauricular pit, branchial cleft cysts, and renal cysts.
CHARGE syndrome **(Fig. 1.161)**	Findings on CT include hypoplasia of vestibules, aplasia or hypoplasia of semicircular canals, abnormal cochlea (IP-II), anomalous position of CN VII (tympanic portion), and stenosis or atresia of oval window.	Syndrome consisting of coloboma, heart anomaly, atresia choanae, retardation, genital hypoplasia, and ear abnormalities, secondary to mutations of the *CHD7* gene on 8q12.1 or *SEMA3E* gene on 7q21.11. Incidence: 1/12,000.
Hemifacial microsomia (Goldenhar syndrome, oculoauriculovertebral spectrum) **(Fig. 1.162)**	Findings include facial asymmetry from unilateral and/ or bilateral hypoplasia of the mandible and zygomatic arches, atresia or stenosis of the external auditory canals, hypoplasia of the middle ear, malformations and/or fusion of the ossicles, oval window atresia, and abnormal position of CN VII.	Asymmetric abnormal development of the first and second branchial arches related to autosomal dominant mutation of the *TCOF1* gene on chromosome 5q32-q33.1. Results in deafness/hearing loss and airway narrowing.

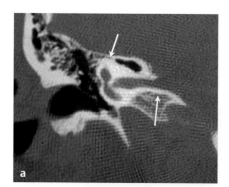 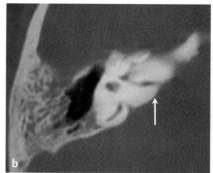 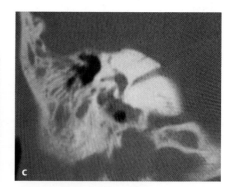

Fig. 1.158 **(a)** Hypoplasia of the right internal auditory canal in a 22-year-old man with CHARGE syndrome as seen on coronal CT (*lower arrow*). Note also the lack of formation of the semicircular canals (*upper arrow*). **(b,c)** A 12-year-old male with hemifacial microsomia (Goldenhar syndrome) who has a very small right internal auditory canal (*arrow*), as seen on axial **(b)** and coronal **(c)** CT.

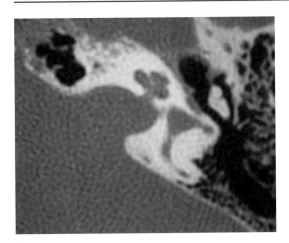

Fig. 1.159 Dilated right internal auditory canal in a 56-year-old woman with mild conductive hearing loss.

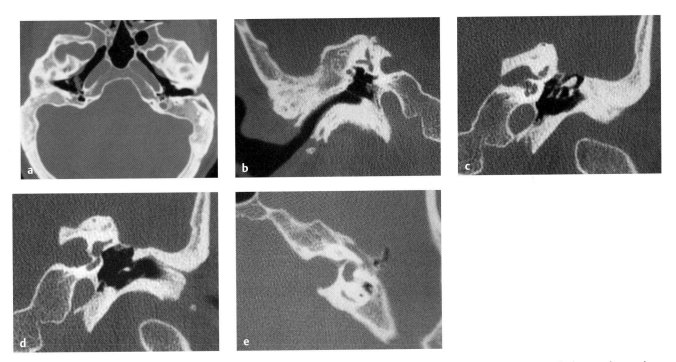

Fig. 1.160 Branchiootorenal syndrome in a 41-year-old man. **(a)** Axial CT image shows bilateral, dilated, air-filled eustachian tubes. **(b)** Coronal CT shows narrowing of the right external auditory canal. **(c)** Hypoplastic left middle ear with malformed and fused ossicles are seen on coronal CT. **(d)** Coronal and **(e)** axial CT shows hypoplasia of the lateral semicircular canal and widened and flared left internal auditory canal.

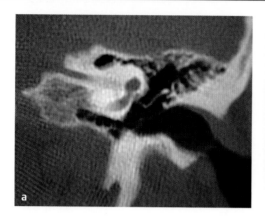
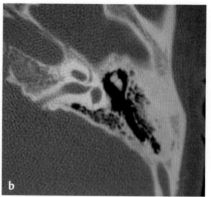

Fig. 1.161 A 22-year-old man with CHARGE syndrome. **(a)** Coronal and **(b)** axial CT images of the left temporal bone show hypoplasia of the vestibule, aplasia of the semicircular canals, and anomalous position of CN VII (tympanic portion), which is positioned over an atretic, bone-covered oval window.

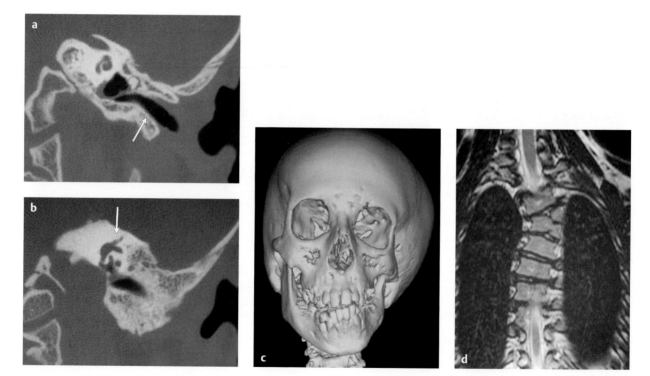

Fig. 1.162 Hemifacial microsomia (Goldenhar syndrome, oculoauriculovertebral spectrum) in a 12-year-old male. **(a,b)** Coronal CT shows stenosis of the left external auditory canal (*arrow* in **a**), hypoplasia of the middle ear with malformed ossicles, abnormal position of CN VII, and hypoplasia of the superior semicircular canal (*arrow* in **b**). **(c)** Coronal 3D/volume-rendered CT shows facial asymmetry from unilateral hypoplasia of the left mandible and left zygomatic arch. **(d)** Coronal T2-weighted imaging shows thoracic scoliosis from a hemivertebral segmentation anomaly in this patient.

Table 1.7   Acquired lesions involving the external auditory canal (EAC)

- Tumorlike Lesions
  - Keratosis obturans
  - Medial canal fibrosis
  - Epidermoid/cholesteatoma
  - Osteoma
  - Exostoses
  - Fibrous dysplasia
- Neoplasms
  - Squamous cell carcinoma
  - Metastatic disease
- Infection
  - Acute external otitis
  - Necrotizing (malignant) otitis externa
- Inflammation (noninfectious)
  - Langerhans' cell histiocytosis
  - Granulomatosis with polyangiitis
  - Sarcoidosis

Table 1.7   Acquired lesions involving the external auditory canal (EAC)

Lesions	Imaging Findings	Comments
Tumorlike Lesions		
Keratosis obturans (**Fig. 1.163**)	*CT:* Zone of soft tissue attenuation within the medial portion of the EAC, ± medial retraction of the tympanic membrane, usually no erosion of adjacent bone of the EAC. *MRI:* Low-intermediate signal on T1-weighted imaging and heterogeneous low- intermediate signal on T2-weighted imaging, ± peripheral rim gadolinium contrast enhancement.	Keratin plug with peripheral granulation tissue fills the medial portion of the EAC, usually in patients < 40 years old. Can be bilateral and painful, as well as associated with chronic sinusitis or bronchiectasis.

(continued on page 110)

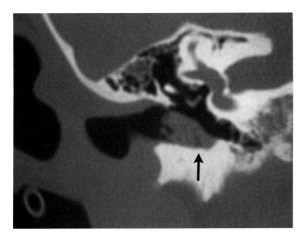

Fig. 1.163   Keratosis obturans in an 11-year-old female. Coronal CT shows a zone of soft tissue attenuation (*arrow*) within the medial portion of the external auditory canal.

Table 1.7 *(cont.)* Acquired lesions involving the external auditory canal (EAC)

Lesions	Imaging Findings	Comments
Medial canal fibrosis **(Fig. 1.164)**	*CT:* Lesions are located in the medial portion of the EAC adjacent to the tympanic membrane and have low-intermediate attenuation. There is no erosion of adjacent bone. *MRI:* Low signal on T1-weighted imaging and heterogeneous low-intermediate signal on T2-weighted imaging and diffusion-weighted imaging, ± gadolinium contrast enhancement.	Chronic inflammation at the medial portion of the EAC can result in progressive fibrosis of localized granulation tissue. Often occurs in middle-aged patients (mean age = 50 years), in males more than in females, and bilaterally in 50%. Surgery is usually indicated if there is associated otorrhea or conductive hearing loss.
Epidermoid/cholesteatoma **(Fig. 1.165)**	*CT:* Lesions have low-intermediate attenuation. Usually associated with erosion or disruption of adjacent bone, ± bone fragments within lesion. *MRI:* Low signal on T1-weighted imaging, heterogeneous intermediate signal on FLAIR, and high signal on T2-weighted imaging and diffusion-weighted imaging, but no contrast enhancement.	Usually unilateral epidermal inclusion cyst in the EAC associated with osseous erosion, ± sinus tracts. Often occurs in patients > 40 years old.
Osteoma **(Fig. 1.166)**	*CT:* Lesions typically have diffuse high attenuation similar to dense cortical bone. *MRI:* Low signal on T1- and T2-weighted imaging, and no contrast enhancement.	Solitary, benign, dense, mature bone lesions that can protrude and narrow the EAC.
Exostoses **(Fig. 1.167)**	*CT:* Osseous lesions typically have diffuse high attenuation similar to dense cortical bone. Causes circumferential narrowing of the osseous EAC. *MRI:* Abnormality has low signal on T1- and T2-weighted imaging similar to cortical bone. No gadolinium contrast enhancement.	Mature, dense bony overgrowths that occur from multiple episodes of prolonged exposure to cold temperatures (deep sea diving), or from chemical or mechanical irritation. Typically are bilateral, with circumferential osseous narrowing of the external auditory canal.
Fibrous dysplasia **(Fig. 1.168)**	*CT:* Expansion of bone that can have a ground-glass appearance, ± radiolucent cystic changes, ± associated aneurysmal bone cysts. *MRI:* Features depend on the proportions of bony spicules, collagen, fibroblastic spindle cells, hemorrhagic and/or cystic changes, and associated pathologic fracture, if present. Lesions are usually well circumscribed and have low or low-intermediate signal on T1-weighted imaging and proton density-weighted imaging. On T2-weighted imaging, lesions have variable mixtures of low, intermediate, and/or high signal, often surrounded by a low-signal rim of variable thickness. Internal septations and cystic changes are seen in a minority of lesions. Bone expansion with thickened and/or thinned cortex can be seen. Lesions show gadolinium contrast enhancement that varies in degree and pattern.	Benign medullary fibro-osseous lesion of bone, most often sporadic, involving a single site, referred to as monostotic fibrous dysplasia, or multiple locations (polyostotic fibrous dysplasia). Results from developmental failure in the normal process of remodeling primitive bone to mature lamellar bone, with resultant zone or zones of immature trabeculae within dysplastic fibrous tissue. Accounts for ~ 10% of benign bone lesions. Patients range in age from < 1 year to 76 years; 75% of cases occur before the age of 30 years.

(continued on page 112)

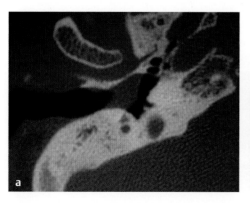
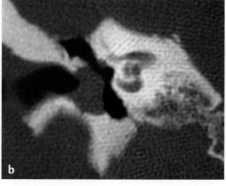

Fig. 1.164 Medial canal fibrosis in a 56-year-old man. **(a)** Axial and **(b)** coronal CT images show soft tissue attenuation adjacent to the outer wall of the tympanic membrane that fills the medial portion of the external auditory canal. The outer margin of the lesion has a crescent shape.

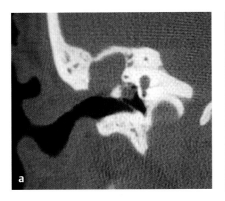

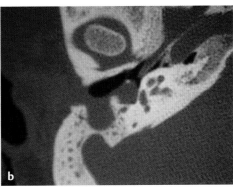

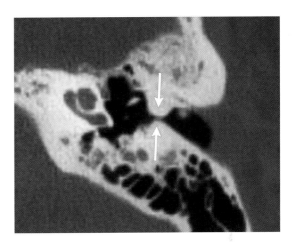

Fig. 1.165 A 76-year-old woman with an epidermoid/cholesteatoma originating in the middle ear and extending into bone at the upper medial external auditory canal (EAC), resulting in an automastoidectomy, which caused extrusion of eroded ossicles out of the external auditory canal. (a) Coronal and (b) axial CT images show absence of the ossicular chain in the middle ear, residual cholesteatoma deep to the tympanic membrane, and bony erosion at the epitympanum and upper medial wall of the right EAC.

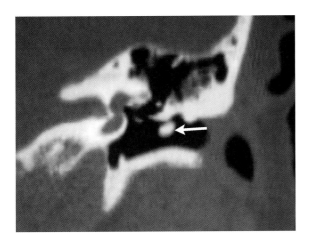

Fig. 1.166 Coronal CT shows an osteoma at the upper margin of the left external auditory canal (*arrow*).

Fig. 1.167 Axial CT images show bilateral exostoses narrowing the osseous portions of the external auditory canals (*arrows*).

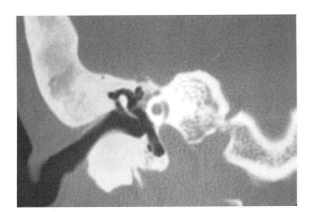

Fig. 1.168 A 3-year-old female with fibrous dysplasia involving the external auditory canal (EAC), with thickened bone that has a ground-glass appearance, causing narrowing of the EAC, as seen on coronal CT.

Table 1.7 *(cont.)*   Acquired lesions involving the external auditory canal (EAC)

Lesions	Imaging Findings	Comments
Neoplasms		
Squamous cell carcinoma (**Fig. 1.169**)	*CT:* Soft tissue attenuation tumor within the EAC associated with bone invasion and destruction. *MRI:* Tumors often have low-intermediate signal on T1-weighted imaging, intermediate to slightly high signal on T2-weighted imaging, and usually show gadolinium contrast enhancement.	Most common malignancy involving the EAC. Often associated with chronic ear infection. Can spread to middle ear. More common in women, with a 5-year mortality of 50% when limited to EAC, 27% if extension into the middle ear occurs. Other tumors that less frequently involve the EAC include basal cell carcinoma, adenoid cystic carcinoma, melanoma, ceruminous adenocarcinoma, and lymphoma.
Metastatic disease (**Fig. 1.170**)	*CT:* Single or multiple well-circumscribed or poorly defined infiltrative lesions involving the marrow, associated with cortical destruction and extraosseous extension. *MRI:* Lesions often have low-intermediate signal on T1-weighted imaging and low, intermediate, and/or high signal on T2-weighted imaging and fat-suppressed T1-weighted imaging, and usually show gadolinium contrast enhancement. Cortical destruction and tumor extension into the extraosseous soft tissues frequently occur.	Metastatic lesions typically occur in the marrow from hematogenous dissemination and are often associated with bone destruction and extraosseous tumor extension.
Infection		
Acute external otitis (**Fig. 1.171**)	*CT:* Zones with soft-tissue attenuation in the EAC. *MRI:* Poorly defined zones of soft tissue thickening with low-intermediate signal on T1-weighted imaging, slightly high to high signal on T2-weighted imaging, and gadolinium contrast enhancement within the EAC.	Most common external ear infection (caused by *Pseudomonas aeruginosa* and *Staphylococcus aureus*, and by fungi in diabetics). Patients often present with pain and swelling, ± conductive hearing loss.
Necrotizing (malignant) otitis externa (**Fig. 1.172**)	*CT:* Zones with soft tissue attenuation in the EAC, ± bone destruction. *MRI:* Poorly defined zones of soft tissue thickening with low-intermediate signal on T1-weighted imaging, slightly high to high signal on T2-weighted imaging, and gadolinium contrast enhancement within the EAC, ± bone invasion and destruction, ± extension into the skull base or intracranially, with involvement of the dura, brain, venous sinuses, nasopharynx, and/or infratemporal fossa.	Aggressive infection of the EAC and adjacent soft tissues in immunocompromised patients and diabetics. *Pseudomonas aeruginosa* is the most common pathogen. Patients present with severe otalgia and otorrhea. Infection can spread from the EAC via the fissures of Santorini into the soft tissues under the skull base, resulting in neuropathies involving CN VII and IX–XII. Also extension of the infection intracranially can occur, resulting venous sinus thrombosis, empyemas, meningitis, and brain infarction. High morbidity and mortality if not adequately treated.

(continued on page 114)

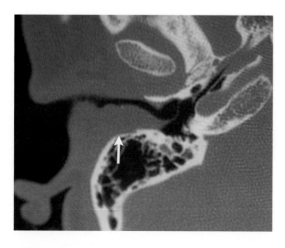

Fig. 1.169 Squamous cell carcinoma. Axial CT image shows the tumor with soft tissue attenuation extending along the membranous and osseous portions of the right external auditory canal (*arrow*).

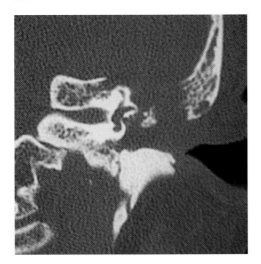

Fig. 1.170 Metastatic disease causing osseous destruction at the left temporal bone, with extension into and filling the left external auditory canal and middle ear.

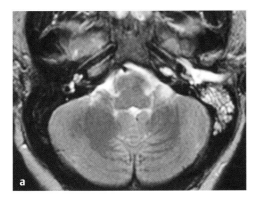

Fig. 1.171 **(a)** A 30-year-old woman with acute external otitis that has high signal on T2-weighted imaging filling the left external auditory canal as well as the left mastoid air cells, left middle ear, and pneumatized left petrous apex air cells. **(b)** Mild peripheral gadolinium contrast enhancement is seen along the left external auditory canal (*arrows*) on coronal fat-suppressed T1-weighted imaging.

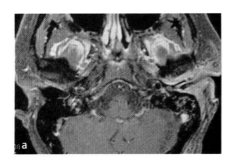

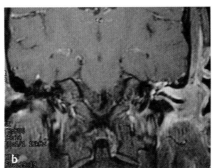

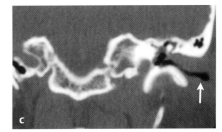

Fig. 1.172 Necrotizing (malignant) otitis externa in a 29-year-old man with poorly controlled diabetes. Poorly defined zones of gadolinium contrast enhancement are seen within the left external auditory canal (EAC), with evidence of extension into the left middle ear, skull base and superficial soft tissue, as seen on **(a)** axial and **(b)** coronal fat-suppressed T1-weighted imaging. **(c)** Abnormal soft tissue attenuation is seen in the left EAC on coronal CT (*arrow*).

Table 1.7 *(cont.)* Acquired lesions involving the external auditory canal (EAC)

Lesions	Imaging Findings	Comments
Inflammation (noninfectious)		
Langerhans' cell histiocytosis **(Fig. 1.173)**	Focal intramedullary osseous lesion associated with trabecular and cortical bone destruction. *CT:* Lesions usually have low-intermediate attenuation, + contrast enhancement, ± enhancement of the adjacent dura. *MRI:* Lesions typically have low-intermediate signal on T1-weighted imaging and heterogeneous slightly high to high signal on FLAIR, T2-weighted imaging (T2WI), and fat-suppressed (FS) T2WI. Poorly defined zones of high signal on T2WI and FS T2WI are usually seen in the marrow and soft tissues peripheral to the lesions secondary to inflammatory changes. Extension of lesions from the marrow into adjacent soft tissues through areas of cortical disruption are commonly seen as well. Lesions typically show prominent gadolinium contrast enhancement in marrow and extraosseous soft tissue portions.	Benign tumorlike lesions consisting of Langerhans' cells (histiocytes) and variable amounts of lymphocytes, polymorphonuclear cells, and eosinophils. Account for 1% of primary bone lesions and 8% of tumorlike lesions. Occur in patients with median age = 10 years (average age = 13.5 years). Peak incidence is between 5 and 10 years; 80 to 85% occur in patients < 30 years old.
Granulomatosis with polyangiitis	*CT:* Zones with soft tissue attenuation in the EAC, ± bone destruction. *MRI:* Poorly defined zones of soft tissue thickening with low-intermediate signal on T1-weighted imaging, slightly high to high signal on T2-weighted imaging, and gadolinium contrast enhancement within the EAC, ± bone invasion and destruction, ± extension into the skull base and intracranially, with involvement of the dura, brain, venous sinuses, nasopharynx, and/or infratemporal fossa.	Multisystem disease with necrotizing granulomas in the respiratory tract, focal necrotizing angiitis of small arteries and veins of various tissues, and glomerulonephritis. Can involve the paranasal sinuses, orbits, and occasionally the temporal bone. Typically, positive immunoreactivity to cytoplasmic antineutrophil cytoplasmic antibody (c-ANCA). Treatment includes corticosteroids, cyclophosphamide, and anti-TNF agents.
Sarcoidosis	*CT:* Intraosseous lesions usually appear as intramedullary radiolucent zones, rarely are sclerotic with high attenuation. *MRI:* Lesions often have low to intermediate signal on T1-weighted imaging and slightly high to high signal on T2-weighted imaging (T2WI) and fat-suppressed (FS) proton density-weighted imaging and FS T2WI. Erosions and zones of destruction involving adjacent bony cortex can occur with extraosseous extension of the granulomatous process. After gadolinium contrast administration, lesions typically show moderate to prominent enhancement.	Chronic systemic granulomatous disease of unknown etiology in which noncaseating granulomas occur in various tissues and organs, including bone.

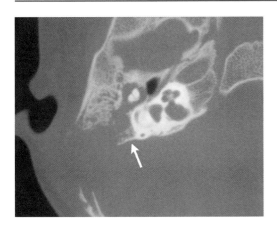

Fig. 1.173 Axial CT of Langerhans' cell histiocytosis in a 1-year-old male. An eosinophilic granuloma involving the right mastoid bone has caused osseous destruction and has extended into the right epitympanum and right external auditory canal (*arrow*).

Table 1.8 Lesions involving the middle ear

- Tumorlike lesions
  - Acquired cholesteatoma
  - Congenital cholesteatoma
  - Cholesterol granuloma
  - Fibrous dysplasia
- Neoplasms
  - Schwannoma
  - Paraganglioma: Glomus tympanicum, Glomus jugulotympanicum
  - Adenoma
  - Carcinoid
  - Adenocarcinoma
  - Squamous cell carcinoma
  - Metastatic disease
  - Meningioma

- Infection
  - Acute otitis media
  - Chronic otitis media/tympanosclerosis
  - Viral infection
- Inflammation (noninfectious)
  - Bell's palsy/neuritis
  - Langerhans' cell histiocytosis
  - Granulomatosis with polyangiitis
- Traumatic Lesions
  - Longitudinal fracture
  - Transverse fracture
  - Complex fracture
  - Cephalocele
- Vascular Lesions
  - Aberrant position of the internal carotid artery
  - Persistent stapedial artery (PSA)
  - Dehiscence of the jugular vein bulb

Table 1.8 Lesions involving the middle ear

Lesions	Imaging Findings	Comments
Tumorlike lesions		
Acquired cholesteatoma (**Fig. 1.174, Fig. 1.175,** and **Fig. 1.176**)	*CT:* Soft tissue attenuation material is seen in Prussak's space, ± osseous erosions of the scutum, ossicular chain, and inner ear (labyrinthine fistula). *MRI:* Lesions often have low-intermediate signal on T1-weighted imaging, intermediate to high signal on T2-weighted imaging, and high signal on diffusion-weighted imaging. Lesions typically show no gadolinium contrast enhancement. MRI can show epidural extension related to osseous erosion at the attic.	Expansile lesion in the middle ear consisting of an enlarging collection of exfoliated keratin debris adjacent to keratinized stratified squamous epithelium (keratoma). More common in men than in women. These nonneoplastic acquired lesions may arise from retraction pockets, perforations, or ingrowth of outer epithelial cells of the tympanic membrane into the inner surface adjacent to the middle ear due to trauma, rapid air pressure changes, or infection. Eighty-two percent of lesions occur at the inner surface of the pars flaccida portion of the tympanic membrane, with progressive filling of Prussak's space, epitympanum, mastoid antrum, and other portions of the middle ear. Eighteen percent of lesions involve the pars tensa. Lesions can erode the ossicular chain and inner ear structures, causing labyrinthine fistulas, tegmen tympani demineralization and disruption, and widening of the aditus ad antrum.
Congenital cholesteatoma (**Fig. 1.177**)	*CT:* Soft tissue attenuation material is seen in the middle ear, ± osseous erosions of the ossicular chain and/or inner ear. *MRI:* Lesions often have low-intermediate signal on T1-weighted imaging, intermediate to slightly high signal on T2-weighted imaging, and high signal on diffusion-weighted imaging. Lesions typically show no gadolinium contrast enhancement. MRI can show epidural extension related to osseous erosion at the attic.	Uncommon type of cholesteatoma (epidermoid) representing only 2% of middle ear cholesteatomas. Etiology attributed to retained epithelial cell rests in the middle ear. Occur medial to an intact tympanic membrane without history of otitis media, otorrhea, or prior surgery. Progressive expansion results in conductive hearing loss, with presentation at 4–6 years of age. Commonly occur in the anterosuperior quadrant of the mesotympaum adjacent to the manubrium of the malleus.
Cholesterol granuloma	*CT:* Lesions usually have low attenuation. *MRI:* Lesions usually have high signal on T1-weighted imaging (T1WI) and fat-suppressed T1WI. Lesions may have high, intermediate and/or low signal on T2-weighted imaging (T2WI) and fat-suppressed T2WI. A peripheral rim of low signal on T2WI may also be seen from hemosiderin.	Lesions occur in young and middle-aged adults and occur when there is obstruction of mucosa-lined air cells in the temporal bone. Multiple cycles of hemorrhage and granulomatous reaction result in accumulation of cholesterol granules, chronic inflammatory cells including multinucleated giant cells, red blood cells, hemosiderin, fibrous tissue, and debris. The lesions are lined by fibrous connective tissue. Cholesterol granulomas occur less frequently as isolated lesions in the middle ear related to eustachian tube dysfunction that results in chronic middle ear effusions complicated by episodes of hemorrhage and blood breakdown products. Can be a cause of idiopathic hemotympanum.
Fibrous dysplasia (**Fig. 1.178**)	*CT:* Expansile bone changes with mixed intermediate and high attenuation, often in a ground-glass appearance. Can show contrast enhancement. *MRI:* Features depend on the proportions of bony spicules, collagen, fibroblastic spindle cells, hemorrhagic and/or cystic changes, and associated pathologic fracture, if present. Lesions are usually well circumscribed and have low or low-intermediate signal on T1-weighted imaging and proton density-weighted imaging. On T2-weighted imaging, lesions have variable mixtures of low, intermediate, and/or high signal, often surrounded by a low signal rim of variable thickness. Internal septations and cystic changes are seen in a minority of lesions. Bone expansion with thickened and/ or thinned cortex can be seen. Lesions show gadolinium contrast enhancement that varies in degree and pattern.	Benign medullary fibro-osseous lesion that can involve a single site (monostotic) or multiple locations (polyostotic). Thought to occur from developmental failure in the normal process of remodeling primitive bone to mature lamellar bone, with resultant zone or zones of immature trabeculae within dysplastic fibrous tissue. Accounts for ~ 10% of benign bone lesions. Patients range in age from < 1 year to 76 years; 75% of cases occur before the age of 30 years.

(continued on page 118)

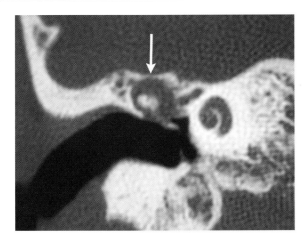

Fig. 1.174 Coronal CT of a 37-year-old man shows a cholesteatoma (*arrow*) in the right middle ear filling Prussak's space and the epitympanum; the lesion is associated with erosion of the scutum.

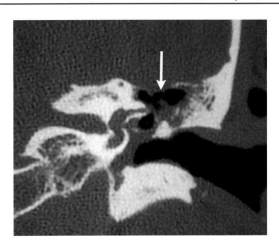

Fig. 1.175 Cholesteatoma seen on coronal CT as soft tissue attenuation within the hypotympanum, mesotympanum, and epitympanum is associated with erosion of bone, including the tegmen tympani (*arrow*). Demineralization of the osseous margin of the lateral semicircular canal is also seen.

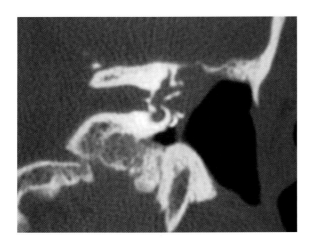

Fig. 1.176 Recurrent cholesteatoma after mastoidectomy seen on coronal CT as soft tissue attenuation within the middle ear displacing an ossicular prosthesis inferiorly. The recurrent cholesteatoma is associated with erosion of the lateral semicircular canal, causing a labyrinthine fistula. Erosion of the tegmen tympani is also seen.

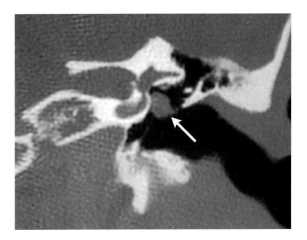

Fig. 1.177 Congenital cholesteatoma in a 16-year-old female. Coronal CT shows a lesion with soft tissue attenuation located deep to the intact tympanic membrane at the anterosuperior quadrant of the mesotympanum adjacent to the manubrium of the malleus (*arrow*).

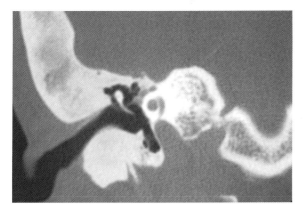

Fig. 1.178 Coronal CT shows fibrous dysplasia in the right temporal bone with diffuse osseous expansion and a ground-glass pattern of increased attenuation resulting in narrowing of the external auditory canal and middle ear.

Table 1.8 *(cont.)*   Lesions involving the middle ear

Lesions	Imaging Findings	Comments
Neoplasms		
Schwannoma (**Fig. 1.179, Fig. 1.180**, and **Fig. 1.181**)	*CT:* Ovoid or fusiform lesions with low-intermediate attenuation. Lesions can show contrast enhancement. Often erode adjacent bone. *MRI:* Circumscribed, lobulated or fusiform lesions with low-intermediate signal on T1-weighted imaging and intermediate-high signal on T2-weighted imaging, + prominent gadolinium contrast enhancement.	Schwannomas in the middle ear can originate within the tympanic space or result from extension from outside (such as from the inner ear from CN VIII schwannomas; or from the jugular foramen for schwannomas involving CN IX, X, or XI). Schwannomas originating in the middle ear include the CN VII facial nerve–chorda tympani (afferent taste sensation to the nucleus solitarius, and parasympathetic efferent-visceral motor fibers to the submandibular and sublingual glands); the tympanic branch (Jacobson's nerve) of CN IX, which includes sensory and visceral motor fibers; and the auricular branch carrying sensory fibers from the tympanic membrane, and (Arnold's nerve) of CN X. CN VII schwannomas account for most tumors of the middle ear. Multiple schwannomas are seen in neurofibromatosis type 2.

(continued on page 120)

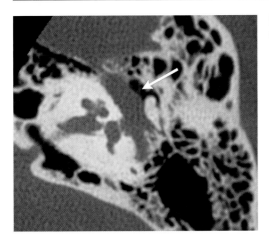

Fig. 1.179 Axial CT shows a fusiform-shaped facial nerve schwannoma (*arrow*) extending posteriorly from the geniculate ganglion passing medial to the malleus.

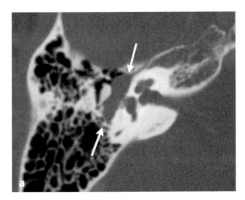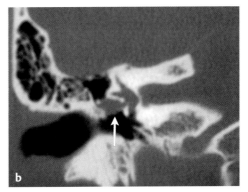

Fig. 1.180 **(a)** Axial and **(b)** coronal CT images show a fusiform-shaped facial nerve schwannoma (*arrows*) medial to the malleus **(a)** and inferior to the lateral semicircular canal (*arrow* in **b**).

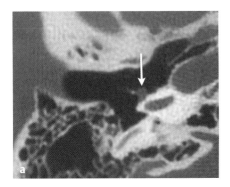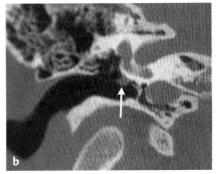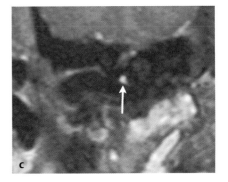

Fig. 1.181 **(a)** Axial and **(b)** coronal CT images show a small schwannoma (*arrows*) involving the tympanic branch of CN IX (Jacobson's nerve) located adjacent to the cochlear promontory. **(c)** The small schwannoma shows gadolinium contrast enhancement on coronal fat-suppressed T1-weighted imaging (*arrow*).

Table 1.8 *(cont.)* Lesions involving the middle ear

Lesions	Imaging Findings	Comments
Paraganglioma: Glomus tympanicum, Glomus jugulotympanicum (**Fig. 1.182** and **Fig. 1.183**)	*CT:* Spheroid or ovoid lesions with low-intermediate attenuation. Lesions can show contrast enhancement. Often erode adjacent bone. Glomus tympanicum tumors/paragangliomas occur where there are glomus bodies. In the middle ear, they are most frequently adjacent to the tympanic branch of CN IX (Jacobson's nerve) at the cochlear promontory. Glomus jugulare tumors extend into the middle ear from the jugular foramen. *MRI:* Circumscribed lesion with intermediate signal on T1-weighted imaging and often heterogeneous intermediate to slightly high signal on T2-weighted imaging, ± small flow voids, + gadolinium contrast enhancement. Can be associated with erosive bone changes.	Benign encapsulated neuroendocrine tumors that arise from neural crest cells associated with autonomic ganglia (paraganglia) throughout the body. Paraganglia cells are chemoreceptors involved in the detection of oxygen, carbon dioxide, and pH. Lesions are also referred to as chemodectomas and are named accordingly (glomus typanicum in the middle ear, glomus jugulare in jugular foramen, etc.). Paragangliomas are the most common tumor of the middle ear. Often immunoreactive to synaptophysin, chromogranin, and neuron-specific enolase. Tumors are typically not immunoreactive to cytokeratins 5 and 7, p63, SMA, and S-100 protein.
Adenoma	*CT:* Soft tissue attenuation tumor within the middle ear. *MRI:* Tumors often have low-intermediate signal on T1-weighted imaging and intermediate to slightly high signal on T2-weighted imaging, and usually show gadolinium contrast enhancement.	Rare benign epithelial neoplasms that arise from the modified respiratory mucosa of the middle ear. Rarely invade and destroy bone and do not metastasize. Subtypes include mucosal adenoma, papillary adenoma, inverted papilloma, and ceruminous adenoma. Mucosal adenomas are immunoreactive to cytokeratins, as well as p63. Ceruminous adenomas are immunoreactive to cytokeratins 5, 6, and 7, S-100 protein, p63, and SMA.
Carcinoid	*CT:* Soft tissue attenuation tumor within the middle ear. *MRI:* Tumors often have low-intermediate signal on T1-weighted imaging and intermediate to slightly high signal on T2-weighted imaging, and usually show gadolinium contrast enhancement.	Rare neuroendocrine tumor that can occur in the middle ear. These epithelial tumors consist of eosinophilic columnar cells with granular cytoplasm and round/oval nuclei. Tumors are immunoreactive to cytokeratin AE1–3, vimentin, and synaptophysin. Tumors are locally invasive and can metastasize.
Adenocarcinoma (**Fig. 1.184**)	*CT:* Soft tissue attenuation tumor within the middle ear. Can be associated with bone destruction. *MRI:* Tumors often have low-intermediate signal on T1-weighted imaging and intermediate to slightly high signal on T2-weighted imaging, and usually show gadolinium contrast enhancement. Tumors can destroy adjacent bone with extraosseous extension.	Very rare locally invasive neoplasm that arises from the middle ear mucosa. Tumors contain cuboidal cells with granular eosinophilic cytoplasm with centrally located nuclei arranged in cords and islands with or without glandular-appearing zones. Immunoreactive to keratin, vimentin, and S-100 protein. Ceruminous adenocarcinomas can appear as an adenoid cystic carcinoma type (imunoreactive to cytokeratins and 7, S-100 protein, p63, and SMA) or as a conventional type (immunoreactive to cytokeratin 7, but lacking reactivity to cytokeratin , S-100 protein, p63, and SMA.)
Squamous cell carcinoma	*CT:* Soft tissue attenuation tumor within the external auditory canal associated with bone invasion and destruction. *MRI:* Tumors often have low-intermediate signal on T1-weighted imaging and intermediate to slightly high signal on T2-weighted imaging, and usually show gadolinium contrast enhancement.	Most common malignancy involving the external auditory canal and middle ear. Often associated with chronic ear infection. More common in women, with a 5-year mortality of 50% when limited to the external auditory canal and 27% if extension into the middle ear occurs.

(continued on page 122)

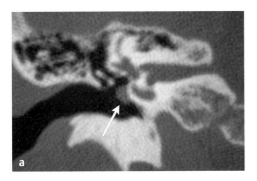

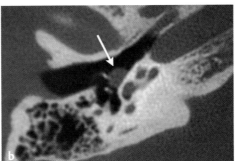

Fig. 1.182 (a) Coronal and **(b)** axial CT images show a small glomus tympanicum (*arrows*) in a 52-year-old woman that is located at the cochlear promontory.

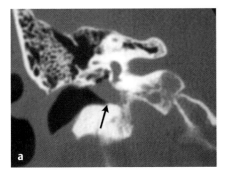

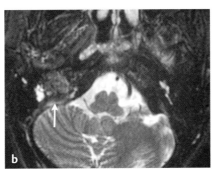

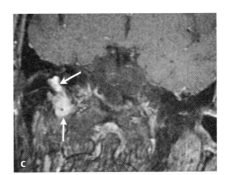

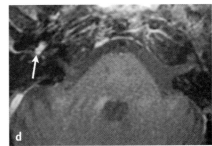

Fig. 1.183   Paraganglioma/glomus jugulotympanicum in a 54-year-old woman. **(a)** Coronal CT image shows a lesion with soft tissue attenuation in the right middle ear adjacent to erosive osseous changes at the jugular foramen (*arrow*). **(b)** The paraganglioma within the right jugular foramen extends into the middle ear and has mixed, intermediate, and slightly high signal with small flow voids on axial fat-suppressed T2-weighted imaging (*arrow*). **(c,d)** The lesion shows prominent gadolinium contrast enhancement on **(c)** coronal and **(d)** axial fat-suppressed T1-weighted imaging (*arrows*).

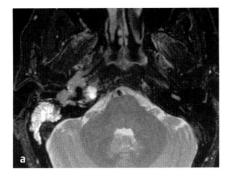

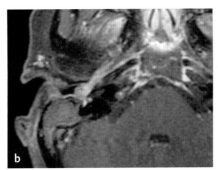

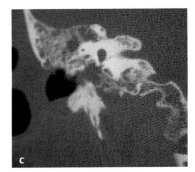

Fig. 1.184   A 61-year-old woman with adenocarcinoma involving the right temporal bone. **(a)** Axial fat-suppressed T2-weighted imaging shows a tumor filling the right middle ear that has intermediate to slightly high signal as well as retained secretions with high signal in the adjacent mastoid air cells and pneumatized petrous apex air cells. **(b)** Tumor in the middle ear shows gadolinium contrast enhancement on axial fat-suppressed T1-weighted imaging. **(c)** Coronal CT shows the tumor in the middle ear and associated destruction of the adjacent bone.

Table 1.8 *(cont.)* Lesions involving the middle ear

Lesions	Imaging Findings	Comments
Metastatic disease (**Fig. 1.185**)	*CT:* Single or multiple well-circumscribed or poorly defined infiltrative lesions involving the marrow and associated with cortical destruction and extraosseous extension. *MRI:* Lesions often have low-intermediate signal on T1-weighted imaging and low, intermediate, and/or high signal on T2-weighted imaging and fat-suppressed T1-weighted imaging, and usually show gadolinium contrast enhancement. Cortical destruction and tumor extension into the extraosseous soft tissues frequently occur.	Metastatic lesions typically occur in the marrow from hematogenous dissemination and are often associated with bone destruction and extraosseous tumor extension.
Meningioma (**Fig. 1.186**)	Extra-axial dura-based lesions that are well circumscribed. Location: supra- > infratentorial, parasagittal > convexity > sphenoid ridge > parasellar > posterior fossa > optic nerve sheath > intraventricular. *CT:* Tumors have intermediate attenuation, usually prominent contrast enhancement, ± calcifications, ± hyperostosis of adjacent bone. *MRI:* Tumors often have intermediate signal on T1-weighted imaging and intermediate to slightly high signal on T2-weighted imaging, and typically show prominent gadolinium contrast enhancement, ± calcifications, ± hyperostosis and/or invasion of adjacent skull. Some meningiomas have high signal on diffusion-weighted imaging.	Benign slow-growing tumors involving cranial and/or spinal dura that are composed of neoplastic meningothelial (arachnoidal or arachnoid cap) cells. Usually solitary and sporadic, but can also occur as multiple lesions in patients with neurofibromatosis type 2. Most are benign, although ~ 5% have atypical histologic features. Anaplastic meningiomas are rare and account for < 3% of meningiomas. Meningiomas account for up to 26% of primary intracranial tumors. Annual incidence is 6 per 100,000. Typically occur in adults (> 40 years old), and in women more than in men. Can result in compression of adjacent brain parenchyma, encasement of arteries, and compression of dural venous sinuses. Rarely, invasive/malignant types occur.
Infection		
Acute otitis media (**Fig. 1.187** and **Fig. 1.188**)	*CT:* Zones with fluid and/or soft tissue attenuation in the middle ear. *MRI:* Poorly defined zones of with low-intermediate signal on T1-weighted imaging, slightly high to high signal on T2-weighted imaging, and gadolinium contrast enhancement within the middle ear.	Infection of the middle ear and mastoid air cells, often caused by organisms like *Staphylococcus pneumoniae, Staphylococcus aureus,* and *Haemophilus influenzae.* Most cases of acute otitis media resolve. Symptoms include facial and ear pain. Complications include meningitis, brain abscess, and intracranial venous sinus thrombosis.

(continued on page 124)

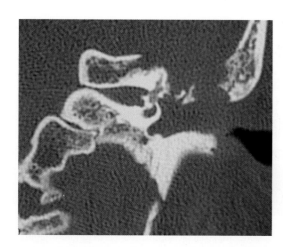

Fig. 1.185 Metastatic skeletal disease causing osseous destruction at the left temporal bone with extension into, and filling of, the left external auditory canal and left middle ear.

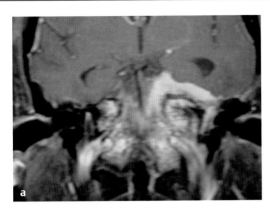
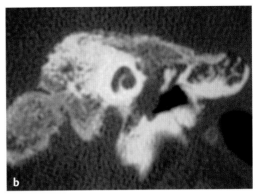

Fig. 1.186 **(a)** A 44-year-old woman with a gadolinium-enhancing meningioma at the inferior left middle cranial fossa on coronal fat-suppressed T1-weighted imaging that invades the petrous apex and tegmen typani of the left temporal bone and extends into the middle ear. **(b)** Coronal CT image shows thickening of the tegmen tympani from the invading meningioma, which also fills most of the middle ear.

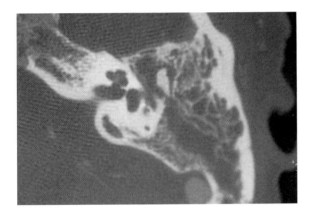

Fig. 1.187 Acute otitis media. Axial CT shows soft tissue attenuation filling the left middle ear and the mastoid air cells.

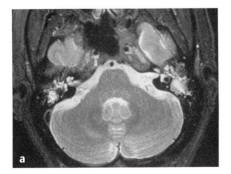
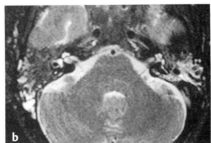
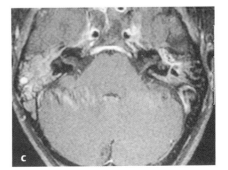

Fig. 1.188 Acute otitis media. **(a,b)** Axial fat-suppressed T2-weighted imaging in two different patients shows abnormal high T2 signal filling the mastoid air cells and middle ears. **(c)** Mild abnormal gadolinium contrast enhancement is seen bilaterally within both middle ears and mastoid air cells on axial fat-suppressed T1-weighted imaging, which corresponds to findings in **(b)**.

Table 1.8 *(cont.)*   Lesions involving the middle ear

Lesions	Imaging Findings	Comments
Chronic otitis media/ tympanosclerosis (**Fig. 1.189** and **Fig. 1.190**)	*CT:* Soft tissue attenuation granulation tissue and debris within the middle ear are typically seen. Osteolysis of mastoid septa can progress to an intramastoid empyema (coalescent mastoiditis). Calcifications within granulation tissue and debris within the middle ear may also occur (tympanosclerosis). *MRI:* Poorly defined zones of soft tissue thickening with low-intermediate signal on T1-weighted imaging, slightly high to high signal on T2-weighted imaging, and gadolinium contrast enhancement within the middle ear and mastoid air cells.	Chronic otitis media usually results from eustachian dysfunction and/or multiple prolonged episodes of infection, with inflammatory cellular infiltration of the mucoperiosteum of the middle ear, associated hyperemia, edema, and bone erosion by polypoid granulation tissue. Tympanosclerosis with calcified debris and granulation tissue in the middle ear can occur from hyalinization of collagen and fibro-osseous sclerosis.
Viral infection (**Fig. 1.191**)	*MRI:* Gadolinium (Gd) contrast enhancement can be seen in the intratympanic, mastoid, and geniculate portions of CN VII, ± Gd contrast enhancement of CN VII and VIII within the internal auditory canal, as well as Gd contrast enhancement involving the vestibule, cochlea, and/or semicircular canals (labyrinthitis).	Reactivation of the varicella-zoster virus (clinically referred to as herpes zoster) in the geniculate ganglion can result in acute onset of painful vesicles involving the tympanic membrane, external auditory canal, and pinna. Associated with facial paralysis or paresis secondary to neuritis involving CN VII, ± hearing loss and tinnitus from involvement of CN VIII.

(continued on page 126)

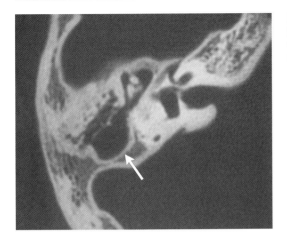

Fig. 1.189 Chronic otitis media in a 12-year-old female. Axial CT shows opacification of the right middle ear and mastoid air cells. The mastoid is small, with zones of lysis of mastoid bone septa related to an intramastoid empyema (referred to as coalescent mastoiditis) (*arrow*).

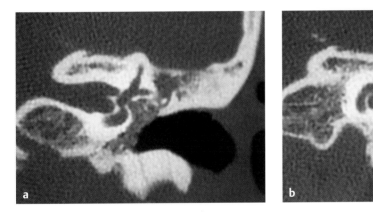

Fig. 1.190 Chronic otitis media/tympanosclerosis in a 21-year-old woman. **(a,b)** Coronal CT images show irregular calcifications within granulation tissue and debris in the left middle ear.

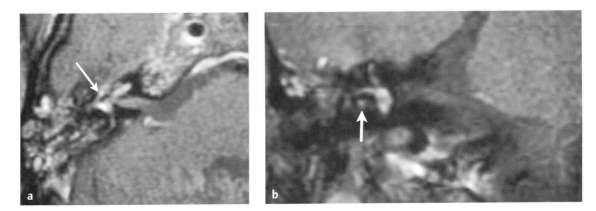

Fig. 1.191 A 41-year-old man with reactivation of latent varicella-zoster virus in the geniculate ganglion (Ramsay-Hunt syndrome; herpes zoster oticus). **(a)** Axial and **(b)** coronal fat-suppressed T1-weighted imaging show abnormal gadolinium contrast enhancement of the geniculate ganglion (*arrow* in **a**), intratympanic and mastoid portions of the facial nerve (*arrow* in **b**), cochlea, vestibule, and semicircular canals secondary to labyrinthitis, as well as CN VII and CN VIII within the internal auditory canal. Abnormal gadolinium contrast enhancement is also seen within the middle ear and mastoid air cells from superimposed otomastoiditis.

Table 1.8 *(cont.)* Lesions involving the middle ear

Lesions	Imaging Findings	Comments
Inflammation (noninfectious)		
Bell's palsy/neuritis **(Fig. 1.192)**	*MRI:* Gadolinium (Gd) contrast enhancement can be seen in the intratemporal, geniculate, intratympanic, and/or mastoid portions of CN VII without focal nodular enlargement, ± Gd contrast enhancement of CN VII in the fundal portion of the internal auditory canal.	Acute onset of idiopathic lower motor neuron facial paralysis that occurs in the absence of abnormalities involving the central nervous system, temporal bone, parotid gland, or other infratemporal sites. Other symptoms include altered taste sensation, ear pain, and facial numbness. May be preceded by a viral illness.
Langerhans' cell histiocytosis **(Fig. 1.193)**	Single or multiple circumscribed soft tissue lesions in the marrow of the skull associated with focal bony destruction/erosion and extension extra- or intracranially or both. *CT:* Lesions usually have low-intermediate attenuation, + contrast enhancement, ± enhancement of the adjacent dura. *MRI:* Lesions typically have low-intermediate signal on T1-weighted imaging and heterogeneous slightly high to high signal on FLAIR, T2-weighted imaging (T2WI), and fat-suppressed (FS) T2WI. Poorly defined zones of high signal on T2WI and FS T2WI are usually seen in the marrow and soft tissues peripheral to the lesions secondary to inflammatory changes. Extension of lesions from the marrow into adjacent soft tissues through areas of cortical disruption are commonly seen as well. Lesions typically show prominent gadolinium contrast enhancement in marrow and extraosseous soft tissue portions.	Single lesions are commonly seen in males more than in females and in patients < 20 years old. There is proliferation of histiocytes in medullary bone with localized destruction of cortical bone and extension into adjacent soft tissues. Multiple lesions are associated with Letterer-Siwe disease (lymphadenopathy hepatosplenomegaly) in children < 2 years old, and Hand-Schüller-Christian disease (lymphadenopathy, exophthalmos, diabetes insipidus) in children 5–10 years old.
Granulomatosis with polyangiitis	*CT:* Zones with soft tissue attenuation ± bone destruction. *MRI:* Poorly defined zones of soft tissue thickening with low-intermediate signal on T1-weighted imaging, slightly high to high signal on T2-weighted imaging, and gadolinium contrast enhancement within the middle ear and external auditory canal, ± bone invasion and destruction, ± extension into the skull base and intracranially, with involvement of the dura, brain, venous sinuses, nasopharynx, and/or infratemporal fossa.	Multisystem disease with necrotizing granulomas in the respiratory tract, focal necrotizing angiitis of small arteries and veins of various tissues, and glomerulonephritis. Typically, positive immunoreactivity to cytoplasmic antineutrophil cytoplasmic antibody (c-ANCA). Commonly involves the paranasal sinuses and occasionally the orbits. Involvement of temporal bone in 40–70% of cases. Peak prevalence is in the fifth decade. Treatment includes corticosteroids, cyclophosphamide, and anti-TNF agents.
Traumatic Lesions		
Longitudinal fracture **(Fig. 1.194)**	*CT: Anterior subtype of longitudinal fracture* extends from anterior squamosa to the petrous apex, ± tegmen tympani, facial nerve canal, and glenoid fossa, ± epidural hematoma. Blood/fluid present within the middle ear and mastoid air cells. *Posterior subtype of longitudinal fracture* extends from the posterior squamosa/mastoid bone to the foramen lacerum, ± ossicular chain disruption, hemotympanum. Blood/fluid present within the middle ear and mastoid air cells.	Fractures oriented parallel to the long axis of the petrous bone along the petrotympanic fissure that often occur from laterally oriented trauma. Account for up to 90% of temporal bone fractures. Fracture plane often extends anteromedial to the petrous apex, sparing the otic capsule. Can involve the ossicular chain (incudostapedial joint derangement more common than malleoincudal joint derangement) resulting in conductive hearing loss. Increased risk for eventual development of acquired cholesteatoma.
Transverse fracture **(Fig. 1.195)**	*CT:* Fractures extend from the foramen magnum or jugular foramen to the middle cranial fossa, ± involvement of the otic capsule, vestibular aqueduct, stapes footplate, and fundus of the internal auditory canal. Blood/fluid present within the middle ear and mastoid air cells.	Transverse fractures are oriented perpendicular to the long axis of the petrous bone from frontally or occipitally oriented trauma. Less common than longitudinal fractures, they account for < 10% of temporal bone fractures. Can involve the otic capsule, resulting in sensorineural hearing loss. Increased risk for perilymphatic fistula.

(continued on page 128)

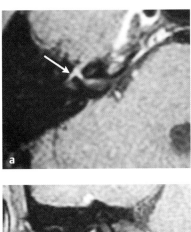
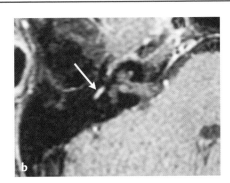
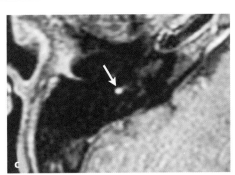
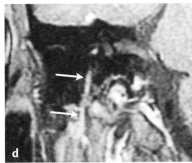

Fig. 1.192 Bell's palsy/neuritis in a 36-year-old man. **(a–c)** Abnormal gadolinium contrast enhancement is seen in the labyrinthine, geniculate, tympanic, and mastoid portions of the facial nerve (*arrows*) on axial and **(d)** coronal fat-suppressed T1-weighted imaging (*arrows*).

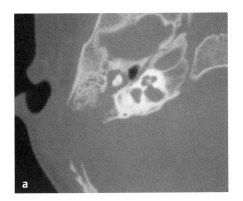
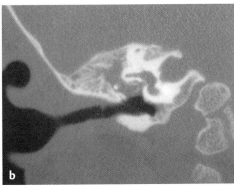

Fig. 1.193 Langerhans' cell histiocytosis in a 1-year-old male. An eosinophilic granuloma involving the right mastoid bone has caused osseous destruction and has extended into the right epitympanum and right external auditory canal, as seen on **(a)** axial and **(b)** coronal CT.

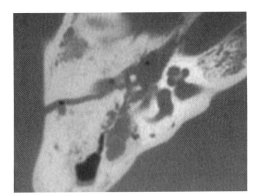

Fig. 1.194 Axial CT image shows a longitudinal fracture involving the right temporal bone oriented parallel to the long axis of the petrous bone along the petrotympanic fissure. The fracture plane extends anteromedial to the petrous apex, sparing the otic capsule. The fracture involves the ossicular chain, with malleoincudal dislocation.

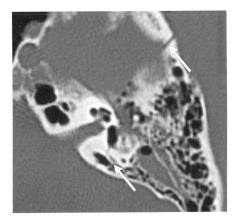

Fig. 1.195 Sensorineural hearing loss from a transverse fracture oriented perpendicular to the long axis of the petrous bone and which extends through the vestibule (*arrows*), with air present in the inner ear. Blood is present in the middle ear and mastoid air cells.

Table 1.8 *(cont.)*   Lesions involving the middle ear

Lesions	Imaging Findings	Comments
Complex fracture	*CT:* Fracture plane oriented transverse, longitudinal, and/or oblique to the long axis of the petrous bone, ± involvement of the ossicular chain, otic capsule, and tegmen tympani. Blood/fluid present within the middle ear and mastoid air cells.	Fractures that are oriented transverse, longitudinal, and/or oblique to the long axis of the petrous bone, ± ossicular chain disruption resulting in conductive hearing loss, ± otic capsule involvement with sensorineural hearing loss, ± facial nerve injury, ± increased risk for perilymphatic fistula, cholesteatoma.
Cephalocele **(Fig. 1.196)**	*CT:* Osseous defect in the tegmen tympani, with soft tissue attenuation in the middle ear from the cephalocele, ± CSF otorrhea. Fluid often present in mastoid air cells. *MRI:* Inferior herniation of meninges with or without brain tissue through an osseous defect of the tegmen tympani.	Defects in temporal bone with inferior protrusion of meninges without brain tissue (meningocele) or with brain tissue (meningoencephalocele). Osseous defects can result from mastoid surgery, traumatic fracture, cholesteatoma, mastoiditis, benign intracranial hypertension, and congenital tegmen defect. Can be associated with meningitis and CSF otorrhea.
Vascular Lesions		
Aberrant position of the internal carotid artery **(Fig. 1.197)**	Abnormal position of the internal carotid artery (ICA), which enters the middle ear posteriorly through an enlarged inferior tympanic canaliculus lateral to the expected site of the petrous carotid canal. The anomalous artery courses anteriorly over the cochlear promontory to connect with the horizontal petrous ICA via a dehiscent carotid bone plate. The aberrant ICA within the middle ear is usually smaller in caliber than the contralateral normal ICA.	Congenital arterial variation related to altered formation of the extracranial ICA resulting from agenesis of the normal first embryonic segment of the ICA. A collateral alternative developmental pathway occurs where the proximal ICA originates from the ascending pharyngeal artery connecting to the inferior tympanic artery, which extends superiorly through the inferior tympanic canal into the middle ear where it anastomoses with the caroticotympanic artery, which connects to the lateral petrous portion of the ICA. As a result, the ICA is positioned laterally within the middle ear cavity. Also, a characteristic narrowing of the inferior tympanic artery occurs as it passes through the inferior tympanic canal at the skull base. Often an incidental finding, with surgical planning implications.
Persistent stapedial artery (PSA) (See **Fig. 1.138**)	Commonly occurs as an anomalous small artery associated with an aberrant internal carotid artery (ICA) or as an isolated anomaly. Findings include an absent ipsilateral foramen spinosum. The small tubular PSA extends from the ICA along the cochlear promontory through the stapes and then adjacent to the tympanic segment of CN VII to an enlarged tympanic facial nerve canal, where it enters the middle cranial fossa as the middle meningeal artery.	Rare vascular anomaly that is often associated with an aberrant ICA. Results from lack of normal evolution of the embryonic hyoid artery (from the second anterior embryonic aortic arch) into the stapedial artery with eventual formation of the branches of the external carotid artery (ECA) supplying the orbits, meninges, and lower face, as well as the small caroticotympanic and superior tympanic arteries. Lack of normal involution of the stapedial artery results in a persistent stapedial artery that extends from the ICA into the middle ear, passing through the stapes near the course of the tympanic portion of CN VII and extending intracranially to supply the middle meningeal artery. As a result, the middle meningeal artery is not supplied by the ECA and internal maxillary artery. There is no ipsilateral foramen spinosum.
Dehiscence of the jugular vein bulb **(Fig. 1.198)**	Protrusion of the jugular bulb into the posteroinferior portion of the middle ear related to deficient or absent bone at the jugular plate.	Venous variant anatomy, with the jugular bulb extending superiorly and laterally into the middle ear through localized bone deficiency/dehiscence of the jugular plate. May be associated with pulsatile tinnitus, Ménière disease, and hearing loss. Important to report for surgical planning.

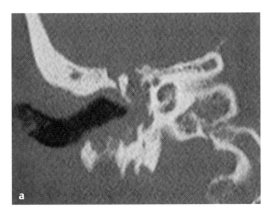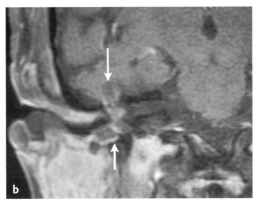

Fig. 1.196 Posttraumatic encephalocele with CSF otorhea. **(a)** Coronal CT shows a defect of the tegmen tympani with fluid filling the middle ear and mastoid air cells. **(b)** Coronal T1-weighted imaging after gadolinium contrast administration shows herniation of brain tissue and meninges inferiorly through a skull defect (*arrows*).

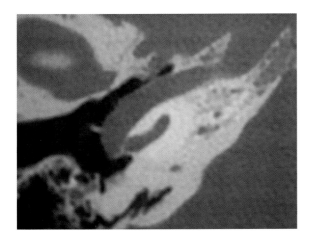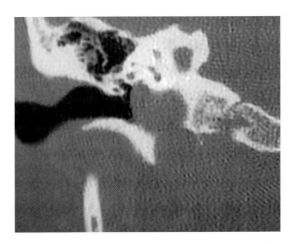

Fig. 1.197 Axial CT image shows the right internal carotid artery passing through the middle ear and positioned lateral to the basal turn of the cochlea.

Fig. 1.198 High-riding jugular bulb with extension into the middle ear, as seen on coronal CT. There is bony dehiscence where the jugular vein protrudes into the right middle ear.

Table 1.9 Acquired lesions involving the inner ear

- Tumorlike lesions
  - Cholesteatoma/Labyrinthine fistula
  - Dehiscence of the superior semicircular canal
  - Cholesterol granuloma
- Neoplasms
  - Schwannoma
  - Intratemporal benign vascular tumor/ Hemangioma
  - Metastatic disease

- Inflammatory Diseases
  - Acute/subacute labyrinthitis
  - Labyrinthitis ossificans
  - Bell's palsy/Neuritis
  - Langerhans' cell histiocytosis
  - Granulomatosis with polyangiitis
- Traumatic Lesions
  - Transverse fracture
  - Complex fracture
- Osseous Abnormalities
  - Otosclerosis
  - Osteogenesis imperfecta (OI)
  - Fibrous dysplasia
  - Paget disease
  - Renal osteodystrophy

Table 1.9 Acquired lesions involving the inner ear

Lesions	MRI Findings	Comments
Tumorlike lesions		
Cholesteatoma/ Labyrinthine fistula (**Fig. 1.199**)	*CT:* Soft tissue attenuation material is seen in the middle ear, ± osseous erosions of the scutum, ossicular chain, and inner ear (labyrinthine fistula). *MRI:* Lesions often have low-intermediate signal on T1-weighted imaging, intermediate to high signal on T2-weighted imaging, and high signal on diffusion-weighted imaging. Lesions typically show no gadolinium contrast enhancement. MRI can show epidural extension related to osseous erosion at the attic.	Expansile lesion in the middle ear consisting of an enlarging collection of exfoliated keratin debris adjacent to keratinized stratified squamous epithelium (keratoma). Lesions can erode the ossicular chain and inner ear structures, causing labyrinthine fistulas, tegmen tympani defects, and widening of the aditus ad antrum.
Dehiscence of the superior semicircular canal (**Fig. 1.200**)	Lack of bone covering the superior semicircular canal seen on high-resolution CT.	Developmental absence or severe thinning of bone covering the superior semicircular canal that can result in abnormal flow dynamics of endolymph in the semicircular canals. Can result in disequilibrium, oscillopsia, and/or Tulio phenomenon (vertigo with or without nystagmus caused by sound).
Cholesterol granuloma	*CT:* Lesions usually have low attenuation. *MRI:* Lesions usually have high signal on T1-weighted imaging (T1WI) and fat-suppressed (FS) T1WI. Lesions may have high, intermediate, and/or low signal on T2-weighted imaging (T2WI) and FS T2WI. A peripheral rim of low signal on T2WI may also be seen from hemosiderin.	Lesions occur in young and middle-aged adults and occur when there is obstruction of mucosa-lined air cells in the temporal bone. Multiple cycles of hemorrhage and granulomatous reaction result in accumulation of cholesterol granules, chronic inflammatory cells including multinucleated giant cells, red blood cells, hemosiderin, fibrous tissue, and debris. The lesions are lined by fibrous connective tissue. Cholesterol granulomas can erode the osseous margins of the inner ear.
Neoplasms		
Schwannoma (**Fig. 1.201** and **Fig. 1.202**)	*MRI:* Circumscribed spheroid, ovoid, or fusiform lesions with low-intermediate signal on T1-weighted imaging, high signal on T2-weighted imaging (T2WI) and fat-suppressed T2WI, and usually prominent gadolinium contrast enhancement. *CT:* Ovoid or fusiform lesions with intermediate attenuation, + contrast enhancement. Large lesions can have cystic degeneration and/or hemorrhage, ± erosion of adjacent bone.	Schwannomas are benign encapsulated tumors that contain differentiated neoplastic Schwann cells. Multiple schwannomas are often associated with neurofibromatosis type 2, which is an autosomal dominant disease involving a gene at chromosome 22q12. Intralabyrinthine schwannomas can involve both the internal auditory canal (IAC) and cochlea (transmodiolar), or IAC and vestibule (transmacular), or IAC, inner ear, and middle ear (transotic). Schwannomas can also be isolated to the inner ear.

(continued on page 132)

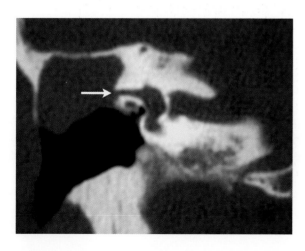

Fig. 1.199 Coronal CT shows a recurrent cholesteatoma with soft tissue attenuation in the right mastoidectomy site and epitympanum. The lesion is associated with erosion of the bone covering the lateral semicircular canal, resulting in a labyrinthine fistula (*arrow*).

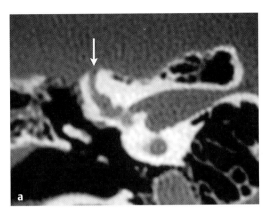
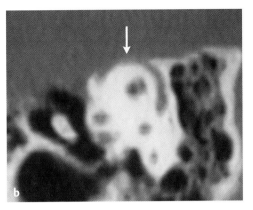

Fig. 1.200 **(a)** Coronal and **(b)** sagittal CT images show dehiscence of the bone covering the superior semicircular canal (*arrows*).

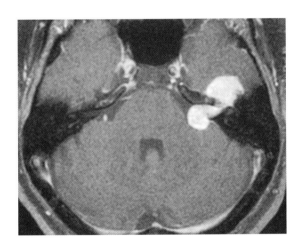

Fig. 1.201 Schwannoma of CN VII in a 54-year-old man. Gadolinium contrast enhancement is seen involving the schwannoma of the left CN VII at the left cerebellopontine angle cistern, left internal auditory canal, and left geniculate ganglion, with associated erosion of the left petrous apex on axial fat-suppressed T1-weighted imaging.

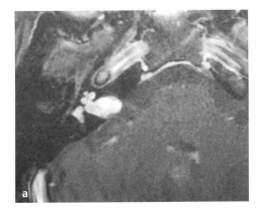
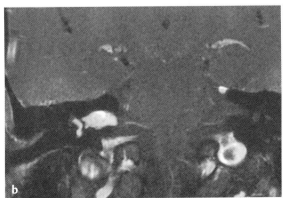

Fig. 1.202 Schwannoma of CN VIII in a 49-year-old man. Gadolinium contrast enhancement is seen involving the schwannoma of the right CN VIII in the right internal auditory canal and extending into the cochlea and vestibule of the right inner ear on **(a)** axial and **(b)** coronal fat-suppressed T1-weighted imaging.

Table 1.9 *(cont.)* Acquired lesions involving the inner ear

Lesions	MRI Findings	Comments
Intratemporal benign vascular tumor/ Hemangioma **(Fig. 1.203)**	*CT:* Radiolucent zone with low-intermediate attenuation containing small bone spicules within the temporal bone in the region of the geniculate ganglion, usually showing contrast enhancement. *MRI:* Lesions have intermediate signal on T1-weighted imaging, slightly high to high signal on T2-weighted imaging, and gadolinium contrast enhancement.	Benign lesions composed of thin-walled vascular spaces within the temporal bone along the course of the facial nerve, often at or near the geniculate ganglion. The lesions grow within bone and are usually radiolucent, containing bone spicules. Lesions can be associated with slowly progressive or recurrent facial paralysis.
Metastatic disease **(Fig. 1.204)**	*CT:* Single or multiple well-circumscribed or poorly defined infiltrative lesions involving the marrow associated with cortical destruction and extraosseous extension. *MRI:* Lesions often have low-intermediate signal on T1-weighted imaging (T1WI), low, intermediate, and/or high signal on T2-weighted imaging and fat-suppressed T1WI, and usually gadolinium contrast enhancement. Cortical bone destruction and tumor extension into the extraosseous soft tissues frequently occur.	Metastatic lesions typically occur in the marrow from hematogenous dissemination and are often associated with bone destruction and extraosseous tumor extension.
Inflammatory Diseases		
Acute/subacute labyrinthitis **(Fig. 1.205** and **Fig. 1.206)**	*MRI:* Typical findings include abnormal gadolinium (Gd) contrast enhancement of the cochlea, vestibule, and/or semicircular canals. Gd contrast enhancement of the labyrinthine portion of CN VII can be seen with herpes zoster oticus (Ramsay-Hunt syndrome). Lack of resolution of acute labyrinthitis can result in fibroblastic and osteoblastic proliferation, with decreased signal in the inner ear on T2-weighted imaging.	Inflammatory disorder of the inner ear involving the membranous labyrinth and perilymphatic spaces. Often associated with sensorineural hearing loss and vertigo. Inflammation can result from viral or bacterial infections or occur as an autoimmune disorder. Viral labyrinthitis is the most common type and is often related to an upper respiratory infection with hematogenous spread to the inner ear. Symptoms from viral labyrinthitis are usually transient. Bacterial labyrinthitis usually results from pyogenic bacterial infection (*Streptococccus pneumoniae, Haemophilus influenzae,* etc.) of the inner ear from hematogenous spread, or as a complication of otitis media, meningitis, trauma, or surgery. Facial nerve symptoms are more common with bacterial labyrinthitis than viral labyrinthitis. Autoimmune labyrinthitis is uncommon, is diagnosed with a positive lymphocyte transformation test, and responds to steroids. Cogan's syndrome includes autoimmune labyrinthitis as well as interstitial keratitis, orbital pseudotumor, uveitis, and/or aortitis.

(continued on page 134)

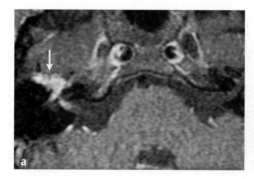 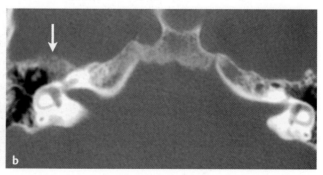

Fig. 1.203 **(a)** Axial fat-suppressed T1-weighted imaging shows gadolinium contrast enhancement involving the geniculate ganglion of the right facial nerve (*arrow*), representing an intratemporal benign vascular tumor/hemangioma in a 40-year-old man. **(b)** On axial CT, the partially radiolucent lesion (*arrow*) contains bone spicules.

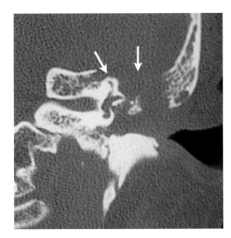

Fig. 1.204 Coronal CT shows metastatic skeletal disease causing osseous destruction at the left temporal bone with extension into, and filling the left external auditory canal and left middle ear (*arrows*).

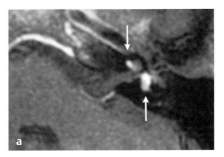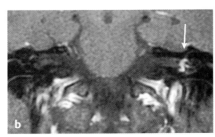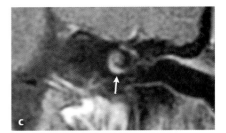

Fig. 1.205 **(a)** Axial and **(b,c)** coronal fat-suppressed T1-weighted images show abnormal gadolinium contrast enhancement involving the cochlea, vestibule, and semicircular canals (*arrows*) in a patient with labyrinthitis.

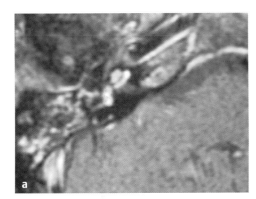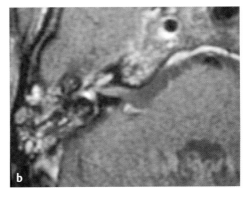

Fig. 1.206 A 41-year-old man with Ramsay-Hunt syndrome. **(a,b)** Abnormal gadolinium contrast enhancement is seen involving the right inner ear (cochlea, vestibule, and semicircular canals), CN VII, middle ear, and mastoid air cells on axial fat-suppressed T1-weighted imaging.

Table 1.9 *(cont.)* Acquired lesions involving the inner ear

Lesions	MRI Findings	Comments
Labyrinthitis ossificans (**Fig. 1.207** and **Fig. 1.208**)	*CT:* Focal and/or diffuse ossifications within portions or all of the inner ear. Complete ossification is referred to labyrinthitis obliterans. *MRI:* Lack of resolution of acute labyrinthitis can result in fibroblastic and osteoblastic proliferation, with decreased signal in the inner ear on T2-weighted imaging, ± gadolinium contrast enhancement.	Lack of resolution of acute/subacute labyrinthitis can result in chronic labyrinthitis with fibroblastic and osteoblastic proliferation leading to ossifications within the inner ear, severely damaging the membranous labyrinth.
Bell's palsy/Neuritis (**Fig. 1.209**)	*MRI:* Gadolinium (Gd) contrast enhancement can be seen involving the intratemporal, geniculate, intratympanic, and/or mastoid portions of CN VII without focal nodular enlargement, ± Gd contrast enhancement of CN VII in the fundal portion of the internal auditory canal.	Acute onset of idiopathic lower motor neuron facial paralysis that occurs in the absence of abnormalities involving the central nervous system, temporal bone, parotid gland, or other infratemporal sites. Other symptoms include altered taste sensation, ear pain, and facial numbness. May be preceded by a viral illness.
Langerhans' cell histiocytosis	Single or multiple circumscribed soft tissue lesions in the marrow of the skull associated with focal bony destruction/erosion and extension extra- or intracranially or both. *CT:* Lesions usually have low-intermediate attenuation, + contrast enhancement, ± enhancement of the adjacent dura. *MRI:* Lesions typically have low-intermediate signal on T1-weighted imaging and heterogeneous slightly high to high signal on FLAIR, T2-weighted imaging (T2WI), and fat-suppressed (FS) T2WI. Poorly defined zones of high signal on T2WI and FS T2WI are usually seen in the marrow and soft tissues peripheral to the lesions, secondary to inflammatory changes. Extension of lesions from the marrow into adjacent soft tissues through areas of cortical disruption are commonly seen as well. Lesions typically show prominent gadolinium contrast enhancement in marrow and extraosseous soft tissue portions.	Single lesions are commonly seen in males more than in females, and in patients < 20 years old. Proliferation of histiocytes in medullary bone with localized destruction of cortical bone and extension into adjacent soft tissues. Multiple lesions are associated with Letterer-Siwe disease (lymphadenopathy hepatosplenomegaly) in children < 2 years old, and Hand-Schüller-Christian disease (lymphadenopathy, exophthalmos, diabetes insipidus) in children 5–10 years old.
Granulomatosis with polyangiitis	*CT:* Zones with soft tissue attenuation ± bone destruction. *MRI:* Poorly defined zones of soft tissue thickening with low-intermediate signal on T1-weighted imaging, slightly high to high signal on T2-weighted imaging, and gadolinium contrast enhancement within the middle ear and external auditory canal, ± bone invasion and destruction, ± extension into the skull base and intracranially, with involvement of the dura, brain, venous sinuses, nasopharynx, and/or infratemporal fossa.	Multisystem disease with necrotizing granulomas in the respiratory tract, focal necrotizing angiitis of small arteries and veins of various tissues, and glomerulonephritis. Typically, positive immunoreactivity to cytoplasmic antineutrophil cytoplasmic antibody (c-ANCA). Commonly involves the paranasal sinuses and occasionally the orbits. Involvement of the temporal bone in 40% of cases. Peak prevalence is in the fifth decade. Treatment includes corticosteroids, cyclophosphamide, and anti-TNF agents.

(continued on page 136)

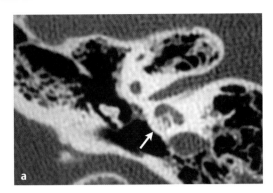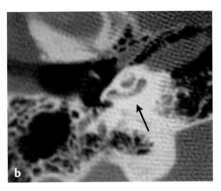

Fig. 1.207 Labyrinthitis ossificans. **(a)** Coronal and **(b)** axial CT images show ossifications within the right cochlea (*arrows*).

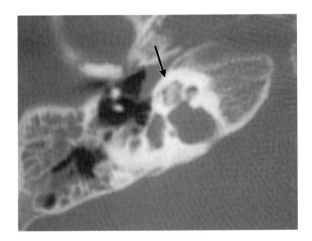

Fig. 1.208 Labyrinthitis ossificans. Axial CT shows ossifications (*arrow*) within the right cochlea.

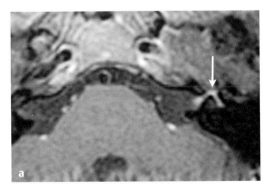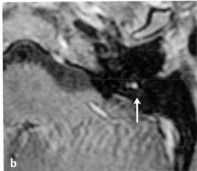

Fig. 1.209 Bell's palsy/neuritis in a 25-year-old woman. **(a,b)** Abnormal gadolinium contrast enhancement is seen in the labyrinthine, tympanic (*arrow* in **a**), and mastoid (*arrow* in **b**) segments of the left facial nerve (*arrows*) on axial fat-suppressed T1-weighted imaging.

Table 1.9 *(cont.)* Acquired lesions involving the inner ear

Lesions	MRI Findings	Comments
Traumatic Lesions		
Transverse fracture (**Fig. 1.210**)	*CT:* Fractures extend from the foramen magnum or jugular foramen to the middle cranial fossa, ± involvement of the otic capsule, vestibular aqueduct, stapes footplate, and fundus of the internal auditory canal. Blood/fluid present within the middle ear and mastoid air cells.	Transverse fractures are oriented perpendicular to the long axis of the petrous bone from frontally or occipitally oriented trauma. Less common than longitudinal fractures, they account for < 10% of temporal bone fractures. Can involve the otic capsule, resulting in sensorineural hearing loss. Increased risk for perilymphatic fistula.
Complex fracture	*CT:* Fracture plane oriented transverse, longitudinal, and/or oblique to the long axis of the petrous bone, ± involvement of the ossicular chain, otic capsule, and tegmen tympani. Blood/fluid present within the middle ear and mastoid air cells.	Fractures that are oriented transverse, longitudinal, and/or oblique to the long axis of the petrous bone, ± ossicular chain disruption resulting in conductive hearing loss, ± otic capsule involvement with sensorineural hearing loss, ± facial nerve injury, ± increased risk for perilymphatic fistula, cholesteatoma.
Osseous Abnormalities		
Otosclerosis (**Fig. 1.211, Fig. 1.212**, and **Fig. 1.213**)	*CT:* Radiolucent zones at the otic capsule adjacent to the oval window (fenestral type). Can progress and extend around the cochlea (cochlear type), forming a *double ring sign*. *MRI:* Small zones with gadolinium contrast enhancement may be seen at the involved sites.	Progressive conductive or mixed hearing loss that occurs in adults resulting from spongiotic-lytic bone changes of unknown etiology in the otic capsule. Often bilateral. Fenestral type is more common (85%) and is associated with conductive hearing loss from fixation of the stapes footplate. The cochlear type of otosclerosis occurs in 15% and often presents with both conductive and sensorineural hearing loss.
Osteogenesis imperfecta (OI) (See **Fig. 1.241**)	*CT:* Diffuse osteopenia, with undermineralized thickened bone around the otic capsule. Can appear similar to otosclerosis. *MRI:* Perichochlear bandlike zones of gadolinium contrast enhancement can be seen corresponding to the sites of demineralization seen on CT.	Also referred to as brittle bone disease, OI has four to seven types. OI is a hereditary disorder with abnormal type I fibrillar collagen production and osteoporosis resulting from mutations of the *COL1A1* gene on chromosome 17q21.31-q22.05 and the *COL1A2* gene on chromosome 7q22.1. Results in fragile bone prone to repetitive microfractures and remodeling.

(continued on page 138)

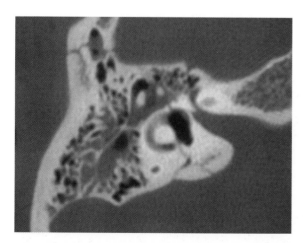

Fig. 1.210 Axial CT shows a transverse fracture through the right temporal bone with air in the vestibule.

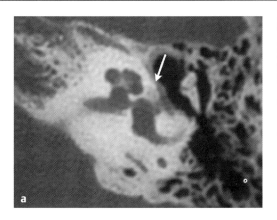
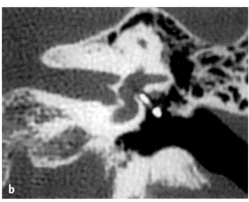

Fig. 1.211 Fenestral otosclerosis. **(a)** Axial CT image shows a small zone of demineralization anterior to the oval window (*arrow*). **(b)** Coronal CT shows treatment of fixation of the stapes caused by otosclerosis with a stapes prosthesis.

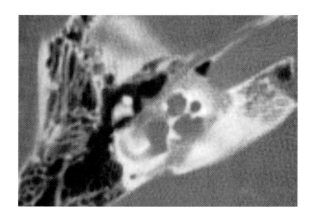

Fig. 1.212 Axial CT image shows irregular zones of demineralization adjacent to the oval window, vestibule, and cochlea caused by otosclerosis.

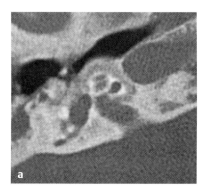
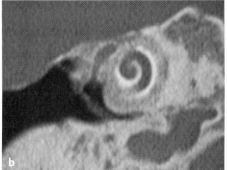
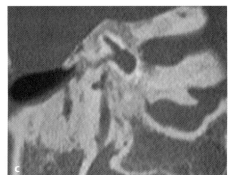

Fig. 1.213 **(a)** Axial and **(b,c)** coronal CT images show extensive otosclerosis with zones of demineralization adjacent to the oval window, vestibule, semicircular canals, and cochlea (*double ring sign*).

Table 1.9 *(cont.)* Acquired lesions involving the inner ear

Lesions	MRI Findings	Comments
Fibrous dysplasia (See **Fig. 1.237**)	*CT:* Expansile bone changes with mixed intermediate and high attenuation, often in a ground-glass appearance. Can show contrast enhancement. *MRI:* Features depend on the proportions of bony spicules, collagen, fibroblastic spindle cells, hemorrhagic and/or cystic changes, and associated pathologic fracture, if present. Lesions are usually well circumscribed and have low or low-intermediate signal on T1-weighted imaging and FLAIR imaging. On T2-weighted imaging, lesions have variable mixtures of low, intermediate, and/or high signal. Bone expansion with thickened and/or thinned cortex can be seen. Lesions show gadolinium contrast enhancement that varies in degree and pattern.	Benign medullary fibro-osseous lesion that can involve a single site (monostotic) or multiple locations (polyostotic). Results from developmental failure in the normal process of remodeling primitive bone to mature lamellar bone, with resultant zone or zones of immature trabeculae within dysplastic fibrous tissue. Accounts for ~ 10% of benign bone lesions. Patients range in age from < 1 year to 76 years; 75% of cases occur before the age of 30 years.
Paget disease (See **Fig. 1.238**)	*CT:* Lesions often have mixed intermediate and high attenuation. Irregular/indistinct borders between marrow and inner margins of the outer and inner tables of the skull. *MRI:* Most cases involving the skull are the late or inactive phases. Findings include osseous expansion and cortical thickening with low signal on T1- and T2-weighted imaging. The inner margins of the thickened cortex can be irregular and indistinct. Zones of low signal on T1- and T2-weighted imaging can be seen in the diploic marrow secondary to thickened bony trabeculae. Marrow in late or inactive phases of Paget disease can have signal similar to normal marrow, contain focal areas of fat signal, have low signal on T1- and T2-weighted imaging secondary to regions of sclerosis, have areas of high signal on fat-suppressed T2-weighted imaging caused by edema or persistent fibrovascular tissue.	Paget disease is a chronic skeletal disease in which there is disordered bone resorption and woven bone formation, resulting in osseous deformity. A paramyxovirus may be the etiologic agent. Paget disease is polyostotic in up to 66% of patients. Paget disease is associated with a risk of less than 1% for developing secondary sarcomatous changes. Occurs in 2.5 to 5% of Caucasians older than 55 years and 10% of those over the age of 85 years. Can result in narrowing of neuroforamina, with cranial nerve compression and basilar impression, ± compression of the brainstem.
Renal osteodystrophy (See **Fig. 1.239**)	*CT:* Trabecular bone resorption with a *salt-and-pepper appearance* caused by mixed osteolysis and osteosclerosis, osteitis fibrosa cystica, cortical thinning, coarsened trabecular pattern, and osteolytic lesions/brown tumors. Another pattern is ground-glass appearance with indistinct corticomedullary borders. *MRI:* Zones of low signal on T1- and T2-weighted imaging corresponding to regions of bone sclerosis. Circumscribed zones with high signal on T2-weighted imaging are due to osteolytic lesions or brown tumors.	Osteoblastic and osteoclastic changes that occur in bone as a result of chronic end-stage renal disease, secondary hyperparathyroidism (hyperplasia of parathyroid glands), and osteomalacia (abnormal vitamin D metabolism). Can result in pathologic fracture. Unlike in secondary hyperparathyroidism, diffuse or patchy bone sclerosis infrequently occurs in primary hyperparathyroidism.

Table 1.10   Lesions involving the petrous apex

- Acquired Abnormalities
  - Retained secretions in pneumatized petrous apex air cells
  - Cholesterol granuloma
  - Epidermoid/cholesteatoma
  - Petrous apex mucocele
  - Petrous apex cephalocele
- Inflammatory Lesions
  - Petrous apicitis
  - Osteomyelitis
  - Langerhans' cell histiocytosis
  - Granulomatosis with polyangiitis
  - Sarcoidosis
- Vascular Abnormalities
  - Carotid artery aneurysm/ pseudoaneurysm
- Benign Tumors
  - Meningioma
  - Schwannoma
  - Paraganglioma
  - Endolymphatic sac cystadenoma
  - Intratemporal benign vascular tumor/hemangioma
- Malignant Tumors
  - Metastatic disease
  - Myeloma/plasmacytoma
  - Lymphoma
  - Chordoma
  - Chondrosarcoma
  - Osteosarcoma
  - Invasive pituitary adenoma
  - Sinonasal squamous cell carcinoma
  - Nasopharyngeal carcinoma
  - Adenoid cystic carcinoma
  - Rhabdomyosarcoma
- Osseous Abnormalities
  - Fibrous dysplasia
  - Paget disease
  - Renal osteodystrophy
  - Otosclerosis
  - Osteogenesis imperfecta (OI)
  - Osteopetrosis
  - Cleidocranial dysplasia (CCD)
- Traumatic Lesions
  - Transverse fracture
  - Complex fracture

Table 1.10   Lesions involving the petrous apex

Lesions	Imaging Findings	Comments
Acquired Abnormalities		
Retained secretions in pneumatized petrous apex air cells (**Fig. 1.214**)	*CT:* Low-attenuation fluid present in multiple petrous apex air cells with or without fluid and inflammatory changes in the middle ear and/or mastoid air cells. No bone destruction or expansion. *MRI:* Zones with low signal on T1-weighted imaging and high signal on T2-weighted imaging, and no gadolinium contrast enhancement.	The petrous apex is normally pneumatized in ~ 33% of patients. Retained secretions in these mucosa-lined air cells can occur as isolated findings or in association with otitis media and/or mastoiditis. Often are asymptomatic incidental findings.

(continued on page 140)

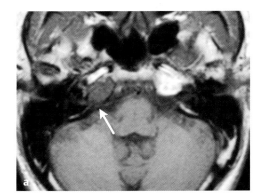 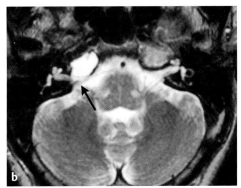

Fig. 1.214   A 48-year-old man with retained secretions in pneumatized right petrous apex air cells, which have low-intermediate signal on **(a)** axial T1-weighted imaging (*arrow*) and high signal on **(b)** axial T2-weighted imaging (*arrow*). Fatty marrow within the left petrous apex has high signal on T1-weighted imaging and intermediate signal on axial T2-weighted imaging.

Table 1.10 *(cont.)* Lesions involving the petrous apex

Lesions	Imaging Findings	Comments
Cholesterol granuloma (**Fig. 1.215**)	Circumscribed lesion measuring between 2 and 4 cm in the marrow of the petrous bone, often associated with mild bone expansion. *CT:* Lesions usually have low attenuation. *MRI:* Lesions usually have high signal on T1-weighted imaging (T1WI) and fat-suppressed T1WI, low, intermediate, and/or high signal on T2-weighted imaging, and no gadolinium contrast enhancement. A peripheral rim of low signal on T2-weighted imaging may also be seen due to hemosiderin.	Most common lesion in petrous apex. Other sites include the mastoid bone and middle ear. Lesions occur in young and middle-aged adults and occur when there is obstruction of mucosa-lined air cells in the petrous bone. Multiple cycles of hemorrhage and granulomatous reaction result in accumulation of cholesterol granules, chronic inflammatory cells, red blood cells, hemosiderin, fibrous tissue, and debris.
Epidermoid/ cholesteatoma (**Fig. 1.216**)	*CT:* Well-circumscribed spheroid ectodermal-inclusion cystic lesions within or adjacent to the skull associated with chronic bone erosion, low-intermediate attenuation, and no contrast enhancement. *MRI:* Lesions have low-intermediate signal on T1-weighted imaging, and ADC, high signal on T2-weighted imaging, FLAIR, and diffusion-weighted imaging, and no gadolinium contrast enhancement.	Accounts for 4–9% of lesions involving the petrous apex, and arises from trapped ectoderm during embryogenesis. Nonneoplastic lesions with peripheral layer of stratified squamous epithelium surrounding internal contents of desquamated cells and keratinaceous debris. Bone expansion and thinning commonly occur. Intracranial extra-axial epidermoids can also erode into the temporal bone.
Petrous apex mucocele (**Fig. 1.217**)	*CT:* Circumscribed expansile lesion within the petrous apex that has variable low, intermediate, and/or high signal attenuation depending on mucus, inspissated mucus, and protein concentration in retained fluid. Typically associated with expansion and thinning of bone margins at the petrous apex. *MRI:* Lesions usually have low-intermediate signal on T1-weighted imaging (T1WI) and diffusion-weighted imaging and high signal on T2-weighted imaging (T2WI). Increased signal on T1WI and decreased signal on T2WI can occur when there is increased protein concentration in the retained fluid/ inspissated secretions. Lesions usually have peripheral gadolinium contrast enhancement.	Uncommon lesions that occur from chronic obstruction of the ostia from pneumatized petrous apex air cells to the mastoid air cells and/or middle ear. Progressive accumulation of retained secretions from the sinus mucosa results in thinning and outward expansion of the osseous margins. Mucoceles occur most commonly in the frontal sinuses, followed by the ethmoid, maxillary, and sphenoid sinuses.

(continued on page 142)

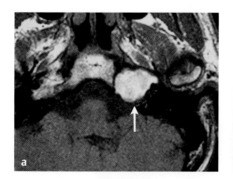
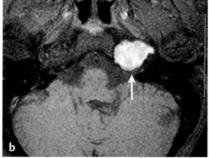
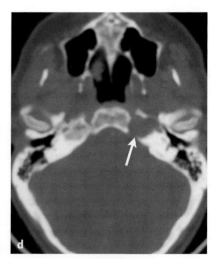
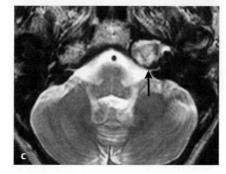

Fig. 1.215 A 40-year-old man with a cholesterol granuloma involving an expanded left petrous apex that has high signal on **(a)** axial T1-weighted imaging (*arrow*) and **(b)** fat-suppressed T1-weighted imaging (*arrow*). **(c)** The lesion has mixed low, intermediate and high signal on axial T2-weighted imaging (*arrow*). **(d)** The lesion is radiolucent, with expanded and thinned bony margins on axial CT (*arrow*).

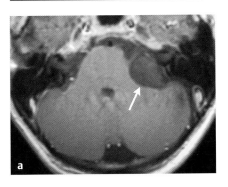

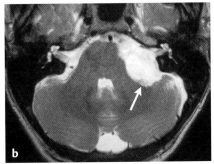

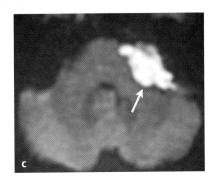

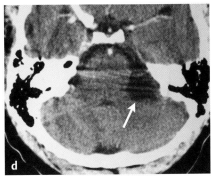

Fig. 1.216 A 30-year-old man with an extra-axial epidermoid in the left cerebellopontine angle cistern, which erodes the endocranial surface of the petrous portion of the left temporal bone. The lesion has **(a)** low-intermediate signal on T1-weighted imaging (*arrow*) and **(b)** high signal on axial T2-weighted imaging (*arrow*) and **(c)** diffusion-weighted imaging (*arrow*). **(d)** The epidermoid has low attenuation on axial CT (*arrow*).

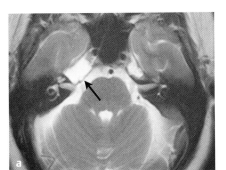

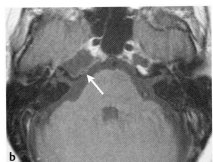

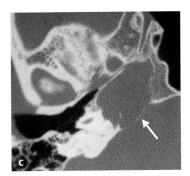

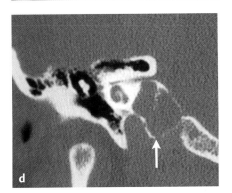

Fig. 1.217 A 50-year-old woman with a right petrous apex mucocele. The circumscribed expansile abnormality involving the right petrous apex has **(a)** high signal on axial T2-weighted imaging (*arrow*) and **(b)** low signal on postcontrast axial fat-suppressed T1-weighted imaging (*arrow*). There is associated thinning, erosion, and expansion of the adjacent bony margins, as seen on **(c)** axial and **(d)** coronal CT (*arrows*).

Table 1.10 *(cont.)* Lesions involving the petrous apex

Lesions	Imaging Findings	Comments
Petrous apex cephalocele (**Fig. 1.218**)	*CT:* Zones with CSF attenuation within enlarged trigeminal nerve cisterns/Meckel's caves associated with chronic erosion and protusion into the petrous apices. *MRI:* Zones with low signal on T1-weighted imaging, FLAIR, and diffusion-weighted imaging and high signal on T2-weighted imaging similar to CSF signal. No gadolinium contrast enhancement.	Rare lesions that consist of protrusions of dura and arachnoid from the trigeminal nerve cisterns/Meckel's cave into the petrous apices, usually bilateral. Associated with chronic raised intracranial pressure (pseudotumor cerebri, Usher syndrome), with empty sella configurations.
Inflammatory Lesions		
Petrous apicitis (**Fig. 1.219**)	*CT:* Retained fluid in the petrous apex air cells with or without trabecular bone disruption. *MRI:* Zones with low-intermediate signal on T1-weighted imaging and high signal on T2-weighted imaging (T2WI) and fat-suppressed T2WI, ± high signal on diffusion-weighted imaging and low signal on ADC. Usually heterogeneous gadolinium contrast enhancement, ± adjacent intracranial dural contrast enhancement, abnormal high T2 signal and contrast enhancement of brain tissue/abscess formation.	Infection of the petrous apex can occur within pneumatized petrous apex air cells (petrous apicitis) or nonpneumatized petrous apex air cells (petrous apex osteomyelitis). Petrous apicitis usually occurs from medial extension of otitis media, often from organisms like *Staphylococcus pneumoniae, Staphylococcus aureus,* and *Haemophilus influenzae.* Symptoms of facial and ear pain in concert with sixth cranial nerve palsy can occur from petrous apicitis, referred to as the Gradenigo triad. Other complications include meningitis, brain abscess, and intracranial venous sinus thrombosis.
Osteomyelitis (**Fig. 1.220**)	*CT:* Zones of abnormal decreased attenuation and focal sites of bone destruction, ± complications, including subgaleal empyema, epidural empyema, subdural empyema, meningitis, cerebritis, intra-axial abscess, and venous sinus thrombosis. *MRI:* Zones with low-intermediate signal on T1-weighted imaging, and high signal on T2-weighted imaging (T2WI) and fat-suppressed T2WI, ± high signal on diffusion-weighted imaging and low signal on ADC. Usually shows heterogeneous gadolinium (Gd) contrast enhancement, ± adjacent intracranial dural and/or leptomeningeal Gd contrast enhancement, ± abnormal high T2 signal and contrast enhancement of brain tissue/abscess formation.	Osteomyelitis (bone infection) of the skull can result from surgery, trauma, hematogenous dissemination from another source of infection, or direct extension of infection from an adjacent site, such as the paranasal sinuses, nasal cavity, petrous apex air cells, and/or mastoid air cells and middle ear.
Langerhans' cell histiocytosis	Single or multiple circumscribed soft tissue lesions in the marrow of the skull associated with focal bony destruction/erosion and extension extra- or intracranially or both. *CT:* Lesions usually have low-intermediate attenuation, + contrast enhancement, ± enhancement of the adjacent dura. *MRI:* Lesions typically have low-intermediate signal on T1-weighted imaging and heterogeneous slightly high to high signal on FLAIR, T2-weighted imaging (T2WI), and fat-suppressed (FS) T2WI. Poorly defined zones of high signal on T2WI and FS T2WI are usually seen in the marrow and soft tissues peripheral to the lesions, secondary to inflammatory changes. Extension of lesions from the marrow into adjacent soft tissues through areas of cortical disruption are commonly seen as well. Lesions typically show prominent gadolinium contrast enhancement in marrow and extraosseous soft tissue portions.	Single lesions are commonly seen in males more than in females and in patients < 20 years old. There is proliferation of histiocytes in medullary bone with localized destruction of cortical bone and extension into adjacent soft tissues. Multiple lesions are associated with Letterer-Siwe disease (lymphadenopathy hepatosplenomegaly) in children < 2 years old, and Hand-Schüller-Christian disease (lymphadenopathy, exophthalmos, diabetes insipidus) in children 5–10 years old.

(continued on page 144)

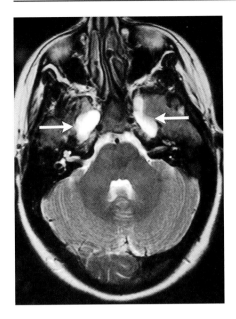

Fig. 1.218 A 25-year-old woman with bilateral petrous apex cephaloceles (*arrows*), which are dilated CSF collections involving both trigeminal cisterns/Meckel's caves. The lesions have high signal on T2-weighted imaging. There is mild erosion of the adjacent petrous apices.

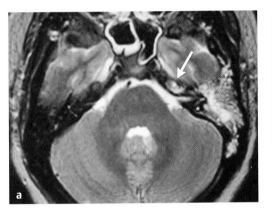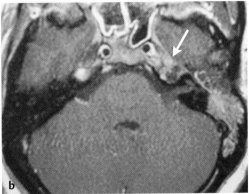

Fig. 1.219 A 30-year-old woman with left petrous apicitis. Zones with **(a)** abnormal high signal on axial T2-weighted imaging and **(b)** heterogeneous gadolinium contrast enhancement on axial fat-suppressed T1-weighted imaging are seen filling the left petrous apex (*arrows*), as well as the left middle ear, and left mastoid air cells caused by infectious exudates.

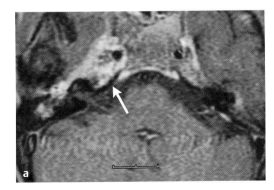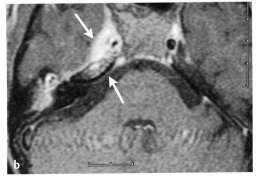

Fig. 1.220 **(a,b)** Osteomyelitis with abnormal gadolinium contrast enhancement on axial fat-suppressed T1-weighted imaging involving the right petrous apex and extending into the right cavernous sinus (*arrows*), resulting in narrowing of the flow void of the right internal carotid artery. Abnormal contrast enhancement is also seen in the right middle ear.

Table 1.10 *(cont.)*   Lesions involving the petrous apex

Lesions	Imaging Findings	Comments
Granulomatosis with polyangiitis (**Fig. 1.221**)	*CT:* Zones with soft tissue attenuation in the external auditory canal, ± bone destruction. *MRI:* Poorly defined zones of soft tissue thickening with low-intermediate signal on T1-weighted imaging, slightly high to high signal on T2-weighted imaging, and gadolinium contrast enhancement within the external auditory canal, ± bone invasion and destruction, ± extension into the skull base and intracranially, with involvement of the dura, brain, venous sinuses, nasopharynx, and/or infratemporal fossa.	Multisystem disease with necrotizing granulomas in the respiratory tract, focal necrotizing angiitis of small arteries and veins of various tissues, and glomerulonephritis. Commonly involves the paranasal sinuses and occasionally the orbits. Involvement of temporal bone in 40% of cases. Peak prevalence is in the fifth decade, and annual incidence is 8 per million. Antibodies to neutrophil cytoplasmic antigens (ANCA) occur in 80–90% of patients and play a role in pathogenesis. Treatment includes corticosteroids, cyclophosphamide, and anti-TNF agents.
Sarcoidosis (**Fig. 1.222**)	*CT:* Intraosseous lesions usually appear as intramedullary radiolucent zones, rarely are sclerotic with high attenuation. *MRI:* Lesions often have low to intermediate signal on T1-weighted imaging and slightly high to high signal on T2-weighted imaging (T2WI) and fat-suppressed (FS) proton density-weighted imaging and FS T2WI. Erosions and zones of destruction involving adjacent bone cortex can occur with extraosseous extension of the granulomatous process. After gadolinium contrast administration, lesions typically show moderate to prominent enhancement.	Multisystem noncaseating granulomatous disease of uncertain cause that can involve the CNS in 5–15% of cases and bone in 1–15%. Associated with severe neurologic deficits if CNS lesions are untreated. Diagnosis of neurosarcoid may be difficult when the neurologic complications precede other systemic manifestations in the lungs, lymph nodes, skin, bone, and/or eyes.
Vascular Abnormalities		
Carotid artery aneurysm/ pseudoaneurysm (**Fig. 1.223**)	*CT:* Focal circumscribed lesion with low-intermediate and/or high attenuation. *MRI:* Focal, circumscribed lesion with layers of low, intermediate, and/or high signal on T1-weighted imaging and T2-weighted imaging secondary to layers of thrombus, as well as a signal void representing a patent lumen. *CTA and contrast-enhanced MRA* show contrast enhancement of nonthrombosed portions within lumens of aneurysms.	Abnormal dilatation of artery secondary to acquired/ degenerative cause, connective tissue disease, atherosclerosis, trauma, infection (mycotic), arteriovenous malformation, drugs, or vasculitis.

(continued on page 146)

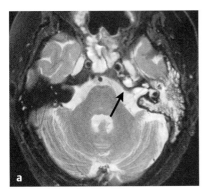
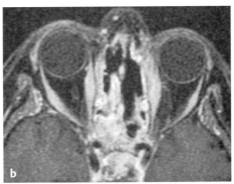
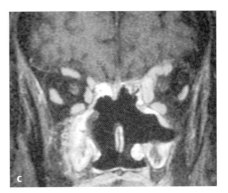

Fig. 1.221 Granulomatosis with polyangiitis in a 65-year-old woman. **(a)** Abnormal high signal on axial fat-suppressed T2-weighted imaging is seen filling the left mastoid air cells, left middle ear, and left petrous apex air cells (*arrow*) secondary to obstruction of the left eustachian tube by gadolinium-enhancing granulomas in the nasopharynx, paranasal sinuses, and nasal cavity, as seen on **(b)** axial and **(c)** coronal fat-suppressed T1-weighted imaging.

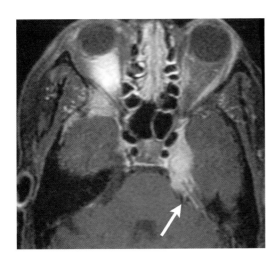

Fig. 1.222 A 55-year-old woman with sarcoidosis and a contrast-enhancing intraosseous lesion involving the left petrous apex and left trigeminal cistern/Meckel's cave, with encasement of the left trigeminal nerve (*arrow*), as seen on axial fat-suppressed T1-weighted imaging. Dural contrast enhancement is seen along the endocranial surface of the left petrous apex. A second contrast-enhancing lesion is seen within the greater wing of the right sphenoid bone.

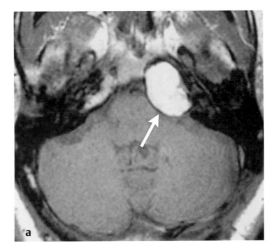
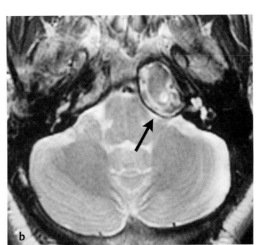

Fig. 1.223 A 35-year-old man with a carotid artery aneurysm in the left petrous apex. **(a)** The aneurysm has mostly high signal on axial T1-weighted imaging (*arrow*). **(b)** The aneurysm has mixed low, intermediate, and high signal on axial T2-weighted imaging (*arrow*).

Table 1.10 *(cont.)* Lesions involving the petrous apex

Lesions	Imaging Findings	Comments
Benign Tumors		
Meningioma **(Fig. 1.224)**	Extra-axial dura-based lesions that are well circumscribed. Location: supra- > infratentorial, parasagittal > convexity > sphenoid ridge > parasellar > posterior fossa > optic nerve sheath > intraventricular. *CT:* Tumors have intermediate attenuation, usually prominent contrast enhancement, ± calcifications, ± hyperostosis of adjacent bone. *MRI:* Tumors often have intermediate signal on T1-weighted imaging, intermediate to slightly high signal on T2-weighted imaging, and typically prominent gadolinium contrast enhancement, ± calcifications, ± hyperostosis and/or invasion of adjacent skull. Some meningiomas have high signal on diffusion-weighted imaging.	Benign slow-growing tumors involving cranial and/or spinal dura that are composed of neoplastic meningothelial (arachnoidal or arachnoid cap) cells. Usually solitary and sporadic, but can also occur as multiple lesions in patients with neurofibromatosis type 2. Most are benign, although ~ 5% have atypical histologic features. Anaplastic meningiomas are rare and account for < 3% of meningiomas. Meningiomas account for up to 26% of primary intracranial tumors. Annual incidence is 6 per 100,000. Typically occur in adults (> 40 years old) and in women more than in men. Can result in compression of adjacent brain parenchyma, encasement of arteries, and compression of dural venous sinuses. Rarely, invasive/malignant types occur.
Schwannoma **(Fig. 1.225, Fig. 1.226, and Fig. 1.227)**	*MRI:* Circumscribed spheroid or ovoid lesions with low-intermediate signal on T1-weighted imaging, high signal on T2-weighted imaging (T2WI) and fat-suppressed T2WI, and usually prominent gadolinium (Gd) contrast enhancement. High signal on T2WI and Gd contrast enhancement can be heterogeneous in large lesions due to cystic degeneration and/or hemorrhage. Schwannomas involving the skull include those from CN V (trigeminal nerve cistern/Meckel's cave), CN VI (Dorello canal), CN VII and CN VIII (internal auditory canal and cerebellopontine angle cistern), CN IX, CN X, and CN XI (jugular foramen). *CT:* Circumscribed spheroid or ovoid lesions with intermediate attenuation, + contrast enhancement. Large lesions can have cystic degeneration and/or hemorrhage, ± erosion of adjacent bone.	Schwannomas are benign encapsulated tumors that contain differentiated neoplastic Schwann cells. Multiple schwannomas are often associated with neurofibromatosis type 2 (NF2), which is an autosomal dominant disease involving a gene mutation at chromosome 22q12. In addition to schwannomas, patients with NF2 can also have multiple meningiomas and ependymomas. Schwannomas represent 8% of primary intracranial tumors and 29% or primary spinal tumors. The incidence of NF2 is 1/37,000 to 1/50,000 newborns. Age at presentation is 22 to 72 years (mean age = 46 years). Peak incidence is in the fourth to sixth decades. Many patients with NF2 present in the third decade with bilateral vestibular schwannomas.

(continued on page 148)

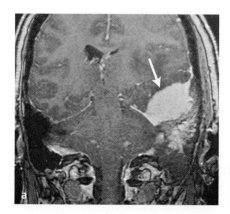 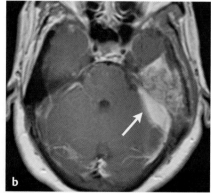 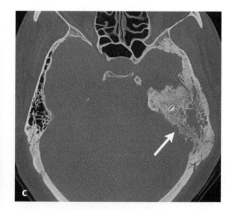

Fig. 1.224 Meningioma in a 46-year-old woman. Gadolinium-enhancing tumor is seen along the floor of the left middle cranial fossa with invasion into the adjacent left temporal bone, as seen on **(a)** coronal (*arrow*) and **(b)** axial (*arrow*) T1-weighted imaging. **(c)** Axial CT shows diffuse hyperostosis of the left temporal bone (*arrow*) from the tumor involvement.

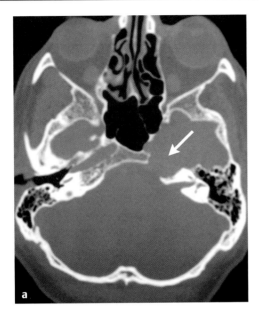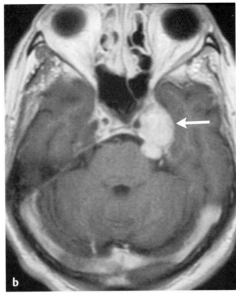

Fig. 1.225 Schwannoma of CN V in a 70-year-old man. **(a)** Axial CT shows erosion of the left petrous apex (*arrow*) caused by **(b)** a contrast-enhancing left trigeminal schwannoma (*arrow*) on axial T1-weighted imaging.

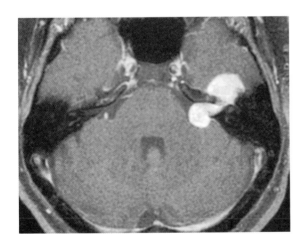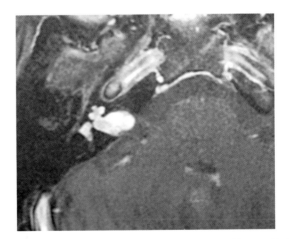

Fig. 1.226 Schwannoma of CN VII in a 54-year-old man. Gadolinium contrast enhancement of a schwannoma is seen involving the left CN VII at the left cerebellopontine angle cistern, left internal auditory canal, and left geniculate ganglion, with associated erosion of the left petrous apex on axial fat-suppressed T1-weighted imaging.

Fig. 1.227 Schwannoma of CN VIII in a 49-year-old man. Gadolinium contrast enhancement of a schwannoma is seen involving the right CN VIII in the right internal auditory canal and extending into the cochlea and vestibule of the inner ear on axial fat-suppressed T1-weighted imaging.

Table 1.10 *(cont.)* Lesions involving the petrous apex

Lesions	Imaging Findings	Comments
Paraganglioma (**Fig. 1.228**)	Ovoid or fusiform lesions with low-intermediate attenuation. *CT:* Lesions can show contrast enhancement. Often erode adjacent bone. *MRI:* Spheroid or lobulated lesion with intermediate signal on T1-weighted imaging (T1WI), intermediate-high signal on T2-weighted imaging (T2WI) and fat-suppressed T2WI, ± tubular zones of flow voids, usually with prominent gadolinium contrast enhancement, ± foci of high signal on T1WI from mucin or hemorrhage, ± peripheral rim of low signal (hemosiderin) on T2WI.	Benign encapsulated neuroendocrine tumors that arise from neural crest cells associated with autonomic ganglia (paraganglia) throughout the body. Lesions, also referred to as chemodectomas, are named according to location (glomus jugulare, tympanicum, vagale). Paragangliomas represent 0.6% of tumors involving the head and neck and 0.03% of all neoplasms.
Endolymphatic sac cystadenoma (**Fig. 1.229**)	Extra-axial retrolabyrinthine lesions involving the posterior petrous bone and extending into the cerebellopontine angle cistern. *CT:* Lesions can have low to intermediate attenuation and can show contrast enhancement. May contain blood products. *MRI:* Lesions often have lobulated margins and contain zones with low, intermediate, and/or high signal on T1- and T2-weighted imaging secondary to methemoglobin, hemosiderin, and cholesterol crystals caused by episodes of hemorrhage. Variable gadolinium contrast enhancement.	Rare solid and/or cystic benign or malignant papillary adenomatous tumors arising from the endolymphatic sac along the dorsal aspect of the temporal bone. Occurs in children and adults. Tumors are slow growing and rarely metastasize. May be sporadic or associated with von Hippel-Lindau disease.
Intratemporal benign vascular tumor/ hemangioma (**Fig. 1.230**)	*CT:* Radiolucent zone with low-intermediate attenuation containing small bone spicules within the temporal bone in the region of the geniculate ganglion. Usually shows contrast enhancement. *MRI:* Lesions have intermediate signal on T1-weighted imaging, slightly high to high signal on T2-weighted imaging, and gadolinium contrast enhancement.	Benign lesions composed of thin-walled vascular spaces within the temporal bone along the course of the facial nerve, often at or near the geniculate ganglion. The lesions grow within bone and are usually radiolucent, containing bone spicules. Lesions can be associated with slowly progressive or recurrent facial paralysis.

(continued on page 150)

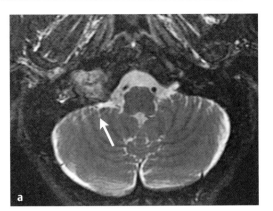
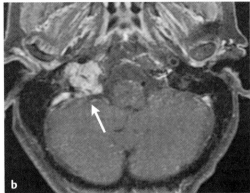

Fig. 1.228 **(a)** A 55-year-old woman with a glomus jugulare at the right jugular foramen that has heterogeneous intermediate and slightly high signal on axial fat-suppressed T2-weighted imaging (*arrow*). Multiple tortuous and punctate zones of signal void are seen that represent intratumoral vessels. **(b)** The tumor shows gadolinium contrast enhancement on axial fat-suppressed T1-weighted imaging (*arrow*).

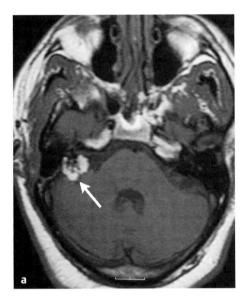
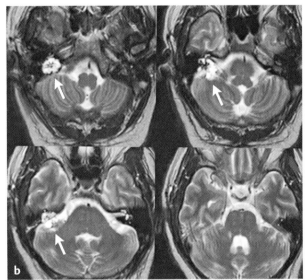

Fig. 1.229 Endolymphatic sac cystadenoma in a 46-year-old man. The lesion has lobulated margins and contains mostly high signal on **(a)** axial T1-weighted imaging (*arrow*) and **(b)** T2-weighted imaging (*arrows*).

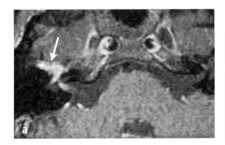
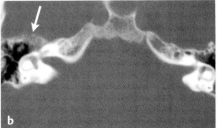
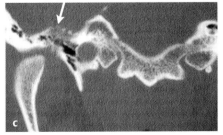

Fig. 1.230 **(a)** Axial fat-suppressed T1-weighted imaging shows gadolinium contrast enhancement in the geniculate ganglion of the right facial nerve and adjacent bone (*arrow*), representing an intratemporal benign vascular tumor/ hemangioma in a 40-year-old man. On **(b)** axial and **(c)** coronal CT, the intraosseous portion of the lesion (*arrows*) is radiolucent and contains bone spicules.

Table 1.10 *(cont.)* Lesions involving the petrous apex

Lesions	Imaging Findings	Comments
Malignant Tumors		
Metastatic disease (**Fig. 1.231**)	Single or multiple well-circumscribed or poorly defined lesions involving the skull, dura, leptomeninges, and/or choroid plexus. *CT:* Intraosseous lesions are usually radiolucent, may also be sclerotic, ± extraosseous tumor extension, usually + contrast enhancement, ± compression of neural tissue or vessels. Leptomeningeal tumor often best seen on postcontrast images. *MRI:* Single or multiple well-circumscribed or poorly defined lesions involving the skull, dura, leptomeninges, and/or choroid plexus with low-intermediate signal on T1-weighted imaging, intermediate-high signal on T2-weighted imaging, and usually gadolinium contrast enhancement, ± bone destruction, ± compression of neural tissue or vessels. Leptomeningeal tumor often best seen on postcontrast images.	Metastatic lesions are proliferating neoplastic cells that are located in sites or organs separated or distant from their origins. Metastatic lesions can disseminate hematogenously via arteries or veins, along CSF pathways, along surgical tracts, and along lymphatic structures. Metastatic carcinoma is the most frequent malignant tumor involving bone. In adults, metastatic lesions to bone occur most frequently from carcinomas of the lung, breast, prostate, kidney, and thyroid, as well as from sarcomas. Primary malignancies of the lung, breast, and prostate account for 80% of bone metastases. Metastatic tumor may cause variable destructive or infiltrative changes in single or multiple sites.
Myeloma/Plasmacytoma (**Fig. 1.232**)	Multiple myeloma or single plasmacytoma are well-circumscribed or poorly defined lesions involving the skull and dura. *CT:* Lesions have low-intermediate attenuation, usually + contrast enhancement, + bone destruction. *MRI:* Well-circumscribed or poorly defined lesions involving the skull and dura with low-intermediate signal on T1-weighted imaging, intermediate-high signal on T2-weighted imaging, and usually gadolinium contrast enhancement, + bone destruction.	Multiple myeloma are malignant tumors composed of proliferating antibody-secreting plasma cells derived from single clones. Multiple myeloma is primarily located in bone marrow. A solitary myeloma or plasmacytoma is an infrequent variant in which a neoplastic mass of plasma cells occurs at a single site of bone or soft tissues. In the United States, 14,600 new cases occur each year. Multiple myeloma is the most common primary neoplasm of bone in adults. Median age at presentation = 60 years. Most patients are more than 40 years old. Tumors occur in the vertebrae > ribs > femur > iliac bone > humerus > craniofacial bones > sacrum > clavicle > sternum > pubic bone > tibia.
Lymphoma	Single or multiple well-circumscribed or poorly defined lesions involving the skull, dura, and/or leptomeninges. *CT:* Lesions have low-intermediate attenuation and may show contrast enhancement, ± bone destruction. Leptomeningeal tumor often best seen on postcontrast images. *MRI:* Lesions have low-intermediate signal on T1-weighted imaging and intermediate to high signal on T2-weighted imaging, + gadolinium contrast enhancement. Can be locally invasive and associated with bone erosion/destruction and intracranial extension with meningeal involvement.	Lymphomas are lymphoid tumors whose neoplastic cells typically arise within lymphoid tissue (lymph nodes and reticuloendothelial organs). Unlike leukemia, lymphomas usually arise as discrete masses. Lymphomas are subdivided into Hodgkin disease (HD) and non-Hodgkin lymphoma (NHL). Distinction between HD and NHL is useful because of differences in clinical and histopathologic features, as well as treatment strategies. HD typically arises in lymph nodes and often spreads along nodal chains, whereas NHL frequently originates at extranodal sites and spreads in an unpredictable pattern. Almost all primary lymphomas of bone are B-cell NHL. Extra-axial lymphoma may cause variable destructive or infiltrative changes in single or multiple sites.

(continued on page 152)

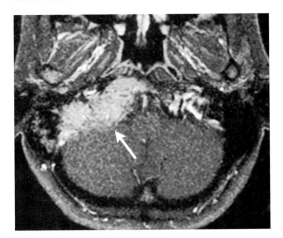

Fig. 1.231 Gadolinium-enhancing metastatic disease (*arrow*) is seen in the right temporal and occipital bones on axial fat-suppressed T1-weighted imaging.

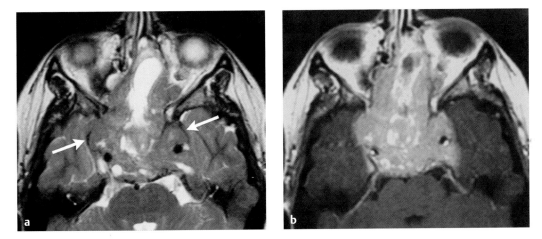

Fig. 1.232 A 28-year-old woman with a plasmacytoma filling the nasal cavity and nasopharynx and extending into the sphenoid bone, cavernous sinuses, and left petrous apex. **(a)** The tumor has mixed intermediate and high signal on axial T2-weighted imaging (*arrows*). **(b)** The tumor shows gadolinium contrast enhancement on axial T1-weighted imaging.

Table 1.10 *(cont.)* Lesions involving the petrous apex

Lesions	Imaging Findings	Comments
Chordoma **(Fig. 1.233)**	Well-circumscribed lobulated lesions along the dorsal surface of the clivus, vertebral bodies, or sacrum, + localized bone destruction. *CT:* Lesions have low-intermediate attenuation, ± calcifications from destroyed bone carried away by tumor, + contrast enhancement. *MRI:* Lesions have low-intermediate signal on T1-weighted imaging and high signal on T2-weighted imaging, + gadolinium contrast enhancement (usually heterogeneous). Can be locally invasive and associated with bone erosion/destruction and encasement of vessels (usually without arterial narrowing) and nerves. Skull base-clivus is a common location, usually in the midline for conventional chordomas that account for 80% of skull base chordomas. Chondroid chordomas tend to be located off midline near skull base synchondroses.	Chordomas are rare, locally aggressive, slow-growing, low to intermediate grade malignant tumors derived from ectopic notochordal remnants along the axial skeleton. Chondroid chondromas (5–15% of all chordomas) have both chordomatous and chondromatous differentiation, Chordomas that contain sarcomatous components (5% of all chordomas) are referred to as dedifferentiated chordomas or sarcomatoid chordoma. Chordomas account for 2–4% of primary malignant bone tumors, 1–3% of all primary bone tumors, and < 1% of intracranial tumors. The annual incidence has been reported to be 0.18 to 0.3 per million. Dedifferentiated chordomas or sarcomatoid chordomas account for less than 5% of all chordomas. For cranial chordomas, patients' mean age = 37 to 40 years.
Chondrosarcoma **(Fig. 1.234)**	Lobulated lesions with bone destruction at synchondroses. *CT:* Lesions have low-intermediate attenuation associated with localized bone destruction, ± chondroid matrix calcifications, + contrast enhancement. *MRI:* Lesions have low-intermediate signal on T1-weighted imaging, high signal on T2-weighted imaging (T2WI), ± matrix mineralization and low signal on T2WI, + gadolinium contrast enhancement (usually heterogeneous). Can be locally invasive and associated with bone erosion/destruction, encasement of vessels and nerves. Skull base petro-occipital synchondrosis is a common location, usually off midline.	Chondrosarcomas are malignant tumors containing cartilage formed within sarcomatous stroma. Chondrosarcomas can contain areas of calcification/mineralization, myxoid material, and/or ossification. Chondrosarcomas rarely arise within synovium. Chondrosarcomas represent 12–21% of malignant bone lesions, 21–26% of primary sarcomas of bone, 9–14% of all bone tumors, 6% of skull base tumors, and 0.15% of all intracranial tumors.
Osteosarcoma	Destructive lesions involving the skull base. *CT:* Tumors have low-intermediate attenuation, usually with matrix mineralization/ossification, and often show contrast enhancement (usually heterogeneous). *MRI:* Tumors often have poorly defined margins and commonly extend from the marrow through destroyed bone cortex into adjacent soft tissues. Tumors usually have low-intermediate signal on T1-weighted imaging. Zones of low signal often correspond to areas of tumor calcification/mineralization and/or necrosis. Zones of necrosis typically have high signal on T2-weighted imaging (T2WI), whereas mineralized zones usually have low signal on T2WI. Tumors can have variable MRI signal on T2WI and fat-suppressed (FS) T2WI depending upon the relative proportions, distributions, and locations of calcified/mineralized osteoid, chondroid, fibroid, and hemorrhagic and necrotic components. Tumors may have low, low-intermediate, and intermediate to high signal on T2WI and FS T2WI. After gadolinium contrast administration, osteosarcomas typically show prominent enhancement in nonmineralized/calcified portions of the tumors.	Osteosarcomas are malignant tumors comprised of proliferating neoplastic spindle cells, which produce osteoid and/or immature tumoral bone. Occur in children as primary tumors, and in adults they are associated with Paget disease, irradiated bone, chronic osteomyelitis, osteoblastoma, giant cell tumor, and fibrous dysplasia.

(continued on page 154)

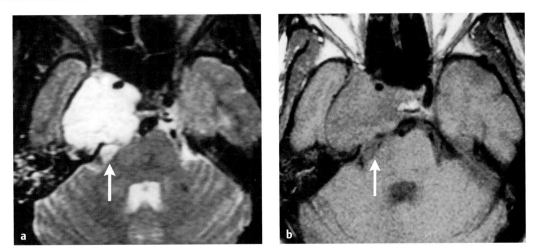

Fig. 1.233 A 21-year-old man with a chondroid chordoma that involves the right petro-occipital synchondrosis with extension into the medial portion of the right middle cranial fossa and right cavernous sinus displacing the right internal carotid artery anteriorly. The tumor has **(a)** high signal on axial T2-weighted imaging (*arrow*) and **(b)** intermediate signal on axial T1-weighted imaging (*arrow*).

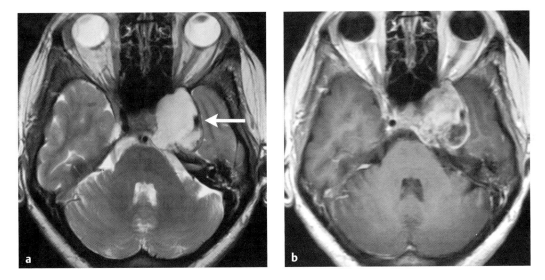

Fig. 1.234 Chondrosarcoma in a 53-year-old woman. The tumor involves the left petro-occipital synchondrosis, with extension into the medial portion of the left middle cranial fossa and left cavernous sinus displacing the left internal carotid artery laterally. **(a)** The tumor (*arrow*) has high signal on axial T2-weighted imaging. **(b)** The tumor shows heterogeneous gadolinium contrast enhancement on axial T1-weighted imaging.

Table 1.10 *(cont.)* Lesions involving the petrous apex

Lesions	Imaging Findings	Comments
Invasive pituitary adenoma or carcinoma (**Fig. 1.235**)	*MRI:* Often have intermediate signal on T1-weighted imaging and T2-weighted imaging, often similar to gray matter, ± necrosis, ± cyst, ± hemorrhage, usually with prominent gadolinium contrast enhancement, extension into suprasellar cistern with waist at diaphragma sella, ± extension into cavernous sinus, ± invasion of skull base and temporal bone.. *CT:* Often have intermediate attenuation, ± necrosis, ± cyst, ± hemorrhage, usually with contrast enhancement, extension into suprasellar cistern with waist at diaphragma sella, ± extension into cavernous sinus. Can invade the skull base.	Pituitary macroadenomas can occasionally have an invasive growth pattern with extension into the sphenoid bone, clivus, ethmoid sinus, orbits, and/ or interpeduncular cistern. Pituitary carcinomas are rare malignant pituitary tumors involving the adenohypophysis. Account for 0.5% of pituitary tumors. In addition to locally invasive disease and subarachnoid tumor dissemination, hematogenous metastatic spread has been reported to bone, liver, lungs, lymph nodes, pancreas, heart, ovaries, and myometrium.
Sinonasal squamous cell carcinoma (See **Fig. 1.44**)	Destructive lesions arising in the nasal cavity and paranasal sinuses, ± intracranial extension via bone destruction or perineural spread. *CT:* Tumors have intermediate attenuation and mild contrast enhancement. Can be large lesions (± necrosis and/or hemorrhage). *MRI:* Destructive lesions in the nasal cavity, paranasal sinuses, and nasopharynx, ± intracranial extension via bone destruction or perineural spread. Intermediate signal on T1-weighted imaging, intermediate-slightly high signal on T2-weighted imaging, often with gadolinium contrast enhancement. Can be large lesions (± necrosis and/or hemorrhage).	Malignant epithelial tumors originating from the mucosal epithelium of the paranasal sinuses (maxillary, 60%; ethmoid, 14%; and sphenoid and frontal sinuses, 1%) and nasal cavity (25%). Include both keratinizing and nonkeratinizing types. Account for 3% of malignant tumors of the head and neck. Occur in adults (usually > 55 years old) and in males more than in females. Associated with occupational or other exposure to tobacco smoke, nickel, chlorophenols, chromium, mustard gas, radium, and material in the manufacture of wood products.
Nasopharyngeal carcinoma	*CT:* Tumors have intermediate attenuation and mild contrast enhancement. Can be large lesions (± necrosis and/or hemorrhage). *MRI:* Invasive lesions in the nasopharynx (lateral wall/ fossa of Rosenmüller, and posterior upper wall), ± intracranial extension via bone destruction or perineural spread. Intermediate signal on T1-weighted imaging, intermediate-slightly high signal on T2-weighted imaging, and often gadolinium contrast enhancement. Can be large lesions (± necrosis and/or hemorrhage).	Carcinomas arising from the nasopharyngeal mucosa with varying degrees of squamous differentiation. Subtypes include squamous cell carcinoma, nonkeratinizing carcinoma (differentiated and undifferentiated), and basaloid squamous cell carcinoma. Occurs at higher frequency in Southern Asia and Africa than in Europe and the Americas. Peak ages: 40–60 years. Occurs two to three times more frequently in men than in women. Associated with Epstein-Barr virus, diets containing nitrosamines, and chronic exposure to tobacco smoke, formaldehyde, chemical fumes, and dust.
Adenoid cystic carcinoma (**Fig. 1.236**)	*CT:* Tumors have intermediate attenuation and variable mild, moderate, or prominent contrast enhancement. *MRI:* Destructive lesions with intracranial extension via bone destruction or perineural spread, intermediate signal on T1-weighted imaging, intermediate-high signal on T2-weighted imaging, and variable mild, moderate, or prominent gadolinium contrast enhancement.	Basaloid tumor composed of neoplastic epithelial and myoepithelial cells. Morphologic tumor patterns include tubular, cribriform and solid. Accounts for 10% of epithelial salivary neoplasms. Most commonly involves the parotid, submandibular, and minor salivary glands (palate, tongue, buccal mucosa, and floor of the mouth, other locations). Perineural tumor spread is common, ± facial nerve paralysis. Usually occurs in adults > 30 years old. Solid type has the worst prognosis. Up to 90% of patients die within 10–15 years of diagnosis.

(continued on page 156)

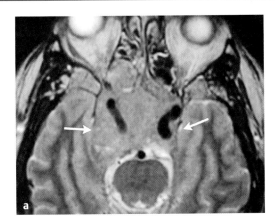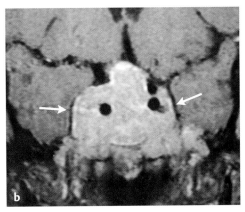

Fig. 1.235   A 44-year-old man with pituitary adenocarcinoma invading the sphenoid bone, posterior ethmoid air cells, cavernous sinuses, and left petrous bone. **(a)** The tumor has slightly high signal on axial T2-weighted imaging (*arrows*). **(b)** The tumor shows gadolinium contrast enhancement on coronal fat-suppressed T1-weighted imaging (*arrows*).

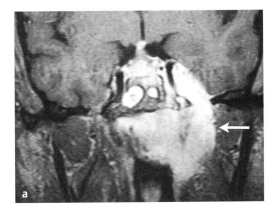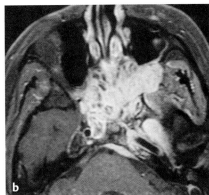

Fig. 1.236   Adenoid cystic carcinoma in a 46-year-old woman. **(a)** Coronal and **(b)** axial fat-suppressed T1-weighted images show gadolinium-enhancing tumor (*arrow* in **a**) extending superiorly from the nasopharynx (*arrow* in **a**) along the third division of the left trigeminal nerve through a widened foramen ovale to involve the left trigeminal cistern/Meckel's cave, left petrous apex, and intracranial dura.

Table 1.10 *(cont.)*   Lesions involving the petrous apex

Lesions	Imaging Findings	Comments
Rhabdomyosarcoma	*CT:* Tumors have soft tissue attenuation and can have circumscribed or irregular margins. Calcifications are uncommon. Tumors can have mixed attenuation, with solid zones of soft tissue attenuation, cystic appearing and/or necrotic zones, and occasional foci of hemorrhage. *MRI:* Tumors are often ovoid and/or lobulated lesions with circumscribed and/or poorly defined margins. Tumors typically have low-intermediate signal on T1-weighted imaging (T1WI) and fat-suppressed (FS) T1WI. Zones of high signal on T1WI may be seen resulting from areas of hemorrhage. Lesions usually have heterogeneous signal (intermediate, slightly high, and/or high signal) on T2-weighted imaging (T2WI) and FS T2WI. Poorly defined zones of edema may occur in the soft tissues adjacent to the tumors. Tumors are often associated with destructive changes in adjacent bone. After gadolinium contrast administration, tumors show variable degrees of enhancement in various patterns.	Malignant mesenchymal tumors with rhabdomyoblastic differentiation that occur primarily in soft tissue and only very rarely in bone. There are three subgroups of rhabdomyosarcoma (embryonal, 50–70%; alveolar, 18–45%; and pleomorphic, 5–10%). Embryonal and alveolar rhabdomyosarcomas occur primarily in children, and pleomorphic rhabdomyosarcomas occur mostly in adults. Embryonal rhabdomyosarcomas have phenotypic and biologic features of embryonal muscle. Alveolar rhabdomyosarcomas are round cell neoplasms that show partial skeletal muscle differentiation. Pleomorphic rhabdomyosarcomas contain bizarre, spheroid, and spindle cells that show skeletal muscle differentiation. Represent ~ 2% of primary malignant soft tissue tumors and < 1% of all primary soft tissue tumors. Account for 19% of soft tissue sarcomas in children. Age at presentation = 2 to 40 years (mean age = 18 years).
Osseous Abnormalities		
Fibrous dysplasia **(Fig. 1.237)**	*CT:* Expansile bone changes with mixed -intermediate and high attenuation, often in a ground-glass appearance. Can show contrast enhancement. *MRI:* Features depend on the proportions of bony spicules, collagen, fibroblastic spindle cells, hemorrhagic and/or cystic changes, and associated pathologic fracture if present. Lesions are usually well circumscribed, and have low or low-intermediate signal on T1-weighted imaging and FLAIR imaging. On T2-weighted imaging, lesions have variable mixtures of low, intermediate, and/or high signal, often surrounded by a low-signal rim of variable thickness. Internal septations and cystic changes are seen in a minority of lesions. Bone expansion with thickened and/or thinned cortex can be seen. Lesions show gadolinium contrast enhancement that varies in degree and pattern.	Benign medullary fibro-osseous lesion that can involve a single site (monostotic) or multiple locations (polyostotic). Results from developmental failure in the normal process of remodeling primitive bone to mature lamellar bone, with resultant zone or zones of immature trabeculae within dysplastic fibrous tissue. Accounts for ~ 10% of benign bone lesions. Patients range in age from < 1 year to 76 years; 75% of cases occur before the age of 30 years.
Paget disease **(Fig. 1.238)**	Expansile sclerotic/lytic process involving the skull. *CT:* Lesions often have mixed intermediate and high attenuation. Irregular/indistinct borders between marrow and inner margins of the outer and inner tables of the skull. *MRI:* The MRI features of Paget disease vary based on the phases of the disease. Most cases involving the skull are the late or inactive phases. Findings include osseous expansion and cortical thickening with low signal on T1- and T2-weighted imaging. The inner margins of the thickened cortex can be irregular and indistinct. Zones of low signal on T1- and T2-weighted imaging can be seen in the marrow secondary to thickened bony trabeculae. Marrow in late or inactive phases of Paget's disease can have signal similar to normal marrow, contain focal areas of fat signal, have low signal on T1- and T2-weighted imaging secondary to regions of sclerosis, have areas of high signal on fat-suppressed T2-weighted imaging from edema or persistent fibrovascular tissue, or have various combinations of the aforementioned.	Paget disease is a chronic skeletal disease in which there is disordered bone resorption and woven bone formation, resulting in osseous deformity. A paramyxovirus may be the etiologic agent. Paget disease is polyostotic in up to 66% of patients. Paget disease is associated with a risk of < 1% for developing secondary sarcomatous changes. Occurs in 2.5 to 5% of Caucasians more than 55 years old and 10% of those over the age of 85 years. Can result in narrowing of neuroforamina, with cranial nerve compression and basilar impression, ± compression of brainstem.

(continued on page 158)

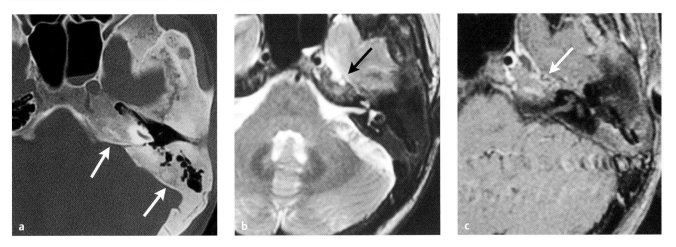

Fig. 1.237   Fibrous dysplasia in a 37-year-old woman. **(a)** Axial CT shows diffuse expansion of the left temporal bone, with a ground-glass pattern of increased attenuation (*arrows*). **(b)** The involved bone has mixed low and intermediate signal on axial T2-weighted imaging (*arrow*) and **(c)** shows heterogeneous gadolinium contrast enhancement on axial fat-suppressed T1-weighted imaging (*arrow*).

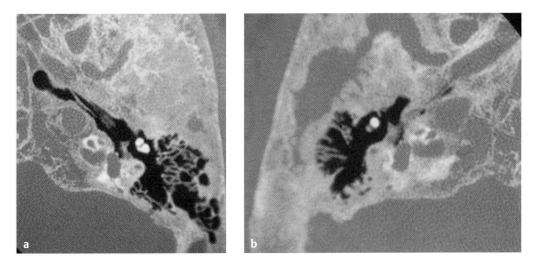

Fig. 1.238   Paget disease involving the skull in an 84-year-old man. **(a,b)** Axial CT images show thickening of bone, with blurring of the borders between the inner and outer tables with the medullary space, as well as mixed zones with osteosclerosis and osteopenia.

Table 1.10 *(cont.)* Lesions involving the petrous apex

Lesions	Imaging Findings	Comments
Renal osteodystrophy (**Fig. 1.239**)	*CT:* Trabecular bone resorption with a salt-and-pepper appearance from mixed osteolysis and osteosclerosis, osteitis fibrosa cystica, cortical thinning, coarsened trabecular pattern, and osteolytic lesions/brown tumors. Another pattern is ground-glass appearance with indistinct corticomedullary borders. *MRI:* Zones of low signal on T1- and T2-weighted imaging corresponding to regions of bone sclerosis. Circumscribed zones with high signal on T2-weighted imaging can be seen due to osteolytic lesions or brown tumors.	Osteoblastic and osteoclastic changes that occur in bone as a result of chronic end-stage renal disease, secondary hyperparathyroidism (hyperplasia of parathyroid glands), and osteomalacia (abnormal vitamin D metabolism). Can result in pathologic fracture. Unlike secondary hyperparathyroidism, diffuse or patchy bone sclerosis infrequently occurs in primary.
Otosclerosis (**Fig. 1.240**)	*CT:* Radiolucent zones at the otic capsule adjacent to the oval window (fenestral type) resulting in fixation of the stapes footplate. Can progress and extend around the cochlea (cochlear type), forming a *double ring sign*. *MRI:* Small zones with gadolinium contrast enhancement may be seen at the involved sites.	Progressive conductive or mixed hearing loss that occurs in adults resulting from spongiotic-lytic bone changes of unknown etiology in the otic capsule. Often bilateral. Fenestral type is more common (85%) and is associated with conductive hearing loss. The cochlear type of otosclerosis occurs in 15% and often presents with both conductive and sensorineural hearing loss.
Osteogenesis imperfecta (OI) (**Fig. 1.241**)	*CT:* Diffuse osteopenia and undermineralized thickened bone around the otic capsule. Can appear similar to otosclerosis. *MRI:* Pericochlear bandlike zones of gadolinium contrast enhancement can be seen that correspond to sites of demineralization seen on CT.	Also referred to as brittle bone disease, OI has four to seven types. OI is a hereditary disorder with abnormal type I fibrillar collagen production and osteoporosis resulting from mutations of the *COL1A1* gene on chromosome 17q21.31-q22.05 and the *COL1A2* gene on chromosome 7q22.1. Results in fragile bone prone to repetitive microfractures and remodeling.

(continued on page 160)

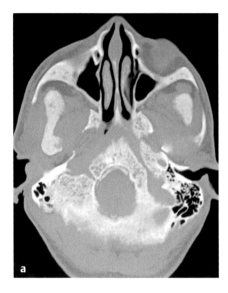

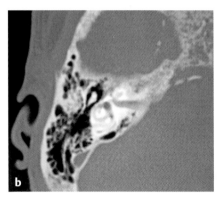

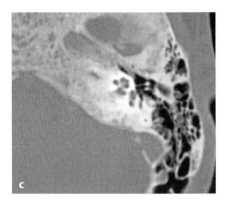

Fig. 1.239 Renal osteodystrophy in a 28-year-old man. **(a–c)** Axial CT images show demineralization at the skull base as well as diffuse sclerosis of the mandibles.

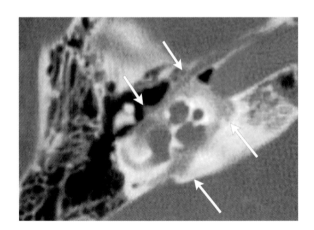

Fig. 1.240 Otosclerosis in a 12-year-old male. Axial CT shows demineralization of the otic capsule (*arrows*) adjacent to the cochlea, oval window, vestibule, and vestibular aqueduct.

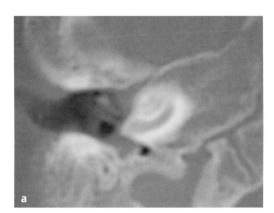

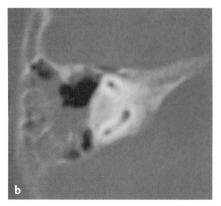

Fig. 1.241 Osteogenesis imperfecta in a 2-year-old male. **(a,b)** Axial CT shows demineralization of the right otic capsule and skull.

Table 1.10 *(cont.)* Lesions involving the petrous apex

Lesions	Imaging Findings	Comments
Osteopetrosis (**Fig. 1.242**)	Findings include generalized bone sclerosis and hyperostosis, resulting in thickening of the skull, as well as narrowing of the foramina and optic canals. *CT:* Osteosclerosis is seen involving the skull base and orbits, followed by the calvarium, with bone thickening and sclerosis. Narrowing of the optic canals and foramina result in blindness and cranial nerve deficits. Other findings are sclerosis at synchondroses and poor pneumatization of paranasal sinuses. *MRI:* Thickened bone containing expanded marrow with intermediate signal on T1- and T2-weighted imaging.	Osteopetrosis is a genetically heterogeneous group of bone diseases with osteoclast failure and impaired bone resorption, also referred to as *marble bone disease*. The typically fatal infantile or malignant type is autosomal recessive, involving mutations of the *OSTM1*, *TCIRG1*, and *ClCN7* genes on chromosomes 6q21, 11q13.4–13.5, and 16p13, seen at birth. Mutations affect the function of the a3 subunit of ATPase, which mediates acidification of the bone-osteoclast interface. Other types include the intermediate autosomal recessive type, which presents in the first decade, and the autosomal dominant type, which occurs in adults. Defective resorption of primary bone spongiosa and mineralized cartilage from osteoclast dysfunction occurs, resulting in failure of conversion of immature woven bone into strong lamellar bone. In the severe autosomal recessive form, medullary crowding from immature sclerotic bone can result in anemia, thrombocytopenia, and immune dysfunction, leading to death.
Cleidocranial dysplasia (CCD) (**Fig. 1.243**)	*CT:* Delayed ossification of membranous > endochondral derived bone. Skull base and calvarium are thickened and can have increased attenuation. Absence or underdevelopment of mastoid air cells and paranasal sinuses. Persistent open cranial sutures and fontanelles, wormian bones, impacted supernumerary teeth.	Autosomal dominant syndrome involving the *RUNX2* gene on chromosome 6p21. Mutations result in haploinsufficiency, which affects osteoblast precursor cell differentiation. Loss of one functional gene results in CCD; when both genes are abnormal, lack of osteoblast differentiation. Involves both membranous and endochondral bone formation. Patients have abnormally large and wide-open fontanelles at birth, brachycephalic cranium, shortened stature, midface hypoplasia, abnormal dentition, clavicular aplasia or hypoplasia, and brachydactyly. Patients have normal intellect.
Traumatic Lesions		
Transverse fracture (**Fig. 1.244**)	*CT:* Fractures extend from the foramen magnum or jugular foramen to the middle cranial fossa, ± involvement of the otic capsule, vestibular aqueduct, stapes footplate, and the fundus of the internal auditory canal. Blood/fluid present within the middle ear and mastoid air cells.	Transverse fractures are oriented perpendicular to the long axis of the petrous bone from frontally or occipitally oriented trauma. Less common than longitudinal fractures, they account for < 10% of temporal bone fractures. Can involve the otic capsule, resulting in sensorineural hearing loss. Increased risk for perilymphatic fistula.
Complex fracture	*CT:* Fracture planes oriented transverse, longitudinal, and/or oblique to the long axis of the petrous bone, ± involvement of the ossicular chain, otic capsule, and tegmen tympani. Blood/fluid present within the middle ear and mastoid air cells.	Fractures that are oriented transverse, longitudinal, and/or oblique to the long axis of the petrous bone, ± ossicular chain disruption resulting in conductive hearing loss, ± otic capsule involvement with sensorineural hearing loss, ± facial nerve inhjury, ± increased risk for perilymphatic fistula, cholesteatoma.

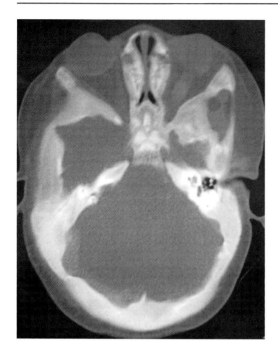

Fig. 1.242 Osteopetrosis in a 5-month-old male. Axial CT shows diffuse thickening and sclerosis of the skull.

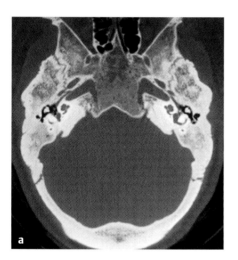

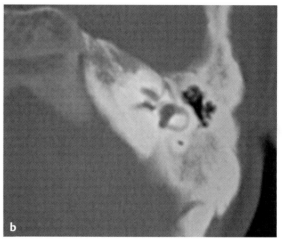

Fig. 1.243 Cleidocranial dysplasia. **(a)** Axial CT shows bone thickening involving the calvarium and skull base, as well as increased osseous attenuation. **(b)** Magnified axial CT shows the same findings at the left temporal bone.

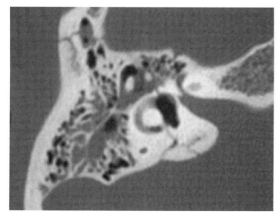

Fig. 1.244 Axial CT shows fractures involving the mastoid and petrous portions of the right temporal bone. Air is seen in the vestibule and lateral semicircular canal secondary to the fracture's involvement of the otic capsule.

Table 1.11 Cerebellopontine angle (CPA) and/or internal auditory canal lesions

- Neoplasms—Extra-Axial
  - Schwannoma (neurinoma)
  - Meningioma
  - Hemangiopericytoma
  - Paraganglioma/glomus jugulare
  - Choroid plexus papilloma
  - Choroid plexus carcinoma
  - Metastatic disease
  - Myeloma
  - Lymphoma
  - Endolymphatic sac adenoma/adenocarcinoma
  - Chordoma
  - Chondrosarcoma
  - Adenoid cystic carcinoma
- Neoplasms—Intra-Axial
  - Ependymoma
  - Glioma of brainstem or cerebellum
  - Hemangioblastoma
  - Medulloblastoma
  - Atypical teratoid/Rhabdoid tumor

- Tumorlike Lesions
  - Epidermoid (congenital cholesteatoma)
  - Dermoid
  - Cholesterol granuloma
  - Lipoma
  - Arachnoid cyst
- Vascular Abnormalities
  - Vertebrobasilar dolichoectasia
  - Arterial aneurysm—Basilar artery/branches, Vertebral arteries
  - Arteriovenous malformations (AVMs)
  - Epidural hematoma
  - Subdural hematoma
  - Subarachnoid hemorrhage
- Inflammation
  - Brainstem/cerebellar abscess
  - Subdural/epidural abscess—Empyema
  - Leptomeningeal infection
  - Dural and/or leptomeningeal noninfectious inflammation
  - Langerhans' cell histiocytosis
- Infection
  - Lyme disease—spirochete infection

Table 1.11 Cerebellopontine angle (CPA) and/or internal auditory canal lesions

Lesions	Imaging Findings	Comments
Neoplasms—Extra-Axial		
Schwannoma (neurinoma) (**Fig. 1.245, Fig. 1.246, Fig. 1.247, and Fig. 1.248**)	*CT:* Ovoid or fusiform lesions with low-intermediate attenuation. Lesions can show contrast enhancement. Often erode adjacent bone. *MRI:* Circumscribed ovoid or fusiformd extra-axial lesions with low-intermediate signal on T1-weighted imaging, high signal on T2-weighted imaging (T2WI) and fat-suppressed T2WI, and usually prominent gadolinium (Gd) contrast enhancement. High signal on T2WI and Gd contrast enhancement can be heterogeneous in large lesions.	Schwannomas are benign encapsulated tumors that contain differentiated neoplastic Schwann cells. Acoustic (vestibular nerve) schwannomas account for 90% of intracranial schwannomas and represent 75% of lesions in the cerebellopontine angle cisterns; trigeminal schwannomas are the next most common intracranial schwannoma, followed by facial nerve schwannomas. Multiple schwannomas are seen in neurofibromatosis type 2.

(continued on page 164)

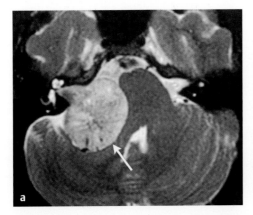 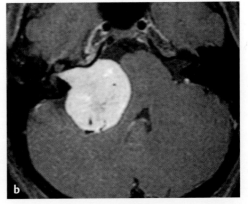

Fig. 1.245 Schwannoma of CN VIII in a 28-year-old woman. **(a)** The tumor is located in the right cerebellopontine angle, with extension into a widened internal auditory canal and has heterogeneous slightly high to high signal on axial T2-weighted imaging (*arrow*). **(b)** The tumor shows prominent gadolinium contrast enhancement on axial fat-suppressed T1-weighted imaging.

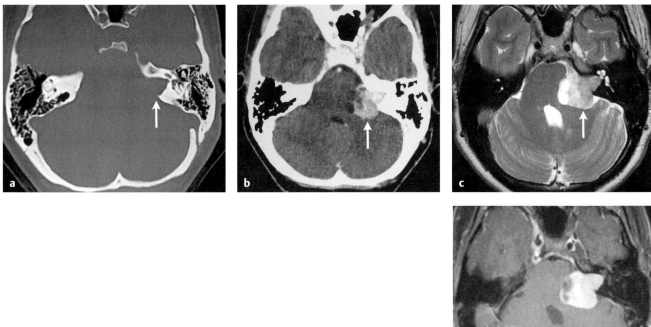

Fig. 1.246 Schwannoma of CN VIII in a 46-year-old woman. **(a)** Axial CT shows a widened left internal auditory canal (*arrow*) caused by **(b)** a contrast-enhancing tumor (*arrow*) in the left cerebellopontine angle. **(c)** The tumor has heterogeneous slightly high to high signal on axial T2-weighted imaging (*arrow*) and **(d)** shows gadolinium contrast enhancement on axial fat-suppressed T1-weighted imaging.

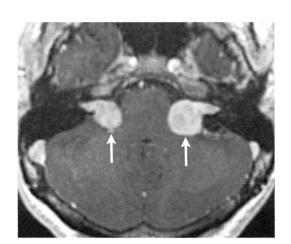

Fig. 1.247 A 25-year-old woman with neurofibromatosis type 2 and bilateral gadolinium-enhancing schwannomas (*arrows*) involving CN VIII, seen on axial T1-weighted imaging.

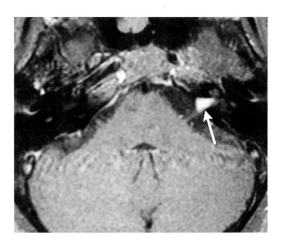

Fig. 1.248 A 38-year-old woman with a gadolinium-enhancing schwannoma (*arrow*) involving the intracanalicular portion of the left CN VII, as seen on axial fat-suppressed T1-weighted imaging.

Table 1.11 *(cont.)* Cerebellopontine angle (CPA) and/or internal auditory canal lesions

Lesions	Imaging Findings	Comments
Meningioma (**Fig. 1.249**)	Extra-axial dura-based lesions that are well circumscribed. Location: supra- > infratentorial. *CT:* Tumors have intermediate attenuation, with or without calcifications, with or without hyperostosis, and usually show prominent contrast enhancement. *MRI:* Intermediate signal on T1-weighted imaging, intermediate-slightly high signal on T2-weighted imaging, and usually prominent gadolinium contrast enhancement, ± calcifications.	Meningiomas are the most common extra-axial tumors and account for up to 26% of primary intracranial tumors. Annual incidence is 6 per 100,000, and they typically occur in adults (> 40 years old) and in women more than in men. Composed of neoplastic meningothelial (arachnoidal or arachnoid cap) cells. Multiple meningiomas are seen in neurofibromatosis type 2 and can result in compression of adjacent brain parenchyma, encasement of arteries, and compression of dural venous sinuses. Rarely, invasive/malignant types occur.
Hemangiopericytoma	*CT:* Tumors have intermediate attenuation, with or without calcifications, and usually show prominent contrast enhancement. *MRI:* Extra-axial mass lesions, often well circumscribed, with intermediate signal on T1-weighted imaging, intermediate-slightly high signal on T2-weighted imaging, and prominent gadolinium contrast enhancement (may resemble meningiomas), ± associated erosive bone changes.	Rare (WHO grade II) neoplasms that account for 0.4% of primary intracranial tumors and are 50 times less frequent than meningiomas. Tumors are composed of closely packed cells with scant cytoplasm and round, ovoid, or elongated nuclei with moderately dense chromatin. Numerous slitlike vascular channels are seen in the tumors that are lined by flattened endothelial cells, ± zones of necrosis. Occur in young adults (males > females). Sometimes referred to as angioblastic meningioma or meningeal hemangiopericytoma, they arise from vascular cells (pericytes). Metastasize more frequently than meningiomas.
Paraganglioma/ glomus jugulare (**Fig. 1.250**)	*CT:* Extra-axial mass lesions located in jugular foramen, often well circumscribed, with intermediate attenuation, + contrast enhancement. Often associated with erosive bone changes and expansion of jugular foramen. *MRI:* Extra-axial mass lesions located in jugular foramen, often well circumscribed, with intermediate signal on T1-weighted imaging, often heterogeneous intermediate-slightly high signal on T2-weighted imaging, ± intratumoral flow voids, + gadolinium contrast enhancement. Often associated with erosive bone changes and expansion of jugular foramen.	These lesions, also referred to as chemodectomas, arise from paraganglia in multiple sites in the body, and are named accordingly (glomus jugulare, tympanicum, vagale, etc.). Paragangliomas are typically well-differentiated neoplasms composed of biphasic collections of chief cells (type I) arranged in nests or lobules (zellballen), surrounded by single layers of sustentacular cells (type II). Present in patients from 24 to 70 years old (mean age = 47 years).
Choroid plexus papilloma (**Fig. 1.251**)	*CT:* Circumscribed and/or lobulated lesions with papillary projections, intermediate attenuation, and usually prominent contrast enhancement, ± calcifications. *MRI:* Tumors often have circumscribed, lobulated margins, intermediate signal on T1-weighted imaging, and intermediate to slightly high signal on T2-weighted imaging, ± calcifications. Tumors usually show prominent gadolinium contrast enhancement.	Rare intracranial neoplasms (WHO grade I) arising in the choroid plexus and composed of a single layer of cuboidal or columnar epithelial cells with round or oval monomorphic nuclei with extremely low mitotic activity overlying fibrovascular connective tissue fronds. Locations: atrium of lateral ventricle > fourth ventricle in children, fourth ventricle > lateral ventricle in adults, and rarely other locations, such as third and fourth ventricles and cerebellopontine angle (CPA). Can be associated with hydrocephalus. Median age for lesions in the lateral and third ventricles = 1.5 years; for the fourth ventricle, median age = 22.5 years; and for the cerebellopontine angle, median age = 35.5 years. Atypical choroid plexus papillomas (WHO grade II) have features similar to choroid plexus papillomas but have two or more mitoses per high-power field.

(continued on page 166)

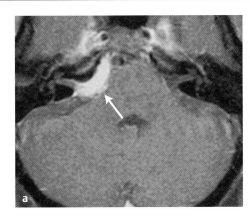
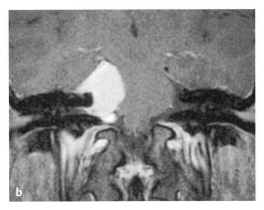

Fig. 1.249 A 42-year-old woman with a gadolinium-enhancing meningioma along the endocranial surface of the right petrous bone extending into the internal auditory canal, as seen on **(a)** axial (*arrow*) and **(b)** coronal fat-suppressed T1-weighted imaging.

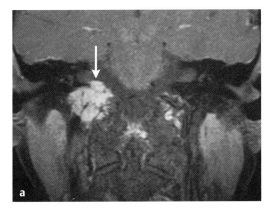
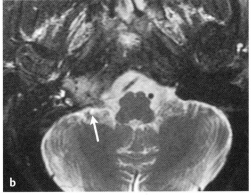

Fig. 1.250 **(a)** Paraganglioma (glomus jugulare) in a 65-year-old woman that is located in the right jugular foramen and that erodes the adjacent bone and extends into the inferior portion of the right internal auditory canal. The tumor shows gadolinium contrast enhancement on coronal fat-suppressed T1-weighted imaging (*arrow*). **(b)** The tumor has intermediate and slightly high signal (*arrow*) as well as several small flow voids on axial fat-suppressed T2-weighted imaging.

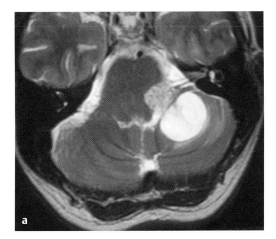
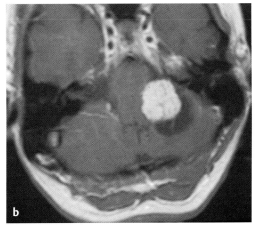

Fig. 1.251 A 46-year-old woman with a choroid plexus papilloma in the left foramen of Luschka and left cerebellopontine angle. **(a)** The solid and cystic tumor has slightly high and high signal on axial T2-weighted imaging. **(b)** The solid portion of the tumor shows prominent gadolinium contrast enhancement on axial T1-weighted imaging.

Table 1.11 *(cont.)* Cerebellopontine angle (CPA) and/or internal auditory canal lesions

Lesions	Imaging Findings	Comments
Choroid plexus carcinoma (**Fig. 1.252**)	*CT:* Large intraventricular lesions with intermediate attenuation, usually prominent contrast enhancement, ± calcifications, ± hemorrhage, ± invasion of adjacent brain tissue, ± disseminated disease. *MRI:* Large intraventricular tumors that often have heterogeneous intermediate signal with zones of high signal from hemorrhage on T1-weighted imaging. Tumors often have heterogeneous intermediate to slightly high signal on T2-weighted imaging as well as zones of low and high signal from hemorrhage, calcifications, and/or necrosis. Tumors usually show heterogeneous gadolinium contrast enhancement, ± contrast enhancement in the leptomeninges caused by disseminated tumor.	Rare malignant intracranial neoplasms (WHO grade III) with sheets of poorly differentiated cells with nuclear pleomorphism, > 5 mitoses per high-power field. Typically occur in young children (median age = 1.8 years). Commonly invade adjacent brain tissue and disseminate along CSF pathways. Carcinomas tend to be larger and have greater amounts of hemorrhage and necrosis than papillomas.
Metastatic disease (**Fig. 1.253** and **Fig. 1.254**)	*CT:* Spheroid lesions in brain that can have various intra-axial locations, often at gray-white matter junctions, with usually low-intermediate attenuation, ± hemorrhage, calcifications, and cysts. Variable contrast enhancement, often with low attenuation peripheral to nodular enhancing lesion representing axonal edema. Metastatic disease involving the meninges can also occur and be seen as abnormal contrast enhancement in the subarachnoid space. *MRI:* Circumscribed spheroid lesions in brain that can have various intra-axial locations, often at gray-white matter junctions, with usually low-intermediate signal on T1-weighted imaging and intermediate-high signal on T2-weighted imaging, ± hemorrhage, calcifications, and cysts. Variable gadolinium enhancement, and often high signal on T2-weighted imaging peripheral to nodular enhancing lesion representing axonal edema. Metastatic disease involving the meninges can also occur and be seen as abnormal contrast enhancement in the subarachnoid space.	Metastatic disease accounts for 33% of intracranial tumors, usually from extracranial primary neoplasm in adults > 40 years old. Primary tumor source: lung > breast > GI > GU > melanoma. Metastatic lesions in the cerebellum can present with obstructive hydrocephalus/neurosurgical emergency.
Myeloma	Multiple myeloma or single plasmacytoma are well-circumscribed or poorly defined lesions involving the skull and dura. *CT:* Lesions have low-intermediate attenuation, usually + contrast enhancement, + bone destruction. *MRI:* Well-circumscribed or poorly defined lesions involving the skull and dura, with low-intermediate signal on T1-weighted imaging, intermediate-high signal on T2-weighted imaging, and usually gadolinium contrast enhancement, + bone destruction.	Multiple myeloma are malignant tumors composed of proliferating antibody-secreting plasma cells derived from single clones. Multiple myeloma is primarily located in bone marrow. A solitary myeloma or plasmacytoma is an infrequent variant in which a neoplastic mass of plasma cells occurs at a single site of bone or soft tissues. In the United States, 14,600 new cases occur each year. Multiple myeloma is the most common primary neoplasm of bone in adults. Median age at presentation = 60 years. Most patients are more than 40 years old.
Lymphoma	Primary CNS lymphoma: Focal or infiltrating lesion located in the basal ganglia, posterior fossa/brainstem. *CT:* Low-intermediate attenuation, ± hemorrhage/necrosis in immunocompromised patients, usually with contrast enhancement. *MRI:* Low-intermediate signal on T1-weighted imaging, intermediate- slightly high signal on T2-weighted imaging, ± hemorrhage/necrosis in immunocompromised patients, usually with gadolinium contrast enhancement. Diffuse leptomeningeal enhancement is another pattern of intracranial lymphoma.	Lymphomas are lymphoid tumors whose neoplastic cells typically arise within lymphoid tissue (lymph nodes and reticuloendothelial organs). Primary CNS lymphoma is more common than secondary, usually occurring in adults > 40 years old, and accounts for 5% of primary brain tumors. Incidence currently ranges from 0.8 to 1.5% of primary intracranial tumors. Prior elevated incidence of 6% in patients with AIDS has been reduced with effective antiviral therapy. B-cell lymphoma is more common than T-cell lymphoma. MRI features of primary and secondary lymphoma of brain overlap. Intracranial lymphoma can involve the leptomeninges in secondary lymphoma > primary lymphoma.

(continued on page 168)

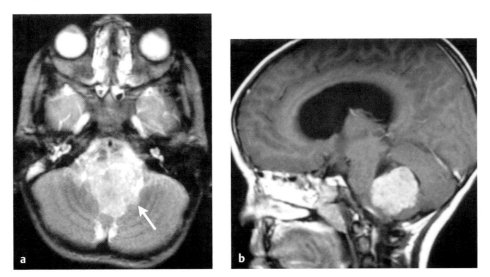

Fig. 1.252   A 3-year-old male with a choroid plexus carcinoma in the fourth ventricle with extension into the left foramen of Luschka and left cerebellopontine angle. **(a)** The tumor (*arrow*) has heterogeneous slightly high and high signal on axial T2-weighted imaging. **(b)** The tumor shows prominent gadolinium contrast enhancement on sagittal T1-weighted imaging.

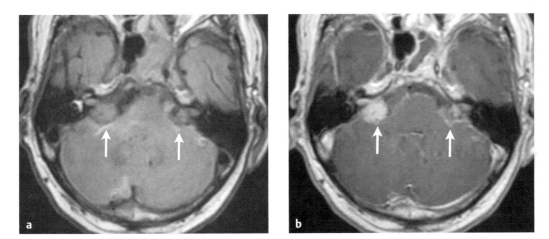

Fig. 1.253   A 71-year-old man with melanoma and disseminated leptomeningeal tumor in both cerebellopontine angles and internal auditory canals. **(a)** The tumor has intermediate signal (*arrows*) on axial FLAIR. **(b)** The lesion shows gadolinium contrast enhancement (*arrows*) on axial T1-weighted imaging.

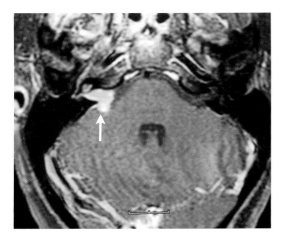

Fig. 1.254   A 42-year-old woman with metastatic disease from breast carcinoma with gadolinium-enhancing leptomeningeal tumor (*arrow*) in the right cerebellopontine angle and internal auditory canal on axial fat-suppressed T1-weighted imaging.

Table 1.11 *(cont.)* Cerebellopontine angle (CPA) and/or internal auditory canal lesions

Lesions	Imaging Findings	Comments
Endolymphatic sac adenoma/adenocarcinoma (**Fig. 1.255**)	Extra-axial retrolabyrinthine lesions involving the posterior petrous bone and extending into the cerebellopontine angle cistern. *CT:* Lesions can have low to intermediate attenuation and can show contrast enhancement. May contain blood products. *MRI:* Lesions often have lobulated margins and contain zones with low, intermediate, and/or high signal on T1- and T2-weighted imaging secondary to methemoglobin, hemosiderin, and cholesterol crystals due to episodes of hemorrhage. Variable gadolinium contrast enhancement.	Rare solid and/or cystic benign or malignant papillary adenomatous tumors arising from the endolymphatic sac along the dorsal aspect of the temporal bone. Occur in children and adults. Tumors are slow growing and rarely metastasize. May be sporadic or associated with von Hippel-Lindau disease.
Chordoma (**Fig. 1.256**)	Well-circumscribed lobulated lesions along the dorsal surface of the clivus, vertebral bodies, or sacrum, + localized bone destruction. *CT:* Lesions have low-intermediate attenuation, ± calcifications from destroyed bone carried away by tumor, + contrast enhancement. *MRI:* Lesion have low-intermediate signal on T1-weighted images, high signal on T2-weighted images, + gadolinium contrast enhancement (usually heterogeneous). Can be locally invasive and associated with bone erosion/destruction and encasement of vessels (usually without arterial narrowing) and nerves. Skull base-clivus is a common location, usually in the midline for conventional chordomas, which account for 80% of skull base chordomas. Chondroid chordomas tend to be located off midline near skull base synchondroses.	Chordomas are rare, locally aggressive, slow-growing, low to intermediate grade malignant tumors derived from ectopic notochordal remnants along the axial skeleton. Chondroid chondromas (5–15% of all chordomas) have both chordomatous and chondromatous differentiation; chordomas that contain sarcomatous components (5% of all chordomas) are referred to as dedifferentiated chordomas or sarcomatoid chordomas. Chordomas account for 2–4% of primary malignant bone tumors, 1–3% of all primary bone tumors, and less than 1% of intracranial tumors. The annual incidence has been reported to be 0.18 to 0.3 per million. Dedifferentiated chordomas or sarcomatoid chordomas account for less than 5% of all chordomas. For cranial chordomas, patients' mean age = 37 to 40 years.
Chondrosarcoma	*CT:* Lobulated lesions with low-intermediate attenuation, ± chondroid matrix mineralization, + contrast enhancement (usually heterogeneous). *MRI:* Lesions often have-intermediate signal on T1-weighted imaging, high signal on T2-weighted imaging, ± matrix mineralization with low signal on T2-weighted imaging, + gadolinium contrast enhancement (usually heterogeneous). Can be locally invasive and associated with bone erosion/destruction and , encasement of vessels and nerves. Skull base petro-occipital synchondrosis is a common location, usually off midline.	Chondrosarcomas involving the skull base are rare, slow-growing, malignant tumors containing cartilage formed within sarcomatous stroma. Chondrosarcomas can contain areas of calcification/mineralization, myxoid material, and/or ossification. Chondrosarcomas rarely arise within synovium. Chondrosarcomas represent 12–21% of malignant bone lesions, 21–26% of primary sarcomas of bone, 9–14% of all bone tumors, 6% of skull-base tumors, and 0.15% of all intracranial tumors.
Adenoid cystic carcinoma (**Fig. 1.257**)	*CT:* Tumors have intermediate attenuation and variable mild, moderate, or prominent contrast enhancement. *MRI:* Destructive lesions in the paranasal sinuses, nasal cavity, and nasopharynx, ± intracranial extension via bone destruction or perineural spread through foramen ovale into trigeminal cistern/intracranially. Intermediate signal on T1-weighted imaging, intermediate-high signal on T2-weighted imaging, and variable mild, moderate, or prominent gadolinium contrast enhancement.	Malignant basaloid tumor comprised of neoplastic epithelial and myoepithelial cells. Morphologic tumor patterns include tubular, cribriform, and solid. Accounts for 10% of epithelial salivary neoplasms. Most commonly involves the parotid, submandibular, and minor salivary glands (palate, tongue, buccal mucosa, and floor of the mouth, other locations). Perineural tumor spread common, ± facial nerve paralysis. Usually occurs in adults > 30 years old. Solid type has the worst prognosis. Up to 90% of patients die within 10–15 years of diagnosis.

(continued on page 170)

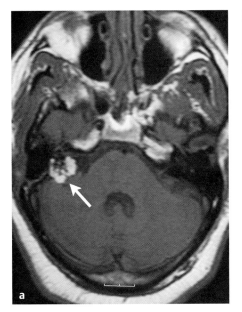

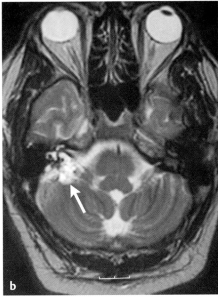

Fig. 1.255 Cystadenoma of the endolymphatic sac in a 46-year-old man. The tumor extends along the endocranial surface of the right temporal bone and has lobulated margins and contains mostly high signal on **(a)** axial T1-weighted imaging (*arrow*) and **(b)** axial T2-weighted imaging (*arrow*).

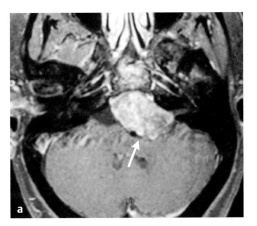

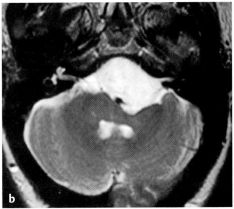

Fig. 1.256 **(a)** A 55-year-old woman with a chordoma along the endocranial surface of the clivus that shows heterogeneous gadolinium contrast enhancement on axial fat-suppressed T1-weighted imaging (*arrow*). **(b)** The tumor has high signal on axial T2-weighted imaging.

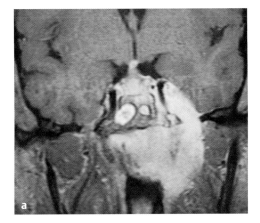

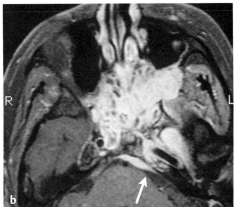

Fig. 1.257 Adenoid cystic carcinoma in a 46-year-old woman. **(a)** Coronal and **(b)** axial fat-suppressed T1-weighted images show gadolinium-enhancing tumor extending superiorly from the nasopharynx along the third division of the left trigeminal nerve through a widened foramen ovale to involve the left trigeminal cistern/Meckel's cave, left petrous apex, and intracranial dura in the left cerebellopontine angle (*arrow* in **b**).

Table 1.11 *(cont.)* Cerebellopontine angle (CPA) and/or internal auditory canal lesions

Lesions	Imaging Findings	Comments
Neoplasms—Intra-Axial		
Ependymoma (**Fig. 1.258** and **Fig. 1.259**)	*CT:* Circumscribed spheroid or lobulated infratentorial lesion, usually in the fourth ventricle, ± cysts and/or calcifications, with low-intermediate attenuation and variable contrast enhancement. *MRI:* Circumscribed spheroid or lobulated infratentorial lesion, usually in the fourth ventricle, ± cysts and/or calcifications, with low-intermediate signal on T1-weighted imaging, intermediate-high signal on T2-weighted imaging, and variable gadolinium contrast enhancement, ± extension through the foramina of Luschka and Magendie.	Slow-growing tumor (WHO grade II) comprised of neoplastic cells with monomorphic round/oval nuclei containing speckled chromatin, perivascular pseudorosettes, and ependymal rosettes. Zones of myxoid degeneration, hyalinization of blood vessels, hemorrhage, and/or calcifications may occur within tumors. Account for 6–12% of intracranial tumors, with an incidence of 0.22 to 0.29 per 100,000. Occur more commonly in children than adults; one-third are supratentorial and two-thirds are infratentorial. Children with infratentorial ependymomas range in age from 2 months to 16 years (mean age = 6.4 years).
Glioma of brainstem or cerebellum (**Fig. 1.260** and **Fig. 1.261**)	*Low-grade astrocytoma* *CT:* Focal lesion with low-intermediate attenuation, usually with prominent contrast enhancement. Lesions located in cerebellum, pons, or brainstem. *MRI:* Focal or diffuse mass lesion, usually located in cerebellar white matter or brainstem, with low-intermediate signal on T1-weighted imaging, high signal on T2-weighted imaging, ± gadolinium contrast enhancement. Minimal associated mass effect. *Juvenile pilocytic astrocytoma* *CT:* Solid/cystic focal lesion with low-intermediate attenuation, usually with prominent contrast enhancement. Lesions located in cerebellum, pons, or brainstem. *MRI:* Solid/cystic focal lesion with low-intermediate signal on T1-weighted imaging, high signal on T2-weighted imaging, usually with prominent gadolinium contrast enhancement. Lesions located in cerebellum and brainstem. *Gliomatosis cerebri* *CT:* Infiltrative lesion with poorly defined margins with mass effect located in the white matter, with low-intermediate attenuation. Usually no contrast enhancement until late in disease. *MRI:* Infiltrative lesion with poorly defined margins and with mass effect, located in the white matter, with low-intermediate signal on T1-weighted imaging, high signal on T2-weighted imaging, and usually no gadolinium contrast enhancement until late in disease. *Anaplastic astrocytoma/glioblastoma* *CT:* Lesion with poorly defined margins and with mass effect, located in the white matter, with low-intermediate attenuation. Variable irregular contrast enhancement. *MRI:* Infiltrative lesion with poorly defined margins and with mass effect, located in the white matter, with low-intermediate signal on T1-weighted imaging, high signal on T2-weighted imaging, and variable irregular gadolinium contrast enhancement. *MRS:* Elevated choline peak, decreased N-acetylaspartate peak, ± lactate peak.	*Low-grade astrocytoma:* Often occurs in children and adults (20–40 years old). Tumors comprised of well-differentiated astrocytes. Association with neurofibromatosis type 1, mean survival 6 to 8 years, and may become malignant. *Juvenile pilocytic astrocytoma:* Common in children, usually favorable prognosis if totally resected. *Gliomatosis cerebri:* Diffusely infiltrating astrocytoma with relative preservation of underlying brain architecture. Imaging appearance may be more prognostic than histologic grade, and approximate 2-year survival. *Anaplastic astrocytoma:* Intermediate between low-grade astrocytoma and glioblastoma multiforme, with approximate 2-year survival.

(continued on page 172)

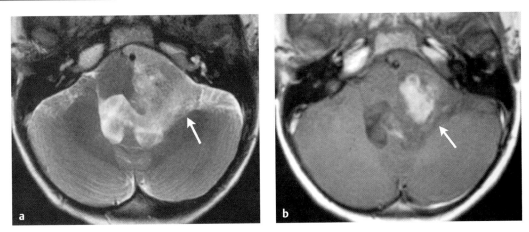

Fig. 1.258   A 5-year-old male with an ependymoma in the left foramen of Luschka extending into the fourth ventricle and left cerebellopontine angle. **(a)** The tumor has heterogeneous slightly high signal on axial T2-weighted imaging (*arrow*). **(b)** The tumor (*arrow*) shows heterogeneous gadolinium contrast enhancement on axial T1-weighted imaging.

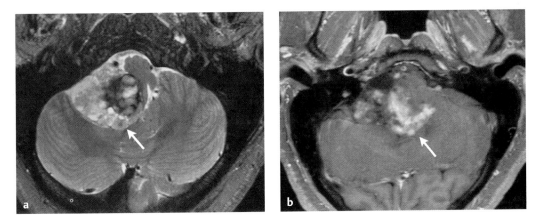

Fig. 1.259   **(a)** A 34 year-old man with an ependymoma in the fourth ventricle extending into the right foramen of Luschka and right cerebellopontine angle that has mixed low, intermediate, slightly high, and high signal on axial T2-weighted imaging (*arrow*). The low signal on T2-weighted imaging is secondary to prior hemorrhage. **(b)** The tumor shows heterogeneous gadolinium contrast enhancement on axial fat-suppressed T1-weighted imaging (*arrow*).

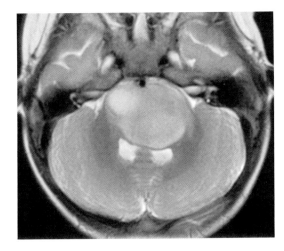

Fig. 1.260   A 15-month-old female with an astrocytoma in the pons that has diffuse high signal on axial T2-weighted imaging with associated mass effect encroaching on the left cerebellopontine angle.

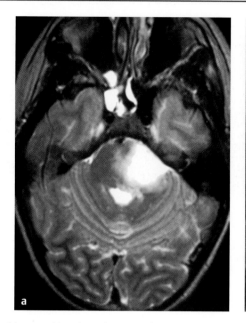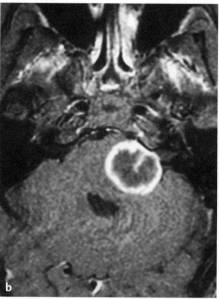

Fig. 1.261 **(a)** An 11-year-old male with an anaplastic astrocytoma involving the pons and left middle cerebellar peduncle that has high signal on axial T2-weighted imaging. **(b)** The tumor shows irregular peripheral gadolinium contrast enhancement on axial fat-suppressed T1-weighted imaging.

Table 1.11 *(cont.)* Cerebellopontine angle (CPA) and/or internal auditory canal lesions

Lesions	Imaging Findings	Comments
Hemangioblastoma **(Fig. 1.262)**	Circumscribed tumors usually located in the cerebellum, brainstem, and/or spinal cord. *CT:* Small contrast-enhancing nodule ± cyst, or larger lesion with prominent heterogeneous enhancement, ± hemorrhage. *MRI:* Small gadolinium-enhancing nodule ± cyst, or larger lesion with prominent heterogeneous enhancement ± flow voids within lesion or at the periphery. Intermediate signal on T1-weighted imaging and intermediate-high signal on T2-weighted imaging, and occasionally lesions have evidence of recent or remote hemorrhage.	Slow-growing, vascular, WHO grade I tumor with large, lipid-containing, vacuolated, neoplastic stromal cells and thin-walled vessels lined by capillary endothelial cells. Sclerosis and hemorrhage are commonly present in the tumors. Tumors are typically located in the cerebellum, brainstem, and spinal cord. Occur in adolescents and young and middle-aged adults. Lesions can be sporadic and solitary. Multiple lesions are typically seen in patients with von Hippel-Lindau disease.
Medulloblastoma	*CT:* Circumscribed or invasive lesions with intermediate-slightly increased attenuation, variable contrast enhancement, and frequent dissemination into the leptomeninges. *MRI:* Circumscribed or invasive lesions with low-intermediate signal on T1-weighted imaging and intermediate-high signal on T2-weighted imaging, ± cystic or necrotic zones. Solid portions can have restricted diffusion, variable gadolinium contrast enhancement, and frequent dissemination into the leptomeninges.	Highly malignant, primitive neuroectodermal tumors (WHO grade IV) located in the cerebellum that frequently disseminate along CSF pathways. Tumors are composed of poorly differentiated or undifferentiated cells with divergent differentiation along neuronal, astrocytic, or ependymal lines. Typically occur in patients from 4 weeks to 20 years old (mean age = 5.5 years).
Atypical teratoid/ Rhabdoid tumor **(Fig. 1.263)**	*CT:* Circumscribed or invasive lesions with low-intermediate attenuation, variable contrast enhancement, and frequent dissemination into the leptomeninges. *MRI:* Circumscribed mass lesions with intermediate signal on T1-weighted imaging, ± zones of high signal from hemorrhage on T1-weighted imaging, and variable mixed low, intermediate, and/or high signal on T2-weighted imaging. Solid portions can have restricted diffusion and usually prominent gadolinium contrast enhancement, ± heterogeneous pattern. Frequent dissemination into the leptomeninges.	Rare malignant tumors involving the CNS usually occurring in the first decade, usually < 3 years. Ki-67/MIB-1 proliferation index is often high, > 50%. Associated with mutations of the *INI1(hSNF5/ SMARCB1)* gene on chromosome 22q11.2. Histologically appear as solid tumors, ± necrotic areas, similar to malignant rhabdoid tumors of the kidney. Associated with a very poor prognosis.

(continued on page 174)

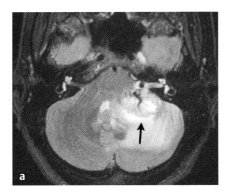
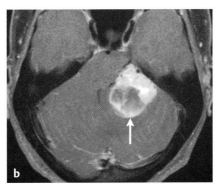
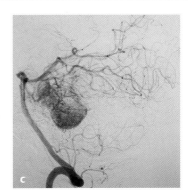

Fig. 1.262 **(a)** A 41-year-old woman with a hemangioblastoma involving the left middle cerebellar peduncle that has slightly high to high signal as well as flow voids on axial T2-weighted imaging (*arrow*). **(b)** The tumor shows irregular peripheral gadolinium contrast enhancement on axial fat-suppressed T1-weighted imaging (*arrow*). **(c)** Lateral view from a conventional arteriogram shows early prominent contrast enhancement of this vascular lesion.

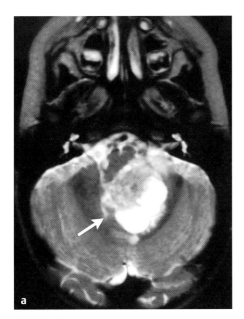
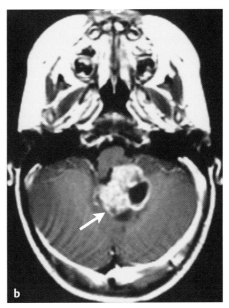

Fig. 1.263 A 2-year-old female with an atypical teratoid/rhabdoid tumor in the fourth ventricle extending through the left foramen Luschka into the left cerebellopontine angle. **(a)** The tumor has heterogeneous slightly high and high signal on axial T2-weighted imaging (*arrow*). **(b)** The tumor shows heterogeneous prominent gadolinium contrast enhancement on axial T1-weighted imaging (*arrow*).

Table 1.11 *(cont.)* Cerebellopontine angle (CPA) and/or internal auditory canal lesions

Lesions	Imaging Findings	Comments
Tumorlike Lesions		
Epidermoid (congenital cholesteatoma) (**Fig. 1.264**)	*CT:* Lesions usually have low-intermediate attenuation and no contrast enhancement, ± bone erosion/destruction. *MRI:* Well-circumscribed spheroid or multilobulated extra-axial ectodermal-inclusion cystic lesions with low-intermediate signal on T1-weighted imaging and high signal on T2-weighted imaging similar to CSF. Mixed low, intermediate, or high signal on FLAIR images, and no gadolinium enhancement. Often insinuate along CSF pathways, with chronic deformation of adjacent neural tissue (brainstem, brain parenchyma), although typically not associated with obstructive hydrocephalus. Commonly located in posterior cranial fossa (cerebellopontine angle cistern) > parasellar/middle cranial fossa.	Nonneoplastic congenital or acquired extra-axial off-midline lesions filled with desquamated cells and keratinaceous debris, usually with mild mass effect on adjacent brain, ± related clinical symptoms, and infratentorial > supratentorial locations. Present in adults, and males and females equally.
Dermoid	*CT:* Circumscribed spheroid or multilobulated extra-axial lesions, with variable low, intermediate, and/or high attenuation and contrast enhancement, ± fluid–fluid or fluid–debris levels. *MRI:* Well-circumscribed spheroid or multilobulated extra-axial lesions, usually with high signal on T1-weighted imaging and variable low, intermediate, and/or high signal on T2-weighted imaging. Typically no gadolinium contrast enhancement, ± fluid–fluid or fluid–debris levels. Can cause chemical meningitis if dermoid cyst ruptures into the subarachnoid space. Commonly located at or near midline, supra- > infra-tentorial.	Nonneoplastic congenital or acquired ectodermal inclusion cystic lesions filled with lipid material, cholesterol, desquamated cells, and keratinaceous debris. Usually have mild mass effect on adjacent brain, ± related clinical symptoms. Present in adults, and in males slightly more than in females.
Cholesterol granuloma (See **Fig. 1.66**)	*CT:* Lesions usually have low attenuation, ± bone erosion, bone expansion. *MRI:* Lesions usually have high signal on T1-weighted imaging (T1WI) and fat-suppressed (FS) T1WI. Lesions may have high, intermediate, and/or low signal on T2-weighted imaging (T2WI) and FS T2WI. A peripheral rim of low signal on T2WI may also be seen due to hemosiderin.	Lesions occur in young and middle-aged adults and occur when there is obstruction of mucosa-lined air cells in the temporal bone. Multiple cycles of hemorrhage and granulomatous reaction result in accumulation of cholesterol granules, chronic inflammatory cells including multinucleated giant cells, red blood cells, hemosiderin, fibrous tissue, and debris. The lesions are lined by fibrous connective tissue.
Lipoma (**Fig. 1.265**)	*CT:* Lipomas have low CT attenuation similar to fat. *MRI:* Lipomas have signal isointense to subcutaneous fat on T1-weighted images (high signal), and on T2-weighted images, signal suppression occurs with frequency-selective fat saturation techniques or with a short time to inversion recovery (STIR) method. Typically there is no gadolinium enhancement or peripheral edema.	Benign fatty lesions resulting from congenital malformation, often located in or near the midline, that may contain calcifications and/or traversing blood vessels.

(continued on page 176)

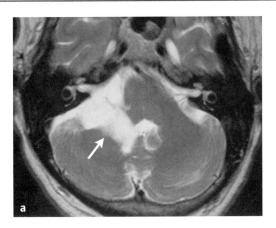
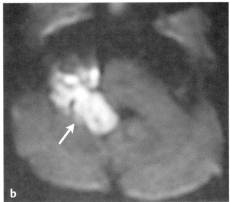

Fig. 1.264   A 66-year-old man with an epidermoid in the right foramen of Luschka and extending into the right cerebellopontine angle that has high signal on **(a)** axial T2-weighted imaging (*arrow*) and **(b)** axial diffusion-weighted imaging (*arrow*) due to restricted diffusion.

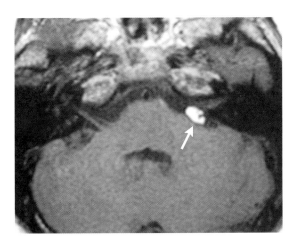

Fig. 1.265   A 52-year-old woman with a small lipoma (*arrow*) that has high signal on axial T1-weighted imaging and that is located at the pial surface of the left middle cerebellar peduncle.

Table 1.11 *(cont.)* Cerebellopontine angle (CPA) and/or internal auditory canal lesions

Lesions	Imaging Findings	Comments
Arachnoid cyst **(Fig. 1.266)**	*CT:* Circumscribed extra-axial lesions with low attenuation equal to CSF and no contrast enhancement. Commonly located: anterior middle cranial fossa > suprasellar/quadrigeminal > frontal convexities > posterior cranial fossa. *MRI:* Circumscribed extra-axial lesions with low signal on T1-weighted imaging and FLAIR imaging, and high signal on T2-weighted imaging similar to CSF, and no gadolinium contrast enhancement. Arachnoid cysts show increased diffusion. Commonly located: anterior middle cranial fossa > suprasellar/quadrigeminal > frontal convexities > posterior cranial fossa.	Nonneoplastic, congenital, developmental or acquired extra-axial lesions filled with CSF, usually with mild mass effect on adjacent brain, ± related clinical symptoms, and in supratentorial > infratentorial locations. Found in males more than in females.

Vascular Abnormalities

Lesions	Imaging Findings	Comments
Vertebrobasilar dolichoectasia **(Fig. 1.267)**	*CT/CTA:* Elongation and tortuosity of dilated vertebral and basilar arteries, ± wall calcifications, ± variable impression on adjacent brainstem. *MRI/MRA:* Elongated and ectatic vertebral and basilar arteries, with variable intraluminal MR signal related to turbulent or slowed blood flow or partial/complete thrombosis.	Abnormal fusiform dilatation of vertebrobasilar arteries secondary to acquired/degenerative etiology, polycystic disease, connective tissue disease, atherosclerosis, chronic hypertension, trauma, infection (mycotic), oncotic, arteriovenous malformation, vasculitis, and drugs.
Arterial aneurysm— Basilar artery/branches, Vertebral arteries **(Fig. 1.268)**	*Saccular aneurysm* *MRI/MRA:* Focal well-circumscribed zone of signal void on T1- and T2-weighted imaging, with variable mixed signal if thrombosed. MRA shows a speroid or ovoid zone of flow signal in non-thrombosed aneurysms. *CT/CTA:* Focal well-circumscribed zone of intermediate-high attenuation, + contrast enhancement in nonthrombosed portion of aneurysm, easily visualized on CTA. *Giant aneurysm* *MRI/MRA:* Focal well-circumscribed structure with layers of low, intermediate, and high signal on T2-weighted imaging secondary to layers of thrombus of different ages, as well as a zone of signal void representing a patent lumen if present. On T1-weighted imaging, layers of intermediate and high signal can be seen as well as a zone of signal void. MRA shows flow signal in lumen of aneurysm. *CT/CTA:* Focal well-circumscribed structure with layers of low, intermediate, and/or high attenuation secondary to layers of thrombus of different ages, as well as a zone of contrast enhancement representing a patent lumen, if present, ± wall calcifications.	Abnormal focal dilatation of artery secondary to acquired/degenerative etiology, polycystic disease, connective tissue disease, atherosclerosis, trauma, infection (mycotic), oncotic, arteriovenous malformation, vasculitis, and drugs. Giant aneurysms are > 2 cm in diameter.

(continued on page 178)

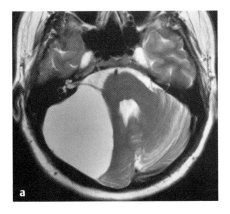
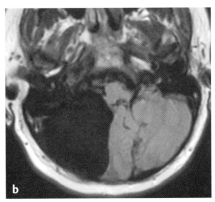
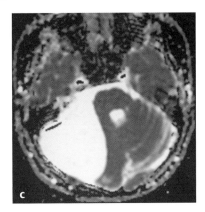

Fig. 1.266 A 33-year-old man with an arachnoid cyst in the lateral portion of the right posterior cranial fossa displacing the right cerebellar hemisphere medially. This extra-axial lesion has signal equal to CSF on **(a)** axial T2-weighted imaging, **(b)** FLAIR, and **(c)** ADC.

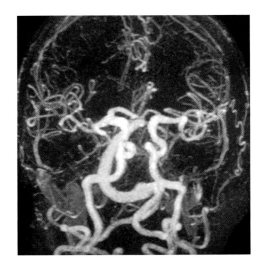

Fig. 1.267 A 61-year-old man with vertebrobasilar dolichoectasia with dilated tortuous basilar artery on coronal gadolinium-enhanced MRA.

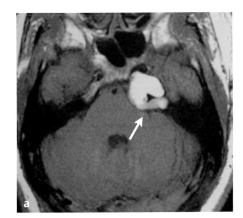
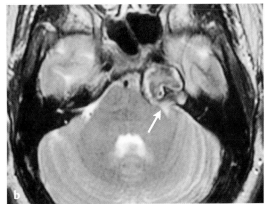

Fig. 1.268 A 35-year-old man with a carotid artery aneurysm in the left petrous apex. The aneurysm has **(a)** mostly high signal on axial T1-weighted imaging (*arrow*) and **(b)** mixed low, intermediate, and high signal on axial T2-weighted imaging (*arrow*).

Table 1.11 *(cont.)* Cerebellopontine angle (CPA) and/or internal auditory canal lesions

Lesions	Imaging Findings	Comments
Arteriovenous malformations (AVMs) (**Fig. 1.269**)	Lesions with irregular margins that can be located in the brain parenchyma/brainstem-pia, dura, or both locations. *CT/CTA:* CTA shows multiple, tortuous, contrast-enhancing vessels, including veins and arteries, ± calcifications, ± hemorrhage. *MRI/MRA:* AVMs contain multiple, tortuous, tubular flow voids on T1- and T2-weighted imaging secondary to patent arteries with high blood flow; as well as thrombosed vessels with variable signal, areas of hemorrhage in various phases, calcifications, and gliosis. The venous portions often show gadolinium contrast enhancement. Gradient echo MRI/MRA shows flow-related enhancement (high signal) in patent arteries and veins of the AVM. Usually not associated with mass effect unless there is recent hemorrhage or venous occlusion.	Supratentorial AVMs occur more frequently than infratentorial AVMs. Annual risk of hemorrhage. AVMs can be sporadic, congenital, or associated with a history of trauma.
Epidural hematoma	Biconvex extra-axial hematoma located between the skull and dura, and displaced dura has low signal on T2-weighted imaging. The signal of the hematoma itself depends on its age, size, hematocrit, and oxygen tension, ± edema (high signal on T2-weighted imaging involving the displaced brain parenchyma), ± subfalcine, uncal herniation. *Hyperacute epidural hematoma* *CT:* Biconvex hematoma with high or mixed intermediate and high attenuation. *MRI:* Intermediate signal on T1-weighted imaging, intermediate-high signal on T2-weighted imaging. *Acute epidural hematoma* *CT:* High or mixed intermediate and high attenuation. *MRI:* Low-intermediate signal on T1-weighted imaging, high signal on T2-weighted imaging. *Subacute epidural hematoma* *CT:* High, or mixed low, intermediate, and/or high attenuation. *MRI:* High signal on T1- and T2-weighted imaging.	Epidural hematomas usually result from trauma/ tearing of an epidural artery or dural venous sinus, ± skull fracture. Epidural hematomas do not cross cranial sutures.

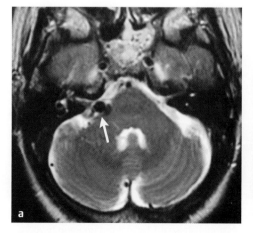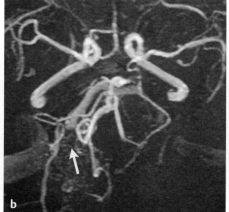

Fig. 1.269 A 64-year-old woman with an arteriovenous malformation in the right cerebellopontine angle, seen as **(a)** abnormal flow voids (*arrow*) on axial T2-weighted imaging and **(b)** a collection of abnormal vessels on axial 3D TOF MRA (*arrow*).

Lesions	Imaging Findings	Comments
Subdural hematoma (**Fig. 1.270**)	Crescentic extra-axial hematoma located in the potential space between the inner margin of the dura and outer margin of the arachnoid membrane. *Hyperacute subdural hematoma* *CT:* High and/or high and intermediate attenuation. *MRI:* Intermediate signal on T1-weighted imaging and intermediate-high signal on T2-weighted imaging. *Acute subdural hematoma* *CT:* High and/or high and intermediate attenuation. *MRI:* Low-intermediate signal on T1-weighted imaging, low signal on T2-weighted imaging. *Subacute subdural hematoma* *CT:* Intermediate attenuation, may be isodense to brain. *MRI:* High signal on T1- and T2-weighted imaging. *Chronic subdural hematoma* *CT:* Variable, often low-intermediate attenuation. *MRI:* Variable, often low-intermediate signal on T1-weighted imaging, high signal on T2-weighted imaging, ± gadolinium contrast enhancement at organizing neomembrane. Mixed MRI signal can result if rebleeding occurs into chronic collection.	Subdural hematomas usually result from trauma/stretching/tearing of cortical veins where they enter the subdural space to drain into dural venous sinuses, ± skull fracture. Subdural hematomas do cross sites of cranial sutures.

(continued on page 180)

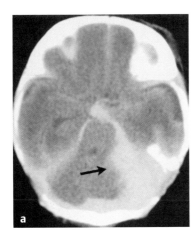 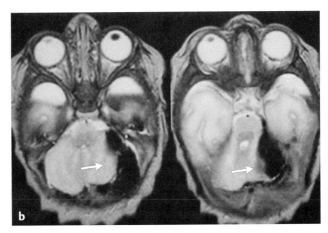

Fig. 1.270 A 3-day-old female with traumatic acute subdural hemorrhage (*arrows*), with **(a)** high-attenuation blood along the tentorium on axial CT (*arrow*) and **(b)** low signal on axial T2-weighted imaging (*arrows*).

Table 1.11 *(cont.)* Cerebellopontine angle (CPA) and/or internal auditory canal lesions

Lesions	Imaging Findings	Comments
Subarachnoid hemorrhage **(Fig. 1.271)**	*CT:* Acute subarachnoid hemorrhage typically appears as poorly defined zones with high attenuation in the leptomeninges within the sulci and basal cisterns. Usually become isodense or hypodense after 1 week unless there is rebleeding. *MRI:* May not be seen on T1- or T2-weighted imaging, although may have intermediate to slightly high signal on FLAIR images.	Extravasated blood in the subarachnoid space can result from ruptured arterial aneurysms or dural venous sinuses, vascular malformations, hypertensive hemorrhages, trauma, cerebral infarcts, coagulopathy, etc.
Inflammation		
Brainstem/ cerebellar abscess **(Fig. 1.272)**	*CT:* Circumscribed lesion with a central zone of low attenuation (± air–fluid level) surrounded by a thin rim of intermediate attenuation, peripheral poorly defined zone of decreased attenuation representing edema, and ringlike contrast enhancement of abscess wall that is sometimes thicker laterally than medially. *MRI:* Circumscribed lesion with low signal on T1-weighted imaging, central zone of high signal on T2-weighted imaging (± air–fluid level) surrounded by a thin rim with T2-weighted imaging that shows ringlike gadolinium contrast enhancement that is sometimes thicker laterally than medially. Peripheral poorly defined zone of high signal on T2-weighted imaging representing edema. Abscess contents typically have restricted diffusion. Mean ADC values for abscesses are significantly lower (0.63 to 1.12×10^{-3} mm²) than for necrotic or cystic neoplasms (2.45×10^{-3} mm²). *MR spectroscopy* shows decreased *N*-acetylaspartate from destruction of neurons, elevated lactate, and amino acid peaks (valine, leucine, and isoleucine) at 0.9 ppm secondary to proteolytic enzymes.	Formation of brain abscess occurs 2 weeks after cerebritis, with liquefaction and necrosis centrally surrounded by a capsule and peripheral edema. Restricted diffusion of abscess contents is related to the combination of the high protein content and viscosity of pus, necrotic debris, and bacteria. Can be multiple, but more than 50% are solitary. Complication from meningitis and/or sinusitis, septicemia, trauma, surgery, cardiac shunt. Accounts for 2% and 8% of intra-axial mass lesions in developed and developing countries, respectively.
Subdural/epidural abscess—Empyema	*CT:* Epidural or subdural collections with low attenuation and linear peripheral zones of contrast enhancement. *MRI:* Epidural or subdural collections with low signal on T1-weighted imaging, high signal on T2-weighted imaging, and thin linear peripheral zones of gadolinium contrast enhancement.	Often results from complications related to sinusitis (usually frontal), meningitis, otitis media, ventricular shunts, or surgery. Can be associated with venous sinus thrombosis and venous cerebral or cerebellar infarctions, cerebritis, or brain abscess. Mortality is 30%.

(continued on page 182)

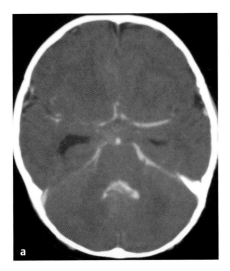
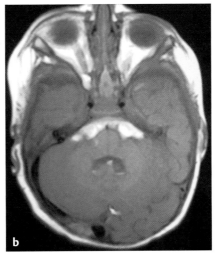

Fig. 1.271 Subarachnoid hemorrhage in the basal cisterns and fourth ventricle, with high attenuation on **(a)** postcontrast axial CT and high signal on **(b)** axial T1-weighted imaging.

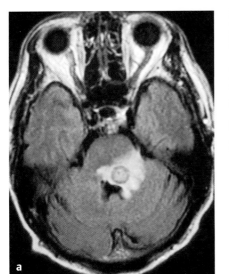
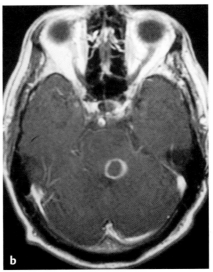
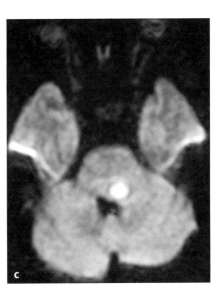

Fig. 1.272 A 70-year-old man with a pyogenic abscess involving the pons and left middle cerebellar peduncle. **(a)** The abscess wall is a thin rim with intermediate-low signal that surrounds a central zone with high signal on axial FLAIR. A poorly defined zone of high signal is also seen surrounding the abscess wall, representing peripheral edema. **(b)** The thin abscess wall shows gadolinium contrast enhancement on axial T1-weighted imaging. **(c)** The abscess contents have restricted diffusion on axial diffusion-weighted imaging.

Table 1.11 *(cont.)* Cerebellopontine angle (CPA) and/or internal auditory canal lesions

Lesions	Imaging Findings	Comments
Leptomeningeal infection **(Fig. 1.273)**	*CT:* Single or multiple nodular contrast-enhancing lesions and/or focal or diffuse abnormal subarachnoid enhancement. *MRI:* Single or multiple nodular gadolinium-enhancing lesions and/or focal or diffuse abnormal subarachnoid enhancement. Low-intermediate signal on T1-weighted imaging, intermediate-high signal on T2-weighted imaging. Leptomeningeal infection often best seen on postcontrast images.	Gadolinium contrast enhancement in the intracranial subarachnoid space (leptomeninges) usually is associated with significant pathology (inflammation and/or infection versus neoplasm). Infection of the leptomeninges can result from pyogenic, fungal, or parasitic diseases, as well as tuberculosis.
Dural and/or leptomeningeal noninfectious inflammation **(Fig. 1.274** and **Fig. 1.275)**	*MRI:* Single or multiple nodular gadolinium-enhancing lesions and/or focal or diffuse abnormal subarachnoid enhancement. Low-intermediate signal on T1-weighted imaging, intermediate-high signal on T2-weighted and FLAIR imaging. Leptomeningeal inflammation often best seen on postcontrast images. *CT:* Single or multiple nodular contrast-enhancing lesions and/or focal or diffuse abnormal subarachnoid enhancement.	Neurosarcoid and Langerhans' cell histiocytosis can result in noninfectious granulomatous disease in the leptomeninges, with subarachnoid gadolinium contrast enhancement in patterns similar to infections.
Langerhans' cell histiocytosis	*CT:* Single or multiple circumscribed soft tissue radiolucent lesions in the marrow of the skull associated with focal trabecular and cortical bony destruction/erosion, with extension extra- or intracranially or both. *MRI:* Lesions usually have low-intermediate signal on T1-weighted imaging, mixed intermediate-slightly high signal on T2-weighted imaging, + gadolinium contrast enhancement, ± enhancement of the adjacent dura.	Benign tumorlike lesions consisting of Langerhans' cells (histiocytes) and variable amounts of lymphocytes, polymorphonuclear cells, and eosinophils. Single lesions are commonly seen in males more than in females and in patients < 20 years old. Proliferation of intraosseous histiocytes in medullary cavity with localized destruction of bone and extension into adjacent soft tissues. Multiple lesions are associated with Letterer-Siwe disease (lymphadenopathy hepatosplenomegaly) in children < 2 years old, and Hand-Schüller-Christian disease (lymphadenopathy, exophthalmos, diabetes insipidus) in children 5–10 years old.
Infection		
Lyme disease—spirochete infection	*CT:* Foci of decreased attenuation in cerebral and/or cerebellar white matter, ± contrast enhancement. *MRI:* Foci (2 to 8 mm) with high signal on T2-weighted imaging and FLAIR in cerebral and/or cerebellar white matter, ± restricted diffusion, ± contrast enhancement of intra-axial lesions and/or leptomeninges and CN III, V, and/or VII.	CNS manifestations presumed to occur from immune-related demyelination caused by Lyme disease (infection by a spirochete, *Borrelia burgdorferi*) transmitted to humans via bites from Ixodes ticks that have been infected by primary hosts (mice and deer). Most cases in the United States occur in the Mid-Atlantic region. Patients can present with headaches, malaise, fevers, myalgias, erythema migrans, and/or facial palsy from facial neuritis.

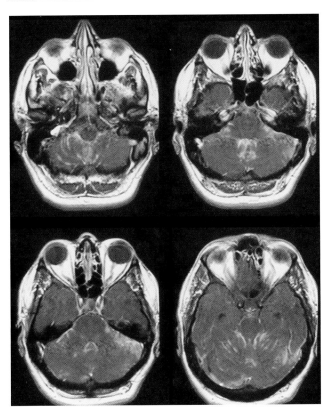

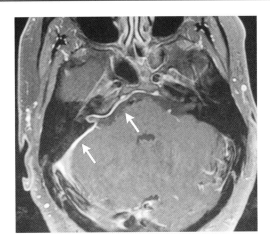

Fig. 1.274 Neurosarcoid with abnormal gadolinium contrast enhancement involving the dura (*arrows*) along the clivus and endocranial surface of the right petrous bone and with extension into the right internal auditory canal, seen on axial fat-suppressed T1-weighted imaging.

Fig. 1.273 A 40-year-old man immunocompromised by HIV infection has cryptococcal meningitis, seen as diffuse gadolinium contrast enhancement in the leptomeninges and fourth ventricle on axial T1-weighted imaging.

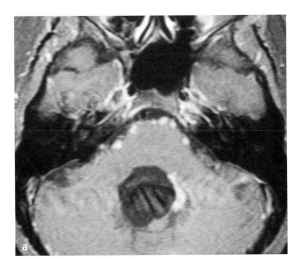

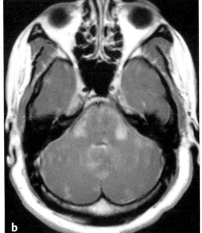

Fig. 1.275 Neurosarcoid in two patients seen as abnormal gadolinium contrast enhancement involving the leptomeninges and fourth ventricle on **(a)** axial fat-suppressed T1-weighted imaging and **(b)** axial T1-weighted imaging.

References

Aberrant Internal Carotid Artery

1. Celebi I, Oz A, Yildirim H, Bankeroglu H, Basak M. A case of an aberrant internal carotid artery with a persistent stapedial artery: association of hypoplasia of the A1 segment of the anterior cerebral artery. Surg Radiol Anat 2012;34(7):665–670

2. Dedhia K, Yellon RF, Branstetter BF, Egloff AM. Anatomic variants on computed tomography in congenital aural atresia. Otolaryngol Head Neck Surg 2012;147(2):323–328

3. Ito S, Miyazaki H, Iino N, Shiokawa Y, Saito I. Unilateral agenesis and hypoplasia of the internal carotid artery: a report of three cases. Neuroradiology 2005;47(5):311–315

4. McEachen JC, Obrzut M, Bokhari SJ. A rare combination of carotid artery congenital abnormalities: understanding the embryology and clinical associations. Emerg Radiol 2009;16(5):411–414

5. Sauvaget E, Paris J, Kici S, et al. Aberrant internal carotid artery in the temporal bone: imaging findings and management. Arch Otolaryngol Head Neck Surg 2006;132(1):86–91

6. Silbergleit R, Quint DJ, Mehta BA, Patel SC, Metes JJ, Noujaim SE. The persistent stapedial artery. AJNR Am J Neuroradiol 2000; 21(3):572–577

7. Tasar M, Yetiser S, Yildirim D, et al. Preoperative evaluation of the congenital aural atresia on computed tomography; an analysis of the severity of the deformity of the middle ear and mastoid. Eur J Radiol 2007;62(1):97–105

8. Thiers FA, Sakai O, Poe DS, Curtin HD. Persistent stapedial artery: CT findings. AJNR Am J Neuroradiol 2000;21(8):1551–1554

9. Watanabe A, Miyashima H, Kobashi T, Take K. CT findings of bilateral congenital absence of the long process of the incus. Neuroradiology 2004;46(10):859–861

10. Yilmaz T, Bilgen C, Savas R, Alper H. Persistent stapedial artery: MR angiographic and CT findings. AJNR Am J Neuroradiol 2003;24(6):1133–1135

Alexander disease

11. van der Knaap MS, Valk J. Alexander disease. In: Magnetic Resonance of Myelination and Myelin Disorders. 3rd ed. Berlin: Springer; 2005:416–435

Anatomy and Development of the Temporal Bone

12. Ahuja AT, Yuen HY, Wong KT, Yue V, van Hasselt AC. Computed tomography imaging of the temporal bone—normal anatomy. Clin Radiol 2003;58(9):681–686

13. Curtin HD, Gupta R, Bergeron RT. Embryology, anatomy, and imaging of the temporal bone. In: Som P and Curtin H, eds. Head and Neck Imaging. 5th ed. St. Louis, MO: Elsevier Mosby; 2011:1053–1096

14. Jackler RK, Luxford WM, House WF. Congenital malformations of the inner ear: a classification based on embryogenesis. Laryngoscope 1987;97(3 Pt 2, Suppl 40):2–14

15. Nayak S. Segmental anatomy of the temporal bone. Semin Ultrasound CT MRI 2001;22:184–218

16. Sennaroglu L, Saatci I. Unpartitioned versus incompletely partitioned cochleae: radiologic differentiation. Otol Neurotol 2004;25(4): 520–529, discussion 529

17. Whitfield TT. Development of the inner ear. Curr Opin Genet Dev 2015;32:112–118

Apert Syndrome

18. Raybaud C, Di Rocco C. Brain malformation in syndromic craniosynostoses, a primary disorder of white matter: a review. Childs Nerv Syst 2007;23(12):1379–1388

Atretic Cephaloceles

19. Brunelle F, Baraton J, Renier D, et al. Intracranial venous anomalies associated with atretic cephalocoeles. Pediatr Radiol 2000; 30(11):743–747

Branchio-Oto-Renal Syndrome

20. Carter MT, Blaser S, Papsin B, et al. Middle and inner ear malformations in mutation-proven branchio-oculo-facial (BOF) syndrome: case series and review of the literature. Am J Med Genet A 2012; 158A(8):1977–1981

21. Ceruti S, Stinckens C, Cremers CWRJ, Casselman JW. Temporal bone anomalies in the branchio-oto-renal syndrome: detailed computed tomographic and magnetic resonance imaging findings. Otol Neurotol 2002;23(2):200–207

22. Kemperman MH, Koch SMP, Joosten FBM, Kumar S, Huygen PLM, Cremers CWRJ. Inner ear anomalies are frequent but nonobligatory features of the branchio-oto-renal syndrome. Arch Otolaryngol Head Neck Surg 2002;128(9):1033–1038

23. Kochhar A, Fischer SM, Kimberling WJ, Smith RJH. Branchio-oto-renal syndrome. Am J Med Genet A 2007;143A(14):1671–1678

24. O'Brien BM, Meyers SP, Crane BT. Brachio-oto-renal syndrome: CT imaging and intraoperative diagnostic findings. Otol Neurotol 2015;36(6):e110–e111

25. Propst EJ, Blaser S, Gordon KA, Harrison RV, Papsin BC. Temporal bone findings on computed tomography imaging in branchio-oto-renal syndrome. Laryngoscope 2005;115(10):1855–1862

Canavan disease

26. van der Knaap MS, Valk J. Canavan disease. In: Magnetic Resonance of Myelination and Myelin Disorders. 3rd ed. Springer 2005:326–333.

Cephaloceles

27. Alonso RC, de la Peña MJ, Caicoya AG, Rodriguez MR, Moreno EA, de Vega Fernandez VM. Spontaneous skull base meningoencephaloceles and cerebrospinal fluid fistulas. Radiographics 2013;33(2):553–570

28. Kanev PM. Congenital malformations of the skull and meninges. Otolaryngol Clin North Am 2007;40(1):9–26, v

29. Nishiike S, Miyao Y, Gouda S, et al. Brain herniation into the middle ear following temporal bone fracture. Acta Otolaryngol 2005; 125(8):902–905

30. Lim ZM, Friedland PL, Boeddinghaus R, Thompson A, Rodrigues SJ, Atlas M. Otitic meningitis, superior semicircular canal dehiscence, and encephalocele: a case series. Otol Neurotol 2012;33(4):610–612

CHARGE Syndrome

31. Arndt S, Laszig R, Beck R, et al. Spectrum of hearing disorders and their management in children with CHARGE syndrome. Otol Neurotol 2010;31(1):67–73

32. Jyonouchi S, McDonald-McGinn DM, Bale S, Zackai EH, Sullivan KE. CHARGE (coloboma, heart defect, atresia choanae, retarded growth and development, genital hypoplasia, ear anomalies/deafness) syndrome and chromosome 22q11.2 deletion syndrome: a comparison of immunologic and nonimmunologic phenotypic features. Pediatrics 2009;123(5):e871–e877

33. Lalani SR, Hefner MA, Belmont JW, Davenport SLH. CHARGE syndrome. GeneReviews 2006

34. Morimoto AK, Wiggins RH III, Hudgins PA, et al. Absent semicircular canals in CHARGE syndrome: radiologic spectrum of findings. AJNR Am J Neuroradiol 2006;27(8):1663–1671

Cholesteatoma

35. Akkari M, Gabrillargues J, Saroul N, et al. Contribution of magnetic resonance imaging to the diagnosis of middle ear cholesteatoma: analysis of a series of 97 cases. Eur Ann Otorhinolaryngol Head Neck Dis 2014;131(3):153–158

36. Corrales CE, Blevins NH. Imaging for evaluation of cholesteatoma: current concepts and future directions. Curr Opin Otolaryngol Head Neck Surg 2013;21(5):461–467

37. Karandikar A, Loke SC, Goh J, et al. Evaluation of cholesteatoma: our experience with DW propeller imaging. Acta Radiol 2015; 56(9):1108–1112

38. Lincot J, Veillon F, Riehm S, et al. Middle ear cholesteatoma: Compared diagnostic performances of two incremental MRI protocols including non-echo planar diffusion-weighted imaging acquired on 3T and 1.5T scanners. J Neuroradiol 2015;42(4):193–201

39. Li PM, Linos E, Gurgel RK, Fischbein NJ, Blevins NH. Evaluating the utility of non-echo-planar diffusion-weighted imaging in the preoperative evaluation of cholesteatoma: a meta-analysis. Laryngoscope 2013;123(5):1247–1250

40. Richter GT, Lee KH. Contemporary assessment and management of congenital cholesteatoma. Curr Opin Otolaryngol Head Neck Surg 2009;17(5):339–345

41. Tada A, Inai R, Tanaka T, et al. The difference in congenital cholesteatoma CT findings based on the type of mass. Diagn Interv Imaging 2016;97(1):65–69

Cleidocranial Dysplasia

42. Cohen MM Jr. Biology of RUNX2 and cleidocranial dysplasia. J Craniofac Surg 2013;24(1):130–133
43. Gonzalez GE, Caruso PA, Small JE, Jyung RW, Troulis MJ, Curtin HD. Craniofacial and temporal bone CT findings in cleidocranial dysplasia. Pediatr Radiol 2008;38(8):892–897
44. Lloret I, Server A, Taksdal I. Calvarial lesions: a radiological approach to diagnosis. Acta Radiol 2009;50(5):531–542

Cochleovestibular Malformations

45. Adunka OF, Roush PA, Teagle HFB, et al. Internal auditory canal morphology in children with cochlear nerve deficiency. Otol Neurotol 2006;27(6):793–801
46. Atkin JS, Grimmer JF, Hedlund G, Park AH. Cochlear abnormalities associated with enlarged vestibular aqueduct anomaly. Int J Pediatr Otorhinolaryngol 2009;73(12):1682–1685
47. Campbell AP, Adunka OF, Zhou B, Qaqish BF, Buchman CA. Large vestibular aqueduct syndrome: anatomic and functional parameters. Laryngoscope 2011;121(2):352–357
48. Chadha NK, James AL, Gordon KA, Blaser S, Papsin BC. Bilateral cochlear implantation in children with anomalous cochleovestibular anatomy. Arch Otolaryngol Head Neck Surg 2009;135(9):903–909
49. Giesemann AM, Goetz F, Neuburger J, Lenarz T, Lanfermann H. Appearance of hypoplastic cochlea in CT and MRI: a new subclassification. Neuroradiology 2011;53(1):49–61
50. Giesemann AM, Goetz F, Neuburger J, Lenarz T, Lanfermann H. From labyrinthine aplasia to otocyst deformity. Neuroradiology 2010;52(2):147–154
51. Jackler RK, Luxford WM, House WF. Congenital malformations of the inner ear: a classification based on embryogenesis. Laryngoscope 1987;97(3 Pt 2, Suppl 40):2–14
52. Joshi VM, Navlekar SK, Kishore GR, Reddy KJ, Kumar ECVCT. CT and MR imaging of the inner ear and brain in children with congenital sensorineural hearing loss. Radiographics 2012;32(3):683–698
53. Ma H, Han P, Liang B, et al. Multislice spiral computed tomography imaging in congenital inner ear malformations. J Comput Assist Tomogr 2008;32(1):146–150
54. Miyasaka M, Nosaka S, Morimoto N, Taiji H, Masaki H. CT and MR imaging for pediatric cochlear implantation: emphasis on the relationship between the cochlear nerve canal and the cochlear nerve. Pediatr Radiol 2010;40(9):1509–1516
55. Mylanus EAM, Rotteveel LJC, Leeuw RL. Congenital malformation of the inner ear and pediatric cochlear implantation. Otol Neurotol 2004;25(3):308–317
56. Ozgen B, Oguz KK, Atas A, Sennaroglu L. Complete labyrinthine aplasia: clinical and radiologic findings with review of the literature. AJNR Am J Neuroradiol 2009;30(4):774–780
57. Papsin BC. Cochlear implantation in children with anomalous cochleovestibular anatomy. Laryngoscope 2005;115(1 Pt 2, Suppl 106):1–26
58. Phillips GS, LoGerfo SE, Richardson ML, Anzai Y. Interactive Web-based learning module on CT of the temporal bone: anatomy and pathology. Radiographics 2012;32(3):E85–E105
59. Romo LV, Casselman JW, Robson CD. Congenital anomalies of the temporal bone. In: Som P and Curtin H, eds. Head and Neck Imaging. 5th ed. St. Louis, MO: Elsevier Mosby; 2011:1097–1165
60. Satar B, Mukherji SK, Telian SA. Congenital aplasia of the semicircular canals. Otol Neurotol 2003;24(3):437–446
61. Sennaroglu L, Saatci I. Unpartitioned versus incompletely partitioned cochleae: radiologic differentiation. Otol Neurotol 2004;25(4):520–529, discussion 529
62. Song JJ, Choi HG, Oh SH, Chang SO, Kim CS, Lee JH. Unilateral sensorineural hearing loss in children: the importance of temporal bone computed tomography and audiometric follow-up. Otol Neurotol 2009;30(5):604–608
63. Swartz JD, Mukherji SK. The inner ear otodystrophies. In: Imaging of the Temporal Bone. 4th ed. New York: Thieme; 2008:298–411
64. Vrabec JT, Lin JW. Inner ear anomalies in congenital aural atresia. Otol Neurotol 2010;31(9):1421–1426
65. Walther LE, Nath V, Krombach GA, Di Martino E. Bilateral posterior semicircular canal aplasia and atypical paroxysmal positional vertigo: a case report. Acta Otorhinolaryngol Ital 2008;28(2):79–82

Congenital Hydrocephalus

66. Morón FE, Morriss MC, Jones JJ, Hunter JV. Lumps and bumps on the head in children: use of CT and MR imaging in solving the clinical diagnostic dilemma. Radiographics 2004;24(6):1655–1674
67. Moritake K, Nagai H, Nagasako N, Yamasaki M, Oi S, Hata T. Diagnosis of congenital hydrocephalus and delivery of its patients in Japan. Brain Dev 2008;30(6):381–386

Craniosynostosis

68. Attaya H, Thomas J, Alleman A. Imaging of craniosynostosis from diagnosis through reconstruction. Neurographics 2011;1:121–128
69. Currarino G. Sagittal synostosis in X-linked hypophosphatemic rickets and related diseases. Pediatr Radiol 2007;37(8):805–812
70. Jezela-Stanek A, Krajewska-Walasek M. Genetic causes of syndromic craniosynostoses. Eur J Paediatr Neurol 2013;17(3):221–224
71. Kirmi O, Lo SJ, Johnson D, Anslow P. Craniosynostosis: a radiological and surgical perspective. Semin Ultrasound CT MR 2009;30(6):492–512
72. Murthy AS. X-linked hypophosphatemic rickets and craniosynostosis. J Craniofac Surg 2009;20(2):439–442

Craniovertebral Abnormalities

73. Bertozzi JC, Rojas CA, Martinez CR. Evaluation of the pediatric craniocervical junction on MDCT. AJR Am J Roentgenol 2009;192(1):26–31
74. Borges A. Imaging of the central skull base. Neuroimaging Clin N Am 2009;19(3):441–468
75. Chang W, Alexander MT, Mirvis SE. Diagnostic determinants of craniocervical distraction injury in adults. AJR Am J Roentgenol 2009;192(1):52–58
76. Chen YF, Liu HM. Imaging of craniovertebral junction. Neuroimaging Clin N Am 2009;19(3):483–510
77. Debernardi A, D'Aliberti G, Talamonti G, Villa F, Piparo M, Collice M. The craniovertebral junction area and the role of the ligaments and membranes. Neurosurgery 2011;68(2):291–301
78. Deliganis AV, Baxter AB, Hanson JA, et al. Radiologic spectrum of craniocervical distraction injuries. Radiographics 2000;20(Spec No):S237–S250
79. Menezes AH. Specific entities affecting the craniocervical region: Down's syndrome. Childs Nerv Syst 2008;24(10):1165–1168
80. Menezes AH. Craniocervical developmental anatomy and its implications. Childs Nerv Syst 2008;24(10):1109–1122
81. Raybaud C, Di Rocco C. Brain malformation in syndromic craniosynostoses, a primary disorder of white matter: a review. Childs Nerv Syst 2007;23(12):1379–1388
82. Rojas CA, Bertozzi JC, Martinez CR, Whitlow J. Reassessment of the craniocervical junction: normal values on CT. AJNR Am J Neuroradiol 2007;28(9):1819–1823
83. Rojas CA, Hayes A, Bertozzi JC, Guidi C, Martinez CR. Evaluation of the C1-C2 articulation on MDCT in healthy children and young adults. AJR Am J Roentgenol 2009;193(5):1388–1392
84. Smoker WRK. Craniovertebral junction: normal anatomy, craniometry, and congenital anomalies. Radiographics 1994;14(2):255–277
12. Smoker WRK, Khanna G. Imaging the craniocervical junction. Childs Nerv Syst 2008;24(10):1123–1145
85. Utz M, Khan S, O'Connor D, Meyers S. MDCT and MRI evaluation of cervical spine trauma. Insights Imaging 2014;5(1):67–75

Crouzon Syndrome

86. Glass RBJ, Fernbach SK, Norton KI, Choi PS, Naidich TP. The infant skull: a vault of information. Radiographics 2004;24(2):507–522
87. Tokumaru AM, Barkovich AJ, Ciricillo SF, Edwards MS. Skull base and calvarial deformities: association with intracranial changes in craniofacial syndromes. AJNR Am J Neuroradiol 1996;17(4):619–630

CSF Leak

88. Brainard L, Chen DA, Aziz KM, Hillman TA. Association of benign intracranial hypertension and spontaneous encephalocele with cerebrospinal fluid leak. Otol Neurotol 2012;33(9):1621–1624
89. Rao AK, Merenda DM, Wetmore SJ. Diagnosis and management of spontaneous cerebrospinal fluid otorrhea. Otol Neurotol 2005;26(6):1171–1175

Dyke-Davidoff-Masson Syndrome

90. Chand G, Goel R, Kapur R. Dyke-Davidoff-Masson syndrome. Arch Neurol 2010;67(8):1026–1027

91. Tasdemir HA, Incesu L, Yazicioglu AK, Belet U, Güngör L. Dyke-Davidoff-Masson syndrome. Clin Imaging 2002;26(1):13–17

External Auditory Canal Atresia

92. Gassner EM, Mallouhi A, Jaschke WR. Preoperative evaluation of external auditory canal atresia on high-resolution CT. AJR Am J Roentgenol 2004;182(5):1305–1312

93. Giesemann AM, Neuburger J, Lanfermann H, Goetz F. Aberrant course of the intracranial facial nerve in cases of atresia of the internal auditory canal (IAC). Neuroradiology 2011;53(9):681–687

94. Tasar M, Yetiser S, Yildirim D, et al. Preoperative evaluation of the congenital aural atresia on computed tomography; an analysis of the severity of the deformity of the middle ear and mastoid. Eur J Radiol 2007;62(1):97–105

External Auditory Canal Cholesteatoma

95. Chawla A, Bosco JIE, Lim TC, Shenoy JN, Krishnan V. Computed tomography features of external auditory canal cholesteatoma: a pictorial review. Curr Prob Diagn Radiol published online 2015. doi:10.1067/j.cpradiol.2015.05.001

96. Darr EA, Linstrom CJ. Conservative management of advanced external auditory canal cholesteatoma. Otolaryngol Head Neck Surg 2010;142(2):278–280

97. Dubach P, Häusler R. External auditory canal cholesteatoma: reassessment of and amendments to its categorization, pathogenesis, and treatment in 34 patients. Otol Neurotol 2008;29(7):941–948

98. Heilbrun ME, Salzman KL, Glastonbury CM, Harnsberger HR, Kennedy RJ, Shelton C. External auditory canal cholesteatoma: clinical and imaging spectrum. AJNR Am J Neuroradiol 2003;24(4):751–756

External Auditory Canal: Exostoses

99. House JW, Wilkinson EP. External auditory exostoses: evaluation and treatment. Otolaryngol Head Neck Surg 2008;138(5):672–678

100. Kozin ED, Remenschneider AK, Shah PV, Reardon E, Lee DJ. Endoscopic transcanal removal of symptomatic external auditory canal exostoses. Am J Otolaryngol 2015;36(2):283–286

External Auditory Canal: Keratosis Obturans

101. Park SY, Jung YH, Oh JH. Clinical characteristics of keratosis obturans and external auditory canal cholesteatoma. Otolaryngol Head Neck Surg 2015;152(2):326–330

External Auditory Canal: Osteoma

102. Bahgat M, Bahgat Y, Bahgat A, Aly S. External auditory canal osteoma. BMJ Case Rep 2012;2012:20–12

External Auditory Canal: Malignant Tumors

103. Chang CH, Shu MT, Lee JC, Leu YS, Chen YC, Lee KS. Treatments and outcomes of malignant tumors of external auditory canal. Am J Otolaryngol 2009;30(1):44–48

104. Chatra PS. Lesions in the external auditory canal. Indian J Radiol Imaging 2011;21(4):274–278

105. Gowthami C, Kumar P, Ravikumar A, Joseph LD, Rajendiran S. Malignant melanoma of the external auditory canal. J Clin Diagn Res 2014;8(8):FD04–FD06

106. Gu FM, Chi FL, Dai CF, Chen B, Li HW. Surgical outcomes of 43 cases with adenoid cystic carcinoma of the external auditory canal. Am J Otolaryngol 2013;34(5):394–398

107. Lim LHY, Goh YH, Chan YM, Chong VFH, Low WK. Malignancy of the temporal bone and external auditory canal. Otolaryngol Head Neck Surg 2000;122(6):882–886

108. Oztürkcan S, Oztürkcan S. Dermatologic diseases of the external ear. Clin Dermatol 2014;32(1):141–152

External Auditory Canal: Medial Canal Fibrosis

109. Suzukawa K, Karino S, Yamasoba T. Surgical treatment of medial meatal fibrosis. Report of four cases. Auris Nasus Larynx 2007;34(3):365–368

110. Ghani A, Smith MCF. Postinflammatory medial meatal fibrosis: early and late surgical outcomes. J Laryngol Otol 2013;127(12):1160–1168

111. Lin VYW, Chee GH, David EA, Chen JM. Medial canal fibrosis: surgical technique, results, and a proposed grading system. Otol Neurotol 2005;26(5):825–829

Hemimegalencephaly

112. Broumandi DD, Hayward UM, Benzian JM, Gonzalez I, Nelson MD. Best cases from the AFIP: hemimegalencephaly. Radiographics 2004;24(3):843–848

113. Di Rocco C, Battaglia D, Pietrini D, Piastra M, Massimi L. Hemimegalencephaly: clinical implications and surgical treatment. Childs Nerv Syst 2006;22(8):852–866

114. Manoranjan B, Provias JP. Hemimegalencephaly: a fetal case with neuropathological confirmation and review of the literature. Acta Neuropathol 2010;120(1):117–130

115. Sato N, Yagishita A, Oba H, et al. Hemimegalencephaly: a study of abnormalities occurring outside the involved hemisphere. AJNR Am J Neuroradiol 2007;28(4):678–682

Inflammation/Infection of the Middle Ear

116. Luntz M, Bartal K, Brodsky A, Shihada R. Acute mastoiditis: the role of imaging for identifying intracranial complications. Laryngoscope 2012;122(12):2813–2817

117. Minks DP, Porte M, Jenkins N. Acute mastoiditis—the role of radiology. Clin Radiol 2013;68(4):397–405

118. Swartz JD. The middle ear and mastoid. In: Swartz JD, Loevner LA, eds. Imaging of the Temporal Bone. 4th ed. New York: Thieme Publishers; 2008:58–246

119. Vazquez E, Castellote A, Piqueras J, et al. Imaging of complications of acute mastoiditis in children. Radiographics 2003;23(2):359–372

Intraosseous Meningioma

120. Ilica AT, Mossa-Basha M, Zan E, et al. Cranial intraosseous meningioma: spectrum of neuroimaging findings with respect to histopathological grades in 65 patients. Clin Imaging 2014;38(5):599–604

Jugular Bulb Abnormalities

121. Friedmann DR, Eubig J, Winata LS, Pramanik BK, Merchant SN, Lalwani AK. Prevalence of jugular bulb abnormalities and resultant inner ear dehiscence: a histopathologic and radiologic study. Otolaryngol Head Neck Surg 2012;147(4):750–756

122. Friedmann DR, Eubig J, Winata LS, Pramanik BK, Merchant SN, Lalwani AK. A clinical and histopathologic study of jugular bulb abnormalities. Arch Otolaryngol Head Neck Surg 2012;138(1):66–71

Lesions at the Cerebellopontine Angle Cisterns and/or Internal Auditory Canals

123. Bonneville F, Savatovsky J, Chiras J. Imaging of cerebellopontine angle lesions: an update. Part 1: enhancing extra-axial lesions. Eur Radiol 2007;17(10):2472–2482

124. Bonneville F, Savatovsky J, Chiras J. Imaging of cerebellopontine angle lesions: an update. Part 2: intra-axial lesions, skull base lesions that may invade the CPA region, and non-enhancing extra-axial lesions. Eur Radiol 2007;17(11):2908–2920

125. Glastonbury CM. The vestibulocochlear nerve, wih an emphasis on the normal and disease internal auditory canal and cerebellopontine angle. In: Swartz JD, Loevner LA, eds. Imaging of the Temporal Bone. 4th ed. New York: Thieme; 2008:480–558

126. Guermazi A, De Kerviler E, Zagdanski AM, Frija J. Diagnostic imaging of choroid plexus disease. Clin Radiol 2000;55(7):503–516

127. Hildenbrand P, Craven DE, Jones R, Nemeskal P. Lyme neuroborreliosis: manifestations of a rapidly emerging zoonosis. AJNR Am J Neuroradiol 2009;30(6):1079–1087

128. Meyers SP, Khademian ZP, Chuang SH, Pollack IF, Korones DN, Zimmerman RA. Choroid plexus carcinomas in children: MRI features and patient outcomes. Neuroradiology 2004;46(9):770–780

129. Meyers SP. Eosinophilic granuloma. In: MRI of Bone and Soft Tissue Tumors and Tumorlike Lesions, Differential Diagnosis and Atlas. Stuttgart, New York: Thieme; 2008:406–412

130. Meyers SP. Meningioma. In: MRI of Bone and Soft Tissue Tumors and Tumorlike Lesions, Differential Diagnosis and Atlas. Stuttgart, New York: Thieme; 2008:596–600

131. Meyers SP. Paraganglioma. In: MRI of Bone and Soft Tissue Tumors and Tumorlike Lesions, Differential Diagnosis and Atlas. Stuttgart, New York: Thieme; 2008:720–725

132. Meyers SP. Schwannoma. In: MRI of Bone and Soft Tissue Tumors and Tumorlike Lesions, Differential Diagnosis and Atlas. Stuttgart, New York: Thieme; 2008:745–752

133. Naeini RM, Yoo JH, Hunter JV. Spectrum of choroid plexus lesions in children. AJR Am J Roentgenol 2009;192(1):32–40

134. Paulus W, Brander S. Choroid plexus tumours. In: Louis DN, Ohgaki H, Wiestler OD, Cavanee WK, eds. WHO Classification of Tumours of the Central Nervous System. 3rd ed. IARC; 2007:82–85

Lesions Involving the Inner Ear

135. Swartz JD, Mukherji S. The inner ear and otodystrophies. In: Swartz JD, Loevner LA, eds. Imaging of the Temporal Bone. 4th ed. New York: Thieme; 2009:298–411

Leukemia

136. Loevner LA, Tobey JD, Yousem DM, Sonners AI, Hsu WC. MR imaging characteristics of cranial bone marrow in adult patients with underlying systemic disorders compared with healthy control subjects. AJNR Am J Neuroradiol 2002;23(2):248–254

137. Seok JH, Park J, Kim SK, Choi JE, Kim CC. Granulocytic sarcoma of the spine: MRI and clinical review. AJR Am J Roentgenol 2010; 194(2):485–489

138. Zha Y, Li M, Yang J. Dynamic contrast enhanced magnetic resonance imaging of diffuse spinal bone marrow infiltration in patients with hematological malignancies. Korean J Radiol 2010;11(2):187–194

Leukoencephalopathy with Vanishing White Matter

139. van der Knaap MS, Valk J. Leukoencephalopathy with vanishing white matter. In: Magnetic Resonance of Myelination and Myelin Disorders. 3rd ed. Berlin: Springer; 2005:481–495

Luckenschadel Skull

140. Coley BD. Ultrasound diagnosis of Luckenschadel (lacunar skull). Pediatr Radiol 2000;30(2):82–84

141. Vigliani MB. Luckenschadel skull: a forgotten entity. Obstet Gynecol 2008;111(2 Pt 2):562–565

Microcephaly

142. Basel-Vanagaite L, Dobyns WB. Clinical and brain imaging heterogeneity of severe microcephaly. Pediatr Neurol 2010;43(1):7–16

143. Vermeulen RJ, Wilke M, Horber V, Krägeloh-Mann I. Microcephaly with simplified gyral pattern: MRI classification. Neurology 2010;74(5):386–391

Middle Ear Tumors

144. Aydin K, Maya MM, Lo WWM, Brackmann DE, Kesser B. Jacobson's nerve schwannoma presenting as middle ear mass. AJNR Am J Neuroradiol 2000;21(7):1331–1333

145. Bierry G, Riehm S, Marcellin L, Stierlé JL, Veillon F. Middle ear adenomatous tumor: a not so rare glomus tympanicum-mimicking lesion. J Neuroradiol 2010;37(2):116–121

146. Elhefnawy NG. Aggressive low grade middle ear adenocarcinoma with multiple recurrences: a case report. Diagn Pathol 2011;6:62

147. Fundakowski CE, Chapman JR, Thomas G. Middle ear carcinoid with distant osseous metastasis. Laryngoscope 2013;123(3):779–782

148. Gurgel RK, Karnell LH, Hansen MR. Middle ear cancer: a population-based study. Laryngoscope 2009;119(10):1913–1917

149. Kim CW, Han DH, Kim CH, Cho SJ, Rho YS. Primary middle ear schwannoma. Am J Otolaryngol 2007;28(5):342–346

150. Lott Limbach AA, Hoschar AP, Thompson LD, Stelow EB, Chute DJ. Middle ear adenomas stain for two cell populations and lack myoepithelial cell differentiation. Head Neck Pathol 2012;6(3):345–353

151. Okada K, Ito K, Yamasoba T, Ishii M, Iwasaki S, Kaga K. Benign mass lesions deep inside the temporal bone: imaging diagnosis for proper management. Acta Otolaryngol Suppl 2007;127(559):71–77

152. Salzman R, Stárek I, Tichá V, Skálová A, Kučera J. Metastasizing middle ear carcinoid: an unusual case report, with focus on ultrastructural and immunohistochemical findings. Otol Neurotol 2012;33(8):1418–1421

153. Thompson LD, Bouffard JP, Sandberg GD, Mena H. Primary ear and temporal bone meningiomas: a clinicopathologic study of 36 cases with a review of the literature. Mod Pathol 2003;16(3):236–245

Neurofibromatosis Type 1

154. Alwan S, Armstrong L, Joe H, Birch PH, Szudek J, Friedman JM. Associations of osseous abnormalities in neurofibromatosis 1. Am J Med Genet A 2007;143A(12):1326–1333

155. Alwan S, Tredwell SJ, Friedman JM. Is osseous dysplasia a primary feature of neurofibromatosis 1 (NF1)? Clin Genet 2005;67(5):378–390

156. Leskelä HV, Kuorilehto T, Risteli J, et al. Congenital pseudarthrosis of neurofibromatosis type 1: impaired osteoblast differentiation and function and altered *NF1* gene expression. Bone 2009;44(2):243–250

157. Schindeler A, Little DG. Recent insights into bone development, homeostasis, and repair in type 1 neurofibromatosis (NF1). Bone 2008;42(4):616–622

Ossicular Anomalies

158. Lemmerling MM, Stambuk HE, Mancuso AA, Antonelli PJ, Kubilis PS. CT of the normal suspensory ligaments of the ossicles in the middle ear. AJNR Am J Neuroradiol 1997;18(3):471–477

159. Park K, Choung YH. Isolated congenital ossicular anomalies. Acta Otolaryngol 2009;129(4):419–422

Ossicular Injuries

160. Maroldi R, Farina D, Palvarini L, et al. Computed tomography and magnetic resonance imaging of pathologic conditions of the middle ear. Eur J Radiol 2001;40(2):78–93

161. Noujaim D, Juliano A, Moonis G. Lesions of the middle ear ossicles: acquired, traumatic, congenital, and postsurgical pathology. Neurographics 2014;4:176–182

162. Wang EY, Shatzkes D, Swartz JD. Temporal bone trauma. In: Swartz JD, Loevner LA, eds. Imaging of the Temporal Bone. 4th ed. New York: Thieme Publishers; 2008:412–443

Osteogenesis Imperfecta

163. Alkadhi H, Rissmann D, Kollias SS. Osteogenesis imperfecta of the temporal bone: CT and MR imaging in Van der Hoeve-de Kleyn syndrome. AJNR Am J Neuroradiol 2004;25(6):1106–1109

164. Barkova E, Mohan U, Chitayat D, et al. Fetal skeletal dysplasias in a tertiary care center: radiology, pathology, and molecular analysis of 112 cases. Clin Genet 2015;87(4):330–337

165. Renaud A, Aucourt J, Weill J, et al. Radiographic features of osteogenesis imperfecta. Insights Imaging 2013;4(4):417–429

Osteopetrosis

166. Cheow HK, Steward CG, Grier DJ. Imaging of malignant infantile osteopetrosis before and after bone marrow transplantation. Pediatr Radiol 2001;31(12):869–875

167. Costelloe CM, Eftekhari F, Petropoulos D. Radiography of successful bone marrow transplantation for osteopetrosis. Skeletal Radiol 2007;36(Suppl 1):S34–S37

168. Curé JK, Key LL, Goltra DD, VanTassel P. Cranial MR imaging of osteopetrosis. AJNR Am J Neuroradiol 2000;21(6):1110–1115

169. Del Fattore A, Cappariello A, Teti A. Genetics, pathogenesis and complications of osteopetrosis. Bone 2008;42(1):19–29

170. Elster AD, Theros EG, Key LL, Chen MYM. Cranial imaging in autosomal recessive osteopetrosis. Part I. Facial bones and calvarium. Radiology 1992;183(1):129–135

171. Steward CG. Neurological aspects of osteopetrosis. Neuropathol Appl Neurobiol 2003;29(2):87–97

172. Tolar J, Teitelbaum SL, Orchard PJ. Osteopetrosis. N Engl J Med 2004;351(27):2839–2849

Paget Disease

173. Smith SE, Murphey MD, Motamedi K, Mulligan ME, Resnik CS, Gannon FH. From the archives of the AFIP. Radiologic spectrum of Paget disease of bone and its complications with pathologic correlation. Radiographics 2002;22(5):1191–1216

174. Whitten CR, Saifuddin A. MRI of Paget's disease of bone. Clin Radiol 2003;58(10):763–769

Parietal Foramina

175. Lerner A, Lu DA, Allison SK, et al. Calvarial lesions and pseudolesions: differential diagnosis and pictorial review of pathologuc entities presenting with focal calvarial abnormalities. Neurographics 2013;3:108–117

176. Mavrogiannis LA, Taylor IB, Davies SJ, Ramos FJ, Olivares JL, Wilkie AO. Enlarged parietal foramina caused by mutations in the homeobox genes ALX4 and MSX2: from genotype to phenotype. Eur J Hum Genet 2006;14(2):151–158

Petrous Apex Lesions

177. Chan JKC, Bray F, McCarron P, et al. Nasopharyngeal carcinoma. In: Barnes L, Eveson JW, Reichart P, Sidaransky D, eds. World Health Organization Classification of Tumours. Pathology and Genetics of Head and Neck Tumors. Lyon, France: IARC Press; 2005:85–97

178. Chapman PR, Shah R, Curé JK, Bag AK. Petrous apex lesions: pictorial review. AJR Am J Roentgenol 2011; 196(3, Suppl):WS26–WS37, Quiz S40–S43

179. Connor SEJ, Leung R, Natas S. Imaging of the petrous apex: a pictorial review. Br J Radiol 2008;81(965):427–435

180. El-Naggar AK, Huvos AG. Adenoid cystic carcinoma. In: Barnes L, Eveson JW, Reichart P, Sidaransky D, eds. World Health Organization Classification of Tumours. Pathology and Genetics of Head and Neck Tumors. Lyon, France: IARC Press; 2005:221–222

181. Isaacson B, Kutz JW, Roland PS. Lesions of the petrous apex: diagnosis and management. Otolaryngol Clin North Am 2007;40(3):479–519, viii

182. Pilch BZ, Bouquot J, Thompson LDR. Squamous cell carcinoma. In: Barnes L, Eveson JW, Reichart P, Sidaransky D, eds. World Health Organization Classification of Tumours. Pathology and Genetics of Head and Neck Tumors. Lyon, France: IARC Press; 2005:15–17

183. Razek AA, Huang BY. Lesions of the petrous apex: classification and findings at CT and MR imaging. Radiographics 2012;32(1):151–173

184. Thompson LDR, Fanburg-Smith JC. Malignant soft tissue tumours. In: Barnes L, Eveson JW, Reichart P, Sidaransky D, eds. World Health Organization Classification of Tumours. Pathology and Genetics of Head and Neck Tumors. Lyon, France: IARC Press; 2005:35–42

Plagiocephaly

185. Kalra R, Walker ML. Posterior plagiocephaly. Childs Nerv Syst 2012; 28(9):1389–1393

186. Sze RW, Hopper RA, Ghioni V, et al. MDCT diagnosis of the child with posterior plagiocephaly. AJR Am J Roentgenol 2005;185(5):1342–1346

Positional Plagiocephaly

187. Glass RBJ, Fernbach SK, Norton KI, Choi PS, Naidich TP. The infant skull: a vault of information. Radiographics 2004;24(2):507–522

Rheumatoid Arthritis

188. Krauss WE, Bledsoe JM, Clarke MJ, Nottmeier EW, Pichelmann MA. Rheumatoid arthritis of the craniovertebral junction. Neurosurgery 2010;66(3, Suppl):83–95

Sickle Cell Disease

189. Saito N, Nadgir RN, Flower EN, Sakai O. Clinical and radiologic manifestations of sickle cell disease in the head and neck. Radiographics 2010;30(4):1021–1034

Sinonasal Undifferentiated Carcinoma

190. Frierson HF. Sinonasal undifferentiated carcinoma. In: Barnes L, Eveson JW, Reichart P, Sidransky D, eds. World Health Organization Classification of Tumours. Pathology and Genetics of Head and Neck Tumors. Lyon, France: IARC Press; 2005:19

Sinus Pericranii

191. Gandolfo C, Krings T, Alvarez H, et al. Sinus pericranii: diagnostic and therapeutic considerations in 15 patients. Neuroradiology 2007;49(6):505–514

192. Glass RBJ, Fernbach SK, Norton KI, Choi PS, Naidich TP. The infant skull: a vault of information. Radiographics 2004;24(2):507–522

193. Park SC, Kim SK, Cho BK, et al. Sinus pericranii in children: report of 16 patients and preoperative evaluation of surgical risk. J Neurosurg Pediatr 2009;4(6):536–542

Skull Lesions

193. Bahrami S, Yim CM. Quality initiatives: blind spots at brain imaging. Radiographics 2009;29(7):1877–1896

194. Lerner A, Lu DA, Shiroshi MS, et al. Calvarial lesions and pseudolesions: differential diagnosis and pictorial review of pathologic entities presenting with focal calvarial abnormaloities. Neurographics 2013;3:108–117

Squamous Cell Carcinoma

195. Frierson HF. Sinonasal undifferentiated carcinoma. In: Barnes L, Eveson JW, Reichart P, Sidransky D, eds. World Health Organization Classification of Tumours. Pathology and Genetics of Head and Neck Tumors. Lyon, France: IARC Press; 2005:15–17

Superior Semicircular Canal Dehiscence

196. Curtin HD. Superior semicircular canal dehiscence syndrome and multi-detector row CT. Radiology 2003;226(2):312–314

Thalassemia

197. Basu S, Kumar A. Hair-on-end appearance in radiograph of skull and facial bones in a case of beta thalassaemia. Br J Haematol 2009; 144(6):807

198. Tyler PA, Madani G, Chaudhuri R, Wilson LF, Dick EA. The radiological appearances of thalassaemia. Clin Radiol 2006;61(1):40–52

Wormian Bones

199. Marti B, Sirinelli D, Maurin L, Carpentier E. Wormian bones in a general paediatric population. Diagn Interv Imaging 2013;94(4):428–432

200. Sanchez-Lara PA, Graham JM Jr, Hing AV, Lee J, Cunningham M. The morphogenesis of wormian bones: a study of craniosynostosis and purposeful cranial deformation. Am J Med Genet A 2007; 143A(24):3243–3251

X-Linked Stapes Gusher

201. Kumar G, Castillo M, Buchman CA. X-linked stapes gusher: CT findings in one patient. AJNR Am J Neuroradiol 2003;24(6):1130–1132

Chapter 2
Orbit

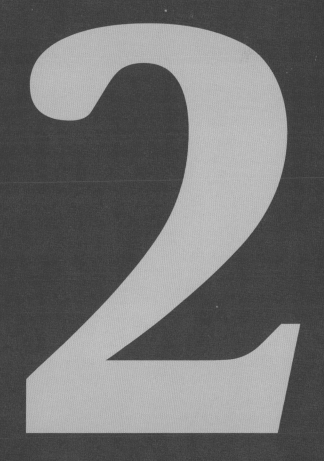

2 Orbit

Introduction

Bony Orbit

The bony orbit is a four-sided pyramidal structure within which are the eye (globe), fat, extraocular muscles, nerves, and blood vessels.[1,2,3,4,5] The *medial orbital wall* is composed of the frontal process of the maxilla, lacrimal bone, lamina papyracea, and sphenoid bone (**Fig. 2.1**). The *lateral orbital wall* is composed of the zygoma, frontal bone, and greater wing of the sphenoid bone (**Fig. 2.2**). The *orbital floor* is composed of the zygoma and orbital plate of the maxilla. At the posterolateral aspect of the orbital floor is the inferior orbital fissure, which the second division of the trigeminal nerve traverses. The V2 nerve enters the orbit from the pterygopalatine fossa. The V2 nerve is located in a sulcus along the posterior orbital floor, where it eventually enters the infraorbital canal and emerges from the infraorbital foramen. Other structures that pass through the inferior orbital fissure are the inferior ophthalmic vein, infraorbital branch of the maxillary artery, and autonomic branches of the pterygopalatine ganglion. The *orbital roof* is composed mostly of the frontal bone, as well as the lesser wing of the sphenoid bone posteriorly.

Superior Orbital Fissure

The superior orbital fissure is located between the greater and lesser sphenoid wings (**Fig. 2.3**). The superior orbital fissure is a passage through which nerves from the cavernous sinus (**Fig. 2.4**) enter the orbits, including the ophthalmic (V1) division of the trigeminal nerve, trochlear nerve (CN IV), oculomotor nerve (CN III), abducens nerve (CN VI), and sympathetic nerve fibers. The annulus of Zinn (annulus tendineus communis) at the superior orbital fissure is a fibrous ring to which the extraocular muscles attach. The superior ophthalmic vein also crosses through the superior orbital fissure.

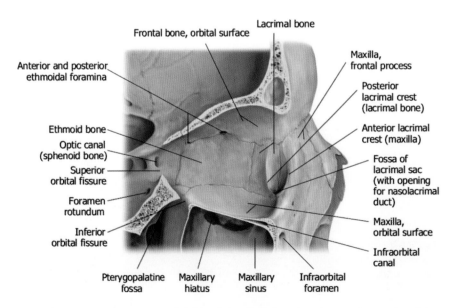

Fig. 2.1 Illustration showing the osseous components of the medial wall of the orbit. From THIEME Atlas of Anatomy: Head and Neuro-anatomy, © Thieme 2007, Illustration by Karl Wesker.

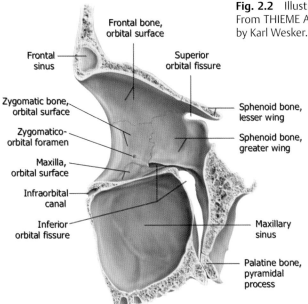

Fig. 2.2 Illustration showing the osseous components of the lateral wall of the orbit. From THIEME Atlas of Anatomy: Head and Neuroanatomy, © Thieme 2007, Illustration by Karl Wesker.

Frontal bone, orbital surface

Frontal sinus

Superior orbital fissure

Zygomatic bone, orbital surface

Zygomatico-orbital foramen

Maxilla, orbital surface

Infraorbital canal

Inferior orbital fissure

Sphenoid bone, lesser wing

Sphenoid bone, greater wing

Maxillary sinus

Palatine bone, pyramidal process

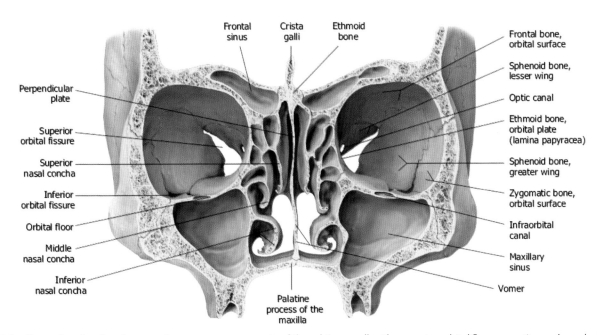

Frontal sinus

Crista galli

Ethmoid bone

Frontal bone, orbital surface

Sphenoid bone, lesser wing

Optic canal

Ethmoid bone, orbital plate (lamina papyracea)

Sphenoid bone, greater wing

Zygomatic bone, orbital surface

Infraorbital canal

Maxillary sinus

Vomer

Perpendicular plate

Superior orbital fissure

Superior nasal concha

Inferior orbital fissure

Orbital floor

Middle nasal concha

Inferior nasal concha

Palatine process of the maxilla

Fig. 2.3 Illustration showing the posterior osseous components of the orbits as well as the superior orbital fissures, optic canals, and adjacent nasal cavity and paranasal sinuses. From THIEME Atlas of Anatomy: Head and Neuroanatomy, © Thieme 2007, Illustration by Karl Wesker.

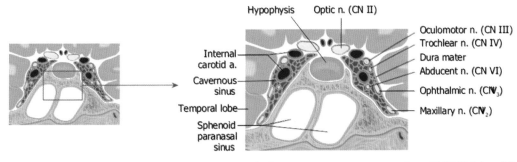

Hypophysis

Optic n. (CN II)

Oculomotor n. (CN III)

Trochlear n. (CN IV)

Dura mater

Abducent n. (CN VI)

Ophthalmic n. (CN V_1)

Maxillary n. (CN V_2)

Internal carotid a.

Cavernous sinus

Temporal lobe

Sphenoid paranasal sinus

Fig. 2.4 Coronal view of the contents of the cavernous sinuses and adjacent anatomic structures. From THIEME Atlas of Anatomy: Head and Neuroanatomy, © Thieme 2007, Illustration by Karl Wesker.

Orbital Apex

The orbital apex is located posteriorly and contains the superior orbital fissure between the lateral orbital wall and orbital roof, the optic canal in the lesser wing of the sphenoid bone, and the inferior orbital fissure (**Fig. 2.5**).

Optic Canal

The optic canal is located within the lesser wing of the sphenoid bone and is medial to the anterior clinoid process and superomedial to the superior orbital fissure. A thin bone wall separates the optic canal and superior orbital fissure. The optic canal contains the optic nerve and ophthalmic artery.

Extraocular Muscles

The extraocular muscles include the medial, lateral, superior, and inferior rectus muscles that originate from the annulus of Zinn and course through orbital fat before inserting onto their respective positions on the globe (**Fig. 2.6**). The superior oblique muscle also originates from the annulus of Zinn and courses anteriorly to the trochlea, where its tendon turns to insert on the posterolateral margin of the globe. The inferior oblique muscle originates from the periorbita at the inferomedial aspect of the globe and courses anteriorly, where its

tendon inserts on the inferolateral aspect of the globe. The seventh extraocular muscle, the levator palpebrae superioris, originates from the lesser sphenoid wing and extends anteriorly to become the aponeurosis, which inserts onto the tarsal plate and eyelid skin. CN III innervates the levator palpebrae superioris and inferior oblique muscles, as well as the medial, superior, and inferior rectus muscles. The motor nucleus of CN III is located in the dorsal portion of the midbrain ventral to the periaqueductal gray at the level of the superior colliculi. CN VI innervates the lateral rectus muscle, and CN IV innervates the superior oblique muscle.

Sensory Nerves

The ophthalmic division of CN V within the lateral wall of the cavernous sinus divides into three branches (lacrimal, frontal, and nasociliary nerves), which then enter the orbit through the superior orbital fissure. The lacrimal nerve provides postganglionic secretomotor fibers to the lacrimal gland and sensory fibers in the conjunctiva and skin. The frontal nerve is located in the upper orbit between the levator palpebrae and periorbita and provides sensory input from the forehead and medial eyelid. The nasociliary nerve passes between the superior oblique and medial rectus muscles and divides into anterior and posterior ethmoidal nerves, nerve branches to the ciliary ganglion, and the infratrochlear nerve, which receives sensory input from the globe, medial upper eyelid, and forehead.

Branches from the maxillary division of CN V enter the inferior orbital fissure from the pterygomaxillary fossa and

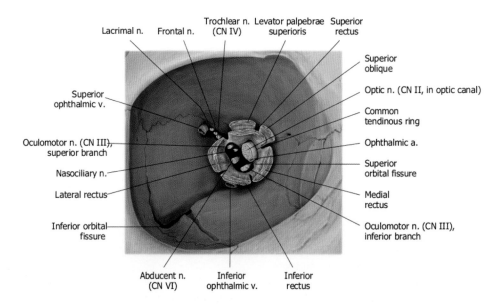

Fig. 2.5 Coronal view of the anatomic relationship of structures at the orbital apex. From THIEME Atlas of Anatomy: Head and Neuroanatomy, © Thieme 2007, Illustration by Karl Wesker.

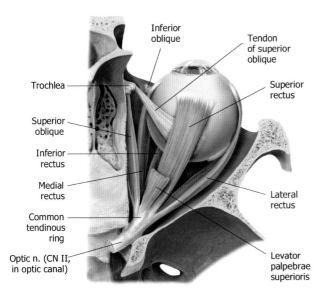

Fig. 2.6 Axial view of the extraocular muscles and their anatomic relationships to adjacent structures. From THIEME Atlas of Anatomy: Head and Neuroanatomy, © Thieme 2007, Illustration by Karl Wesker.

pass anteriorly through the orbit in the infraorbital canal to receive sensory input from the lower eyelid, conjunctiva, cheek, and upper lip. A branch of the infraorbital nerve is the superior alveolar nerve, which receives sensory input from the upper anterior teeth. The zygomatic V2 branch of CN V enters the inferior orbital fissure and receives sensory input from the skin at the lateral orbit and supplies additional secretomotor fibers to the lacrimal gland.

Periorbita, Tenon's Capsule, and Orbital Fat

Along the inner bony walls of the orbit is a fibrous lining referred to as the *periorbita* that is tightly attached to bone at the orbital margins anteriorly (orbital septum), suture lines and fissures, and anterior lacrimal crest. *Tenon's capsule* is a fascial sheath that surrounds the eye, separating the globe from the adjacent orbital fat. This fascial sheath fuses anteriorly with the sclera at the scleral–corneal junction and bulbar conjunctiva. Structures that extend through Tenon's capsule include the tendons of the extraocular muscles, optic nerve, ciliary nerves, and veins from the choroid and sclera (vortex veins). The potential space that can occur between the sclera and Tenon's capsule is referred to as the episcleral or Tenon's space, which is a site where infection, inflammation, and neoplasms can enter. *Orbital fat* surrounds the globe, extraocular muscles, and optic nerve. Connective tissue septa separate the intraconal fat deep to extraocular muscles from the extraconal fat.

Eye

The eye (globe) has three primary layers (sclera, uveal tract, and retina; **Fig. 2.7**).

The *sclera* is the outermost layer, which consists of the transparent cornea anteriorly and a fibrous opaque portion that extends posteriorly where it fuses with the dural sheath of the optic nerve.

The *uveal tract* is a pigmented vascular layer between the sclera and retina. The uveal tract includes the iris, ciliary body, and choroid. The *choroid* extends from the optic nerve to the ora serrata (anterior-most margin of the retina). The choroid has firm attachments to the adjacent sclera anteriorly at the ora serrata/ciliary body and posteriorly where the vortex veins exit the eye. Between the choroid and the retina is an acellular layer referred to a Bruch's membrane. The *iris* is a pigmented contractile structure consisting of smooth muscles (sphincter and dilator pupillae) with a central opening (pupil) that separates the anterior chamber containing aqueous humor from the posterior chamber, which contains vitreous humor. The *dilator pupillae muscles* are innervated by sympathetic fibers from the superior cervical ganglion, and the *sphincter pupillae* are innervated the parasympathetic fibers from CN III that connect to the Edinger-Westphal nucleus located dorsomedial to the motor nucleus of CN III in the posterior portion of the midbrain at the level of the superior colliculi. The outer posterior margins of the iris attach to the base of the ring-shaped *ciliary body*. The ciliary body at its periphery posteriorly merges with the choroid at the ora serrata. The inner margins of the ciliary body attach to the lens via suspensory ligaments.

The *retina* is a 250-micron-thick layer of the eye located deep to the choroid and consists of nine anatomic layers, including inner photoreceptor sensory layers containing first- and second-order neurons and neuroglial elements, and an outer thin layer of cells that borders Bruch's membrane of the choroid. The retina is firmly adherent anteriorly at the ora serrata and posteriorly at the optic disc. The center of the retina (macula) is also the thinnest portion and is located 3.5 mm lateral to the optic disc. The optic disc is referred to as the blind spot because it lacks rod and cone light receptors. The central retinal artery, which is a branch of the ophthalmic artery, provides blood to the central retina. Choroidal capillaries provide blood to the rods and cones.

Visual Pathway

Light that passes through the cornea, lens, and vitreous interacts with the retina, causing action potentials that are transmitted to the optic nerve and visual pathway[6,7,8] (**Fig. 2.8**). The optic nerve (CN II) is derived from the diencephalon and contains retinal ganglion cells, oligodendrocytes, and astrocytes. The optic nerve is considered part of

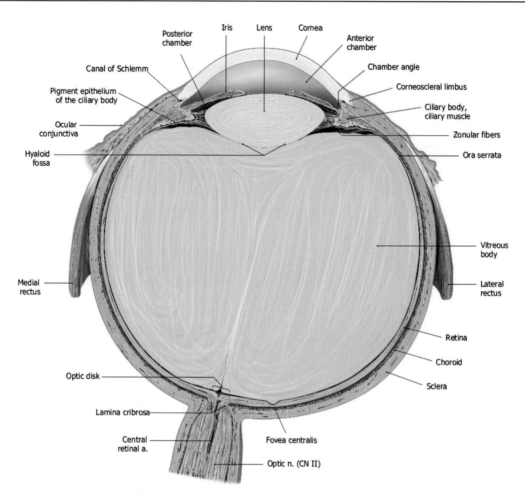

Fig. 2.7 The anatomic structures of the eye. From THIEME Atlas of Anatomy: Head and Neuroanatomy, © Thieme 2007, Illustration by Karl Wesker.

the central nervous system because it is myelinated by oligodendrocytes, instead of the Schwann cells for peripheral nerves, and it is covered by dura and arachnoid contiguous with the intracranial meninges. The optic nerve has four segments (intraocular, intraorbital, intracanalicular, and intracranial portions). The intracanalicular segment of the optic nerve passes through the optic canal to continue as the intracranial segment to the optic chiasm in the suprasellar cistern. At the optic chiasm, retinal nerve fibers from the medial (nasal) halves of both retinas cross to the contralateral side, whereas nerve fibers from the lateral portions of the retinas continue on to the ipsilateral optic tracts. The optic tracts represent posterior extensions of the visual pathway from the optic chiasm to the lateral geniculate bodies (nuclei) of the thalamus. Postsynaptic efferent axons from lateral geniculate bodies extend posteriorly as the optic radiations to the primary visual cortex at the medial occipital lobes.

2.1 Congenital and Developmental Abnormalities

Development of the Eye

At 3 weeks of gestation, two indentations (diverticula) begin to form at the ectodermal margins of the diencephalon (forebrain) lateral to the neural groove. These diverticula progress to form the optic vesicles at 4 weeks.[9,10] The superficial wall of each optic vesicle invaginates, resulting in an optic cup, the inner wall of which eventually forms the retina and the outer wall of which forms the retinal pigment epithelium. Surface ectoderm covering the optic vesicle thickens to form the lens. Constriction of the inner portion of each optic vesicle progressively forms the optic stalk, through which mesenchyme enters with the hyaloid artery through the choroid fissure.

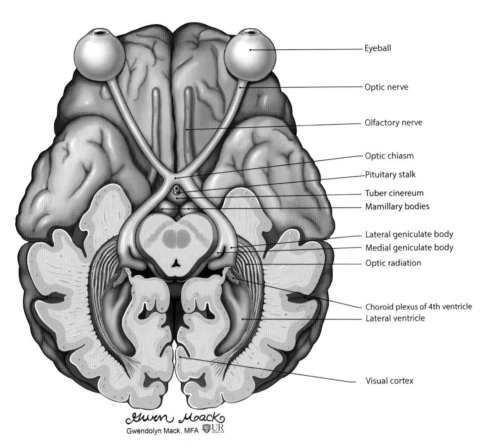

The Visual Pathway

- Eyeball
- Optic nerve
- Olfactory nerve
- Optic chiasm
- Pituitary stalk
- Tuber cinereum
- Mamillary bodies
- Lateral geniculate body
- Medial geniculate body
- Optic radiation
- Choroid plexus of 4th ventricle
- Lateral ventricle
- Visual cortex

Gwendolyn Mack, MFA

Fig. 2.8   Axial view of the components of the visual pathway.

Mesenchyme at the margins of the optic cup forms the ciliary muscles, suspensory ligaments of the lens, choroid, hyaloid artery, extraocular muscles, and orbital bone. Surface ectoderm forms the cornea, lacrimal glands, and duct. The eyelids and vitreous derive from both ectoderm and mesoderm.

References

1. Burns NS, Iyer RS, Robinson AJ, Chapman T. Diagnostic imaging of fetal and pediatric orbital abnormalities. AJR Am J Roentgenol 2013; 201(6):W797–W808
2. Mafee MF, Karimi A, Shah J, Rapoport M, Ansari SA. Anatomy and pathology of the eye: role of MR imaging and CT. Neuroimaging Clin N Am 2005;15(1):23–47
3. Malhotra A, Minja FJ, Crum A, Burrowes D. Ocular anatomy and cross-sectional imaging of the eye. Semin Ultrasound CT MR 2011; 32(1):2–13
4. René C. Update on orbital anatomy. Eye (Lond) 2006;20(10):1119–1129
5. Tantiwongkosi B, Hesselink JR. Imaging of the ocular motor pathway. Neuroimaging Clin N Am 2015;25(3):425–438
6. Tantiwongkosi B, Mafee MF. Imaging of optic neuropathy and chiasmal syndromes. Neuroimaging Clin N Am 2015;25(3):395–410
7. Tantiwongkosi B, Salamon N. Imaging of retrochiasmal and higher cortical visual disorders. Neuroimaging Clin N Am 2015;25(3):411–424
8. YU F. Duang T, Tantiwongkosi B. Advence MR imaging of the visual pathway. Neuroimaging Clin N Am 2015;25:383–393
9. Edward DP, Kaufman LM. Anatomy, development, and physiology of the visual system. Pediatr Clin North Am 2003;50(1):1–23
10. Mafee MF. The eye. In: Mafee MF, Valvassori GE, Becker M, eds. Imaging of the Head and Neck. 2nd ed. New York: Thieme; 2005:137–139

Table 2.1 Congenital and developmental abnormalities

- Anophthalmia/microphthalmia
- Persistent hyperplastic primary vitreous (PHPV)
- Norrie's disease
- Retinopathy of prematurity
- Coloboma
- Morning glory disc
- Staphyloma
- Coats' disease (primary retinal telangiectasia)
- Marfan syndrome
- Cephalocele
- Holoprosencephaly

- Septo-optic dysplasia (de Morsier syndrome)
- Craniosynostosis
- Hemifacial microsomia (Goldenhar syndrome, oculoauriculovertebral spectrum)
- Neurofibromatosis type 1 (NF1)
- von Hippel-Lindau disease
- Tuberous sclerosis
- Sturge-Weber syndrome
- Optic nerve head drusen
- Orbital infantile hemangioma
- Congenital hemangioma
- Orbital venolymphatic malformation
- Orbital epidermoid
- Orbital dermoid

Table 2.1 Congenital and developmental abnormalities

Abnormality	Imaging Findings	Comments
Anophthalmia/ microphthalmia **(Fig. 2.9)**	*Primary anophthalmia:* Absence of eye, extraocular muscles, and optic nerve. Usually bilateral. *Secondary anophthalmia:* Absence of eye, but optic nerves and extraocular muscles are present. Can be unilateral or bilateral. *Microphthalmia:* Small, malformed eye can be associated with persistent hyperplastic primary vitreous.	Complete (anophthalmia) or partial (microphthalmia) absence of ocular tissue in the orbit. Can be due to mutation causing lack of development of the optic vesicle at 4 weeks of gestation (primary type), resulting in absence of both globes and optic nerves, or due to the more common secondary type, which results from degeneration (infection, toxin, trauma, or ischemia) during the fourth week of gestation. The optic nerves and extraocular muscles can be present in the secondary type of anophthalmia.
Persistent hyperplastic primary vitreous (PHPV) **(Fig. 2.10** and **Fig. 2.11)**	*CT:* Microphthalmos, with increased attenuation in vitreous. *MRI:* Flattened, deformed lens with narrow anterior chamber. Subretinal exudates can have high signal on T1-weighted imaging and slightly high to high signal on T2-weighted imaging (T2WI). A centrally located stalk with low signal on T2WI can be seen within the eye, with a flared anterior retrolental portion, ± tubular, cylindrical, or triangular gadolinium contrast enhancement in the vitreous, retrolental soft tissue, and anterior chamber.	Leukocoria in a microphthalmic eye, which occurs from failure of normal involution of the embryonic hyaloid vascular system of the primary vitreous and capillary network around the lens. Replacement of the primary vitreous with the secondary vitreous normally occurs by the sixth month of gestation. PHPV is unilateral in 80% of sporadic cases, may be bilateral in Norrie's disease. Treatment options include vitrectomy and lensectomy with intraocular prosthetic lens.
Norrie's disease **(Fig. 2.11)**	*CT:* Bilateral microphthalmia, vitreoretinal hemorrhage with slightly high to high attenuation, retinal detachment, cataracts, small dense lens, and phthisis bulbi. *MRI:* Bilateral microphthalmia, small and/or malformed lenses, partial or complete retinal detachment, persistent hyperplastic primary vitreous, chronic subretinal or vitreous hemorrhage with high signal on T1- and T2-weighted imaging, and optic nerve atrophy.	X-linked recessive disorder (also referred to as congenital progressive oculoacousticocerebral degeneration) with clinical findings of retinal malformation, mental retardation, sensorineural hearing loss, and deafness. Ocular abnormalities occur in infants and typically progess to bilateral blindness.
Retinopathy of prematurity	Bilateral microphthalmia, shallow anterior chambers of eyes, retinal detachment, and occasional calcifications, ± persistent hyaloid vascular system.	Occurs in low-birth-weight premature infants with prolonged exposure to supplemental oxygen therapy, which results in abnormal vascular changes.

(continued on page 198)

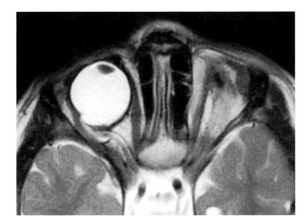

Fig. 2.9 A 5-year-old female with left anophthalmia, secondary type.

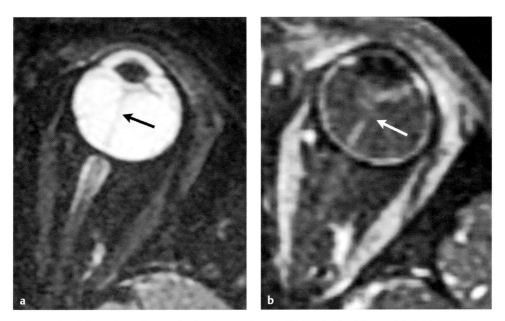

Fig. 2.10 A 9-year-old male with persistent hyperplastic primary vitreous (PHPV) in the left eye. **(a)** Axial STIR shows a centrally located stalk with low signal (*arrow*) within the high-signal vitreous. **(b)** Postcontrast axial fat-suppressed T1-weighted imaging shows gadolinium contrast enhancement of the stalk (*arrow*) as well as in the flared zone anteriorly behind the lens.

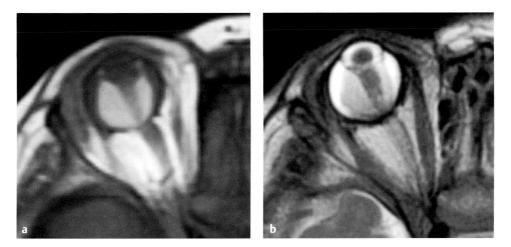

Fig. 2.11 An 18-month-old female with Norrie's disease. **(a)** Axial T1-weighted imaging and **(b)** axial T2-weighted imaging show microph-thalmia, persistent hyperplastic primary vitreous, and vitreous hemorrhage with high signal on T1-weighted imaging and intermediate to high signal on T2-weighted imaging.

Table 2.1 *(cont.)* Congenital/developmental abnormalities

Abnormality	Imaging Findings	Comments
Coloboma (**Fig. 2.12**, **Fig. 2.13**, and **Fig. 2.14**)	*MRI and CT:* *Normal-size eyes:* Circumscribed, protruding defect of the eye that often occurs at the inferonasal portion of the globe but can occur anywhere along the path of the embryonic optic fissure, including the optic disc and optic nerve. Fluid within the defect has low signal on T1-weighted imaging and FLAIR and high signal on T2-weighted imaging similar to vitreous. *Microphthalmic eye:* Small, dysplastic eye with a scleral defect through which there is herniation of dysplastic neuroepithelial tissue into an extraocular cyst, which can be larger than the globe. The colobomatous cyst may or may not show an obvious connection to the dysplastic globe on MRI or CT. The contents of the cyst have CT and MRI findings similar to CSF.	Defect in the eye from incomplete closure of the embryonic optic fissure at weeks 5–6 of gestation. The embryonic optic fissure develops from invagination of the optic disc and normally extends from the iris to the optic nerve. Colobomas can occur anywhere along the optic fissure. Can be bilateral in up to 50% of cases. Involved eye can be normal size or microphthalmic. Associated with decreased visual acuity, strabismus, and nystagmus. Can be associated with CHARGE syndrome, VATER syndrome, Aicardi's syndrome, Warburg's syndrome, branchio-oculo-facial syndrome, trisomy 13, trisomy 18, oculocerebrocutaneous syndrome, and focal dermal hypoplasia.
Morning glory disc (**Fig. 2.15** and **Fig. 2.16**)	*MRI:* Funnel-shaped defect in the fundus at the level of the optic disc and optic nerve, ± elevation of adjacent retinal tissue, enlargement of the distal optic nerve/optic nerve head, ± high signal on T1-weighted imaging at the anterior optic nerve, ± gadolinium contrast enhancement. Other findings can include cleft palate, basal cephalocele, enlarged persistent craniopharyngeal canal, corpus callosal dysgenesis, arterial stenosis, and vascular anomalies.	Sporadic congenital optic nerve disorder with funnel-shaped excavation of the posterior fundus, including the optic disc, surrounded by chorioretinal pigment deposition and radially oriented blood vessels. The excavated disc looks like a morning glory flower on ophthalmoscopic examination. Usually unilateral, and two times more common in females than males. Usually associated with midline craniofacial and skull-base defects (cleft palate, basal cephalocele, enlarged craniopharyngeal canal), vascular abnormalities (arterial hypoplasia/aplasia, arterial stenosis), and corpus callosal dysgenesis. Patients can present with endocrinologic deficiency (hypopituitarism), seizures, and cerebral ischemia.

(continued on page 200)

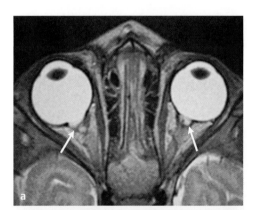

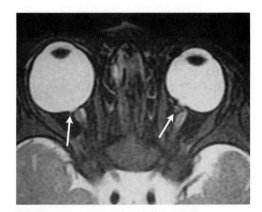

Fig. 2.13 A 15-month-old male with CHARGE syndrome and small bilateral colobomas (*arrows*) on axial fat-suppressed T2-weighted imaging.

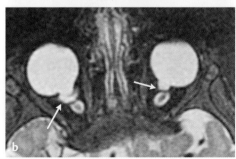

Fig. 2.12 An 8-month-old male with bilateral colobomas on **(a)** axial T2-weighted imaging (*arrows*) and **(b)** axial STIR (*arrows*).

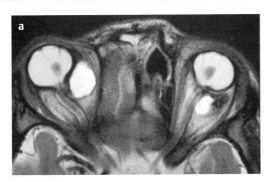
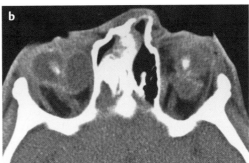

Fig. 2.14 Patient with branchio-oculo-facial syndrome. **(a)** Axial T2-weighted imaging shows small, dysplastic eyes and extraocular cysts that resulted from herniation of dysplastic neuroepithelial tissue through small scleral defects. These colobomatous cysts did not show obvious connections to the dysplastic globes on MRI or CT. **(b)** The contents of the cyst have MRI and CT findings similar to CSF. Both calcified and dysplastic lenses are in abnormal locations dorsal to the anterior chambers.

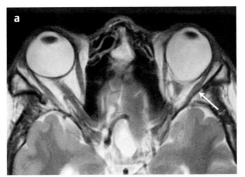
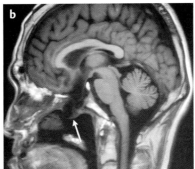
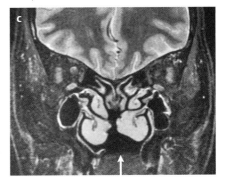

Fig. 2.15 **(a)** A 40-year-old man with a morning glory disc anomaly involving the left eye seen as a funnel-shaped defect in the fundus at the level of the optic disc and optic nerve on axial T2-weighted imaging (*arrow*). **(b)** Associated skull-base defect with a basal cephalocele (*arrow*) on sagittal T1-weighted imaging and **(c)** midline craniofacial anomaly of a cleft palate (*arrow*) on coronal T2-weighted imaging are also seen.

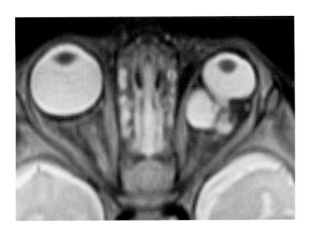

Fig. 2.16 A 6-month-old female with a morning glory disc anomaly. Axial T2-weighted imaging shows a small left eye with funnel-shaped defect in the fundus at the level of the optic disc and optic nerve, and extraocular pseudocysts dorsal to the eye.

Table 2.1 *(cont.)* Congenital and developmental abnormalities

Abnormality	Imaging Findings	Comments
Staphyloma **(Fig. 2.17)**	Symmetric enlargement of the eye without a focal wall defect.	Ectasia and thinning of intact scleral and uveal layers of the eye without a focal defect. Staphylomas can result from degeneration, glaucoma, trauma, prior infection, inflammation, radiation treatment, or surgery.
Coats' disease (primary retinal telangiectasia) **(Fig. 2.18)**	*CT:* Subretinal homogeneous exudates have attenuation slightly higher than the vitreous, ± linear contrast enhancement at the anterior margin of the subretinal exudates. Typically no calcifications are present. *MRI:* Subretinal exudates often contain lipids and cholesterol, which result in slightly high to high signal on T1- and T2-weighted imaging. The subretinal exudates typically do not show gadolinium (Gd) contrast enhancement, which allows distinction from retinoblastoma. A thin zone of Gd contrast enhancement may be seen at the border between the subretinal exudate and vitreous secondary to the vascular abnormalities of the displaced/detached retina.	Progressive idiopathic disorder of telangiectatic and aneurysmal retinal blood vessels that are associated with subretinal exudates and lipoproteinaceous material from leakage that causes retinal detachment. Usually occurs in males less than 20 years old (peak ages = 6 to 8 years). Unilateral in 90% of cases. Presents as leukocoria, strabismus, and painful glaucoma. Treatment is surgery, cryotherapy, or diathermy.
Marfan syndrome **(Fig. 2.19)**	*MRI and CT:* Lens ectopia occurs in 50–80% of patients with Marfan syndrome. Minor trauma can cause lens dislocations.	Caused by autosomal dominant mutation of the *FBN1* gene on chromosome 15q21.1 that normally encodes for the extracellular matrix protein fibrillin 1. Defective fibrillin 1 protein is associated with aortic root aneurysms/dissections, ectopia lentis with predisposition to traumatic lens dislocations, tall stature, scoliosis, arachnodactyly, and spontaneous pneumothorax. Incidence is 1–3/10,000 live births.
Cephalocele (See **Fig. 2.15b**)	Defect in skull through which there is herniation of either meninges and CSF (meningocele) or meninges, CSF, and brain tissue (meningoencephalocele).	Congenital malformation involving lack of separation of neuroectoderm from surface ectoderm, with resultant localized failure of bone formation. Occipital location is most common in patients in the Western hemisphere, and a frontoethmoidal location is most common in Southeast Asians. Other sites include the parietal and sphenoid bones and between the frontal and nasal bones. Cephaloceles can also result from trauma or surgery.

(continued on page 202)

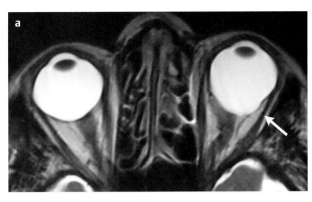
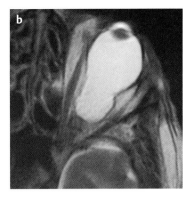

Fig. 2.17   Axial T2-weighted images of **(a)** a 70-year-old woman (*arrow*) and **(b)** an 83-year-old woman show staphylomas, which are seen as enlargement of the left eye without focal wall defects.

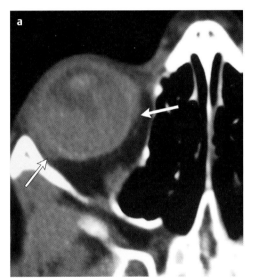
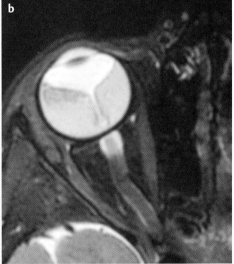

Fig. 2.18   A 6-year-old female with Coats' disease. **(a)** Axial CT shows subretinal homogeneous exudates that have attenuation slightly higher than the vitreous (*arrows*). **(b)** The subretinal exudates have slightly high to high signal on axial T2-weighted imaging.

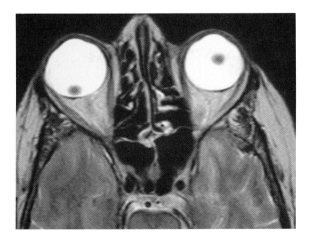

Fig. 2.19   Patient with Marfan syndrome who has dislocated lenses bilaterally on axial T2-weighted imaging.

Table 2.1 *(cont.)* Congenital and developmental abnormalities

Abnormality	Imaging Findings	Comments
Holoprosencephaly (**Fig. 2.20**)	*Alobar:* Large monoventricle with posterior midline cyst, lack of hemisphere formation, with absence of falx, corpus callosum, and septum pellucidum. Fused thalami. Can be associated with facial anomalies (facial clefts, arhinia, hypotelorism, cyclops). *Semilobar:* Anterior frontal portions of brain are fused across the midline and lack the interhemispheric fissure anteriorly. Partial formation of interhemispheric fissure posteriorly and occipital and temporal horns of ventricles, as well as partially fused thalami. Absent corpus callosum anteriorly but splenium is present. Absent septum pellucidum. Associated with mild craniofacial anomalies. *Lobar:* Near-complete formation of interhemispheric fissure and ventricles. Fused inferior portions of frontal lobes, dysgenesis of corpus callosum with formation of posterior portion without anterior portion, malformed frontal horns of lateral ventricles, absence of septum pellucidum, separate thalami, and neuronal migration disorders. *Syntelencephaly (middle interhemispheric variant):* Partial formation of interhemispheric fissure in the anterior and posterior regions, with fusion of the portions of the upper frontal and/or parietal lobes. Genu and splenium of the corpus callosum can be observed with localized absence/defect of the central body of the corpus callosum. Septum pellucidum is often absent.	Holoprosencephaly (HPE) is a spectrum of diverticulation disorders that occur during weeks 4–6 of gestation and that are characterized by absent or partial cleavage and differentiation of the embryonic forebrain cerebrum (prosenecephalon) into hemispheres and lobes. Causes include maternal diabetes, teratogens, and fetal genetic abnormalities, such as trisomy 16 (Patau syndrome) and trisomy 18 (Edwards syndrome). Familial HPE can be due to mutations of *HPE1* on chromosome 21q22.3, *HPE2* on 2p21, *HPE3* on 7q36, *HPE4* on 18p, *HPE5* on 13q32, *HPE6* on 2q37, *HPE7* on 9q22.3, *HPE8* on 14q13, and *HPE9* on 2q14. These genes are related to ventral and dorsal induction of the prosencephalon. *ZIC2* mutations are also associated with HPE. Clinical manifestations depend on severity of malformation and include early death, seizures, mental retardation, facial dysmorphism, and developmental delay. Patients with syntelencephaly often have mild to moderate cognitive dysfunction, spasticity, and mild visual impairment.
Septo-optic dysplasia (de Morsier syndrome) (**Fig. 2.21**)	Dysgenesis/hypoplasia or agenesis of septum pellucidum, optic nerve hypoplasia, and squared frontal horns. There is an association with schizencephaly in 50% of cases. Optic canals are often small. May be associated with gray matter heterotopia and polymicrogyria.	Patients can have nystagmus, decreased visual acuity, hypothalamic-pituitary disorders (decreased thyroid-stimulating hormone and/or growth hormone). Clinical exam shows small optic discs. May be sporadic, caused by in utero insults, or may be due to abnormal genetic expression caused by mutations (*HESX1* gene on chromosome 3p21.1–3p21.2 accounts for less than 1% of cases) during formation of the basal prosencephalon. Some findings overlap those of mild lobar holoprosencephaly.

(continued on page 204)

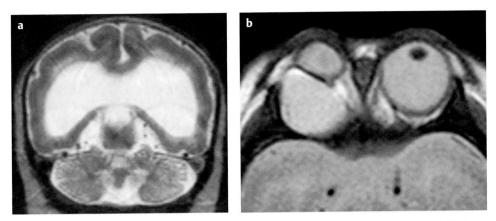

Fig. 2.20 **(a)** A 5-day-old female with holoprosencephaly, as seen on coronal T2-weighted imaging, and **(b)** hypotelorism and right microphthalmia with colobomatous cyst on axial T2-weighted imaging.

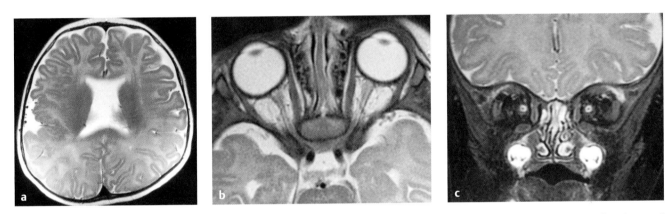

Fig. 2.21 Septo-optic dysplasia in a 5-month-old male. **(a)** Axial T2-weighted imaging shows absence of the septum pellucidum and polymicrogyria involving the right cerebral hemisphere. **(b)** Axial T2-weighted imaging and **(c)** coronal STIR show very small optic nerves bilaterally.

Table 2.1 *(cont.)*   Congenital and developmental abnormalities

Abnormality	Imaging Findings	Comments
Craniosynostosis **(Fig. 2.22** and **Fig. 2.23)**	*Coronal suture:* Premature closure, ~ 10% of cases, results in a vertically elongated skull that is asymmetric from the anterior to posterior portions of the skull (brachycephaly) and hypertelorism. *Unilateral coronal suture:* Premature closure results in cranial asymmetry from left to right sides (plagiocephaly) and orbital asymmetry.	Premature closure of cranial suture resulting from developmental anomaly (primary synostosis) due to intrauterine or postnatal trauma, toxins, drugs (aminopterin, dilantin, retinoic acid, valproic acid), metabolic disorders (hyperthyroidism, hypercalcemia, hypophosphatasia, rickets, mucopolysaccharidoses, hydrocephalus, etc.), or lack of brain growth/microcephaly. Sagittal suture closure is the most common (60%), followed by unilateral or bilateral closure of the coronal suture (25%). Premature closure of the metopic suture, resulting in trigonocephaly, occurs in 15%. Only 2–3% have premature closure of the lambdoid suture. Most cases are sporadic. Eight percent of coronal craniosynostosis and 2% of sagittal craniosynostosis are related to X-linked hypophosphatemic rickets. Premature sutural closure can result from chromosomal abnormalities (Apert syndrome, mutation on chromosome 10; Saethre-Chotzen syndrome, mutation at chromosome 7p21.2; Pfeiffer syndrome, mutation on chromosome 10; Crouzon syndrome, mutation on chromosome 10).
Hemifacial microsomia (Goldenhar syndrome, oculoauriculovertebral spectrum) **(Fig. 2.24)**	Findings include facial and orbital asymmetry from unilateral and/or bilateral hypoplasia of the mandible and zygomatic arches, atresia or stenosis of the external auditory canals, hypoplasia of the middle ear, malformations and/or fusion of the ossicles, oval window atresia, and abnormal position of CN VII.	Asymmetric abnormal development of the first and second branchial arches related to autosomal dominant mutation of the *TCOF1* gene on chromosome 5q32-q33.1. Results in deafness/hearing loss and airway narrowing.

(continued on page 206)

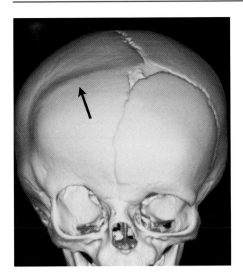

Fig. 2.22 Volume-rendered CT shows craniosynostosis from premature fusion of the right coronal suture (*arrow*), resulting in plagiocephaly and asymmetry of the orbits.

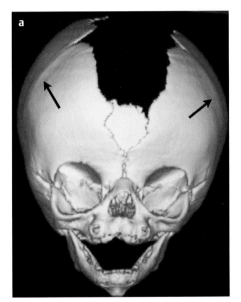

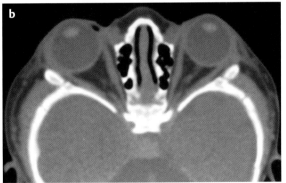

Fig. 2.23 A 5-month-old child with Apert syndrome. **(a)** Coronal volume-rendered CT shows craniosynostosis consisting of premature closure of the coronal suture (*arrows*), resulting in a widened sagittal suture. Also seen is midface hypoplasia/underdevelopment. **(b)** Axial CT shows hypertelorism.

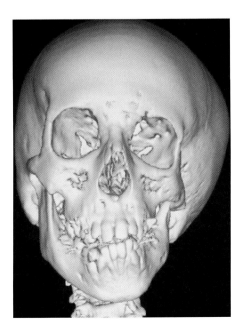

Fig. 2.24 A 12-year-old male with hemifacial microsomia (Goldenhar syndrome, oculoauriculovertebral spectrum). Coronal volume-rendered CT shows facial and orbital asymmetry from unilateral hypoplasia of the left maxilla, left zygomatic arch, and left mandible, resulting in malformation of the left orbit.

Table 2.1 *(cont.)*   Congenital and developmental abnormalities

Abnormality	Imaging Findings	Comments
Neurofibromatosis type 1 (NF1) **(Fig. 2.25, Fig. 2.26,** and **Fig. 2.27)**	NF1 is associated with focal ectasia of intracranial dura, dural and frontal or temporal lobe protrusion into orbit through bony defect, bony hypoplasia of greater sphenoid wing, bone malformation or erosion from plexiform neurofibromas, or optic glioma.	Autosomal dominant disorder (1/2500 births) from mutations involving the neurofibromin gene on chromosome 17q11.2. Represents the most common type of neurocutaneous syndrome. Neurofibronin is a GTPase-activating protein (Ras-GTP) that negatively activates the intracellular signaling protein p21-ras (Ras). Haploinsufficiency or complete deficiency in NF1 results in elevation of Ras activity, which alters cellular proliferation and differentiation of different cell types. Clinical features include café-au-lait spots (skin), axillary freckles, and cutaneous neurofibromas. Osseous lesions include malformations of the sphenoid bone (greater wing hypoplasia/aplasia—usually unilateral), vertebrae, and long bones (tibia/fibula). More than 50% of osseous malformations of the sphenoid greater wing are associated with NF1. Bony defects can also occur at the lambdoid and sagittal sutures.
von Hippel-Lindau disease **(Fig. 2.28)**	Circumscribed tumors usually located in the cerebellum and/or brainstem; small lesions may be seen involving the optic nerve or retina. *MRI:* Small gadolinium-enhancing nodule ± cyst, with intermediate signal on T1-weighted imaging and intermediate-high signal on T2-weighted imaging. Occasionally, lesions have evidence of recent or remote hemorrhage. *CT:* Small contrast-enhancing nodule ± cyst, ± hemorrhage.	Slow-growing, vascular tumors—hemangioblastomas (WHO grade I)—that involve the cerebellum, brainstem, spinal cord, optic nerves, and retina. Tumors consist of numerous thin-walled vessels as well as large, lipid-containing vacuolated stromal cells that have variably sized hyperchromatic nuclei. Mitotic figures are rare. Sporadic mutations of the *VHL* gene or autosomal dominant germline mutation of the *VHL* gene on chromosome 3p25–26 results in von Hippel-Lindau (VHL) disease. In VHL disease, multiple CNS hemangioblastomas occur, as well as clear-cell renal carcinoma, pheochromocytoma, endolymphatic sac tumor, neuroendocrine tumor, adenoma of the pancreas, and epididymal cystadenoma. VHL disease occurs in adolescents and young and middle-aged adults.

(continued on page 208)

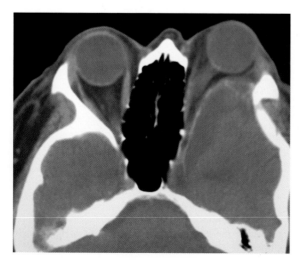

Fig. 2.25   A 10-year-old female with neurofibromatosis type 1. Axial CT shows absent greater wing of the left sphenoid bone, with dural and temporal lobe protrusion into left orbit through the bony defect.

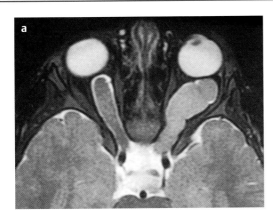
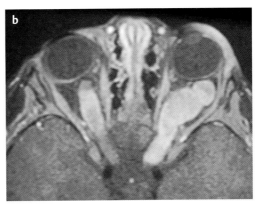

Fig. 2.26 A 3-year-old female with neurofibromatosis type 1. **(a)** Axial fat-suppressed T2-weighted imaging shows bilateral optic nerve gliomas, which have slightly high signal. **(b)** The gliomas show gadolinium contrast enhancement on axial fat-suppressed T1-weighted imaging.

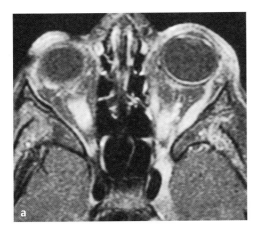
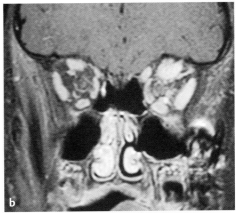

Fig. 2.27 A 7-year-old male with neurofibromatosis type 1. **(a)** Axial and **(b)** coronal fat-suppressed T1-weighted images show irregular zones of contrast enhancement in the left orbit and left superior and inferior orbital fissures from a plexiform neurofibroma.

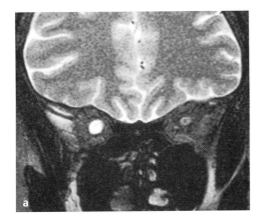
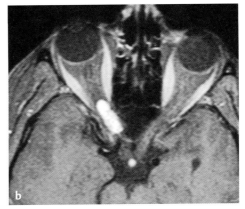

Fig. 2.28 **(a)** A 43-year-old woman with von Hippel-Lindau disease who has a hemangioblastoma involving the right optic nerve that has high signal on coronal fat-suppressed T2-weighted imaging and **(b)** shows gadolinium contrast enhancement on axial fat-suppressed T1-weighted imaging.

Table 2.1 *(cont.)*   Congenital and developmental abnormalities

Abnormality	Imaging Findings	Comments
Tuberous sclerosis	*MRI: Giant cell astrocytomas* of the retina can have intermediate signal on T1- and T2-weighted imaging and FLAIR; calcification and gadolinium contrast enhancement are common. Retinal astrocytic hamartomas may appear as small zones of thickening along the retina.	Tuberous sclerosis is an autosomal dominant disorder associated with hamartomas in multiple organs. In the brain, cortical hamartomas (tubers), subcortical glioneuronal hamartomas, subependymal glial hamartomas (nodules), and subependymal giant cell astrocytomas are nonmalignant lesions associated with tuberous sclerosis. In the eye, multiple retinal nodular astrocytic hamartomas can occur, and rarely giant cell astrocytomas. Extraneural lesions include retinal astrocytic hamartomas, cutaneous angiofibromas (adenoma sebaceum), subungual fibromas, visceral cysts, renal angioleiomyomas, intestinal polyps, cardiac rhabdomyomas, and pulmonary lymphangioleiomyomatosis. Caused by mutations of the *TSC1* gene on 9q or the *TSC2* gene on 16p. Prevalence of 1 in 6,000 newborns.
Sturge-Weber syndrome **(Fig. 2.29)**	*MRI:* Prominent, localized, unilateral leptomeningeal gadolinium contrast enhancement, usually in parietal and/or occipital regions in children, ± gyral enhancement, mild localized atrophic changes in brain with decreased signal on T2-weighted imaging adjacent to the pial angioma, ± prominent medullary and/or subependymal veins, ± ipsilateral prominence of choroid plexus. Diffuse choroidal hemangiomas typically show thickened prominent gadolinium contrast enhancement of the posterior inner wall of the eye ipsilateral to the enhancing pial angioma. *CT:* Localized encephalomalacia adjacent to gyral calcifications > 2 years, progressive cerebral atrophy in region of pial angioma.	Also known as encephalotrigeminal angiomatosis, Sturge-Weber syndrome is a neurocutaneous syndrome associated with ipsilateral port wine cutaneous lesion and seizures. It results from persistence of primitive leptomeningeal venous drainage (pial angioma) and developmental lack of normal cortical veins, producing chronic venous congestion and ischemia. Diffuse choroidal hemangioma can be seen in up to 50% of patients ipsilateral to the enhancing pial angioma. The choroidal hemangioma can be associated with exudates that cause retinal or choroidal detachments. Clinical findings include vision loss and visual field deficits, glaucoma, and vascular malformations of the conjunctiva and episclera.
Optic nerve head drusen **(Fig. 2.30)**	*CT:* Discrete, focal, rounded zone with high density or calcification at the optic nerve head.	At the optic nerve head, acellular deposition of protein can occur and can eventually calcify. May result from accumulation of axoplasmic derivatives of degenerating retinal nerve fibers. Can be bilateral. Ophthalmoscopic evaluation can appear similar to papilledema. Usually is asymptomatic.

(continued on page 210)

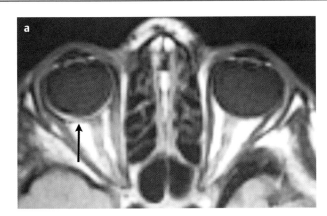
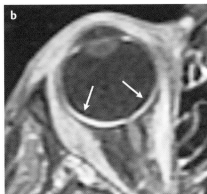

Fig. 2.29 A 5-year-old male with Sturge-Weber syndrome. **(a)** Axial T1-weighted and **(b)** thin-section fat-suppressed T1-weighted images show a diffuse choroidal hemangioma in the right eye, which is seen as thickened prominent gadolinium contrast enhancement of the posterior inner wall of the eye (*arrows*) and is ipsilateral to an enhancing pial angioma (not shown).

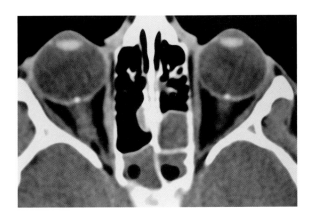

Fig. 2.30 Axial CT shows small, focal, rounded, calcified zones at both optic disc heads representing bilateral optic nerve head drusens.

Table 2.1 *(cont.)* Congenital and developmental abnormalities

Abnormality	Imaging Findings	Comments
Orbital infantile hemangioma (**Fig. 2.31**)	*MRI:* During the proliferative phase, lesions have intermediate signal on T1-weighted imaging (T1WI) and slightly high signal on T2-weighted imaging (T2WI), as well as intralesional flow voids. Typically show prominent gadolinium (Gd) contrast enhancement. Involuting hemangiomas have heterogeneous signal on T1WI and T2WI, lack of intralesional flow voids, and heterogeneous Gd contrast enhancement. *CT:* Proliferating lesions have intermediate attenuation and show contrast enhancement, ± intralesional fatty changes.	Hemangiomas are lesions that contain vascular spaces with varying sizes and shapes. Hemangiomas can be classified as capillary or cavernous based on the sizes of the vascular spaces. Hemangiomas can occur in soft tissue or bone and can be small or large, solitary circumscribed, or infiltrative. Infantile hemangiomas (also referred to as hemangioma of infancy, common infantile hemangioma, or juvenile hemangioma) are the most common congenital lesions in the head and neck. The infantile/juvenile capillary hemangioma contains small vascular spaces lined by small, densely packed, round endothelial cells and pericyte clusters. May present as small lesions at birth, but more commonly present during the first year. Typically increase in size over 10 months (proliferative phase), with subsequent involution over 6–10 years. Usually treated conservatively except for large lesions associated with clinical problems. Can occur in association with the PHACE (posterior fossa anomalies, neonatal hemangiomas, arterial abnormalities, aortic coarctation, cardiac and eye abnormalities) or LUMBAR (lower body hemangiomas, urogenital anomalies, ulceration, myelopathy, bone deformities, anorectal malformations, and arterial and renal anomalies) syndromes.
Congenital hemangioma	*MRI:* Lesions have intermediate signal on T1-weighted imaging (T1WI) and slightly high to high signal on T2-weighted imaging (T2WI). Typically show prominent gadolinium (Gd) contrast enhancement. Involuting hemangiomas have heterogeneous signal on T1WI and T2WI, lack of intralesional flow voids, and heterogeneous Gd contrast enhancement. *CT:* Lesions have intermediate attenuation and show contrast enhancement, ± intralesional fat.	Uncommon, solitary, vascular lesions that are present at birth and do not undergo significant enlargement after birth. There are two types of congenital hemangiomas. The rapidly involuting type of congenital hemangioma regresses by 14 months or earlier. The noninvoluting congenital hemangioma usually shows growth in proportion to the rest of the body. Treatment of these lesions can be done with percutaneous injection of sclerosing agents.
Orbital venolymphatic malformation (**Fig. 2.32**)	Can be circumscribed lesions or may occur in an infiltrative pattern, with extension within soft tissue and between muscles. *MRI:* Often contain single or multiple cystic zones, which can be large (macrocystic type) or small (microcystic type), which have predominantly low signal on T1-weighted imaging (T1WI) and high signal on T2-weighted imaging (T2WI) and fat-suppressed T2WI. Fluid–fluid levels and zones with high signal on T1WI and variable signal on T2WI may result from cysts containing hemorrhage, high protein concentration, and/or necrotic debris. Septa between the cystic zones can vary in thickness and gadolinium (Gd) contrast enhancement. Nodular zones within the lesions can have variable degrees of Gd contrast enhancement. Microcystic type typically shows more Gd contrast enhancement than the macrocystic type. *CT:* The macrocystic type is usually a low-attenuation cystic lesion (10–25 HU) separated by thin walls, ± intermediate or high attenuation, which can result from hemorrhage or infection, ± fluid–fluid levels.	Benign vascular anomalies (also referred to as lymphangioma or cystic hygroma) that primarily result from abnormal lymphangiogenesis. Up to 75% occur in the head and neck. Can be observed in utero with MRI or sonography, at birth (50–65%), or within the first 5 years. Approximately 85% are detected by age 2. Lesions are composed of endothelium-lined lymphatic ± venous channels interspersed within connective tissue stroma. Account for less than 1% of benign soft tissue tumors and 5.6% of all benign lesions of infancy and childhood. Can occur in association with Turner syndrome and Proteus syndrome.

(continued on page 212)

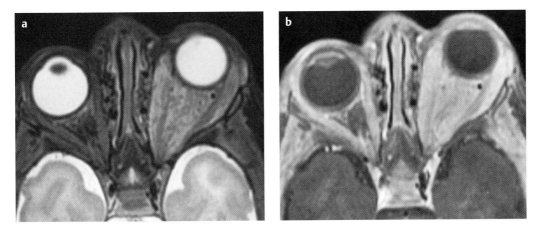

Fig. 2.31 **(a)** A 6-week-old female with an infantile hemangioma in the left orbit that has diffuse, slightly high signal on fat-suppressed T2-weighted imaging with several flow voids. **(b)** The hemangioma also shows diffuse gadolinium contrast enhancement on axial fat-suppressed T1-weighted imaging. The hemangioma causes left proptosis.

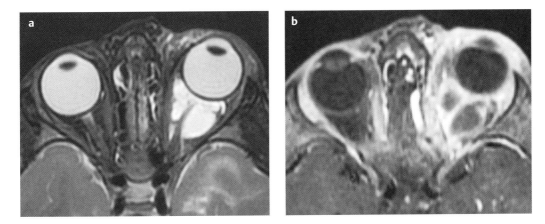

Fig. 2.32 A 2-year-old male with a venolymphatic malformation in the left orbit. **(a)** Axial fat-suppressed T2-weighted imaging shows multiple cystic zones with high signal. **(b)** Axial fat-suppressed T1-weighted imaging shows gadolinium contrast enhancement of the septae between cystic zones.

Table 2.1 *(cont.)* Congenital and developmental abnormalities

Abnormality	Imaging Findings	Comments
Orbital epidermoid (**Fig. 2.33**)	*MRI:* Well-circumscribed spheroid or multilobulated extra-axial ectodermal-inclusion cystic lesions with low-intermediate signal on T1-weighted imaging and high signal on T2- and diffusion-weighted imaging. Mixed low, intermediate, or high signal on FLAIR images, and no gadolinium contrast enhancement. *CT:* Well-circumscribed spheroid or multilobulated extra-axial ectodermal-inclusion cystic lesions with low-intermediate attenuation. Can be associated with bone erosion.	Nonneoplastic congenital or acquired ectodermal inclusion cysts filled with desquamated cells and keratinaceous debris, usually with mild mass effect on adjacent orbital structures, ± related clinical symptoms. Equal sex distribution. Often located adjacent to the frontozygomatic and frontoethmoidal sutures.
Orbital dermoid (**Fig. 2.34**)	*MRI:* Well-circumscribed spheroid or multilobulated extra-axial lesions, usually with high signal on T1-weighted imaging and variable low, intermediate, and/or high signal on T2-weighted imaging. No gadolinium contrast enhancement, ± fluid–fluid or fluid–debris levels. *CT:* Well-circumscribed spheroid or multilobulated extra-axial lesions, usually with low attenuation, ± fat–fluid or fluid–debris levels. Can be associated with bone erosion.	Nonneoplastic congenital or acquired ectodermal-inclusion cystic lesions filled with lipid material, cholesterol, desquamated cells, keratinaceous debris, skin appendages (hair follicles and sebaceous and sweat glands). Usually have mild mass effect on adjacent brain, ± related clinical symptoms. Occur in adults, and in males slightly more often than in females. Often located adjacent to the frontozygomatic and frontoethmoidal sutures.

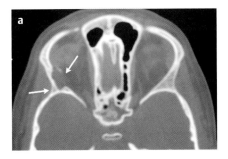 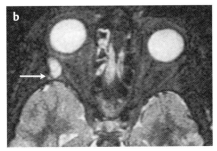 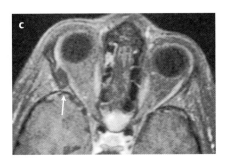

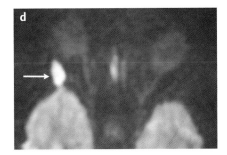

Fig. 2.33 **(a)** Axial CT of a 9-year-old female with an epidermoid (*arrows*) at the posterolateral portion of the right orbit that has low attenuation and is associated with bone erosion. **(b)** The lesion has high signal on fat-suppressed T2-weighted imaging (*arrow*), **(c)** low signal on postcontrast axial fat-suppressed T1-weighted imaging (*arrow*), and **(d)** restricted diffusion on axial diffusion-weighted imaging (*arrow*).

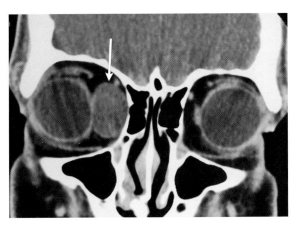

Fig. 2.34 Coronal CT shows a circumscribed dermoid (*arrow*) with low-intermediate attenuation at the medial portion of the right orbit.

Table 2.2   Acquired lesions involving the eye

- Malignant Neoplasms
  - Retinoblastoma
  - Ocular melanoma
  - Ocular metastases
  - Medulloepithelioma
  - Intraocular lymphoma
  - Intraocular leukemia
- Benign Neoplasms
  - Choroidal hemangioma
  - Retinal astrocytoma
  - Choroidal osteoma

- Infection
  - Endophthalmitis
  - *Toxocara* endophthalmitis
  - Uveitis from infection
  - Conjunctivitis
- Inflammation
  - Idiopathic orbital inflammatory pseudotumor
  - Noninfectious uveitis
  - Posterior scleritis
- Traumatic Abnormalities
  - Globe trauma
  - Retinal detachment
  - Choroidal detachment
- Degeneration
  - Phthisis bulbi
  - Cataract

Table 2.2 Acquired lesions involving the eye

Lesion	Imaging Findings	Comments
Malignant Neoplasms		
Retinoblastoma (**Fig. 2.35** and **Fig. 2.36**)	*CT:* Intraocular lesion with soft tissue attenuation, and up to 95% have variably sized calcifications related to necrosis of tumor cells. Tumors typically show contrast enhancement. *MRI:* Intraocular lesions can arise from the inner retinal layers and grow into the vitreous (endophytic type) with or without separated tumor cell clusters (vitreous seeding), or they can arise in the outer retinal layers and grow into the subretinal space (exophytic type), often in association with retinal detachment and subretinal exudates containing tumor cells. Combined endophytic and exophytic types can also occur. Rarely, tumors can have a diffuse, infiltrative, plaquelike pattern. Tumors often have intermediate to slightly high signal on T1-weighted imaging and low to intermediate signal on T2-weighted imaging, ± restricted diffusion. Tumors usually show prominent gadolinium contrast enhancement. Contrast-enhanced MRI can show tumor invasion of the choroid, sclera, optic disc (prelaminar involvement), and/or optic nerve (postlaminar involvement). Metastatic disease is associated with extrascleral tumor extension and tumor in the optic nerve posterior to the lamina cribrosa (anatomic site where the optic nerve pierces the sclera).	Most frequent malignant intraocular tumor in children, composed of poorly cohesive primitive neoplastic cells with spheroid basophilic nuclei within scant cytoplasm. Tumors typically have high mitotic activity, zones of ischemic necrosis, and dystrophic calcifications. Retinoblastoma occurs with an incidence of 1.2 per 100,000 children ranging from 0 to 4 years in age, and accounts for 11% of pediatric cancer in the first year, and 6% of cancer in the first 5 years. Unilateral in 70% of cases, with mean age at diagnosis of 2 years, bilateral in remainder, with mean age at diagnosis of 1 year for bilateral (25%) or multifocal (5%) forms (trilateral or tetralateral) associated with midline tumors, such as pineoblastoma and pineal and/or suprasellar PNET. All bilateral and multifocal types have mutation involving the *RB1* gene on chromosome 13q14. Up to 15% of the unilateral type have a similar mutation involving the *RB1* gene. Fundoscopic exam shows a white papillary reflex/leukocoria. Patients can also have strabismus from tumor involving the macula, which disrupts sensory imput for proper alignment of the eyes. With unilateral tumor, small tumors can be treated with laser photocoagulation, cryoablation, chemotherapy, or brachytherapy. Larger tumors can be treated with chemoreduction followed by surgery. Tumors filling more than half of the globe are treated with enucleation. Five-year survival is up to 99%. Prognosis for trilateral tumor, however, is very poor.

(continued on page 216)

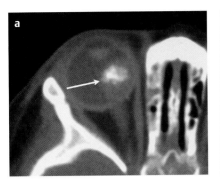
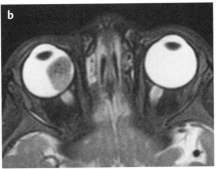
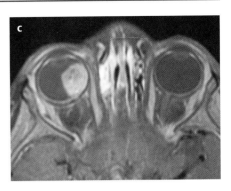

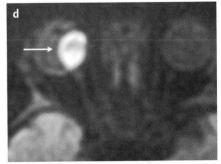

Fig. 2.35 Retinoblastoma in a 5-year-old female. **(a)** An intraocular lesion (*arrow*) with soft tissue attenuation and calcifications is seen in the right eye on axial CT. **(b)** The tumor extends into the vitreous (endophytic type) and has low to intermediate signal on fat-suppressed T2-weighted imaging, **(c)** gadolinium contrast enhancement on axial fat-suppressed T1-weighted imaging, and **(d)** restricted diffusion (*arrow*) on axial diffusion-weighted imaging.

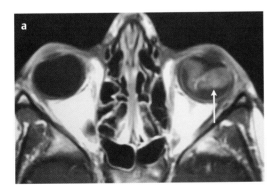
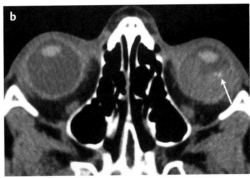

Fig. 2.36 A 6-year-old female with a retinoblastoma within the vitreous that shows **(a)** gadolinium contrast enhancement on axial T1-weighted imaging (*arrow*) and **(b)** intermediate attenuation and a small calcification (*arrow*) on axial CT.

Table 2.2 *(cont.)*   Acquired lesions involving the eye

Lesion	Imaging Findings	Comments
Ocular melanoma (**Fig. 2.37** and **Fig. 2.38**)	*MRI:* Lesions arise in the choroid and can penetrate through Bruch's membrane into the vitreous, resulting in a "collar button" tumor shape. Tumors can also have a crescentic shape involving the choroid. Tumors often have slightly high to high signal on T1-weighted imaging, low-intermediate signal on T2-weighted imaging, and gadolinium contrast enhancement. MRI can show associated retinal detachment as well as scleral infiltration/invasion. *CT:* Tumors have intermediate attenuation, moderate contrast enhancement, and typically no calcifications.	Uveal melanoma is the most frequent intraocular neoplasm in adults (40–60 years old), with an incidence of 5–6/million. Patients present with visual field defects, vision loss, and photopsia. Tumors arise from the outer layers of the choroid, causing localized thickening of the choroid and eventual penetration through Bruch's membrane (acellular structure/barrier between the retina and choroid) into the subretinal space, resulting in a "mushroom" or "collar button" shaped tumor. Within the uvea, 90% of melanomas occur in choroid, 7% occur in the ciliary body, and 3% in the iris. Iris melanomas can be detected and treated early and have high survival rates. Ciliary body and choroid melanomas are associated with metastatic disease (liver in 90% of cases, as well as lungs, bones, kidneys, and brain) in up to 50%. Small uveal melanomas less than 10 mm in thickness can be treated with plaque brachytherapy, proton beam radiation therapy, or thermotherapy. Enucleation is done for ciliary body and choroidal melanomas > 10 mm thick. Five-year survival ranges from 47% for large choroidal melanomas to 84% for large tumors.
Ocular metastases (**Fig. 2.39**)	*MRI:* Lesions commonly occur in the choroid and have intermediate signal on T1-weighted imaging and low-intermediate or slightly high signal on T2-weighted imaging, with gadolinium contrast enhancement. MRI can show scleral infiltration/invasion. *CT:* Tumors have intermediate attenuation and moderate contrast enhancement, ± calcifications.	Usually occur in adults. Most common metastatic tumors to the eye are from malignancies of the breast, lung, and kidneys. Patients can present with vision loss and/or pain. Most ocular metastases result from hematogenous spread to the uvea.
Medulloepithelioma	*MRI:* Tumors commonly occur in the ciliary body and rarely the retina. Solid portions of tumor have intermediate signal on T1-weighted imaging and low-intermediate, or slightly high signal on T2-weighted imaging (T2WI). Cystic zones in tumors have high signal on T2WI. Intratumoral calcifications in the teratoid subtype can have low signal on T2WI. Solid portions of tumor show gadolinium contrast enhancement. MRI can show scleral infiltration/invasion. *CT:* Tumors usually involve the ciliary body and have intermediate attenuation as well as zones of low attenuation related to cystic portions in large lesions. Solid portions of tumors show moderate to prominent contrast enhancement. Calcifications are typically absent from the nonteratoid subtype and can be seen in 30% of the teratoid subtype. Zones of low attenuation from cartilage can be seen in the teratoid type.	Rare embryonal intraocular tumor derived from the primitive neuroectoermal, nonpigmented epithelium of the ciliary body. Typically are unilateral and occur in young children (average age = 5 years). Patients can have poor vision, leukocoria, strabismus, and/or change in eye color. There are two tumor subtypes, nonteratoid and teratoid variants. Both nonteratoid and teratoid tumors contain poorly differentiated neuroepithelial cells within a loose hyaluronic acid-rich mesenchymal background. Teratoid variants (30 to 50% of cases) also contain cartilage and skeletal muscle. Up to 66% have malignant features. Enucleation is commonly done as treatment. Metastatic disease is uncommon. Tumors limited to the globe have a 5-year survival rate of 95% after enucleation.

(continued on page 218)

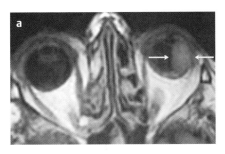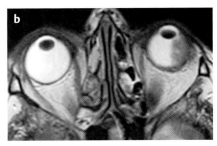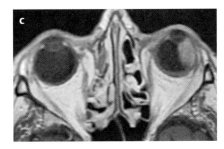

Fig. 2.37 **(a)** A 74-year-old woman with an ocular melanoma that has slightly high signal on axial T1-weighted imaging (*arrows*), **(b)** low-intermediate signal on axial T2-weighted imaging, and **(c)** gadolinium contrast enhancement on axial T1-weighted imaging.

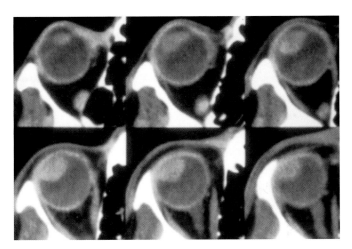

Fig. 2.38 Axial CT shows an ocular melanoma in the right eye that has intermediate attenuation.

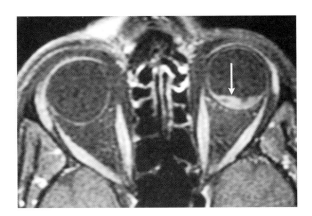

Fig. 2.39 A 52-year woman with breast carcinoma and gadolinium-enhancing metastatic tumor (*arrow*) involving choroid in the left eye on axial fat-suppressed T1-weighted imaging.

Table 2.2 *(cont.)*   Acquired lesions involving the eye

Lesion	Imaging Findings	Comments
Intraocular lymphoma	*MRI:* Poorly defined or circumscribed intraocular lesions with intermediate signal on T1-weighted imaging and low-intermediate or slightly high signal on T2-weighted imaging, + gadolinium contrast enhancement. *CT:* Lesions often have intermediate attenuation.	Primary intraocular lymphoma (PIOL) is a subset of primary central nervous system lymphoma (PCNSL) involving the brain. Up to 33% of patients with PIOL will have concurrent PCNSL at presentation, and up to 90% will eventually develop PCNSL at 29 months. PIOL usually occurs in adults from the third to eighth decades. Most PIOLs are B-cell lymphomas. Can occur in immunocompetent and immunocompromised patients. Can present with decreased vision, diplopia, chronic vitreitis, or posterior uveitis. Treatment includes radiation therapy and intravenous or intravitreal administration of methotrexate or rituximab.
Intraocular leukemia (**Fig. 2.40**)	*MRI:* Poorly defined or circumscribed intraocular lesions with intermediate signal on T1-weighted imaging and low-intermediate or slightly high signal on T2-weighted imaging, + gadolinium contrast enhancement, ± serous or hemorrhagic retinal detachment. Can involve the retina, choroid, and/or optic nerve. *CT:* Lesions often have intermediate attenuation.	Malignant neoplasms of hematopoietic stem cells within bone marrow and blood. Can infiltrate the uvea, anterior segment, retina, and/or optic nerve. Ocular and orbital involvement is more common with acute leukemias than with the chronic types. Optic nerves can be involved from extension of intracranial neoplastic cells into the optic nerve sheath.
Benign Neoplasms		
Choroidal hemangioma (**Fig. 2.41** and **Fig. 2.42**)	*MRI:* Small, circumscribed lesions in the choroid that have intermediate signal on T1-weighted imaging, slightly high to high signal on T2-weighted imaging, and gadolinium contrast enhancement. *CT:* Lesions have intermediate attenuation, + contrast enhancement, – calcifications. *Ultrasound:* Localized thickening of choroid with echogenicity similar to adjacent normal choroid.	Choroidal hemangiomas are rare, benign, hamartomatous vascular lesions that can occur as circumscribed lesions or as a diffuse form in Sturge-Weber syndrome. Lesions are composed of endothelium-lined vascular channels. Usually diagnosed between the second and fourth decades. On ophthalmoscopic exam, circumscribed choroidal hemangioma typically occurs in the posterior pole and appears as a discrete, solitary, orange-red lesion measuring up to 6 mm in thickness. Usually asymptomatic, although uncommonly causes visual disturbances when associated with exudative retinal detachment (in less than 10% of cases). Treatment options for symptomatic cases include photodynamic therapy, laser photocoagulation, and/or transpupillary thermotherapy.
Retinal astrocytoma	*MRI:* Small lesion near the optic nerve with intermediate signal on T1-weighted imaging and low-intermediate or slightly high signal on T2-weighted imaging, ± retinal detachment. *CT:* Small lesion with intermediate attenuation, ± calcification.	Benign slow-growing tumor of the retina often associated with neurofibromatosis type 1 or tuberous sclerosis. May be associated with exudative retinal detachment.
Choroidal osteoma (**Fig. 2.43**)	*CT:* dense nodular zone of calcification/ossification in the choroid ranging in size from 2 to 22 mm in diameter and up to 25 mm in thickness.	Benign, slow-growing, small lesion composed of mature bone that can occur in the choroid between the macula and juxtapapillary region. Unilateral in 75%. Can occur in children and adults (median age = 35 years), with a female predominance. On ophthalmoscopic exam, lesions are yellow-white or orange-red, with variable thinning of the overlying retina. Can be asymptomatic or associated with serous retinal detachment, which may or may not be associated with a subretinal neovascularized membrane. Subretinal neovascularization can be treated with laser ablation.

(continued on page 220)

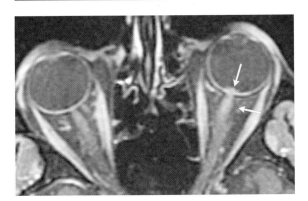

Fig. 2.40 A 27-year-old man with acute lymphoblastic leukemia with gadolinium-enhancing neoplastic involvement of the anterior optic nerve sheath and optic nerve head (*arrows*) on axial fat-suppressed T1-weighted imaging.

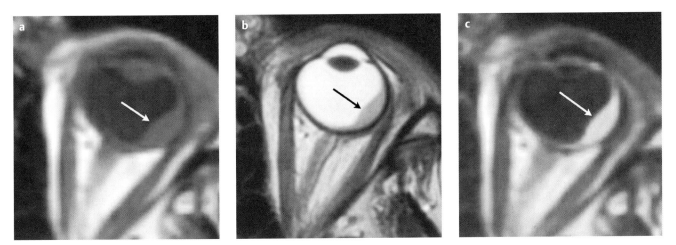

Fig. 2.41 **(a)** A choroidal hemangioma has intermediate signal on axial T1-weighted imaging (*arrow*), **(b)** slightly high signal on axial T2-weighted imaging (*arrow*), and **(c)** gadolinium contrast enhancement on axial T1-weighted imaging (*arrow*).

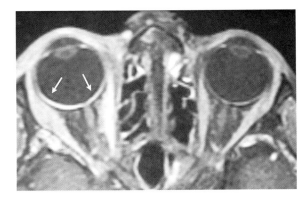

Fig. 2.42 A 5-year-old male with Sturge-Weber syndrome who has a diffuse choroidal hemangioma (*arrows*) in the right eye that is seen as thickened prominent gadolinium contrast enhancement of the posterior inner wall of the eye on axial fat-suppressed T1-weighted imaging.

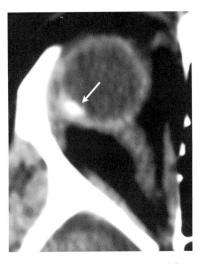

Fig. 2.43 A 56-year-old woman with a choroidal osteoma that is seen as a dense nodular zone of calcification/ossification in the choroid (*arrow*) on axial CT.

Table 2.2 *(cont.)* Acquired lesions involving the eye

Lesion	Imaging Findings	Comments
Infection		
Endophthalmitis (**Fig. 2.44** and **Fig. 2.45**)	*CT:* Endophthalmitis shows increased attenuation in the vitreous with scleral and uveal thickening and associated contrast enhancement. *MRI:* Endophthalmitis shows increased signal of the vitreous on T1-weighted imaging and FLAIR; restricted diffusion involving the vitreous, anterior chamber, and/or choroid; and abnormal thickening of the sclera and choroid. Gadolinium contrast enhancement of the vitreous, anterior chamber, sclera, and/or uvea can be seen. Subchoroid or subretinal infected collections may be present.	Endophthalmitis (infection of the vitreous chamber) most commonly occurs as a complication of cataract surgery, trauma, corneal ulcer, or periocular infection (exogeneous type), or occasionally (< 10%) from hematogenous spread to the choroid (endogenous type). Patients can present with ocular pain, vision loss, diplopia, chemosis, and/or proptosis. Common etiologic organisms include bacteria, such as *Staphylococcus aureus, Klebsiella pneumoniae,* and group B *Streptococcus,* and fungi, such as *Candida, Aspergillus,* and *Histoplasma* species. Urgent treatment with intravenous antibiotics is necessary.
Toxocara endophthalmitis	*CT:* Normal-size eye, with subretinal exudates with intermediate to slightly high attenuation, without calcifications. Posterior choroid pole granuloma may be calcified, ± thickend sclera. *MRI:* Central vitreous lesion with low-intermediate signal on T1-weighted imaging (T1WI) and slightly high to high signal on T2-weighted imaging (T2WI). Posterior pole granuloma can have low signal on T2WI and can show gadolinium contrast enhancement. ± Retinal detachment with subretinal exudates, which can have variable signal on T1WI and T2WI.	Hypersensitivity immune response and T-cell granulomatous reaction with eosinophilic inflammatory changes involving the human vitreous and/or uvea from dying larvae of the nematode parasites *Toxocara canis* (definitive host = dogs) and *Toxocara cati* (definitive host = felines) via oral-fecal exposures. Ingested larvae penetrate the intestinal wall, enter the bloodstream, and hematogenously disseminate to various tissues, such as the liver, lungs, brain, and choroid of the eye. Results in sclerosing choroidal inflammation, diffuse endophthalmitis, and posterior pole granulomas, with or without tractional retinal detachment. Most commonly occurs in children (5–10 years old). Patients can present with unilateral visual impairment, strabismus, redness, and pain. Treatment is with anthelmintic drugs, ± vitrectomy. Lack of treatment can lead to blindness.
Uveitis from infection (**Fig. 2.46**)	*CT:* Thickening and contrast enhancement of all or portions of the uveal tract. *MRI:* Thickening of the choroid and sclera, with gadolinium (Gd) contrast enhancement of all or portions of the uveal tract, ± anterior uveitis. With posterior uveitis, Gd contrast enhancement can also be seen in the dorsal episcleral soft tissue and Tenon's capsule.	The uvea consists of the choroid, ciliary body, and iris. Uveitis is categorized based on location. Anterior uveitis involves the anterior chamber including the iris (iritis) and/or ciliary body (cyclitis). Intermediate uveitis involves the vitreous and anterior retina (posterior cyclitis, hyalitis). Posterior uveitis involves the choroid and retina (chorioretinitis) Viruses associated with anterior uveitis include herpes simplex virus-1 (HSV), varicella-zoster virus (VZV), cytomegalovirus (CMV), and rubella virus. Intermediate uveitis occurs in Lyme disease and toxocariasis. Posterior uveitis is caused by HSV, VZV, CMV, toxoplasmosis, tuberculosis, syphilis, and bacterial or fungal infections. Anterior uveitis can result in cataract and/or glaucoma. Acyclovir is used to treat HSV/VZV, and ganciclovir is used for CMV.

(continued on page 222)

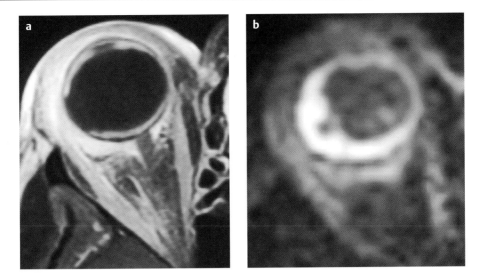

Fig. 2.44 A 52-year-old man with endophthalmitis. **(a)** Abnormal gadolinium contrast enhancement of the uvea, vitreous, anterior chamber, sclera, and extraocular soft tissues is seen on axial fat-suppressed T1-weighted imaging. **(b)** Restricted diffusion involving the uvea, vitreous, and anterior chamber is seen on axial diffusion-weighted imaging.

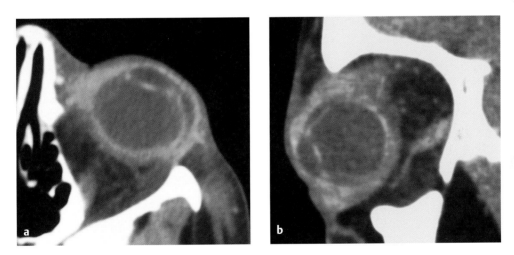

Fig. 2.45 A 79-year-old man with *Enterococcus* endophthalmitis. **(a)** Axial and **(b)** sagittal images show scleral and uveal thickening, with subchoroid and subretinal infected collections.

Fig. 2.46 Uveitis from infection. **(a)** Axial fat-suppressed T1-weighted imaging shows thickening of the choroid and sclera with gadolinium contrast enhancement of all or portions of the uveal tract, as well as the dorsal episcleral soft tissue and Tenon's capsule (*arrow*). **(b)** Axial CT shows thickening of the sclera and choroid, as well as slightly increased attenuation of the vitreous.

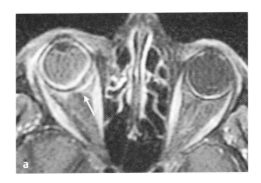

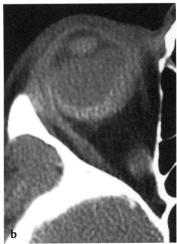

Table 2.2 *(cont.)*　Acquired lesions involving the eye

Lesion	Imaging Findings	Comments
Conjunctivitis **(Fig. 2.47)**	*CT:* Irregular thickening of the eyelid and conjunctiva, with variable contrast enhancement. *MRI:* Irregular soft tissue thickening involving the eyelid and conjunctiva, with poorly defined high signal on T2-weighted imaging (T2WI) and fat-suppressed T2WI and gadolinium contrast enhancement.	Common cause of red eye. Most common cause is infection. In children, bacterial infection is more common than viral infection. In adults, viral infections are the most common cause, followed by bacteria, allergens, fungi, and toxins. Bacterial infections commonly result from *Streptococcus, Staphylococcus,* and *Pseudomonas* species. Neonatal infections by *Neisseria gonorrhoeae* and *Chlamydia* require prompt treatment to avoid permanent eye damage. Treatment for bacterial infections includes an appropriate antibiotic. Viral conjunctivitis is self-limited and is treated with topical antihistamines and non-antibiotic lubricating drops. Allergic conjunctivitis is treated with antihistamine drops.
Inflammation		
Idiopathic orbital inflammatory pseudotumor **(Fig. 2.48)**	*CT:* Thickening of the uvea and sclera, with contrast enhancement and blurring of the optic nerve junction. *MRI:* Thickening and gadolinium contrast enhancement of the uvea, sclera, and Tenon's capsule.	Nonspecific, benign proliferative disorder of unknown etiology with accumulation of polymorphous inflammatory cells, lymphocytes, histiocytes, plasma cells, and eosinophils within the orbital soft tissues. Usually has an abrupt onset. Can occur as localized or diffuse forms. Can involve the anterior orbit (eye including the uvea), lacrimal gland (idiopathic dacryoadenitis), extraocular muscles (myositic pseudotumor), and/or posterior orbit/orbital apex. Equal sex distribution, with peak incidence in fourth to fifth decades. Can be unilateral or bilateral. Treatment often consists of corticosteroids or other immunosuppressive medication. Anterior ocular disease often involves the globe, uvea, Tenon's capsule, sclera, and periscleral soft tissues. Patients present with proptosis, eye pain, diplopia, and decreased vision.

(continued on page 224)

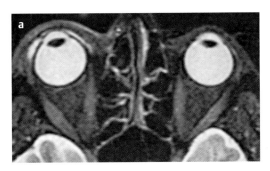
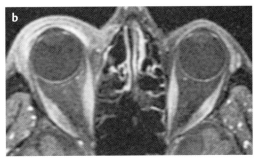

Fig. 2.47   A 47-year-old man with conjunctivitis. **(a)** Axial STIR shows soft tissue thickening involving the right eyelid and conjunctiva, with poorly defined high signal and **(b)** corresponding gadolinium contrast enhancement on axial fat-suppressed T1-weighted imaging.

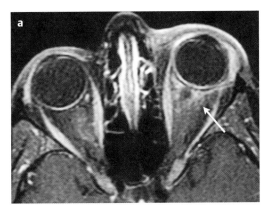
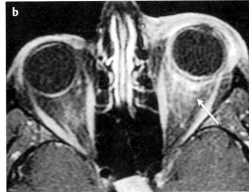

Fig. 2.48   **(a,b)** A 37-year-old man with idiopathic orbital inflammatory pseudotumor involving the left orbit seen as poorly defined zones of abnormal gadolinium contrast enhancement in the posterior episcleral soft tissues and intraconal fat (*arrows*) on axial fat-suppressed T1-weighted imaging.

Table 2.2 *(cont.)* Acquired lesions involving the eye

Lesion	Imaging Findings	Comments
Noninfectious uveitis **(Fig. 2.49** and **Fig. 2.50)**	*CT:* Thickening of the uvea and sclera, with contrast enhancement and blurring of the optic nerve junction. *MRI:* Thickening and gadolinium contrast enhancement of the uvea and sclera, ± Tenon's capsule.	Anterior uveitis involves the anterior chamber, including the iris and/or ciliary body, and can occur with ankylosing spondylitis, reactive arthritis (formerly referred to as Reiter's syndrome), inflammatory bowel disease, juvenile idiopathic arthritis, multiple sclerosis, Behçet's disease, Fuch's disease, and sarcoidosis. Intermediate uveitis involves the vitreous and anterior retina and can be seen with sarcoidosis, multiple sclerosis, and Behçet's disease. Posterior uveitis involves the choroid and retina and can be seen with sarcoidosis, Behçet's disease, and Vogt-Koyanagi-Harada syndrome (chronic granulomatous uveitis with exudative choroid effusion and nonrhegmatogenous retinal detachment of unknown etiology in association with fever, headaches, vertigo, meningitis, tinnitus, and hearing loss). Other reported inflammatory or autoimmune diseases associated with uveitis include polyartritis nodosa, rheumatoid arthritis, Sjögren's syndrome, systemic lupus erythematosus, and granulomatosis with polyangiitis. Treatment includes corticosteroids, surgically placed steroid implants, and immunosuppressive drugs.
Posterior scleritis **(Fig. 2.51)**	*CT:* Diffuse or nodular thickening of the posterior uvea and sclera, with variable contrast enhancement, ± blurring of the optic nerve junction. *MRI:* Diffuse or nodular thickening and gadolinium contrast enhancement of the uvea and sclera, ± involvement of Tenon's capsule, ± retinal or choroidal detachment.	Uncommon granulomatous inflammatory disorder involving the sclera behind the ora serrata (anterior-most portion of choroid within the eye, where the sensory retina ends), and juxtascleral soft tissue. Can be associated with rheumatoid arthritis, granulomatosis with polyangiitis, or systemic lupus erythematosus, or it may be idiopathic. More common in women than in men. Usually unilateral (70%), can progress to involve the anterior sclera. Clinical findings include eye pain, decreased visual acuity, and referred facial pain, ± exudative retinal or choroidal detachment.

(continued on page 226)

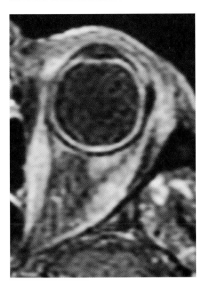

Fig. 2.49 An 89-year-old man with noninfectious uveitis in the left eye seen as diffuse gadolinium contrast enhancement of the slightly thickened uveal tract on axial fat-suppressed T1-weighted imaging.

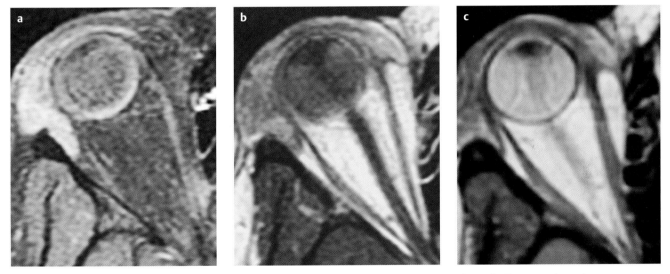

Fig. 2.50 Vogt-Koyanagi-Harada syndrome (chronic granulomatous uveitis with exudative choroid effusion and nonrhegmatogenous retinal detachment of unknown etiology). **(a)** Axial fat-suppressed T1-weighted imaging shows prominent thickening of the uvea, with gadolinium contrast enhancement and blurring of the optic nerve junction. Also seen is retinal detachment with subretinal exudative effusion, which has **(b)** slightly high signal on axial T1-weighted imaging and **(c)** high signal on axial T2-weighted imaging.

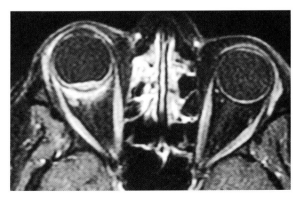

Fig. 2.51 A 36-year-old woman with posterior scleritis, which is seen as thickening and gadolinium contrast enhancement of the dorsal choroidal portion of the uvea and adjacent sclera, as well as Tenon's capsule and bordering posterior episcleral soft tissue.

Table 2.2 *(cont.)*   Acquired lesions involving the eye

Lesion	Imaging Findings	Comments
Traumatic Abnormalities		
Globe trauma (**Fig. 2.52** and **Fig. 2.53**)	*CT and MRI:* Altered shape and decreased size of the eye, scleral discontinuity, intraocular hemorrhage in vitreous or anterior chamber (traumatic hyphema), ± subluxed or displaced lens, ± intraocular air, ± intraocular foreign body, ± retinal or choroid detachment.	Penetrating trauma results in ocular rupture at the site of impact. Blunt trauma often results in rupture of the eye at the weakest portions of the sclera located posterior to the insertions of the extraocular muscles. Globe rupture is an ophthalmologic emergency, with potential for eventual complications like vision loss, sympathetic ophthalmia, endophthalmitis, and/or meningitis. Intraocular foreign bodies can be classified as inorganic (metal alloys, glass, plastic) or organic (wood, plant material, soil), and they vary in attenuation on CT.
Retinal detachment (**Fig. 2.54** and **Fig. 2.55**)	Fluid and/or blood occurs beneath the elevated, thin, linear leaves of the sensory retina, which are still attached to the ora serrata anteriorly and the optic disc posteriorly in a *V-shaped pattern,* with the apex at the optic disc. The subretinal fluid can have low, intermediate, or high attenuation on CT, and variable signal on MRI, depending on the protein or blood content.	Retinal detachment can result from trauma, neoplasms, inflammation, or infection. The retina has firm attachments to the ora serrata, blood vessels and optic disc; and loose attachments elsewhere. Fluid or blood occurs in the potential space beneath the retina and choroid. Rhegmatogenous retinal detachments occur from vitreous fluid entering the subretinal space via a retinal tear. Tractional retinal detachments occur due to separation of the sensory retina from the retinal pigment epithelium caused by neovascularization or fibrovascular tissue resulting from trauma or inflammation.
Choroidal detachment (**Fig. 2.56**)	*CT:* Fluid and/or blood occurs beneath the leaves of the choroid, which are still attached to the ora serrata anteriorly and the vortex veins posteriorly in biconvex or lentiform configuration. The detached choroid leaves do not extend to the optic nerve heads, and have a U shape. Serous subchoroidal fluid has low attenuation, whereas hemorrhagic collections have high attenuation. *MRI:* Serous subchoroidal fluid has low signal on T1-weighted imaging and high signal on T2-weighted imaging, whereas hemorrhagic fluid can have variable signal, depending on the protein and iron content.	The choroid (middle layer of the eye) extends from the optic nerve head posteriorly to the ora serrata anteriorly. The choroid has firm attachments to the adjacent sclera at the ora serrata/ciliary body anteriorly and posteriorly where the vortex veins exit the eye. Trauma can result in ocular hypotony (decreased ocular pressure), with serous fluid, exudates, and/or hemorrhage accumulating in the potential space between the choroid and sclera.

(continued on page 228)

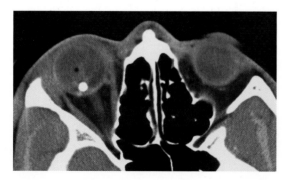

Fig. 2.52 Axial CT shows traumatic injury of the right globe secondary to penetration from a small metallic projectile with high attenuation (bb), as well as associated intraocular air and hemorrhage.

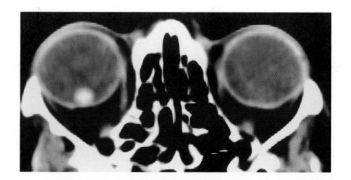

Fig. 2.53 Axial CT shows a dislocated lens with high attenuation in the dependent portion of the right eye.

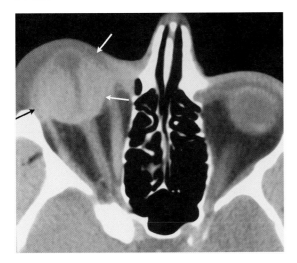

Fig. 2.54 Axial CT shows retinal detachment in the right eye with high-attenuation blood (*arrows*) beneath the elevated, thin, linear leaves of the sensory retina, which are still attached to the optic disc posteriorly.

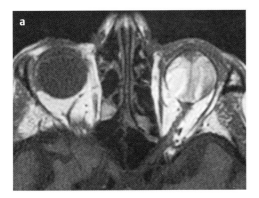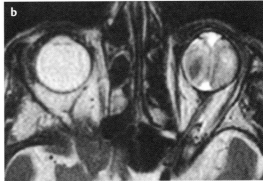

Fig. 2.55 **(a)** Axial T1-weighted imaging shows retinal detachment in the left eye with subretinal blood, which has mostly high signal on axial T1-weighted imaging and **(b)** mixed low and slightly high signal on axial T2-weighted imaging.

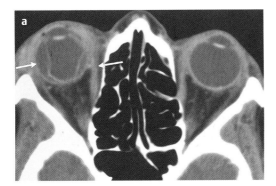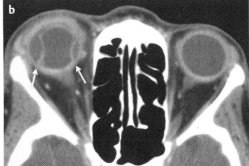

Fig. 2.56 Choroidal detachment in the right eye. **(a,b)** Axial CT shows serous subchoroidal fluid with low-attenuation fluid beneath the leaves of the choroid, which are still attached to the ora serrata anteriorly and the vortex veins posteriorly in a biconvex configuration (*arrows*). The detached choroid leaves do not extend to the optic nerve heads, and have a U shape.

Table 2.2 *(cont.)* Acquired lesions involving the eye

Lesion	Imaging Findings	Comments
Degeneration		
Phthisis bulbi (**Fig. 2.57** and **Fig. 2.58**)	*CT and MRI:* Shrunken, deformed eye, ± calcifications, with variable CT attenuation and MRI signal of internal contents.	Nonfunctional eye secondary to end-stage degenerative changes that can result from inflammation, infection, or trauma.
Cataract (**Fig. 2.59**)	*CT:* Increased attenuation of the native lens.	Opacification and clouding of the native lens from accumulation of intracellular crystalline proteins. Cataracts most often result from aging (senile type). Can also result from radiation exposure or trauma, or they may be congenital. Treatment is surgical removal and replacement with a lens implant.

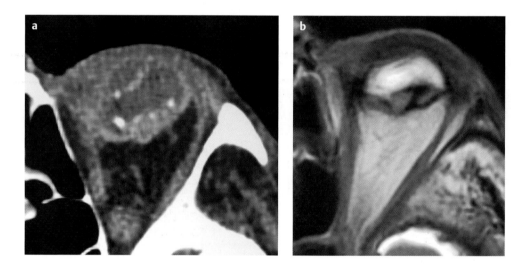

Fig. 2.57 A 80-year-old woman with phthisis bulbi in the left eye. **(a)** Axial CT shows a shrunken, deformed left eye with irregular zones of fluid and soft tissue attenuation as well as dystrophic calcifications. **(b)** The deformed eye has mixed low, intermediate, and high signal on axial T2-weighted imaging.

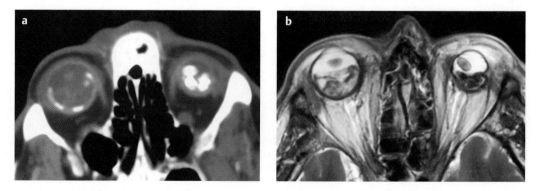

Fig. 2.58 A 50-year-old man with bilateral phthisis bulbi. **(a)** On axial CT, the shrunken deformed eyes contain dystrophic calcifications, and **(b)** they have mixed low, intermediate, and high signal on axial T2-weighted imaging.

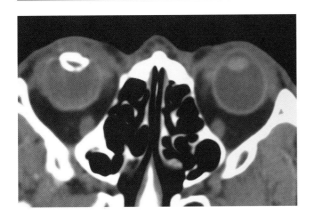

Fig. 2.59 An 80-year-old man with a high-attenuation cataract in the right eye on axial CT.

Table 2.3 Extraocular lesions involving the orbit

- Malignant Neoplasms
  - Metastases
  - Myeloma
  - Lymphoma
  - Leukemia
  - Squamous cell carcinoma
  - Esthesioneuroblastoma
  - Sinonasal undifferentiated carcinoma (SNUC)
  - Rhabdomyosarcoma
  - Osteosarcoma
  - Ewing's sarcoma
  - Chondrosarcoma
  - Lacrimal gland adenoid cystic carcinoma
  - Lacrimal duct malignant tumors
- Benign Neoplasms
  - Optic nerve sheath meningioma
  - Intraosseous meningioma
  - Optic glioma
  - Hemangioblastoma of the optic nerve (von Hippel-Lindau disease)
  - Schwannoma
  - Neurofibroma
  - Lacrimal gland pleomorphic adenoma
- Tumorlike Osseous Lesions
  - Osteoma
  - Fibrous dysplasia
  - Paget disease
  - Arachnoid cyst
  - Epidermoid
  - Dermoid
- Infection
  - Preseptal orbital cellulitis
  - Postseptal orbital cellulitis
  - Mucocele/pyocele
- Inflammation
  - Optic neuritis
  - Idiopathic orbital inflammation (inflammatory pseudotumor)
  - Tolosa-Hunt syndrome
  - IgG4-related systemic disease
  - Thyroid orbitopathy (Graves' disease)
  - Sarcoidosis
  - Langerhans' cell histiocytosis
  - Erdheim-Chester disease
  - Sjögren's syndrome
  - Granulomatosis with polyangiitis
- Vascular Lesions
  - Cavernous hemangioma
  - Orbital infantile hemangioma
  - Orbital venolymphatic malformation
  - Orbital varix
  - Dural arteriovenous malformations (AVMs)
  - Carotid cavernous fistula
- Traumatic Abnormalities
  - Orbital fracture
  - Intraorbital foreign bodies
  - Retinal detachment
  - Choroidal detachment
- Degeneration
  - Phthisis bulbi
  - Pseudotumor cerebri (idiopathic intracranial hypertension)

Table 2.3 Extraocular lesions involving the orbit

Lesion	Imaging Findings	Comments
Malignant Neoplasms		
Metastases (**Fig. 2.60, Fig. 2.61,** and **Fig. 2.62**)	*MRI:* Lesions often have intermediate signal on T1-weighted imaging, low-intermediate, or slightly high signal on T2-weighted imaging, and gadolinium contrast enhancement. MRI can show scleral infiltration/invasion. *CT:* Tumors have intermediate attenuation and moderate contrast enhancement, ± calcifications, ± bone destruction.	Metastatic disease usually occurs in adults. Most common malignancies metastasizing to the orbit, orbital bones, and eye are neoplasms of the breast, lung, and kidneys. In children, neuroblastoma metastases to bone are the most common involving the orbit. Patients can present with diplopia, vision loss, and/or pain. Most ocular metastases result from hematogenous spread to the uvea.
Myeloma (**Fig. 2.63**)	Multiple myeloma or single plasmacytoma are well-circumscribed or poorly defined lesions involving the skull, dura, and/or orbital soft tissue. *CT:* Lesions have low-intermediate attenuation, usually + contrast enhancement, + bone destruction. *MRI:* Well-circumscribed or poorly defined lesions involving the skull and dura, with low-intermediate signal on T1-weighted imaging and intermediate-high signal on T2-weighted imaging. Myeloma usually shows gadolinium contrast enhancement, + bone destruction.	Multiple myeloma is composed of proliferating antibody-secreting plasma cells derived from single clones. Multiple myeloma is primarily located in bone marrow. A solitary myeloma or plasmacytoma is an infrequent variant in which a neoplastic mass of plasma cells occurs at a single site of bone or soft tissues. In the United States, 14,600 new cases occur each year. Multiple myeloma is the most common primary neoplasm of bone in adults. Median age at presentation = 60 years. Most patients are more than 40 years old. Tumors occur in the vertebrae > ribs > femur > iliac bone > humerus > craniofacial bones > sacrum > clavicle > sternum > pubic bone > tibia.

(continued on page 232)

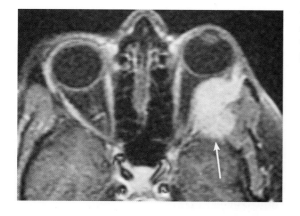

Fig. 2.60 A 44-year-old woman with breast carcinoma and a gadolinium-enhancing destructive metastatic lesion in the lateral wall of the left orbit (*arrow*), with intraorbital and intracranial tumor extension on axial fat-suppressed T1-weighted imaging.

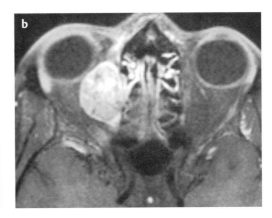

Fig. 2.61 A 44-year-old man with lung carcinoma and a metastatic lesion in the medial portion of the right orbit that has **(a)** heterogeneous intermediate signal on axial T2-weighted imaging (*arrow*) and **(b)** gadolinium contrast enhancement on axial fat-suppressed T1-weighted imaging.

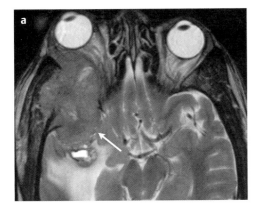
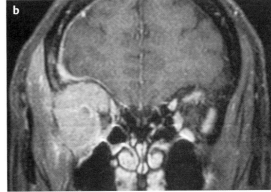

Fig. 2.62 A 7-year-old male with neuroblastoma and a destructive osseous metastasis involving the skull with intraorbital and intracranial tumor extension. The metastasis has **(a)** heterogeneous intermediate signal on axial T2-weighted imaging (*arrow*) and **(b)** gadolinium contrast enhancement on coronal fat-suppressed T1-weighted imaging.

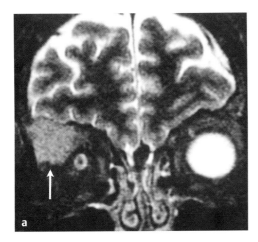
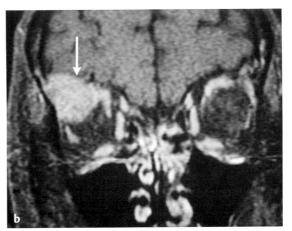

Fig. 2.63 **(a)** Myeloma in the upper portion of the right orbit has slightly high signal on coronal fat-suppressed T2-weighted imaging (*arrow*) and **(b)** shows gadolinium contrast enhancement on coronal fat-suppressed T1-weighted imaging (*arrow*).

Table 2.3 *(cont.)* Extraocular lesions involving the orbit

Lesion	Imaging Findings	Comments
Lymphoma (**Fig. 2.64** and **Fig. 2.65**)	Single or multiple well-circumscribed or poorly defined lesions involving the skull, dura, orbital soft tissues, and/or lacrimal glands. *CT:* Lesions have low-intermediate attenuation and may show contrast enhancement, ± bone destruction. *MRI:* Lesions have low-intermediate signal on T1-weighted imaging and intermediate to high signal on T2-weighted imaging, + gadolinium contrast enhancement, ± associated bony erosion/destruction and intracranial extension with meningeal involvement.	Lymphoma represents a group of lymphoid tumors whose neoplastic cells typically arise within lymphoid tissue (lymph nodes and reticuloendothelial organs). Lymphoma involving the orbit can arise from intraosseous lesions. Almost all primary lymphomas of bone are B-cell non-Hodgkin lymphomas. The MALT (mucosa-associated lymphoid tissue) subtype of NHL is the most common primary orbital lymphoma. Lymphoma can also occur exclusively in the orbital soft tissues, often involving the lacrimal gland. Lacrimal gland lymphoma occurs in older adults (mean age = 62–69 years). May be associated with Sjögren's syndrome.
Leukemia (**Fig. 2.66** and **Fig. 2.67**)	*MRI:* *Soft tissue:* Collections of myelogenous leukemic cells in soft tissues (chloromas/granulocytic sarcomas) have variable MRI findings. Chloromas are more common in acute myelogenous leukemia than in chronic myelogenous leukemia. Lesions may be poorly defined or well circumscribed. Lesions often have low-intermediate signal on T1-weighted imaging (T1WI) and intermediate to high signal on T2-weighted imaging (T2WI) and fat-suppressed T2WI, as well as moderate to marked gadolinium (Gd) contrast enhancement. Chloromas may occur primarily in soft tissue or extend from intraosseous lesions. *Osseous involvement:* Focal or diffuse abnormal signal in the marrow, with low-intermediate signal on T1WI and intermediate-high signal on T2WI, ± Gd contrast enhancement, ± bone destruction. *CT:* ± zones of bone destruction.	Leukemias are neoplastic proliferations of hematopoietic cells. Myeloid sarcomas (also referred to as chloromas, granulocytic sarcomas) are focal tumors composed of myeloblasts and neoplastic granulocyte precursor cells, and they occur in 2% of patients with acute myelogenous leukemia. These lesions can involve the skull marrow, leptomeninges, and/or brain. Intracranial lesions can be solitary or multiple.

(continued on page 234)

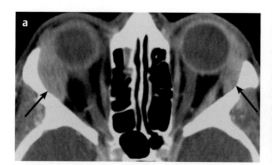
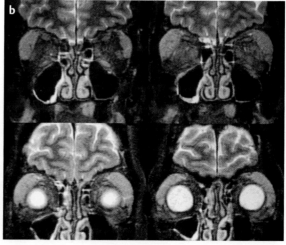

Fig. 2.64 A 65-year-old man with non-Hodgkin lymphoma who has neoplastic infiltration and enlargement of the lacrimal glands, which have **(a)** intermediate attenuation on axial CT (*arrows*) and **(b)** slightly high signal on coronal STIR.

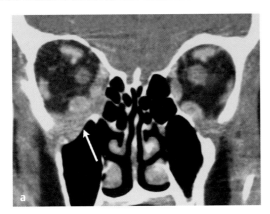
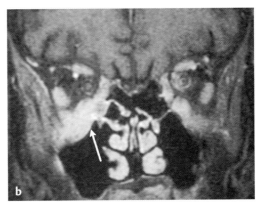

Fig. 2.65 **(a)** An 82-year-old woman with non-Hodgkin lymphoma who has an infiltrative neoplastic lesion at the inferior potion of the right orbit that has intermediate attenuation on coronal CT (*arrow*). **(b)** The tumor shows gadolinium contrast enhancement on coronal fat-suppressed T1-weighted imaging (*arrow*). The tumor involves the inferior and medial rectus muscles and extends into the upper right maxillary sinus through destroyed bone.

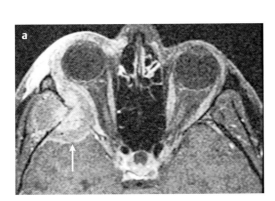
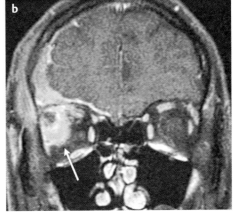

Fig. 2.66 **(a)** Axial and **(b)** coronal fat-suppressed T1-weighted imaging shows gadolinium-enhancing acute lymphoblastic leukemia causing destruction of the right sphenoid bone and with intraorbital, extracranial, and intracranial tumor extension with dural involvement (*arrows*).

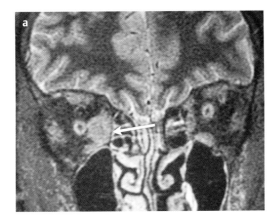
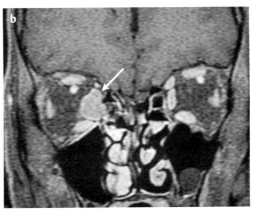

Fig. 2.67 **(a)** A 44-year-old man with a lesion from acute myelogenous leukemia in the medial right orbit that has slightly high signal on coronal STIR (*arrow*). **(b)** The lesion shows gadolinium contrast enhancement on coronal fat-suppressed T1-weighted imaging (*arrow*).

Table 2.3 *(cont.)* Extraocular lesions involving the orbit

Lesion	Imaging Findings	Comments
Squamous cell carcinoma (See **Fig. 1.44**)	*MRI:* Destructive lesions in the nasal cavity, paranasal sinuses, and nasopharynx, ± intracranial and/or introrbital extension via bone destruction or perineural spread. Lesions have intermediate signal on T1-weighted imaging, intermediate to slightly high signal on T2-weighted imaging, and mild gadolinium contrast enhancement, as well as, in large lesions, ± necrosis and/or hemorrhage. *CT:* Tumors have intermediate attenuation and mild contrast enhancement. Large lesions ± necrosis and/or hemorrhage.	Malignant epithelial tumors originating from the mucosal epithelium of the paranasal sinuses (maxillary sinus, 60%; ethmoid sinus, 14%; sphenoid and frontal sinuses,1%) and nasal cavity (25%). There are both keratinizing and nonkeratinizing types. Squamous cell carcinoma accounts for 3% of malignant tumors of the head and neck. Occurs in adults, usually > 55 years old, and in males more than in females. Associated with occupational or other exposure to tobacco smoke, nickel, chlorophenols, chromium, mustard gas, radium, and material in the manufacture of wood products.
Esthesioneuroblastoma (**Fig. 2.68**; see **Fig. 1.45**)	*MRI:* Locally destructive lesions with low-intermediate signal on T1-weighted imaging and intermediate-high signal on T2-weighted imaging, + prominent gadolinium contrast enhancement. Found in superior nasal cavity and ethmoid air cells, with occasional extension into the other paranasal sinuses, orbits, anterior cranial fossa, and cavernous sinuses. *CT:* Tumors have intermediate attenuation and variable mild, moderate, or prominent contrast enhancement. *PET/CT:* FDG is useful for staging of disease and detection of metastases.	Also referred to as olfactory neuroblastoma, these malignant neoplasms of neuroectodermal origin arise from olfactory epithelium in the upper nasal cavity and cribriform region. Tumors consist of immature neuroblasts with variable nuclear pleomorphism, mitoses, and necrosis. Tumor cells occur in a neurofibrillary intercellular matrix. Bimodal occurrence in adolescents (11–20 years old) and adults (50–60 years old). Occurs in males more frequently than in females.
Sinonasal undifferentiated carcinoma (SNUC) (See **Fig. 1.46**)	*MRI:* Locally destructive lesions usually larger than 4 cm, with low-intermediate signal on T1-weighted imaging and intermediate-high signal on T2-weighted imaging, + prominent gadolinium contrast enhancement. Found in superior nasal cavity and ethmoid air cells, with occasional extension into the other paranasal sinuses, orbits, anterior cranial fossa, and cavernous sinuses. *CT:* Tumors have intermediate attenuation and variable mild, moderate, or prominent contrast enhancement.	Malignant tumor composed of pleomorphic neoplastic cells with medium to large nuclei, prominent single nucleoli, and small amounts of eosinophilic cytoplasm. Mitotic activity is typically high and necrosis is common. Immunoreactive to CK7, CK8, CK19, ± p53, epithelial membrane antigen, and neuron-specific enolase. Poor prognosis, with 5-year survival less than 20%.
Rhabdomyosarcoma (**Fig. 2.69** and **Fig. 2.70**)	*MRI:* Tumors can have circumscribed and/or poorly defined margins and typically have low-intermediate signal on T1-weighted imaging and heterogeneous signal (various combinations of intermediate, slightly high, and/or high signal) on T2-weighted imaging (T2WI) and fat-suppressed T2WI. Tumors show variable degrees of gadolinium contrast enhancement, ± bone destruction and invasion. *CT:* Soft tissue lesions that usually can have circumscribed or irregular margins. Calcifications are uncommon. Tumors can have mixed CT attenuation with solid zones of soft tissue attenuation, cystic-appearing and/or necrotic zones, and occasional foci of hemorrhage, ± bone invasion and destruction.	Malignant mesenchymal tumors with rhabdomyoblastic differentiation that occur primarily in soft tissue and only very rarely in bone. There are three subgroups of rhabdomyosarcoma: embryonal (50 to 70%), alveolar (18 to 45%), and pleomorphic (5 to 10%). Embryonal and alveolar rhabdomyosarcomas occur primarily in children less than 10 years old, and pleomorphic rhabdomyosarcomas occur mostly in adults (median age in the sixth decade). Alveolar and pleomorphic rhabdomyosarcomas occur frequently in the extremities. Embryonal rhabdomyosarcomas occur mostly in the head and neck.

(continued on page 236)

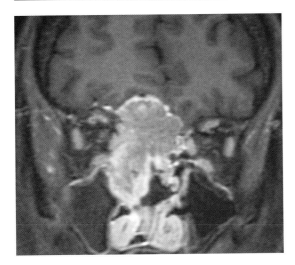

Fig. 2.68 A 30-year-old woman with a gadolinium-enhancing esthesioneuroblastoma in the nasal cavity, right maxillary and ethmoid sinuses on coronal fat-suppressed T1-weighted imaging that extends into the medial portion of the right orbit and intracranially through sites of bone destruction.

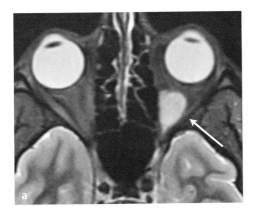

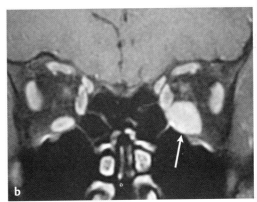

Fig. 2.69 **(a)** A 22-year-old man with a rhabdomyosarcoma involving the inferior rectus muscle in the left orbit that has high signal on axial fat-suppressed T2-weighted imaging (*arrow*). **(b)** The tumor shows gadolinium contrast enhancement on coronal fat-suppressed T1-weighted imaging (*arrow*).

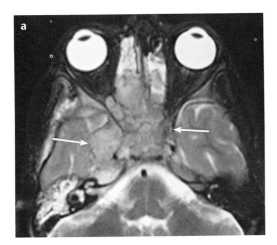

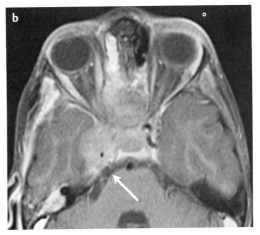

Fig. 2.70 **(a)** A 5-year-old male with rhabdomyosarcoma in the sphenoid and ethmoid sinuses with extension into the right orbit, right cavernous sinus, and medial portion of the right middle cranial fossa. The tumor has heterogeneous intermediate signal on axial fat-suppressed T2-weighted imaging (*arrows*). **(b)** The tumor shows gadolinium contrast enhancement on axial fat-suppressed T1-weighted imaging (*arrow*).

Table 2.3 *(cont.)* Extraocular lesions involving the orbit

Lesion	Imaging Findings	Comments
Osteosarcoma (**Fig. 2.71**)	Destructive lesions involving the skull. *CT:* Tumors have low-intermediate attenuation, usually + matrix mineralization/ossification, and often show contrast enhancement (usually heterogeneous). *MRI:* Tumors often have poorly defined margins and commonly extend from the marrow through destroyed bone cortex into adjacent soft tissues. Tumors usually have low-intermediate signal on T1-weighted imaging. Zones of low signal often correspond to areas of calcification/mineralization and/or necrosis. Zones of necrosis typically have high signal on T2-weighted imaging (T2WI), whereas mineralized zones usually have low signal on T2WI. Tumors can have variable signal on T2WI and fat-suppressed T2WI, depending upon the relative amounts of calcified/mineralized osteoid, chondroid, fibroid, hemorrhagic, and necrotic components. Tumors may have low, low-intermediate, or intermediate to high signal on T2WI and fat-suppressed T2WI. After gadolinium contrast administration, osteosarcomas typically show prominent enhancement in nonmineralized/calcified portions of the tumors.	Osteosarcomas are malignant tumors composed of proliferating neoplastic spindle cells, which produce osteoid and/or immature tumoral bone. They occur in children as primary tumors, and in adults they are associated with Paget disease, irradiated bone, chronic osteomyelitis, osteoblastoma, giant cell tumor, and fibrous dysplasia.
Ewing's sarcoma (**Fig. 2.72**)	*MRI:* Destructive lesions involving the skull, with low-intermediate signal on T1-weighted imaging and mixed low, intermediate, and high signal on T2-weighted imaging, + gadolinium contrast enhancement (usually heterogeneous). *CT:* Destructive lesions involving the skull, with low-intermediate attenuation. They can show contrast enhancement (usually heterogeneous).	Malignant primitive tumor of bone composed of undifferentiated small cells with round nuclei. Ewing's sarcoma accounts for 6 to 11% of primary malignant bone tumors, and 5 to 7% of primary bone tumors. Usually occurs between the ages of 5 and 30, and in males more than in females. Ewing's sarcomas commonly have translocations involving chromosomes 11 and 22: t(11;22) (q24:q12) which results in fusion of the FL1-1 gene at 11q24 to the EWS gene at 22q12. Lesions are locally invasive, with high metastatic potential. Rarely, lesions involve the skull base and are locally invasive, with high metastatic potential.
Chondrosarcoma (**Fig. 2.73**)	Lobulated lesions with bone destruction at synchondroses. *CT:* Lesions have low-intermediate attenuation associated with localized bone destruction, ± chondroid matrix calcifications, + contrast enhancement. *MRI:* Lesions have low-intermediate signal on T1-weighted imaging, high signal on T2-weighted imaging (T2WI), ± matrix mineralization with low signal on T2WI, + gadolinium contrast enhancement (usually heterogeneous). Chondrosarcoma is locally invasive and is associated with bony erosion/destruction and encasement of vessels and nerves. Usually occurs off midline.	Chondrosarcomas are malignant tumors containing cartilage formed within sarcomatous stroma. Chondrosarcomas can contain areas of calcification/mineralization, myxoid material, and/or ossification. Chondrosarcomas rarely arise within synovium. Chondrosarcomas represent from 12 to 21% of malignant bone lesions, 21 to 26% of primary sarcomas of bone, 9 to 14% of all bone tumors, 6% of skull base tumors, and 0.15% of all intracranial tumors.

(continued on page 238)

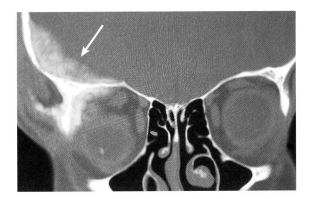

Fig. 2.71 A 10-year-old female with an osteosarcoma involving the right frontal bone, with extraosseous tumor containing malignant mineralized osseous matrix in the upper right orbit and inferior right anterior cranial fossa on coronal CT (*arrow*).

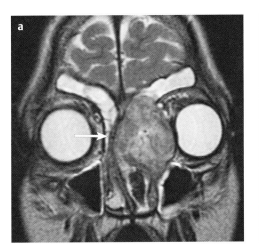
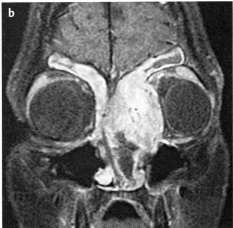

Fig. 2.72 (a) A 12-year-old female with a Ewing's sarcoma in the upper left nasal cavity, left ethmoid, and frontal sinuses associated with bone destruction and extension into the medial portion of the left orbit. The tumor has mixed intermediate and slightly high signal on coronal T2-weighted imaging (*arrow*). (b) The tumor shows gadolinium contrast enhancement on coronal fat-suppressed T1-weighted imaging.

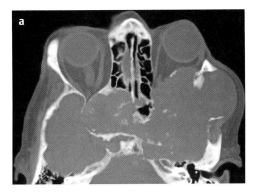
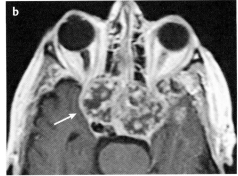

Fig. 2.73 (a) An 81-year-old woman with a large chondrosarcoma involving both middle cranial fossae, the suprasellar cistern, the sphenoid and ethmoid sinuses, and the left orbit. The tumor is associated with bone destruction and has mixed intermediate and low attenuation as well as chondroid calicifications on axial CT. (b) The tumor (*arrow*) has peripheral lobulated and irregular curvilinear gadolinium contrast enhancement on axial T1-weighted imaging.

Table 2.3 *(cont.)* Extraocular lesions involving the orbit

Lesion	Imaging Findings	Comments
Lacrimal gland adenoid cystic carcinoma (**Fig. 2.74**)	*MRI:* Lesions often have ill-defined margins, intermediate signal on T1-weighted imaging, intermediate to slightly high signal on T2-weighted imaging, and, usually, gadolinium contrast enhancement. *CT:* Lesions have mostly intermediate attenuation and usually show contrast enhancement, ± adjacent bone erosion or destruction.	Most common malignant tumor of the lacrimal gland and accounts for up to 5% of primary orbital tumors. Tumors contain neoplastic epithelial cells arranged in nests or cords. Tumors have an infiltrative growth pattern, ± perineural spread. Peak incidence is in the fourth decade. Treatment includes surgery and radiation. Ten-year survival is only 20%.
Lacrimal duct malignant tumors (**Fig. 2.75**)	*MRI:* Lesions often have intermediate signal on T1-weighted imaging, intermediate to slightly high signal on T2-weighted imaging, and, usually, gadolinium contrast enhancement. *CT:* Lesions have mostly intermediate attenuation and usually show contrast enhancement, ± adjacent bone erosion or destruction.	Malignant epithelial tumors of the lacrimal drainage system include squamous cell carcinoma (most common type), adenocarcinoma, mucoepidermoid carcinoma, undifferentiated carcinoma, adenoid cystic carcinoma, and eccrine adenocarcinoma.
Benign Neoplasms		
Optic nerve sheath meningioma (**Fig. 2.76, Fig. 2.77** and **Fig. 2.78**)	Dura-based lesions involving the optic nerve sheath that can appear as a nodular mass extending off the optic nerve sheath, or as circumferential lesions surrounding the optic nerves in a "tram-track" configuration. Can also occur as extensions of intracranial meningiomas via the optic canal along the dural sheath. *MRI:* Tumors often have intermediate signal on T1-weighted imaging, intermediate to slightly high signal on T2-weighted imaging, and, typically, gadolinium contrast enhancement. *CT:* Tumors have intermediate attenuation and show contrast enhancement.	Benign slow-growing tumors involving the dura of the optic nerve sheath and composed of neoplastic meningothelial (arachnoidal or arachnoid cap) cells. Intracranial meningiomas can extend into the orbits via the optic canal or arise as primary lesions along the optic nerve sheath. Usually they are solitary and sporadic, but they can also occur as multiple lesions in patients with neurofibromatosis type 2. Most are benign, although ~ 5% have atypical histologic features. Anaplastic meningiomas are rare and account for less than 3% of meningiomas.
Intraosseous meningioma (**Fig. 2.79**)	*CT:* Intraosseous meningiomas are often associated with enlarged hyperostotic bone changes with high attenuation, and they often show peripheral contrast enhancement. *MRI:* Intraosseous meningiomas have low-intermediate signal on T1-weighted imaging, intermediate signal on T2-weighted imaging, and gadolinium contrast enhancement in the adjacent paraosseous soft tissue.	Meningiomas can invade bone, causing hyperostosis, or occasionally occur as lesions predominantly within bone.

(continued on page 241)

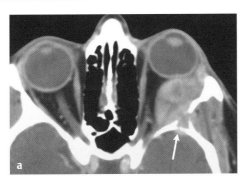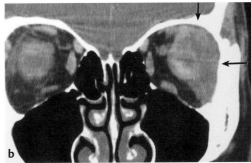

Fig. 2.74 A 51-year-old woman with a large lesion in the superolateral portion of the left orbit from lacrimal gland adenocarcinoma that involves the left superior and lateral rectus muscles and intraconal fat and is associated with bone destruction. The tumor shows irregular contrast enhancement on **(a)** axial and **(b)** coronal CT (*arrows*).

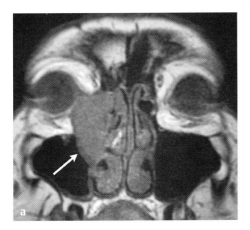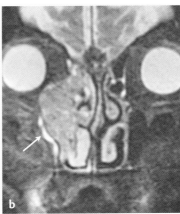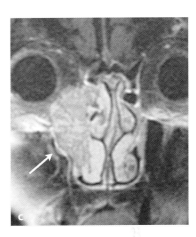

Fig. 2.75 An 87-year-old woman with a squamous cell carcinoma involving the right lacrimal duct that has destroyed the adjacent bone and has invaded the right orbit and right maxillary sinus. **(a)** The tumor has intermediate signal on coronal T1-weighted imaging (*arrow*), **(b)** slightly high to high signal on coronal fat-suppressed T2-weighted imaging (*arrow*), and **(c)** gadolinium contrast enhancement on coronal fat-suppressed T1-weighted imaging (*arrow*).

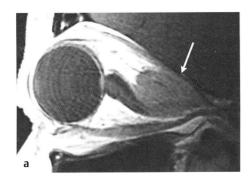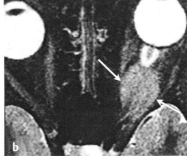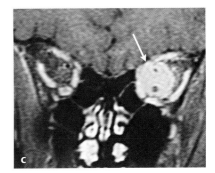

Fig. 2.76 **(a)** A 35-year-old woman with an optic nerve sheath meningioma in the left orbit that has intermediate signal on sagittal T1-weighted imaging (*arrow*), **(b)** slightly high signal on axial STIR (*arrow*), and **(c)** circumferential gadolinium contrast enhancement surrounding the optic nerve on coronal fat-suppressed T1-weighted imaging (*arrow*).

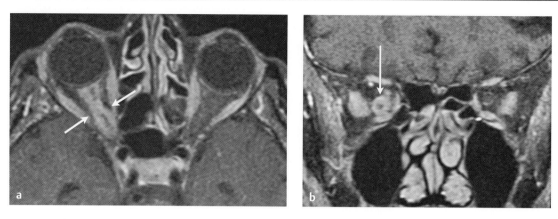

Fig. 2.77 A 77-year-old woman with a meningioma involving the right optic nerve sheath that is seen as circumferential gadolinium contrast enhancement surrounding the optic nerve in a "tram track" pattern on **(a)** axial (*arrows*) and **(b)** coronal fat-suppressed T1-weighted imaging (*arrow*).

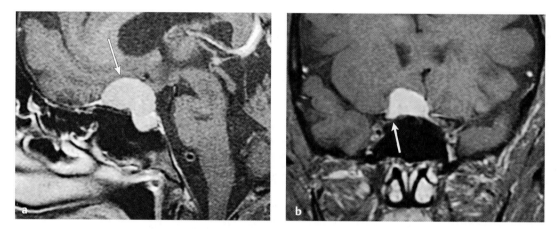

Fig. 2.78 A 48-year-old woman with a gadolinium-enhancing meningioma along the planum sphenoidale on **(a)** sagittal and **(b)** coronal fat-suppressed T1-weighted imaging that extends into the right optic canal and into the suprasellar cistern (*arrow*).

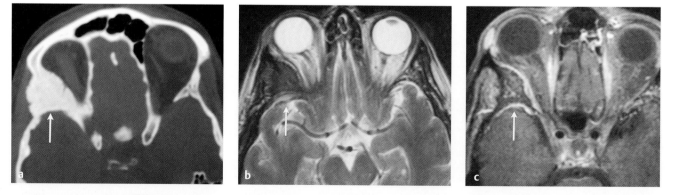

Fig. 2.79 A 52-year-old woman with an intraosseous meningioma. **(a)** Axial CT shows thickening and hyperostosis at the posterolateral wall of the right orbit (*arrow*). **(b)** The intraosseous meningioma has mostly low signal on axial T2-weighted imaging, as well as thin zones of slightly high signal at sites of extraosseous extension (*arrow*). **(c)** The small zones of extraosseous tumor at the lateral orbit and anterior middle cranial fossa show gadolinium contrast enhancement on axial fat-suppressed T1-weighted imaging (*arrow*).

Table 2.3 *(cont.)* Extraocular lesions involving the orbit

Lesion	Imaging Findings	Comments
Optic glioma **(Fig. 2.80)**	*MRI:* Fusiform and/or nodular enlargement of optic chiasm and/or optic nerves. Usually has low-intermediate signal on T1-weighted imaging, intermediate-high signal on T2-weighted imaging, and variable gadolinium contrast enhancement, ± cystic components with large lesions. *CT:* Usually intermediate attenuation, variable or no contrast enhancement, ± cystic components with large lesions.	Most common primary tumor of the optic nerve. In children, usually associated with neurofibromatosis type 1 (~ 10% of patients with NF1), Most tumors are slow-growing grade I astrocytomas (often pilocytic type) and contain spindle-shaped astrocytes with hairlike (pilocytic) structures and linear eosinophilic (Rosenthal) fibers. High signal abnormality on T2-weighted imaging can extend along optic radiations from neoplastic extension.

(continued on page 242)

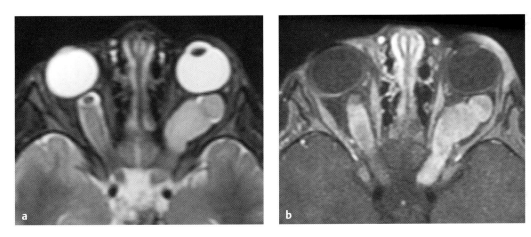

Fig. 2.80 A 3-year-old female with neurofibromatosis type 1. **(a)** Axial fat-suppressed T2-weighted imaging shows bilateral optic nerve gliomas, which have slightly high signal. **(b)** The gliomas show gadolinium contrast enhancement on axial fat-suppressed T1-weighted imaging.

Table 2.3 *(cont.)* Extraocular lesions involving the orbit

Lesion	Imaging Findings	Comments
Hemangioblastoma of the optic nerve (von Hippel-Lindau disease) (**Fig. 2.81**)	Circumscribed tumors usually located in the cerebellum, brainstem, and, rarely, the optic nerve. *MRI:* Gadolinium-enhancing lesion involving the optic nerve with fusiform enlargement. Lesions have intermediate signal on T1-weighted imaging, intermediate-high signal on T2-weighted imaging (T2WI), and high signal on fat-suppressed T2WI and STIR. *CT:* Fusiform enlargement of the optic nerve.	Slow-growing, vascular tumors (WHO grade I) that involve the cerebellum, brainstem, spinal cord, and rarely the optic nerve. Tumors consist of numerous thin-walled vessels as well as large, lipid-containing vacuolated stromal cells that have variably sized hyperchromatic nuclei. Mitotic figures are rare. Stromal cells are immunoreactive to VEGF, vimentin, CXCR4, aquaporin 1, carbonic anhydrase, S-100, CD56, neuron-specific enolase, and D2–40. Vessels typically react to a reticulin stain. Sporadic mutations of the *VHL* gene or autosomal dominant germline mutation of the *VHL* gene on chromosome 3p25–26 causes von Hippel-Lindau (VHL) disease. In VHL disease, multiple CNS hemangioblastomas occur, as well as clear-cell renal carcinoma, pheochromocytoma, endolymphatic sac tumor, neuroendocrine tumor, adenoma of the pancreas, and epididymal cystadenoma. VHL disease occurs in adolescents and young and middle-aged adults.
Schwannoma (**Fig. 2.82**)	*MRI:* Circumscribed spheroid, ovoid, or fusiform lesions, with low-intermediate signal on T1-weighted imaging, high signal on T2-weighted imaging (T2WI) and fat-suppressed T2WI, and usually prominent gadolinium (Gd) contrast enhancement. High signal on T2WI and Gd contrast enhancement can be heterogeneous in large lesions due to cystic degeneration and/or hemorrhage. Schwannomas involving the orbit include those from CN III, CN IV, CN V (trigeminal nerve cistern/Meckel's cave), and CN VI (Dorello canal). *CT:* Circumscribed spheroid, ovoid, or fusiform lesions with intermediate attenuation, + contrast enhancement. Large lesions can have cystic degeneration and/or hemorrhage, ± erosion of adjacent bone.	Schwannomas are benign encapsulated tumors that contain differentiated neoplastic Schwann cells. Multiple schwannomas are often associated with neurofibromatosis type 2 (NF2), which is an autosomal dominant disease involving a gene on chromosome 22q12. In addition to schwannomas, patients with NF2 can also have multiple meningiomas and ependymomas. Schwannomas represent 8% of primary intracranial tumors and 29% of primary spinal tumors. The incidence of NF2 is 1/ 37,000 to 1/50,000 newborns. Age at presentation = 22 to 72 years (mean age = 46 years). Peak incidence is in the fourth to sixth decades. With NF2, many patients present in the third decade with bilateral vestibular schwannomas.
Neurofibroma (**Fig. 2.83**)	*MRI:* *Solitary neurofibromas* are circumscribed spheroid, ovoid, or lobulated extra-axial lesions, with low-intermediate signal on T1-weighted imaging (T1WI) and intermediate-high signal on T2-weighted imaging (T2WI), + prominent gadolinium (Gd) contrast enhancement. High signal on T2WI and Gd contrast enhancement can be heterogeneous in large lesions. *Plexiform neurofibromas* appear as curvilinear and multinodular lesions involving multiple nerve branches. They have low to intermediate signal on T1WI and intermediate or slightly high to high signal on T2WI and fat-suppressed T2WI, with or without bands or strands of low signal. Lesions usually show Gd contrast enhancement. *CT:* Ovoid or fusiform lesions with low-intermediate attenuation. Lesions can show contrast enhancement. Often erode adjacent bone.	Benign nerve sheath tumors that contain mixtures of Schwann cells, perineural-like cells, and interlacing fascicles of fibroblasts associated with abundant collagen. Unlike schwannomas, neurofibromas lack Antoni A and B regions and cannot be separated pathologically from the underlying nerve. Most frequently occur as sporadic, localized, solitary lesions, less frequently as diffuse or plexiform lesions. Multiple neurofibromas are typical in neurofibromatosis type 1 (NF1), which is an autosomal dominant disorder (1/2,500 births) caused by mutations of the neurofibromin gene on chromosome 17q11.2. NF1 represents the most common type of neurocutaneous syndrome, and it is associated with neoplasms of the central and peripheral nervous systems (optic gliomas, astrocytomas, plexiform and solitary neurofibromas) and skin (café-au-lait spots, axillary and inguinal freckling). NF1 is also associated with meningeal and skull dysplasias, as well as hamartomas of the iris (Lisch nodules).

(continued on page 244)

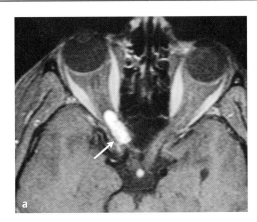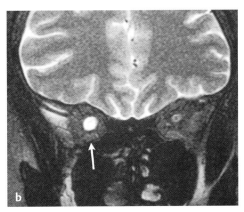

Fig. 2.81   **(a)** A 43-year-old woman with von Hippel-Lindau disease who has a hemangioblastoma involving the right optic nerve that shows gadolinium contrast enhancement on axial fat-suppressed T1-weighted imaging (*arrow*). **(b)** The tumor has high signal on coronal fat-suppressed T2-weighted imaging (*arrow*).

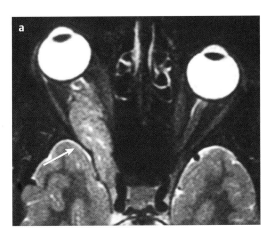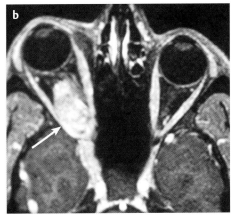

Fig. 2.82   A 28-year-old man with a schwannoma in the right orbit and superior orbital fissure that has **(a)** heterogeneous slightly high signal on axial STIR (*arrow*) and **(b)** gadolinium contrast enhancement on axial T1-weighted imaging (*arrow*).

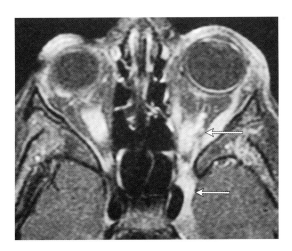

Fig. 2.83   A 5-year-old female with neurofibromatosis type 1 who has an irregular, gadolinium-enhancing, plexiform neurofibroma in the left orbit and superior orbital fissure (*arrows*) on axial fat-suppressed T1-weighted imaging.

Table 2.3 *(cont.)*   Extraocular lesions involving the orbit

Lesion	Imaging Findings	Comments
Lacrimal gland pleomorphic adenoma	*MRI:* Circumscribed lesions, with low-intermediate signal on T1-weighted imaging and slightly high to high signal on T2-weighted imaging, + gadolinium contrast enhancement. Large lesions may contain zones of cystic change and/or hemorrhage. *CT:* Circumscribed lesions with low-intermediate attenuation. Lesions can show contrast enhancement. May be associated with erosion of adjacent bone.	The most common benign neoplasm of the lacrimal gland, pleomorphic adenoma usually occurs in the fourth to fifth decades. Tumors are slow growing and contain low-grade mesenchymal and epithelial neoplastic cells, which may be organized into tubules or nests within stroma containing myxoid material, ± bone or cartilaginous elements. Complete resection is associated with a good prognosis.
Tumorlike Osseous Lesions		
Osteoma **(Fig. 2.84)**	*CT:* Well-circumscribed lesions involving the skull, with high attenuation. *MRI:* Well-circumscribed lesions involving the skull, with low-intermediate signal on T1- and T2-weighted imaging and typically no significant gadolinium contrast enhancement.	Benign primary bone tumors composed of dense, lamellar, woven and/or compact cortical bone, usually located at the surface of the skull or paranasal sinuses (frontal > ethmoid > maxillary > sphenoid) and occasionally involve the orbits. Account for less than 1% of primary benign bone tumors. Present in patients 16 to 74 years old and are most frequent in the sixth decade.
Fibrous dysplasia **(Fig. 2.85)**	*CT:* Lesions involving the skull are often associated with bony expansion. Lesions have variable density and attenuation on radiographs and CT, respectively, depending on the degree of mineralization and the number of bony spicules in the lesions. Attenuation coefficients can range from 70 to 400 Hounsfield units. Lesions can have a ground glass radiographic appearance secondary to the mineralized spicules of immature woven bone in fibrous dysplasia. Sclerotic borders of varying thickness can be seen surrounding parts or all of the lesions. *MRI:* Features depend on the proportions of bony spicules, collagen, fibroblastic spindle cells, and hemorrhagic and/or cystic changes. Lesions are usually well circumscribed and have low or low-intermediate signal on T1-weighted imaging. On T2-weighted imaging, lesions have variable mixtures of low, intermediate, and/or high signal, often surrounded by a low-signal rim of variable thickness. Internal septations and cystic changes are seen in a minority of lesions. Bony expansion is commonly seen. All or portions of the lesions can show gadolinium contrast enhancement in a heterogeneous, diffuse, or peripheral pattern.	Benign medullary fibro-osseous lesion of bone, most often sporadic, involving a single site, referred to as monostotic (80–85%), or in multiple locations (polyostotic fibrous dysplasia). Results from developmental failure in the normal process of remodeling primitive bone to mature lamellar bone, with a resultant zone or zones of immature trabeculae within dysplastic fibrous tissue. These lesions do not mineralize normally and can result in cranial neuropathies from neuroforaminal narrowing, facial deformities, sinonasal drainage disorders, and sinusitis. McCune-Albright syndrome accounts for 3% of polyostotic fibrous dysplasia and may include the presence of pigmented cutaneous macules (sometimes referred to as café-au-lait spots) with irregular indented borders that are ipsilateral to bone lesions, precocious puberty, and/or other endocrine disorders, such as acromegaly, hyperthyroidism, hyperparathyroidism, and Cushing's syndrome. *Leontiasis ossea* is a rare form of polyostotic fibrous dyplasia that involves the craniofacial bones, resulting in facial enlargement and deformity. Age at presentation ranges from < 1 year to 76 years, and 75% occur before the age of 30 years. Median age for monostotic fibrous dysplasia = 21 years; mean and median ages for polyostotic fibrous dysplasia are between 8 and 17 years. Most cases are diagnosed in patients between the ages of 3 and 20 years.

(continued on page 246)

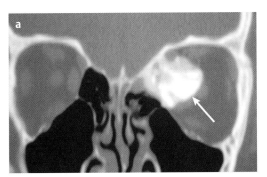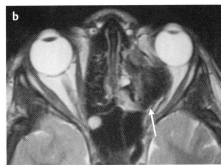

Fig. 2.84 **(a)** A 12-year-old male with an osteoma in the medial portion of the left orbit and left ethmoid sinus that has high attenuation on coronal CT (*arrow*) and **(b)** mostly low signal on axial T2-weighted imaging (*arrow*).

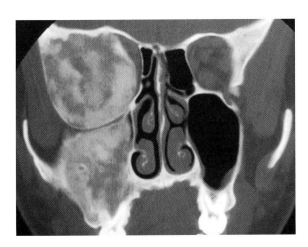

Fig. 2.85 Coronal CT of a 19-year-old man with fibrous dysplasia involving the right sphenoid bone and maxilla, resulting in narrowing of the dimensions of the right orbit and the pneumatized portion of the right maxillary sinus.

Table 2.3 *(cont.)*   Extraocular lesions involving the orbit

Lesion	Imaging Findings	Comments
Paget disease (**Fig. 2.86**)	*CT:* Lesions often have mixed intermediate and high attenuation. Irregular/indistinct borders between marrow and inner margins of the outer and inner tables of the skull. *MRI:* Most cases involving the skull are the late or inactive phases. Findings include osseous expansion and cortical thickening with low signal on T1-weighted imaging (T1WI) and T2-weighted imaging (T2WI). The inner margins of the thickened cortex can be irregular and indistinct. Zones of low signal on T1WI and T2WI can be seen in the diploic marrow secondary to thickened bony trabeculae. Marrow in late or inactive phases of Paget disease can: (1) have signal similar to normal marrow, (2) contain focal areas of fat signal, (3) have low signal on T1WI and T2WI secondary to regions of sclerosis, (4) have areas of high signal on fat-suppressed T2WI from edema or persistent fibrovascular tissue.	Paget disease is a chronic skeletal disease in which there is disordered bone resorption and woven bone formation resulting in osseous deformity. A paramyxovirus may be the etiologic agent. Paget disease is polyostotic in up to 66% of patients. Paget disease is associated with a risk of less than 1% for developing secondary sarcomatous changes. Occurs in 2.5 to 5% of Caucasians more than 55 years old, and in 10% of those older than 85 years. Can result in narrowing of neuroforamina with cranial nerve compression, basilar impression, ± compression of brainstem.
Arachnoid cyst (**Fig. 2.87**)	*MRI:* Well-circumscribed extra-axial lesions with low signal on T1-weighted imaging, FLAIR, and diffusion-weighted imaging, high signal on T2-weighted imaging similar to CSF, and no gadolinium contrast enhancement. Commonly located in anterior middle cranial fossa > suprasellar/quadrigeminal > frontal convexities > posterior cranial fossa. *CT:* Well-circumscribed extra-axial lesions with low attenuation and no contrast enhancement.	Nonneoplastic congenital, developmental, or acquired extra-axial lesions filled with CSF, usually with mild mass effect on adjacent brain. Found in supratentorial more than infratentorial locations, and occur in males more often than in females. Can cause remodeling of adjacent bone, with expansion and thinning of adjacent skull, ± orbital wall modeling, ± related clinical symptoms.
Epidermoid (**Fig. 2.88**)	*MRI:* Well-circumscribed spheroid or multilobulated extra-axial ectodermal-inclusion cystic lesions with low-intermediate signal on T1-weighted imaging, high signal on T2-weighted imaging, mixed low, intermediate, or high signal on FLAIR images, and no gadolinium contrast enhancement. *CT:* Well-circumscribed spheroid or multilobulated extra-axial ectodermal-inclusion cystic lesions with low-intermediate attenuation. Can be associated with bone erosion.	Nonneoplastic congenital or acquired ectodermal inclusion cysts filled with desquamated cells and keratinaceous debris, usually with mild mass effect on adjacent orbital structures, ± related clinical symptoms. Equal sex distribution. Often located adjacent to the frontozygomatic and frontoethmoidal sutures.
Dermoid (**Fig. 2.89**)	*MRI:* Well-circumscribed spheroid or multilobulated extra-axial lesions, usually with high signal on T1-weighted images, variable low, intermediate, and/or high signal on T2-weighted imaging, and no gadolinium contrast enhancement, ± fluid–fluid or fluid–debris levels. *CT:* Well-circumscribed spheroid or multilobulated extra-axial lesions, usually with low attenuation, ± fat–fluid or fluid–debris levels. Can be associated with bone erosion.	Nonneoplastic congenital or acquired ectodermal-inclusion cystic lesions filled with lipid material, cholesterol, desquamated cells, keratinaceous debris, skin appendages (hair follicles and sebaceous and sweat glands), usually with mild mass effect on adjacent brain, ± related clinical symptoms. Occur in adults and in males slightly more often than in females. Often located adjacent to the frontozygomatic and frontoethmoidal sutures.

(continued on page 248)

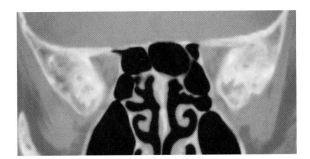

Fig. 2.86 An 84-year-old man with Paget disease involving both sphenoid bones, resulting in osseous expansion narrowing the transverse dimensions of the orbits, as seen on coronal CT.

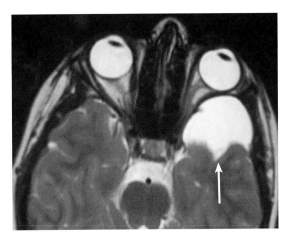

Fig. 2.87 An 11-year-old female with an arachnoid cyst in the anterior portion of the left middle cranial fossa (*arrow*) associated with osseous thinning and expansion anteriorly toward the left orbit on axial T2-weighted imaging.

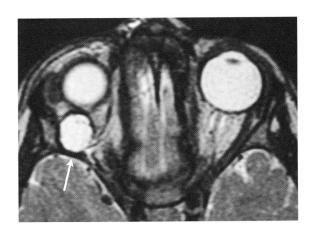

Fig. 2.88 A 2-year-old female with an epidermoid (*arrow*) at the lateral portion of the right orbit that has high signal on axial T2-weighted imaging.

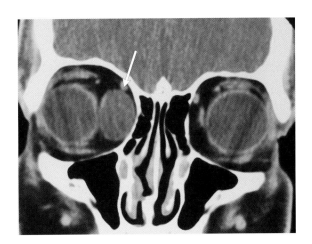

Fig. 2.89 A 33-year-old woman with a dermoid (*arrow*) at the medial portion of the right orbit that has circumscribed margins and low-attenuation contents on coronal CT.

Table 2.3 *(cont.)*   Extraocular lesions involving the orbit

Lesion	Imaging Findings	Comments
Infection		
Preseptal orbital cellulitis (**Fig. 2.90**)	*CT:* Findings of preseptal cellulitis include poorly defined soft tissue thickening and contrast enhancement of the eyelid and superficial periorbital soft tissues without involvement of the orbital fat, extraocular muscles, or optic nerve sheath. *MRI:* Poorly defined infiltrative zones with abnormal increased signal on T2-weighted imaging (T2WI) and fat-suppressed T2WI, as well as gadolinium contrast enhancement of the preseptal soft tissues without involvement of the eye, orbital fat, extraocular muscles, and optic nerve sheath.	The orbital septum is a thin fibrous layer of the eyelids that firmly attaches to the bony margins of the orbits and forms a relative barrier separating superficial infections from more clinically serious postseptal infections. Preseptal orbital cellulitis can result from trauma, adjacent skin infection, or upper respiratory infection. Common pathogens include *Staphylococcus aureus, Streptococcus,* and *Haemophilus influenzae* type B. Preseptal cellulitis, which typically is not associated with endophthalmitis, can be treated with oral antibiotics.
Postseptal orbital cellulitis (**Fig. 2.91, Fig. 2.92**, and **Fig. 2.93**)	*CT:* Findings of postseptal cellulitis include sinusitis, subperiosteal intraorbital abscess, poorly defined infiltrative soft tissue attenuation within the orbital fat, intraorbital muscles, and optic nerve sheath, ± abscess. Findings of endophthalmitis include: increased attenuation of the vitreous, scleral and uveal thickening with contrast enhancement. *MRI:* Findings of postseptal cellulitis include: adjacent paranasal sinusitis, subperiosteal intraorbital abscess, poorly defined infiltrative zones with abnormal increased signal on T2-weighted imaging (T2WI) and fat-suppressed T2WI within the orbital fat, extraocular muscles, and optic nerve sheath, with corresponding gadolinium contrast enhancement, ± abscess. Abscesses typically have restricted diffusion on diffusion-weighted imaging. Findings of endophthalmitis include: increased signal of the vitreous on T1-weighted imaging and FLAIR; restricted diffusion on diffusion-weighted imaging involving the vitreous, anterior chamber, and/or choroid; abnormal thickening of the sclera and choroid; and gadolinium contrast enhancement of the vitreous, anterior chamber, sclera and/or uvea.	Intraorbital infection can result from extension of adjacent sinusitis (60–80%), trauma, or complication from surgery. Infection occurs posterior to the orbital septum—fibrous connective tissue from the tarsal plate (eyelid) and deep to the palpebral section of the orbicularis oculi muscle, which attaches to the anterior bony orbital margins. Infections can involve the orbital fat, extraocular muscles, optic nerve sheath, and rarely the eye. A complication of ethmoid sinusitis is intraorbital subperiosteal abscess with postseptal cellulitis. Postseptal cellulitis usually occurs in children and young adults. In children, *Haemophilus influenzae* is a common cause, whereas in adults *Staphylococcus* and *Streptococcus* are common infectious agents. In immunocompromised or diabetic patients, aspergillosis and *Mucor* spp. can spread into the orbits via direct extension from the paranasal sinuses. Patients present with pain, vision loss, diplopia, chemosis, and/or proptosis. Urgent treatment with intravenous antibiotics is necessary.

(continued on page 250)

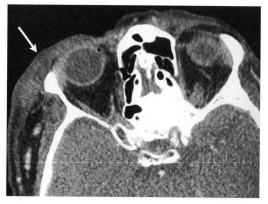

Fig. 2.90   Axial CT of a 62-year-old woman with preseptal cellulitis, which is seen as poorly defined soft tissue thickening involving the eyelid and superficial periorbital soft tissues (*arrow*) without involvement of the orbital fat.

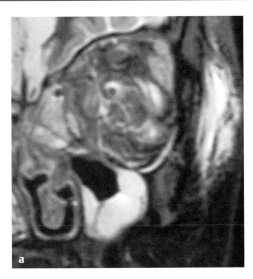
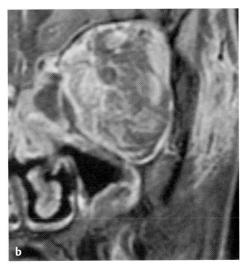

Fig. 2.91 A 14-year-old male with left ethmoid sinusitis associated with postseptal orbital cellulitis seen as **(a)** poorly defined infiltrative zones with abnormal increased signal on coronal fat-suppressed T2-weighted imaging involving the orbital fat and extraocular muscles, with **(b)** corresponding gadolinium contrast enhancement on coronal fat-suppressed T1-weighted imaging.

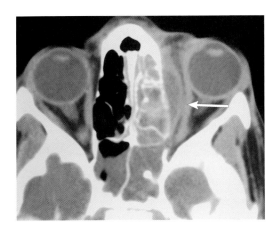

Fig. 2.92 Axial CT of an 11-year-old female with left ethmoid and sphenoid sinusitis resulting in a subperiosteal abscess and postseptal cellulitis in the left orbit (*arrow*).

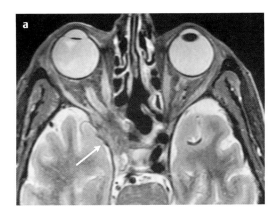
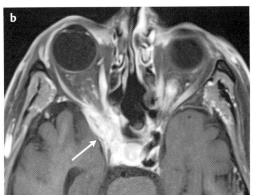

Fig. 2.93 An 84-year-old patient with postseptal fungal cellulitis from aspergillosis. **(a)** Axial STIR shows poorly defined zones with abnormal slightly high signal (*arrow*). **(b)** There is corresponding gadolinium contrast enhancement on axial fat-suppressed T1-weighted imaging involving the right orbital fat, orbital apex, right cavernous sinus, and dura of the anteromedial right middle cranial fossa (*arrow*).

Table 2.3 *(cont.)* Extraocular lesions involving the orbit

Lesion	Imaging Findings	Comments
Mucocele/pyocele **(Fig. 2.94)**	*CT:* Airless expanded sinus with mucus (10–18 HU). *MRI:* Lesion with low signal on T1-weighted imaging (T1WI) and high signal on T2-weighted imaging (T2WI). Mucoceles and pyoceles can have high signal on T1WI and low signal on T2WI due to inspissated secretions with high protein content.	Inflammation/infection of paranasal sinuses can cause obstruction of the sinus ostium, resulting in accumulation of mucus and desquamated epithelium. Progressive remodeling and expansion of sinus bone walls into orbits and cranial compartments. Distribution is frontal sinuses (65%), ethmoid air cells (25%), and maxillary sinuses (10%).
Inflammation		
Optic neuritis **(Fig. 2.95)**	*MRI:* Zone or zones with abnormal high signal on fat-suppressed (FS) T2-weighted imaging (T2WI) and STIR involving the optic nerve. In acute optic neuritis, the involved nerve can be slightly enlarged and can show gadolinium (Gd) contrast enhancement. Late findings include residual high signal on FS T2WI and STIR, localized atrophy, and no Gd contrast enhancement. *CT:* Can show slight localized enlargement of the involved optic nerve sheath.	Acute inflammatory demyelination of the optic nerve(s) without, or in association with, multiple sclerosis (MS) or neuromyelitis optica. Incidence of unilateral optic neuritis is 1–46 per 100,000, and incidence is higher in northern latitudes and higher altitudes. Female predominance of 3 to 1. Presenting symptom in 25% of patients with MS, and occurs in up to 70% of patients with MS. In the acute phase, activated T cells cross the blood–brain/neural barrier and release cytokines and other inflammatory mediators that cause axonal degeneration and neuronal loss. Patients often present with painful loss of vision. Steroids have been used for treatment. The presence of anti-aquaporin 4 (AQP-4) antibodies is specific for neuromyelitis optica, enabling distinction from MS. Aziathioprine and rituximab are used to treat patients with neuromyelitis optica.
Idiopathic orbital inflammation (inflammatory pseudotumor) **(Fig. 2.96** and **Fig. 2.97)**	*MRI:* Poorly defined or localized zone or zones with abnormal high signal on fat-suppressed (FS) T2-weighted imaging (T2WI) and STIR, with gadolinium (Gd) contrast enhancement involving one or more extraocular muscles, including the tendon insertions (orbital myositis), intraconal or extraconal fat, lacrimal gland (dacryoadenitis), optic nerve sheath, uvea/sclera, orbital apex, optic canal, superior orbital fissure, and/or cavernous sinus. Involved extraocular muscles and lacrimal gland are often enlarged. Late findings include residual high signal on FS T2WI and STIR, localized atrophy, and no Gd contrast enhancement. *CT:* Poorly defined or localized zone or zones with abnormal soft tissue attenuation involving the intraconal or extraconal fat. Involved extraocular muscles and lacrimal gland are often enlarged.	Nonspecific, benign proliferative disorder of unknown etiology with accumulation of polymorphous inflammatory cells, polyclonal lymphocytes, histiocytes, plasma cells, and eosinophils within the orbital soft tissues. Varying amounts of fibroconnective tissue are associated with the chronic inflammatory changes. Peak incidence is in the fourth to fifth decades, with equal sex distribution. Common symptoms include acute onset of orbital pain and diplopia. Can occur as localized or diffuse forms. Can involve the anterior orbit (eye including the uvea), lacrimal gland (idiopathic dacryoadenitis), extraocular muscles (myositic pseudotumor), and/or posterior orbit/orbital apex. Can sometimes extend intracranially or into the paranasal sinuses or infratemporal fossa. Treatment often consists of corticosteroids or other immunosuppressive medication.

(continued on page 252)

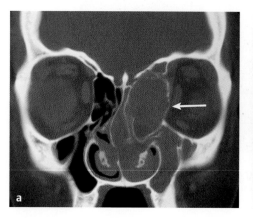
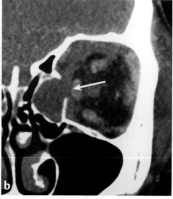

Fig. 2.94 **(a)** Coronal CT shows a mucocele involving a right ethmoid air cell with expanded, thinned, intact bony margins (*arrow*). **(b)** Coronal CT shows a pyocele involving an expanded left ethmoid air cell with osseous defect (*arrow*), as well as extension of infection to involve the soft tissues in the medial and superior portions of the left orbit.

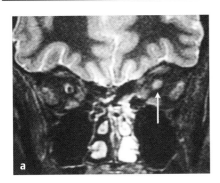
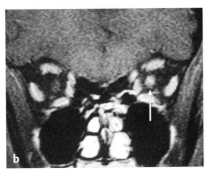
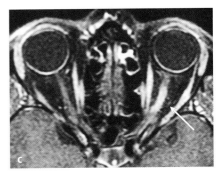

Fig. 2.95 A 30-year-old woman with acute left optic neuritis that has **(a)** high signal on coronal STIR (*arrow*) and gadolinium contrast enhancement on **(b)** coronal (*arrow*) and **(c)** axial (*arrow*) fat-suppressed T1-weighted imaging.

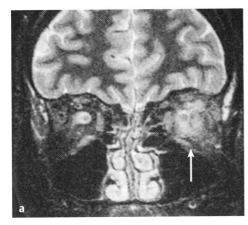
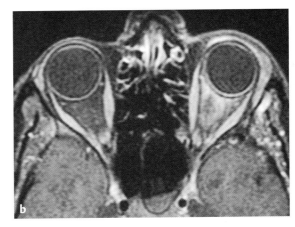

Fig. 2.96 A 45-year-old woman with idiopathic orbital inflammation (inflammatory orbital pseudotumor) involving the intraconal fat of the left orbit with **(a)** poorly defined high signal (*arrow*) on coronal STIR and **(b)** gadolinium contrast enhancement on axial fat-suppressed T1-weighted imaging.

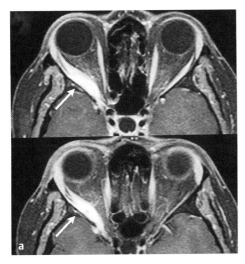
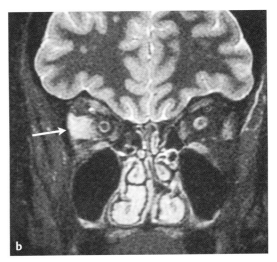

Fig. 2.97 Idiopathic orbital inflammation (inflammatory orbital pseudotumor) involving the lateral rectus muscle of the right orbit (myositis) and its tendons, which are enlarged and show **(a)** increased gadolinium contrast enhancement on axial fat-suppressed T1-weighted imaging (*arrows*) and **(b)** high signal on coronal STIR (*arrow*). The inflamed muscle has irregular margins with the adjacent intraconal fat.

Table 2.3 *(cont.)* Extraocular lesions involving the orbit

Lesion	Imaging Findings	Comments
Tolosa-Hunt syndrome (**Fig. 2.98**)	*MRI:* Poorly defined or localized zone with abnormal high signal on fat-suppressed T2-weighted imaging and STIR, and with associated abnormal gadolinium contrast enhancement involving the orbital apex, optic canal, superior orbital fissure, and cavernous sinus. Narrowing of the flow void of the cavernous portion of the internal carotid artery can occur. *CTA/MRA:* Can show narrowing or occlusion of the cavernous portion of the internal carotid artery.	Variant of idiopathic orbital inflammation with accumulation of noninfectious chronic inflammatory cells within the superior orbital fissure, optic canal, and cavernous sinus. Inflammation in the cavernous sinus can result in paresis/palsy of the motor nerves of the third, fourth, fifth, and/or sixth cranial nerves and oculosympathetic dysfunction from involvement of the second division of CN V, as well as narrowing or thrombosis of the cavernous portion of the internal carotid artery and/or cavernous sinus thrombosis. Patients present with acute onset of painful ophthalomoplegia, which is responsive to steroids.
IgG4-related systemic disease	*MRI:* Poorly defined or localized zone or zones with variable low-intermediate to slightly high signal on fat-suppressed (FS) T2-weighted imaging (T2WI) and STIR, with gadolinium (Gd) contrast enhancement involving one or more extraocular muscles, intraconal or extraconal fat, lacrimal gland, optic nerve sheath, orbital apex, optic canal, superior orbital fissure, cavernous sinus, trigeminal nerve, and/or infraorbital nerves. Involved extraocular muscles, lacrimal glands, and/or infraorbital nerves are often enlarged. Late findings include residual high signal on FS T2WI and STIR, localized atrophy, and no Gd contrast enhancement. *CT:* Poorly defined or localized zone or zones with abnormal soft tissue attenuation involving the intraconal or extraconal fat. Involved extraocular muscles, lacrimal glands, and/or infraorbital nerves are often enlarged.	Systemic autoimmune disorder with diffuse or tumefactive lesions consisting of lymphoplastic infiltrates, IgG4-positive plasma cells, and fibroblasts with storiform fibrosis. Can have elevated serum levels of IgG4 (> 135 mg/dL), and localized tissue accumulation of IgG4-plasma cells. Lesions occur in the orbits, thyroid, salivary glands, aorta, lungs, lymph nodes, pancreas, gallbladder, and kidneys. Treatment with steroids is usually effective.
Thyroid orbitopathy (Graves' disease) (**Fig. 2.99** and **Fig. 2.100**)	*MRI:* Asymmetric enlargement of the extraocular muscles (inferior rectus > medial rectus > superior rectus > lateral rectus) without involvement of the corresponding tendon. Involved muscles have a fusiform shape with circumscribed and/or slightly irregular margins, usually have slightly high signal on fat-suppressed (FS) T2-weighted imaging (T2WI) and STIR, and show slightly increased gadolinium (Gd) contrast enhancement. Intraorbital fat is often increased in volume and can contain poorly defined or linear zones with abnormal high signal on FS T2WI and STIR, with Gd contrast enhancement. These changes result in proptosis and stretching of the optic nerve. In the chronic phase, signal changes and Gd contrast enhancement can progressively diminish due to collagen deposition/fibrosis. *CT:* Proptosis with increased orbital fat volume, as well as asymmetric enlargement of the extraocular muscles (inferior rectus > medial rectus > superior rectus > lateral rectus) without involvement of the corresponding tendon. Bone remodeling and erosion can result from adjacent muscle hypertrophy.	Graves' disease is a common autoimmune disease involving the thyroid gland that results from circulating antibodies that mimic the function of thyroid-stimulating hormone (TSH also referred to as thyrotropin), which binds to and activates the TSH receptors in the thyroid gland. The activated TSH receptor results in increased synthesis and release of thyroid hormones, causing hyperthyroidism and hypertrophy of thyroid follicular cells, resulting in a goiter. Graves' orbitopathy occurs in up to 50% of patients with Graves' disease and is associated with asymmetric extraocular muscle hypertrophy, enlargement and inflammation of orbital fat, and proptosis. It is the most common cause of orbital inflammation in adults (accounts for 60% of cases in patients 21 to 60 years old). Incidence is 14 per 100,000, mean age = 41 years, occurs in women three times more frequently than men. Patients can present with proptosis, reduced visual acuity, diplopia, limitation of eye movements, and swelling of the eyelids. Treatment includes antithyroid drugs (thioamides), radioactive iodine, or surgery.

(continued on page 254)

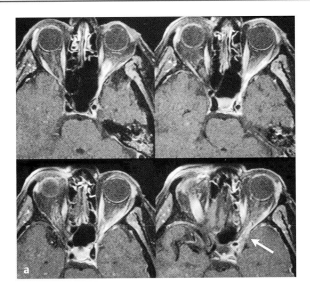
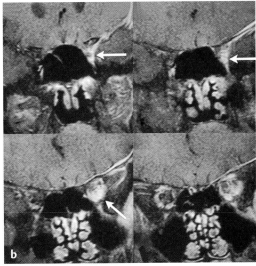

Fig. 2.98 Tolosa-Hunt syndrome. **(a)** Axial and **(b)** coronal fat-suppressed T1-weighted images show poorly defined gadolinium contrast enhancement in the left orbital apex extending posteriorly into the left superior orbital fissure and left cavernous sinus (*arrows*).

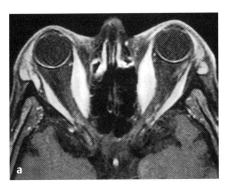
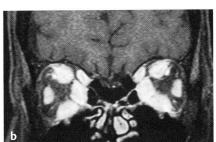
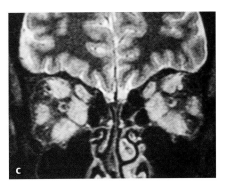

Fig. 2.99 A 53-year-old woman with thyroid orbitopathy and bilateral proptosis. **(a)** Axial and **(b)** coronal fat-suppressed T1-weighted images show increased gadolinium contrast enhancement of asymmetrically enlarged extraocular muscles without involvement of the corresponding tendons in both orbits. **(c)** The involved muscles have fusiform shapes and have slightly high signal on coronal STIR.

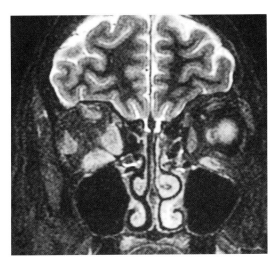

Fig. 2.100 A 64-year-old woman with thyroid orbitopathy and asymmetric enlargement of the extraocular muscles of the right orbit, which have slightly higher signal on coronal STIR than the normal-size extraocular muscles of the left orbit.

Table 2.3 *(cont.)*   Extraocular lesions involving the orbit

Lesion	Imaging Findings	Comments
Sarcoidosis (**Fig. 2.101**; see also **Fig. 1.222**)	*MRI:* Lesions often have low to intermediate signal on T1-weighted imaging and slightly high signal on T2-weighted imaging (T2WI) and fat-suppressed T2WI. After gadolinium (Gd) contrast administration, lesions typically show Gd contrast enhancement. The lacrimal gland is most commonly involved (up to 60%), with resultant diffuse enlargement. Other sites of involvement include the eyelids (20%), optic nerve sheath (20%), extraocular muscles (5%), and other orbital sites (20%). Extension of intraosseous sarcoid into the adjacent orbital soft tissues can also occur. *CT:* Intraorbital lesions have soft tissue attenuation with sharply defined margins in 85% and ill-defined margins in the remainder. Intraosseous sarcoid lesions usually appear as intramedullary radiolucent zones, and rarely are sclerotic or have high attenuation.	Sarcoidosis is a multisystem noncaseating granulomatous disease of uncertain cause that can involve the CNS in 5 to 15% of cases. If untreated, it is associated with severe neurologic deficits, such as encephalopathy, cranial neuropathies, and myelopathy. Sarcoid also involves various orbital structures, such as the eye (uveitis, chorioretinitis, vitreitis), eyelid, conjunctiva, lacrimal gland, extraocular muscles, and/or optic nerve sheath. Sarcoid in bone can also extend into the adjacent extraosseous orbital soft tissues. Diagnosis of neurosarcoid may be difficult when the neurologic complications precede other systemic manifestations involving the lungs, lymph nodes, skin, bone, and/or eyes. Treatment includes oral corticosteroids and surgical debulking.
Langerhans' cell histiocytosis (**Fig. 2.102**)	Single or multiple circumscribed soft tissue lesions in the marrow of the skull associated with focal bony destruction/erosion and extension extra- or intracranially or both. The osseous lesions most commonly occur in the superior or superolateral orbital roof. *CT:* Lesions usually have low-intermediate attenuation, + contrast enhancement, ± enhancement of the adjacent dura. *MRI:* Lesions typically have low-intermediate signal on T1-weighted imaging and heterogeneous slightly high to high signal on T2-weighted imaging (T2WI) and fat-suppressed (FS) T2WI. Poorly defined zones of high signal on T2WI and FS T2WI are usually seen in the marrow and soft tissues peripheral to the lesions secondary to inflammatory changes. Lesions typically show prominent gadolinium contrast enhancement in marrow and extraosseous soft tissue portions.	Disorder of the reticuloendothelial system in which bone marrow–derived dendritic Langerhans' cells infiltrate various organs as focal lesions or in diffuse patterns. Langerhans' cells have eccentrically located ovoid or convoluted nuclei within pale to eosinophilic cytoplasm. Lesions often consist of Langerhans' cells, macrophages, plasma cells, and eosinophils. Lesions are immunoreactive to S-100, CD1a, CD-207, HLA-DR, and β_2-microglobulin. Prevalence of 2 per 100,000 children less than 15 years old; only a third of lesions occur in adults. Localized lesions (eosinophilic granuloma) can be single or multiple in the skull, usually at the skull base and/or orbital roof. Commonly seen in males more than in females, < 20 years old. Proliferation of histiocytes in medullary bone results in localized destruction of cortical bone with extension into adjacent soft tissues. Multiple lesions are associated with Letterer-Siwe disease (lymphadenopathy and hepatosplenomegaly), in children < 2 years old and Hand-Schüller-Christian disease (lymphadenopathy, exophthalmos, and diabetes insipidus) in children 5–10 years old.

(continued on page 256)

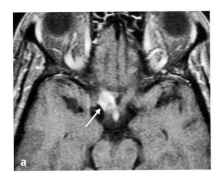
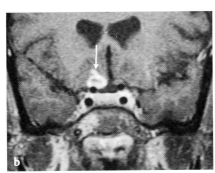
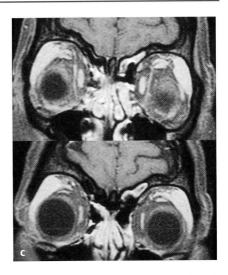

Fig. 2.101   A 42-year-old woman with sarcoidosis who has leptomeningeal gadolinium contrast enhancement surrounding the right side of the optic chiasm and adjacent right optic nerve on **(a)** axial (*arrow*) and **(b)** coronal fat-suppressed T1-weighted imaging. **(c)** A 32-year-old woman with sarcoidosis involving both lacrimal glands, which are diffusely enlarged and show gadolinium contrast enhancement on coronal fat-suppressed T1-weighted imaging.

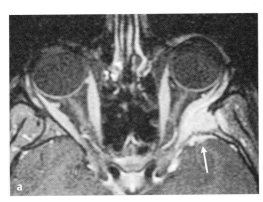
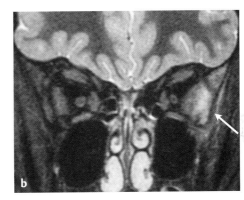

Fig. 2.102   **(a)** A 13-year-old female with Langerhans' cell histiocytosis who has a gadolinium-enhancing destructive lesion in the lateral wall of the left orbit on axial fat-suppressed T1-weighted imaging (*arrow*). The lesion extends into the left orbit and anterior left middle cranial fossa (*arrow*). **(b)** The lesion (*arrow*) has mixed intermediate and high signal on coronal STIR.

Table 2.3 *(cont.)*   Extraocular lesions involving the orbit

Lesion	Imaging Findings	Comments
Erdheim-Chester disease **(Fig. 2.103)**	*MRI:* Lesions can occur in the orbits, brain, choroid plexus, and spinal or cranial dura. Intraorbital lesions can be unilateral or bilateral and are usually intraconal. Lesions have low to intermediate signal on T1-weighted imaging and low, intermediate, and/ or slightly high signal on T2-weighted imaging. After gadolinium (Gd) contrast administration, lesions usually show enhancement. Prolonged Gd contrast enhancement may occur from contrast retention by histiocytes. *CT:* Lesions have intermediate attenuation. Intraorbital lesions can present with exophthalmos.	Rare multisystem non-Langerhans' cell histiocytic disorder of unknown etiology that usually affects adults. Collections of foamy lipid-laden histiocytes with small bland nuclei, Touton-like giant cells, multinucleated giant cells, fibrosis/dense collagen, chronic inflammatory cells (lymphocytes and histiocytes), and occasional scattered eosinophils occur in various tissues. Immunoreactive to the histiocytic antigen CD68 and shows variable or no reactivity to S100. Unlike Langerhans' cell histiocytosis, Erdheim-Chester lesions lack immunoreactivity to CD1a or OKT6. Can involve the CNS (brain, hypothalamic-pituitary axis, and/or meninges, and dentate nuclei) as well as the musculoskeletal, pulmonary, cardiac, and gastrointestinal systems. Age range is 7 to 84 years. Most common in fourth to seventh decades. Prognosis depends on the extent and location of disease. Treatment includes surgical debulking, prednisone, cyclosporine, vincristine, vinblastine, cyclophosphamide, and/or doxorubicin. Radiation treatment may be useful for intracranial lesions in the brain parenchyma and other locations. Immunotherapy with agents like interferon-α_{2a} has also been used. Multisystem disease can result in death from respiratory distress, pulmonary fibrosis, and renal and/or heart failure. Thirty-seven percent of patients had died after a mean follow-up interval of 32 months.
Sjögren's syndrome **(Fig. 2.104)**	*MRI:* Lacrimal glands have heterogeneous low-intermediate signal on T1-weighted imaging (T1WI) and variable mixed low, intermediate, and/or high signal on T2-weighted imaging (T2WI) and fat-suppressed T2WI. In the early phases of disease, the involved glands may be enlarged. Over time, the glands decrease in size from apoptosis, with increased fat deposition resulting in progressive increase in signal on T1WI. Also in the later disease phases, the ADCs of involved glands become lower than those of normal lacrimal glands. *CT:* Lacrimal glands can be enlarged in the early phases of the disease or atrophic in later stages.	Common autoimmune disease in which a mononuclear lymphocyte infiltration can occur in one or more exocrine glands (lacrimal glands and parotid, submandibular, and minor salivary glands), resulting in acinar cell destruction and impaired gland function. Can be a primary disorder or a secondary form associated with other autoimmune diseases, such as rheumatoid arthritis and systemic lupus erythematosus. Patients present with decreased lacrimal and salivary gland function, xerostomia, and keratoconjunctivitis sicca.
Granulomatosis with polyangiitis **(Fig. 2.105)**	*MRI:* Poorly defined zones of soft tissue thickening with low-intermediate signal on T1-weighted imaging, slightly high to high signal on T2-weighted imaging, and gadolinium contrast enhancement within the nasal cavity, paranasal sinuses, orbits, infratemporal fossa, and external auditory canal, ± bone invasion and destruction, ± extension into the skull base. Intracranial involvement of the dura, leptomeninges, brain, or venous sinuses is possible. *CT:* Zones with soft tissue attenuation, ± bone destruction.	Multisystem disease with necrotizing granulomas in the respiratory tract, focal necrotizing angiitis of small arteries and veins of various tissues, and glomerulonephritis. Can involve the paranasal sinuses, orbits, skull base, dura, leptomeninges, and occasionally the temporal bone. Typically, positive immunoreactivity to cytoplasmic antineutrophil cytoplasmic antibody (c-ANCA). Commonly involves the paranasal sinuses and occasionally the orbits. Involvement of temporal bone in 40–70% of cases. Peak prevalence is in the fifth decade. Treatment includes corticosteroids, cyclophosphamide, and anti-TNF agents.

(continued on page 258)

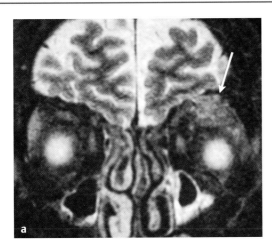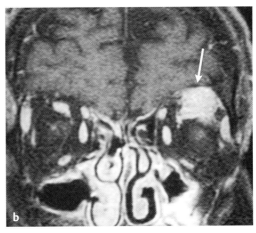

Fig. 2.103 **(a)** A 74-year-old man with Erdheim-Chester disease who has a lesion with ill-defined margins in the upper portion of the left orbit that has heterogeneous intermediate signal on coronal STIR (*arrow*). **(b)** The lesion shows gadolinium contrast enhancement on coronal fat-suppressed T1-weighted imaging (*arrow*).

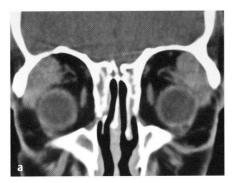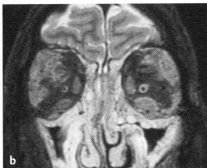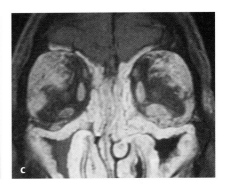

Fig. 2.104 **(a)** Coronal CT of a 58-year-old patient with Sjögren's syndrome who has enlargement of the lacrimal glands in both orbits on coronal CT. Irregular soft tissue with ill-defined margins, is seen within both orbits, which have **(b)** intermediate to slightly high signal on coronal STIR and **(c)** gadolinium contrast enhancement on coronal fat-suppressed T1-weighted imaging. Extensive mucosal thickening in the paranasal sinuses is also present.

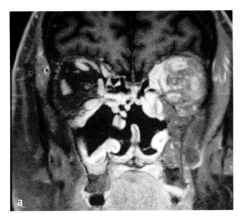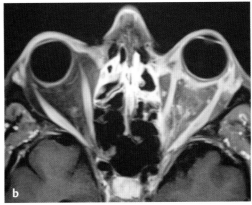

Fig. 2.105 A 51-year-old woman with granulomatosis with polyangiitis. **(a)** Coronal and **(b)** axial fat-suppressed T1-weighted images show irregular, diffuse, abnormal gadolinium contrast enhancement involving the intra- and extraconal soft tissues of the left orbit, including the extraocular muscles and episcleral region. Thickened, irregular contrast enhancement seen in the paranasal sinuses is associated with sites of osseous and nasal septal destruction.

Table 2.3 *(cont.)* Extraocular lesions involving the orbit

Lesion	Imaging Findings	Comments
Vascular Lesions		
Cavernous hemangioma (**Fig. 2.106**)	*MRI:* Circumscribed lesions that have intermediate signal on T1-weighted imaging, slightly high to high signal on T2-weighted imaging, and gadolinium contrast enhancement. *CT:* Lesions have intermediate attenuation, + contrast enhancement, – calcifications.	Hemangiomas are benign hamartomatous vascular lesions that contain endothelium-lined vascular spaces of varying sizes and shapes. Hemangiomas can be classified as capillary or cavernous based on the size of the vascular spaces. Hemangiomas can occur in soft tissue or bone and can be small or large, solitary and circumscribed, or infiltrative. Usually diagnosed between the second and fourth decades.
Orbital infantile hemangioma (**Fig. 2.107**; see **Fig. 2.31**)	*MRI:* During the proliferative phase, lesions have intermediate signal on T1-weighted imaging (T1WI) and slightly high signal on T2-weighted imaging (T2WI), as well as intralesional flow voids. Typically show prominent gadolinium (Gd) contrast enhancement. Involuting hemangiomas have heterogeneous signal on T1WI and T2WI, lack of intralesional flow voids, and heterogeneous Gd contrast enhancement. *CT:* Proliferating lesions have intermediate attenuation and show contrast enhancement, ± intralesional fatty changes.	Infantile hemangioma (also referred to as hemangioma of infancy, common infantile hemangioma, or juvenile hemangioma) is the most common congenital lesion in the head and neck. The infantile/juvenile capillary hemangioma contains small vascular spaces lined by small, densely packed, round endothelial cells and pericyte clusters. May present as small lesions at birth, but more commonly present during the first year. Typically increase in size over 10 months (proliferative phase), with subsequent involution over 6–10 years. Usually treated conservatively except for large lesions associated with clinical problems.
Orbital venolymphatic malformation (See **Fig. 2.32**)	Can be circumscribed lesions or can occur in an infiltrative pattern with extension in soft tissue and between muscles. *MRI:* Often contain single or multiple cystic zones that can be large (macrocystic type) or small (microcystic type) and that have predominantly low signal on T1-weighted imaging (T1WI) and high signal on T2-weighted imaging (T2WI) and fat-suppressed T2WI. Fluid–fluid levels and zones with high signal on T1WI and variable signal on T2WI may result from cysts containing hemorrhage, high protein concentration, and/or necrotic debris. Septa between the cystic zones can vary in thickness and gadolinium (Gd) contrast enhancement. Nodular zones within the lesions can have variable degrees of Gd contrast enhancement. Microcystic type typically shows more Gd contrast enhancement than the macrocystic type. *CT:* The macrocystic type is usually a low-attenuation cystic lesion (10–25 HU) separated by thin walls, ± intermediate or high attenuation resulting from hemorrhage or infection, ± fluid–fluid levels.	Benign vascular anomalies (also referred to as lymphangioma or cystic hygroma) that primarily result from abnormal lymphangiogenesis. Up to 75% occur in the head and neck. Can be observed in utero with MRI or sonography, at birth (50–65%), or within the first 5 years. Approximately 85% are detected by age 2. Lesions are composed of endothelium-lined lymphatic ± venous channels interspersed within connective tissue stroma. Account for less than 1% of benign soft tissue tumors and 5.6% of all benign lesions of infancy and childhood. Can occur in association with Turner syndrome and Proteus syndrome.
Orbital varix (**Fig. 2.108**)	*MRI:* Dilated vein or veins within the orbits that can have variable signal on T1- and T2-weighted imaging, ± fluid–fluid levels. Usually show gadolinium contrast enhancement. *CT:* Dilated tubular structures (veins) with intermediate attenuation, usually show contrast enhancement, ± phleboliths with calcification.	Distensible intraorbital venous lesions that can change size depending on venous pressure, positioning, and Valsalva maneuver. Weakness in venous walls causes dilated venous channels with fibrosis in the walls, with or without phleboliths. Endovascular embolization coiling can be used as a treatment.

(continued on page 260)

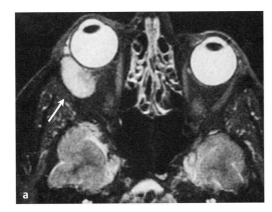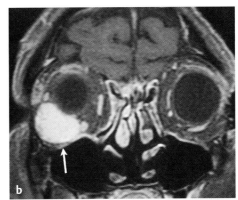

Fig. 2.106 A 70-year-old woman with a cavernous hemangioma in the right orbit that has **(a)** high signal on axial STIR (*arrow*) and **(b)** prominent gadolinium contrast enhancement on coronal fat-suppressed T1-weighted imaging (*arrow*).

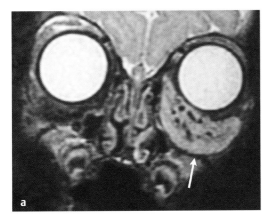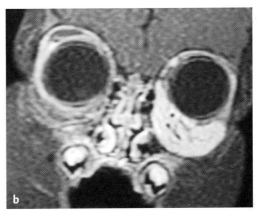

Fig. 2.107 **(a)** A 5-month-old female with an infantile hemangioma in the inferior portion of the left orbit that has slightly high signal on coronal fat-suppressed T2-weighted imaging (*arrow*) as well as intralesional flow voids. **(b)** The hemangioma shows prominent gadolinium contrast enhancement on coronal fat-suppressed T1-weighted imaging.

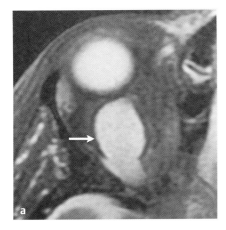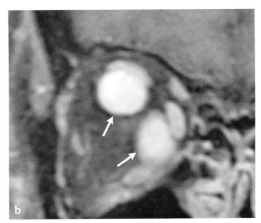

Fig. 2.108 A 72-year-old woman who has an orbital varix in the right orbit that has **(a)** high signal on axial fat-suppressed T2-weighted imaging (*arrow*) and **(b)** gadolinium contrast enhancement on coronal fat-suppressed T1-weighted imaging (*arrows*).

Table 2.3 *(cont.)* Extraocular lesions involving the orbit

Lesion	Imaging Findings	Comments
Dural arteriovenous malformations (AVMs) **(Fig. 2.109)**	*MRI:* Dural AVMs contain multiple, tortuous, tubular flow voids on T1-weighted imaging and T2-weighted imaging. The venous portions often show gadolinium contrast enhancement. Gradient echo MR images and MRA using time-of-flight or phase-contrast techniques show flow signal in patent portions of the vascular malformation. Usually not associated with mass effect unless there is recent hemorrhage or venous occlusion. *CT:* Dural AVMs contain multiple, tortuous, contrast-enhancing vessels on CTA at the site of a recanalizing thrombosed dural venous sinus. Usually not associated with mass effect. *MRA and CTA* can show patent portions of the vascular malformation at sites of recanalization within venous sinus occulsions. Usually not associated with mass effect unless there is recent hemorrhage or venous occlusion. ± venous brain infarction.	Dural AVMs are usually acquired lesions resulting from thrombosis or occlusion of an intracranial venous sinus, with subsequent recanalization resulting in direct arterial to venous sinus communications. Located in transverse and sigmoid venous sinuses > cavernous sinus > straight and superior sagittal sinuses.
Carotid cavernous fistula **(Fig. 2.110)**	*MRI:* Multiple flow voids are seen in dilated cavernous sinuses on T2-weighted imaging. Areas of brain contusion may also be seen. *MRA and CTA* show marked dilatation of the cavernous sinuses as well as the superior and inferior ophthalmic veins and facial veins.	Carotid artery to cavernous sinus fistulas usually occur as a result of blunt trauma causing dissection or laceration of the cavernous portion of the internal carotid artery. Patients can present with pulsating exophthalmos.
Traumatic Abnormalities		
Orbital fracture **(Fig. 2.111, Fig. 2.112,** and **Fig. 2.113)**	*CT:* *Orbital floor fractures* show cortical bone discontinuities with or without displaced bone fragments. Herniation of orbital fat and inferior rectus muscle can occur through the fracture into the maxillary sinus. The normal inferior rectus muscle has a flat shape in the coronal plane. If this muscle has a rounded shape, the fascial sling is injured, predisposing to herniation of orbital fat and the inferior rectus muscle through the fracture. Orbital floor fractures can involve the infraorbital canal, injuring the infraorbital nerve (terminal branch of the maxillary nerve/V2),which provides sensory innervation to the skin and mucous membranes of the midface (injury causes pain and sensory loss in the lower eyelid, upper lip, and/or nasal vestibule). *Medial wall fractures:* Medial concavity of fractured lamina papyracea, increase in orbital volume, and enophthalmos. Can result in restriction of horizontal eye movement. Fractures can extend anteriorly to involve the lacrimal fossa and attachment of the medial canthal tendon, requiring medial canthoplasty to avoid globe malposition. *Orbital roof fractures:* More common in children than in adults. Can involve the frontal sinus and can be associated with pneumocephalus, CSF leaks, intracranial infection, and/or hemorrhage. *Orbital apex fractures:* Angulation of the lateral orbital wall, ± multiple bone fragments, ± zygomaxillary fractures, ± involvement of the optic canal and injury of the optic nerve.	Traumatic fractures involving the orbits can occur in isolation or in combination with other craniofacial fractures. Fractures can involve the medial orbital wall (lamina papyracea), orbital roof, and orbital floor and/or lateral orbital wall (zygomaticomaxillary bones). Fractures involving the orbital floor or medial wall usually result from blunt trauma causing abrupt increase in orbital pressure. Fractures involving the orbital roof result from direct blunt trauma. Orbital apex and external wall fractures result from lateral blunt trauma with or without fractures involving the zygoma and adjacent maxilla. Complex craniofacial fractures involving the orbits include the LeFort II (orbital floor and medial orbital wall) and LeFort III (medial and lateral orbital walls and orbital floor) fractures. Other findings are epidural hematoma, subdural hematoma, subarachnoid hemorrhage, and CSF leakage—rhinorrhea and otorrhea.

(continued on page 263)

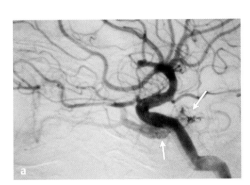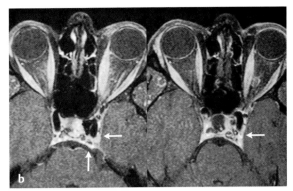

Fig. 2.109 **(a)** A 42-year-old woman with a dural arteriovenous malformation in the left cavernous sinus with a dilated draining vein anteriorly (*lower arrow*) and nidus (*upper arrow*) on a lateral arteriogram. **(b)** Postcontrast axial fat-suppressed T1-weighted imaging shows an enlarged left cavernous sinus, which contains multiple small flow voids (*arrows*).

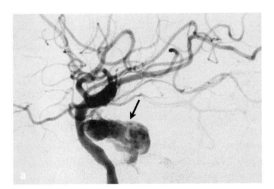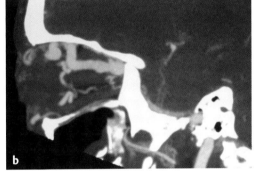

Fig. 2.110 **(a)** An 18-year-old man with a carotid cavernous fistula from trauma, as seen on an early arterial-phase lateral-projection arteriogram (*arrow*). **(b)** Sagittal CTA shows a dilated superior ophthalmic vein due to retrograde blood flow from the carotid cavernous fistula.

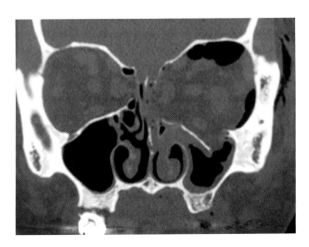

Fig. 2.111 A 47-year-old woman with a left orbital floor fracture as seen on coronal CT.

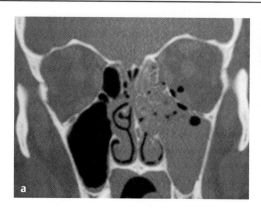

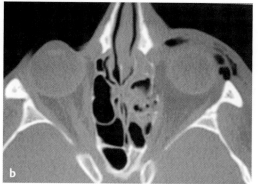

Fig. 2.112 A 24-year-old with fractures involving the medial wall (lamina papyracea) on **(a)** coronal and **(b)** axial CT.

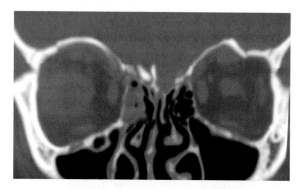

Fig. 2.113 Coronal CT shows a depressed fracture involving the left orbital roof.

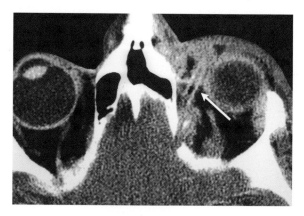

Fig. 2.114 Axial CT shows a wood foreign body in the medial left orbit, which is radiolucent centrally surrounded by a thin layer of soft tissue attenuation (*arrow*).

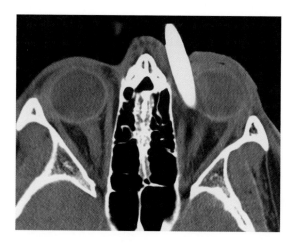

Fig. 2.115 A 16-year-old male with a metal projectile in the medial portion of the left orbit.

Table 2.3 *(cont.)* Extraocular lesions involving the orbit

Lesion	Imaging Findings	Comments
Intraorbital foreign bodies (**Fig. 2.114** and **Fig. 2.115**)	*CT:* Optimal test to safely evaluate for metallic foreign bodies and can detect metal fragments less than 1 mm. Metal fragments have high attenuation and can show streak artifacts. Glass fragments > 1.5 mm can be detected in more than 96% of cases, whereas smaller glass fragments (< 0.5 mm) are detected in ~ 50%. Wood foreign bodies have low attenuation that can be similar to air, although they have geometric shapes with peripheral inflammation that may suggest the diagnosis. *MRI:* Gadolinium contrast enhancement can be seen surrounding nonmetallic foreign bodies.	Intraorbital foreign bodies occur in up to 20% of orbital trauma cases. For metallic foreign bodies, CT should be done prior to MRI because of potential safety issues. Retained foreign bodies can result in impaired vision, cellulitis, and abscess formation.
Retinal detachment (See **Fig. 2.54** and **Fig. 2.55**)	Fluid and/or blood occur beneath the elevated, thin, linear leaves of the sensory retina, which are still attached to the ora serrata anteriorly and the optic disc posteriorly in a *V-shape pattern* with the apex at the optic disc. The subretinal fluid can have low, intermediate, or high attenuation on CT and variable signal on MRI, depending on the protein or blood content.	Retinal detachment can result from trauma, neoplasms, inflammation, or infection. The retina has firm attachments to the ora serrata, blood vessels, and optic disc and loose attachments elsewhere. Fluid or blood occurs in the potential space beneath the retina and choroid. Rhegmatogenous retinal detachments occur from vitreous fluid entering the subretinal space via a retinal tear. Tractional retinal detachments occur from separation of the sensory retina from the retinal pigment epithelium due to neovasculatization or fibrovascular tissue from trauma or inflammation.
Choroidal detachment (See **Fig. 2.56**)	*CT:* Fluid and/or blood occur beneath the leaves of the choroid, which are still attached to the ora serrata anteriorly and the vortex veins posteriorly in a biconvex or lentiform configuration. The detached choroid leaves do not extend to the optic nerve heads, and have a U shape. Serous subchoroidal fluid has low attenuation, whereas hemorrhagic collections have high attenuation. *MRI:* Serous subchoroidal fluid has low signal on T1-weighted imaging and high signal on T2-weighted imaging, whereas hemorrhagic fluid can have variable signal depending on the protein and iron content.	The choroid (middle eye layer) extends from the optic nerve head posteriorly to the ora serrata anteriorly. The choroid has firm attachments anteriorly to the adjacent sclera at the ora serrata/ciliary body and posteriorly where the vortex veins exit the eye. Trauma can result in ocular hypotony (decreased ocular pressure) with serous fluid, exudates, and/or hemorrhage accumulating in the potential space between the choroid and sclera.
Degeneration		
Phthisis bulbi (See **Fig. 2.57** and **Fig. 2.58**)	*CT and MRI:* shrunken deformed eye ± calcifications, variable CT attenuation and MRI signal of internal contents.	Nonfunctional eye secondary to end-stage degenerative changes that can result from inflammation, infection, or trauma.
Pseudotumor cerebri (idiopathic intracranial hypertension) (**Fig. 2.116**)	*MRI:* Normal shaped but small ventricles, ± mild prominence of intracranial subarachnoid spaces, ± empty sella configuration (prevalence up to 70%), enlarged trigeminal cisterns/Meckel's caves without meningoceles (9%), and Meckel's cave/pertous apex meningoceles (11%). Orbital findings include increased fluid in distended optic nerve sheath complexes (67%), flattening of the posterior sclera (prevalance of 80%, specificity of 100%), intraocular protrusion of the optic nerve head (30%), tortuosity of the optic nerves, and/or gadolinium contrast enhancement of the prelaminar optic nerve.	Idiopathic intracranial hypertension is a syndrome with elevated intracranial pressure without evidence of a mass lesion, hydrocephalus, or abnormal CSF composition. MRI with gadolinium contrast has a role in excluding intracranial tumors involving the brain or leptomeninges. MRV is useful to exclude intracranial venous sinus thrombosis or stenosis causing increased intracranial pressure. Treatment includes medications to reduce CSF pressure or CSF diversion procedures/ shunts.

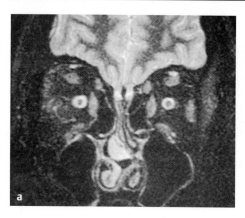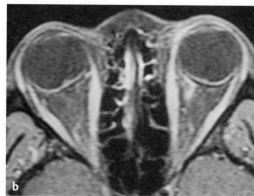

Fig. 2.116 A 26-year-old woman with pseudotumor cerebri. **(a)** Coronal STIR shows dilated optic nerve sheaths with increased CSF. **(b)** Axial postcontrast fat-suppressed T1-weighted imaging shows flattening of the posterior sclera and intraocular protrusion of the optic nerve heads.

References

Branchio-Oculo-Facial Syndrome

1. Milunsky JM, Maher TM, Zhao G, et al. Genotype-phenotype analysis of the branchio-oculo-facial syndrome. Am J Med Genet A 2011;155A(1):22–32

Choroidal Hemangioma

2. Mashayekhi A, Shields CL. Circumscribed choroidal hemangioma. Curr Opin Ophthalmol 2003;14(3):142–149
3. Singh AD, Kaiser PK, Sears JE. Choroidal hemangioma. Ophthalmol Clin North Am 2005;18(1):151–161, ix

Choroidal Melanoma

4. Houle V, Bélair M, Allaire GS. AIRP best cases in radiologic-pathologic correlation: choroidal melanoma. Radiographics 2011; 31(5):1231–1236

Choroidal Osteoma

5. Browning DJ. Choroidal osteoma: observations from a community setting. Ophthalmology 2003;110(7):1327–1334
6. Murthy R, Das T, Gupta A. Bilateral choroidal osteoma with optic atrophy. J AAPOS 2010;14(5):438–440

Coats' Disease and Persistent Hyperplastic Primary Vitreous

7. Apushkin MA, Apushkin MA, Shapiro MJ, Mafee MF. Retinoblastoma and simulating lesions: role of imaging. Neuroimaging Clin N Am 2005;15(1):49–67
8. Edward DP, Mafee MF, Garcia-Valenzuela E, Weiss RA. Coats' disease and persistent hyperplastic primary vitreous. Role of MR imaging and CT. Radiol Clin North Am 1998;36(6):1119–1131, x
9. Küker W, Ramaekers V. Persistent hyperplastic primary vitreous: MRI. Neuroradiology 1999;41(7):520–522
10. Mafee MF, Mafee RF, Malik M, Pierce J. Medical imaging in pediatric ophthalmology. Pediatr Clin North Am 2003;50(1):259–286

Coloboma

11. Kaufman LM, Villablanca JP, Mafee MF. Diagnostic imaging of cystic lesions in the child's orbit. Radiol Clin North Am 1998;36(6): 1149–1163, xi

Endophthalmitis

12. Ala-Kauhaluoma M, Aho I, Ristola M, Karma A. Involvement of intraocular structures in disseminated histoplasmosis. Acta Ophthalmol (Copenh) 2010;88(4):493–496
13. McCourt EA, Hink EM, Durairaj VD, Oliver SCN. Isolated group B streptococcal endogenous endophthalmitis simulating retinoblastoma or persistent fetal vasculature in a healthy full-term infant. J AAPOS 2010;14(4):352–355
14. Rumboldt Z, Moses C, Wieczerzynski U, Saini R. Diffusion-weighted imaging, apparent inversion recovery MR imaging in endophthalmitis. AJNR Am J Neuroradiol 2005;26:1869–1872

Erdheim-Chester Disease

15. Drier A, Haroche J, Savatovsky J, et al. Cerebral, facial, and orbital involvement in Erdheim-Chester disease: CT and MR imaging findings. Radiology 2010;255(2):586–594

Eye Trauma

16. Dunkin JM, Crum AV, Swanger RS, Bokhari SA. Globe trauma. Semin Ultrasound CT MR 2011;32(1):51–56
17. Yuan WH, Hsu HC, Cheng HC, et al. CT of globe rupture: analysis and frequency of findings. AJR Am J Roentgenol 2014;202(5):1100–1107

Hemangioblastoma of the Optic Nerve

18. Plate KH, Vortmeyer AO, Zagzag D, Neumann HPH. Von Hippel-Lindau disease and haemangioblastoma. In: Louis DN, Ohgaki H, Wiestler OD, Cavenee WK, eds. World Health Organization Classification of Tumours of the Central Nervous System. 4th ed. Geneva: IARC Press; 2007:215–217
19. Rubio A, Meyers SP, Powers JM, Nelson CN, de Papp EW. Hemangioblastoma of the optic nerve. Hum Pathol 1994;25(11):1249–1251

Hemangioma

20. Bilaniuk LT. Vascular lesions of the orbit in children. Neuroimaging Clin N Am 2005;15(1):107–120
21. Gemmete JJ, Pandey AS, Kasten SJ, Chaudhary N. Endovascular methods for the treatment of vascular anomalies. Neuroimaging Clin N Am 2013;23(4):703–728
22. Odell E. Haemangioma. In: Barnes L, Eveson JW, Reichart P, Sidransky D, eds. World Health Organization Classification of Tumours. Pathology and Genetics of Head and Neck Tumours. Lyon: IARC Press; 2005:276

Infantile Hemangioma and Venolymphatic Malformations

23. Baer AH, Parmar HA, McKnight CD, et al. Head and neck vascular anomalies in the pediatric population. Neurographics 2014;4:2–19

Infection and Inflammation Involving the Eye

24. Campbell JP, Wilkinson CP. Imaging in the diagnosis and management of ocular toxocariasis. Int Ophthalmol Clin 2012;52(4):145–153
25. Platnick J, Crum AV, Soohoo S, Cedeño PA, Johnson MH. The globe: infection, inflammation, and systemic disease. Semin Ultrasound CT MR 2011;32(1):38–50

Intraocular Leukemia

26. Ou JI, Wheeler SM, O'Brien JM. Posterior pole tumor update. Ophthalmol Clin North Am 2002;15(4):489–501
27. Sharma T, Grewal J, Gupta S, Murray PI. Ophthalmic manifestations of acute leukaemias: the ophthalmologist's role. Eye (Lond) 2004;18(7):663–672

Intraocular Lymphoma

28. Hormigo A, DeAngelis LM. Primary ocular lymphoma: clinical features, diagnosis, and treatment. Clin Lymphoma 2003;4(1):22–29
29. Kim YK, Kim HJ, Woo KI, Kim YD. Intraocular lymphoma after cardiac transplantation: magnetic resonance imaging findings. Korean J Radiol 2013;14(1):122–125
30. Sagoo MS, Mehta H, Swampillai AJ, et al. Primary intraocular lymphoma. Surv Ophthalmol 2014;59(5):503–516

Lacrimal Duct Lesions

31. Ansari SA, Pak J, Shields M. Pathology and imaging of the lacrimal drainage system. Neuroimaging Clin N Am 2005;15(1):221–237

Langerhans' Cell Histiocytosis Involving the Orbits

32. Herwig MC, Wojno T, Zhang Q, Grossniklaus HE. Langerhans cell histiocytosis of the orbit: five clinicopathologic cases and review of the literature. Surv Ophthalmol 2013;58(4):330–340
33. Kiratli H, Tarlan B, Söylemezoglu F. Langerhans cell histiocytosis of the orbit. Eur J Ophthalmol 2013;23(4):578–583

Lymphoproliferative Tumors of the Orbits

34. Demirci H, Shields CL, Karatza EC, Shields JA. Orbital lymphoproliferative tumors: analysis of clinical features and systemic involvement in 160 cases. Ophthalmology 2008;115(9):1626–1631, 1631.e1–1631.e3

Marfan Syndrome

35. LeBlanc SK, Taranath D, Morris S, Barnett CP. Multisegment coloboma in a case of Marfan syndrome: another possible effect of increased TGFb signaling. J AAPOS 2014;18(1):90–92
36. Konradsen TR, Zetterström C. A descriptive study of ocular characteristics in Marfan syndrome. Acta Ophthalmol (Copenh) 2013;91(8):751–755
37. Miraldi Utz V, Coussa RG, Traboulsi EI. Surgical management of lens subluxation in Marfan syndrome. J AAPOS 2014;18(2):140–146

Medulloepithelioma

38. Sansgiri RK, Wilson M, McCarville MB, Helton KJ. Imaging features of medulloepithelioma: report of four cases and review of the literature. Pediatr Radiol 2013;43(10):1344–1356

Morning Glory Optic Anomaly

39. Ellika S, Robson CD, Heidary G, Paldino MJ. Morning glory disc anomaly: characteristic MR imaging findings. AJNR Am J Neuroradiol 2013;34(10):2010–2014
40. Kalra VB, Gilbert JW, Levin F, Malhotra A. Spectrum of MRI findings in morning glory syndrome. Neurographics 2014;4(1):56–60
41. Knape RM, Motamarry SP, Clark CL III, Bohsali KI, Khuddus N. Morning glory disc anomaly and optic nerve coloboma. Clin Pediatr (Phila) 2012;51(10):991–993
42. Magrath GN, Cheeseman EW, Sarrica RA. Morning glory optic disc anomaly. Pediatr Neurol 2013;49(6):517
43. Quah BL, Hamilton J, Blaser S, Héon E, Tehrani NN. Morning glory disc anomaly, midline cranial defects and abnormal carotid circulation: an association worth looking for. Pediatr Radiol 2005;35(5):525–528

Norrie's Disease

44. Cunnane ME, Sepahdari A, Gardiner M, Mafee M. Pathology of the eye and orbit. In: Som PM, Curtin HD, eds. Head and Neck Imaging. 5th ed. St. Louis, MO: Mosby Elsevier; 2011:591–756

Ocular Neoplasms

45. Apushkin MA, Apushkin MA, Shapiro MJ, Mafee MF. Retinoblastoma and simulating lesions: role of imaging. Neuroimaging Clin N Am 2005;15(1):49–67
46. Bonavolontà G, Strianese D, Grassi P, et al. An analysis of 2,480 space-occupying lesions of the orbit from 1976 to 2011. Ophthal Plast Reconstr Surg 2013;29(2):79–86
47. Brennan RC, Wilson MW, Kaste S, Helton KJ, McCarville MB. US and MRI of pediatric ocular masses with histopathological correlation. Pediatr Radiol 2012;42(6):738–749
48. Chung EM, Specht CS, Schroeder JW. Pediatric orbit tumors and tumorlike lesions of the ocular globe and optic nerve. Radiographics 2007;27:1159–1186
49. Mahajan A, Crum A, Johnson MH, Materin MA. Ocular neoplastic disease. Semin Ultrasound CT MR 2011;32(1):28–37
50. Mafee MF, Mafee RF, Malik M, Pierce J. Medical imaging in pediatric ophthalmology. Pediatr Clin North Am 2003;50(1):259–286
51. Shields JA, Shields CL, Scartozzi R. Survey of 1264 patients with orbital tumors and simulating lesions: The 2002 Montgomery Lecture, part 1. Ophthalmology 2004;111(5):997–1008
52. Tailor TD, Gupta D, Dalley RW, Keene CD, Anzai Y. Orbital neoplasms in adults: clinical, radiologic, and pathologic review. Radiographics 2013;33(6):1739–1758

Optic Neuritis

53. Matiello M, Jacob A, Wingerchuk DM, Weinshenker BG. Neuromyelitis optica. Curr Opin Neurol 2007;20(3):255–260
54. Pau D, Al Zubidi N, Yalamanchili S, Plant GT, Lee AG. Optic neuritis. Eye (Lond) 2011;25(7):833–842
55. Toosy AT, Mason DF, Miller DH. Optic neuritis. Lancet Neurol 2014;13(1):83–99
56. Waldman AT, Stull LB, Galetta SL, Balcer LJ, Liu GT. Pediatric optic neuritis and risk of multiple sclerosis: meta-analysis of observational studies. J AAPOS 2011;15(5):441–446

Orbital Infections

57. Sepahdari AR, Aakalu VK, Kapur R, et al. MRI of orbital cellulitis and orbital abscess: the role of diffusion-weighted imaging. AJR Am J Roentgenol 2009;193(3):W244–W250
58. Tovilla-Canales JL, Nava A, Tovilla y Pomar JL. Orbital and periorbital infections. Curr Opin Ophthalmol 2001;12(5):335–341

Orbital Inflammatory Disease

59. Brannan PA. A review of sclerosing idiopathic orbital inflammation. Curr Opin Ophthalmol 2007;18(5):402–404
60. Ginat DT, Freitag SK, Kieff D, et al. Radiographic patterns of orbital involvement in IgG4-related disease. Ophthal Plast Reconstr Surg 2013;29(4):261–266
61. Hagiya C, Tsuboi H, Yokosawa M, et al. Clinicopathological features of IgG4-related disease complicated with orbital involvement. Mod Rheumatol 2013; 10.3109/14397595.2013.844307
62. Heiligenhaus A, Foeldvari I, Edelsten C, et al; Multinational Interdisciplinary Working Group for Uveitis in Childhood. Proposed outcome measures for prospective clinical trials in juvenile idiopathic arthritis-associated uveitis: a consensus effort from the multinational interdisciplinary working group for uveitis in childhood. Arthritis Care Res (Hoboken) 2012;64(9):1365–1372
63. Lutt JR, Lim LL, Phal PM, Rosenbaum JT. Orbital inflammatory disease. Semin Arthritis Rheum 2008;37(4):207–222
64. Mahr MA, Salomao DR, Garrity JA. Inflammatory orbital pseudotumor with extension beyond the orbit. Am J Ophthalmol 2004;138(3):396–400
65. McNab AA, McKelvie P. IgG4-related ophthalmic disease. Part I: Background and pathology. Ophthal Plast Reconstr Surg 2015;31(2):83–88
66. McNab AA, McKelvie P. IgG4-related ophthalmic disease. Part II: Clinical aspects. Ophthal Plast Reconstr Surg 2015;31(3):167–178
67. Pakdaman MN, Sepahdari AR, Elkhamary SM. Orbital inflammatory disease: pictorial review and differential diagnosis. World J Radiol 2014;6(4):106–115

68. Pemberton JD, Fay A. Idiopathic sclerosing orbital inflammation: a review of demographics, clinical presentation, imaging, pathology, treatment, and outcome. Ophthal Plast Reconstr Surg 2012; 28(1):79–83

70. Sa HS, Lee JH, Woo KI, Kim YD. IgG4-related disease in idiopathic sclerosing orbital inflammation. Br J Ophthalmol 2015;99(11):1493–1497

71. Sepahdari AR, Aakalu VK, Kapur R, et al. MRI of orbital cellulitis and orbital abscess: the role of diffusion-weighted imaging. AJR Am J Roentgenol 2009;193(3):W244–W250

72. Takase H, Mochizuki M. The role of imaging in the diagnosis and management of ocular sarcoidosis. Int Ophthalmol Clin 2012; 52(4):113–120

73. Tovilla-Canales JL, Nava A, Tovilla y Pomar JL. Orbital and periorbital infections. Curr Opin Ophthalmol 2001;12(5):335–341

74. Wakabayashi T, Morimura Y, Miyamoto Y, Okada AA. Changing patterns of intraocular inflammatory disease in Japan. Ocul Immunol Inflamm 2003;11(4):277–286

75. Wallace ZS, Khosroshahi A, Jakobiec FA, et al. IgG4-related systemic disease as a cause of "idiopathic" orbital inflammation, including orbital myositis, and trigeminal nerve involvement. Surv Ophthalmol 2012;57(1):26–33

Pseudotumor Cerebri/Idiopathic Intracranial Hypertension

76. Bialer OY, Rueda MP, Bruce BB, Newman NJ, Biousse V, Saindane AM. Meningoceles in idiopathic intracranial hypertension. AJR Am J Roentgenol 2014;202(3):608–613

77. Saindane AM, Bruce BB, Riggeal BD, Newman NJ, Biousse V. Association of MRI findings and visual outcome in idiopathic intracranial hypertension. AJR Am J Roentgenol 2013;201(2):412–418

Orbital Neoplasms

78. Bonavolontà G, Strianese D, Grassi P, et al. An analysis of 2,480 space-occupying lesions of the orbit from 1976 to 2011. Ophthal Plast Reconstr Surg 2013;29(2):79–86

79. Chung EM, Specht CS, Schroeder JW. Pediatric orbit tumors and tumorlike lesions of the ocular globe and optic nerve. Radiographics 2007;27:1159–1186

80. Mafee MF, Mafee RF, Malik M, Pierce J. Medical imaging in pediatric ophthalmology. Pediatr Clin North Am 2003;50(1):259–286

81. Shields JA, Shields CL, Scartozzi R. Survey of 1264 patients with orbital tumors and simulating lesions: The 2002 Montgomery Lecture, part 1. Ophthalmology 2004;111(5):997–1008

82. Tailor TD, Gupta D, Dalley RW, Keene CD, Anzai Y. Orbital neoplasms in adults: clinical, radiologic, and pathologic review. Radiographics 2013;33(6):1739–1758

Pediatric Orbital Diseases

83. Vachha BA, Robson CD. Imaging of Pediatric orbital diseases. Neuroimaging Clin N Am 2015;25(3):477–501

Retinoblastoma

84. Brisse HJ, Guesmi M, Aerts I, et al. Relevance of CT and MRI in retinoblastoma for the diagnosis of postlaminar invasion with normal-size optic nerve: a retrospective study of 150 patients with histological comparison. Pediatr Radiol 2007;37(7):649–656

85. Broaddus E, Topham A, Singh AD. Incidence of retinoblastoma in the USA: 1975–2004. Br J Ophthalmol 2009;93:21–23

86. de Graaf P, Barkhof F, Moll AC, et al. Retinoblastoma: MR imaging parameters in detection of tumor extent. Radiology 2005; 235(1):197–207

87. de Graaf P, van der Valk P, Moll AC, et al. Contrast-enhancement of the anterior eye segment in patients with retinoblastoma: correlation between clinical, MR imaging, and histopathologic findings. AJNR Am J Neuroradiol 2010;31(2):237–245

Sarcoid Involving the Orbits

88. Demirci H, Christianson MD. Orbital and adnexal involvement in sarcoidosis: analysis of clinical features and systemic disease in 30 cases. Am J Ophthalmol 2011;151(6):1074–1080.e1

89. Mavrikakis I, Rootman J. Diverse clinical presentations of orbital sarcoid. Am J Ophthalmol 2007;144(5):769–775

Scleritis

90. Okhravi N, Odufuwa B, McCluskey P, Lightman S. Scleritis. Surv Ophthalmol 2005;50(4):351–363

91. Wakefield D, Di Girolamo N, Thurau S, Wildner G, McCluskey P. Scleritis: Immunopathogenesis and molecular basis for therapy. Prog Retin Eye Res 2013;35:44–62

Sjögren's Syndrome

92. de Sousa Gomes P, Juodzbalys G, Fernandes MH, Guobis Z. Diagnostic approaches to Sjogren's syndrome: a literature review and our own clinical experience. J Oral Maxillofac Res. 2012;3(1):e3

93. Kawai Y, Sumi M, Kitamori H, Takagi Y, Nakamura T. Diffusion-weighted MR microimaging of the lacrimal glands in patients with Sjogren's syndrome. AJR Am J Roentgenol 2005;184(4):1320–1325

94. Niemelä RK, Takalo R, Pääkkö E, et al. Ultrasonography of salivary glands in primary Sjogren's syndrome. A comparison with magnetic resonance imaging and magnetic resonance sialography of parotid glands. Rheumatology (Oxford) 2004;43(7):875–879

Sturge-Weber Syndrome

95. Griffiths PD, Boodram MB, Blaser S, et al. Abnormal ocular enhancement in Sturge-Weber syndrome: correlation of ocular MR and CT findings with clinical and intracranial imaging findings. AJNR Am J Neuroradiol 1996;17(4):749–754

Thyroid Orbitopathy

96. Menconi F, Marcocci C, Marinò M. Diagnosis and classification of Graves' disease. Autoimmun Rev 2014;13(4-5):398–402

97. Müller-Forell W, Kahaly GJ. Neuroimaging of Graves' orbitopathy. Best Pract Res Clin Endocrinol Metab 2012;26(3):259–271

98. Gonçalves AC, Gebrim EMMS, Monteiro MLR. Imaging studies for diagnosing Graves' orbitopathy and dysthyroid optic neuropathy. Clinics (Sao Paulo) 2012;67(11):1327–1334

Tolosa-Hunt Syndrome

99. Cakirer S. MRI findings in Tolosa-Hunt syndrome before and after systemic corticosteroid therapy. Eur J Radiol 2003;45(2):83–90

100. Schuknecht B, Sturm V, Huisman TAGM, Landau K. Tolosa-Hunt syndrome: MR imaging features in 15 patients with 20 episodes of painful ophthalmoplegia. Eur J Radiol 2009;69(3):445–453

Traumatic Abnormalities of the Orbits

101. Caranci F, Cicala D, Cappabianca S, Briganti F, Brunese L, Fonio P. Orbital fractures: role of imaging. Semin Ultrasound CT MR 2012; 33(5):385–391

102. Hu KS, Kwak HH, Song WC, et al. Branching patterns of the infraorbital nerve and topography within the infraorbital space. J Craniofac Surg 2006;17(6):1111–1115

103. Kubal WS. Imaging of orbital trauma. Radiographics 2008; 28(6):1729–1739

104. Ong HS, Qatarneh D, Ford RL, Lingam RK, Lee V. Classification of orbital fractures using the AO/ASIF system in a population surveillance cohort of traumatic optic neuropathy. Orbit 2014;33(4):256–262

105. Pinto A, Brunese L, Daniele S, et al. Role of computed tomography in the assessment of intraorbital foreign bodies. Semin Ultrasound CT MR 2012;33(5):392–395

Tuberous Sclerosis

106. Jung CS, Hubbard GB, Grossniklaus HE. Giant cell astrocytoma of the retina in one month infant. J Pediatr Ophthalmol Strabismus 2009; 10.3928/01913913-20091019-05

107. Martin K, Rossi V, Ferrucci S, Pian D. Retinal astrocytic hamartoma. Optometry 2010;81(5):221–233

108. Rosser T, Panigrahy A, McClintock W. The diverse clinical manifestations of tuberous sclerosis complex: a review. Semin Pediatr Neurol 2006;13(1):27–36

Uveitis from Infection

109. Hsu D, Sandborg C, Hahn JS. Frontal lobe seizures and uveitis associated with acute human parvovirus B19 infection. J Child Neurol 2004;19(4):304–306

110. Jap A, Chee SP. Viral anterior uveitis. Curr Opin Ophthalmol 2011; 22(6):483–488

111. Jap A, Chee SP. Emerging forms of viral uveitis in the developing world. Int Ophthalmol Clin 2010;50(2):155–171

112. Mandelcorn ED. Infectious causes of posterior uveitis. Can J Ophthalmol 2013;48(1):31–39

113. Nakajima H, Tani H, Kobayashi T, Kimura F. Chronic herpes simplex virus type 2 encephalitis associated with posterior uveitis. BMJ Case Rep 2014; 10.1136/bcr-2013-201586

114. Newman H, Gooding C. Viral ocular manifestations: a broad overview. Rev Med Virol 2013;23(5):281–294

Noninfectious Uveitis

115. Allegri P, Rissotto R, Herbort CP, Murialdo U. CNS diseases and uveitis. J Ophthalmic Vis Res 2011;6(4):284–308

116. Heiligenhaus A, Foeldvari I, Edelsten C, et al; Multinational Interdisciplinary Working Group for Uveitis in Childhood. Proposed outcome measures for prospective clinical trials in juvenile idiopathic arthritis-associated uveitis: a consensus effort from the multinational interdisciplinary working group for uveitis in childhood. Arthritis Care Res (Hoboken) 2012;64(9):1365–1372

117. Menezo V, Lobo A, Yeo TK, du Bois RM, Lightman S. Ocular features in neurosarcoidosis. Ocul Immunol Inflamm 2009;17(3):170–178

118. Messenger W, Hildebrandt L, Mackensen F, et al. Characteristics of uveitis in association with multiple sclerosis. Br J Ophthalmol 2014; 10.1136/brjophthamol-2014-305518

119. Pan J, Kapur M, McCallum R. Noninfectious immune-mediated uveitis and ocular inflammation. Curr Allergy Asthma Rep 2014;14(1):409

120. Rabinovich CE. Treatment of juvenile idiopathic arthritis-associated uveitis: challenges and update. Curr Opin Rheumatol 2011; 23(5):432–436

Vascular Abnormalities of the Orbits

121. Gujar SK, Gandhi D. Congenital malformations of the orbit. Neuroimaging Clin N Am 2011;21(3):585–602, viii

122. Hwang CS, Lee S, Yen MT. Optic neuropathy following endovascular coiling of an orbital varix. Orbit 2012;31(6):418–419

123. Rootman J, Heran MKS, Graeb DA. Vascular malformations of the orbit: classification and the role of imaging in diagnosis and treatment strategies. Ophthal Plast Reconstr Surg 2014;30(2):91–104

Von Hippel-Lindau Disease

124. Haddad NM, Cavallerano JD, Silva PS. Von Hippel-Lindau disease: a genetic and clinical review. Semin Ophthalmol 2013;28(5–6):377–386

125. Meyerle CB, Dahr SS, Wetjen NM, et al. Clinical course of retrobulbar hemangioblastomas in von Hippel-Lindau disease. Ophthalmology 2008;115(8):1382–1389

126. Toy BC, Agrón E, Nigam D, Chew EY, Wong WT. Longitudinal analysis of retinal hemangioblastomatosis and visual function in ocular von Hippel-Lindau disease. Ophthalmology 2012;119(12):2622–2630

Chapter 3
Paranasal Sinuses and Nasal Cavity

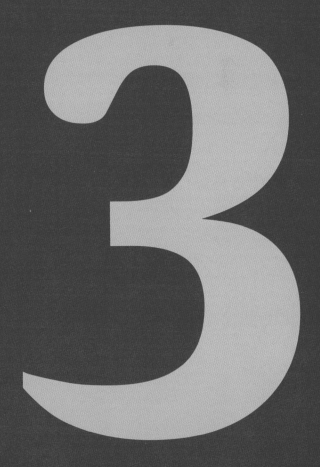

3   Paranasal Sinuses and Nasal Cavity

Table 3.1	Congenital and developmental abnormalities
Table 3.2	Solitary lesions involving the paranasal sinuses and nasal cavity
Table 3.3	Multifocal or diffuse sinonasal disease

Introduction

The nasal cavity is the anatomic compartment located between the roof of the mouth inferiorly, skull base superiorly, nostrils anteriorly, and nasopharynx posteriorly. The nasal cavity is divided into two compartments by the vertically oriented nasal septum. The upper anterior portion of the nasal septum is the septal cartilage, which connects to the perpendicular plate of the ethmoid bone posteriorly and the vomer posteroinferiorly (**Fig. 3.1**). The lateral walls of the nasal cavity are the superior and middle turbinates (concha of the ethmoid bone), inferior turbinate (inferior concha), maxilla anteroinferiorly, perpendicular plate of the palatine bone posteriorly, and the ethmoid bony labyrinth superiorly (**Fig. 3.2**). The anterior portion of the floor of the nasal cavity is formed by the palatine processes of the maxilla, with the small posterior portion contributed by the horizontal processes of the palatine bone.

The paranasal sinuses are air-containing, mucosa-lined structures named for the bones in which they are located. The paranasal include the frontal, ethmoid, maxillary, and sphenoid sinuses (**Fig. 3.3**). The frontal sinuses are located between the inner and outer tables. The frontal sinus drains through the frontonasal recess and duct into the semilunar hiatus and the middle meatus below the middle turbinate. The ethmoid sinuses consist of anterior ethmoid air cells whose ostia drain into the infundibulum, hiatus semilunaris, and the middle meatus. The posterior ethmoid air cells are separated from the anterior ethmoid air cells by the vertical portion of the basal lamella of the middle concha. The ostia of the posterior ethmoid air cells and sphenoid sinus open directly into the superior meatus. Mucosal secretions in the maxillary sinus move to the primary ostium at the upper margin of the uncinate process of the ethmoid bone, which is located lateral to the middle turbinate.

Development of the paranasal sinuses is related to development of the craniofacial bones.

During the fourth month of gestation, the sinuses develop as intraosseous evaginations of nasal mucosa. The maxillary and ethmoid sinuses develop first, followed by the frontal and sphenoid sinuses. At birth, the maxillary sinuses measure up to 8 mm in diameter, whereas the sphenoid and frontal sinuses may not be seen with imaging until after the child is 2 years old. The sinuses progressively develop during the first 3 years, followed by a slower growth pattern until 7 years, after which another accelerated growth phase occurs. The paranasal sinuses reach adult sizes by 12 years.

The nasal cavity is lined by stratified squamous and ciliated respiratory columnar epithelium, with serous and mucinous glands separated by zones of transitional epithelium. At the upper portion of the nasal cavity, olfactory epithelium develops, containing cells with olfactory receptors (neurons) whose axons form the olfactory nerves, which grow into the olfactory bulbs. The paranasal sinuses are lined by ciliated respiratory epithelium. The function of the ciliated epithelial cells is to move mucus with trapped bacteria and environmental particles toward the sinus ostia and into the nasal cavity. The common drainage pathway of the frontal, anterior ethmoid, and maxillary sinuses is referred to as the ostiomeatal unit, which includes each uncinate process of the ethmoid bone, maxillary ostium, ethmoid infundibulum, ethmoid bulla, hiatus semilunaris, and middle meatus (**Fig. 3.4**). The sphenoid sinus and posterior ethmoid air cells drain into the nasal cavity via the sphenoethmoid recess.

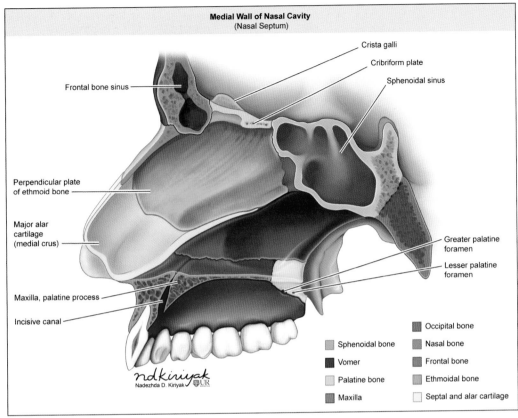

Fig. 3.1 Diagram of the medial portion of the nasal cavity shows the components of the nasal septum and adjacent anatomic structures.

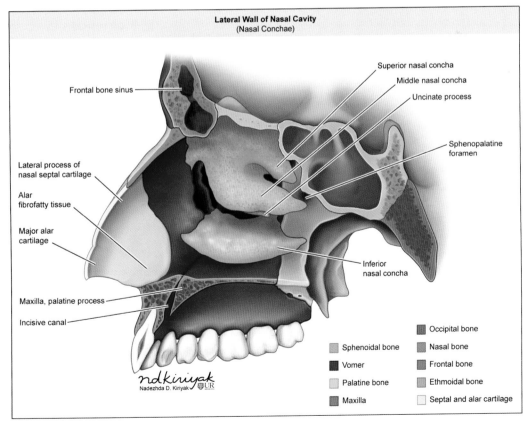

Fig. 3.2 Diagram shows the lateral aspect of the nasal cavity.

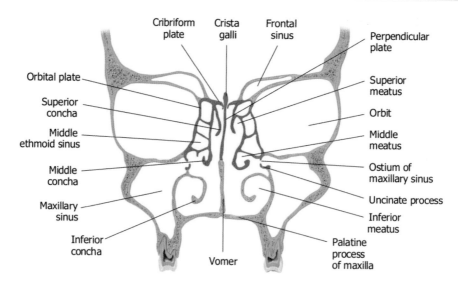

Fig. 3.3 Coronal view diagram shows the osseous structures of the nasal cavity and paranasal sinuses. The ethmoid bone is shown in red. From THIEME Atlas of Anatomy: Head and Neuroanatomy, © Thieme 2007, Illustration by Karl Wesker.

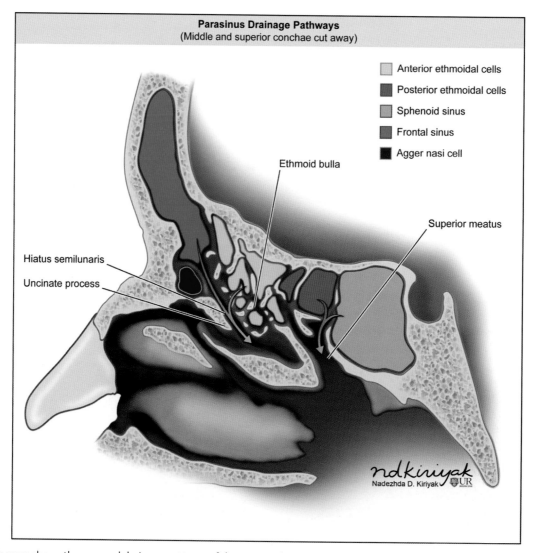

Fig. 3.4 Diagram shows the mucosal drainage patterns of the paranasal sinuses.

Table 3.1 Congenital and developmental abnormalities

- Nasal Cavity
  - Arhinia
  - Frontonasal cephalocele
  - Fronto-ethmoidal cephalocele, nasal glioma, nasal dermoid
  - Neuroglial heterotopia
  - Congenital nasal piriform aperture stenosis
  - Cleft lip with or without cleft palate
  - Nasopalatine duct cyst
  - Nasolabial cyst
  - Dacrocystocele
  - Choanal atresia and stenosis
  - Nasal septum: deviation, perforation, and osteophyes
  - Concha bullosa

- Paranasal Sinuses
  - Sphenoid cephalocele
  - Apert syndrome
  - Crouzon syndrome
  - Hemifacial microsomia (Goldenhar syndrome, oculoauriculovertebral spectrum)
  - Treacher Collins syndrome
  - Silent sinus syndrome
  - Infraorbital air cells (Haller cells)
  - Agger nasi cells
  - Frontoethmoidal (Kuhn) cells
  - Onodi cell

Table 3.1 Congenital and developmental abnormalities

	Imaging Findings	Comments
Nasal Cavity		
Arrhinia (**Fig. 3.5**)	Lack of formation of nose and hypoplasia of nasal cavity, ± cleft palate. Absence of olfactory lobes, olfactory sulci, and olfactory bulbs confirmed on coronal T1- or T2-weighted MRI. Other anomalies may be seen in the corpus callosum, hypothalamus, and pituitary gland.	Arrhinia refers to absence of nose formation, and arrhinencephaly refers to congenital absence of the olfactory lobes. Typically associated with other congenital craniofacial anomalies, such as cleft palate/ lip, hypertelorism, and hypoplasia of the nasal cavity. Considered to result from insult in utero or genetic mutation involving formation of the embryonic prosencephalon and cerebral vesicles at 42 days of gestation.

(continued on page 274)

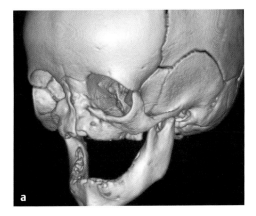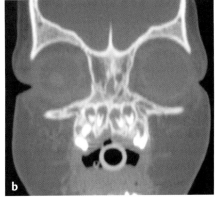

Fig. 3.5 Arrhinia in a neonate. **(a)** Oblique coronal volume-rendered CT image and **(b)** coronal CT image show lack of formation of the nasal bones and nasal cavity.

Table 3.1 *(cont.)* Congenital and developmental abnormalities

	Imaging Findings	Comments
Frontonasal cephalocele (**Fig. 3.6**)	Cephalocele located between the frontal and nasal bones.	Congenital midline mass that results from lack of normal developmental regression of the embryologic fonticulus frontalis between the frontal bone and nasal bone, with herniation of meninges ± brain tissue through the skull defect.
Fronto-ethmoidal cephalocele, nasal glioma, nasal dermoid (**Fig. 3.7**)	Nasoethmoidal cephaloceles are the most common type and occur between the nasal bones and nasal cartilage. A persistent enlarged foramen cecum is usually present. The sinus tract can contain epidermal inclusion cysts. Gadolinium contrast enhancement of the sinus tract can be seen, with superimposed infection with or without intracranial extension.	Congenital midline masses that result from lack of normal developmental regression of an embryologic dural projection through the foramen cecum (between the nasal bone and nasal cartilage). Lack of normal separation of the dural projection from the skin can result in a sinus tract that may eventually contain an epidermal inclusion cyst (dermoid, epidermoid) or extracranial dysplastic brain tissue (nasal glioma) in the nasal cavity or subcutaneous tissue. A nasal dimple is usually present on clinical exam. Sinus tracts can become infected and extend intracranially to cause meningitis, cerebritis, subdural empyema, and/or brain abscess.
Neuroglial heterotopia (See **Fig. 4.21**)	*CT:* Can contain zones with low and intermediate attenuation. *MRI:* Lesions usually have circumscribed margins, and can contain various combinations and proportions of zones with low and/or intermediate signal on T1-weighted imaging, and intermediate, high, and/or low signal on T2-weighted imaging (T2WI) and fat-suppressed T2WI, ± gadolinium contrast enhancement.	Rare congenital lesions that result from encephaloceles that become sequestered on the extracranial side of the skull base and that contain mature neuroglial elements. Can occur in the nasal cavity or nasopharynx with or without neonatal airway obstruction. Can be associated with an osseous defect at the skull base. Typically no communication with intracranial subarachnoid space.
Congenital nasal piriform aperture stenosis (**Fig. 3.8**)	*CT:* Nasal piriform aperture stenosis occurs when the aperture measures < 11 mm (between the medial aspects of the maxilla at the level of the inferior meatus). ± triangular palate, ± bony ridge along the undersurface of the palate from overlapping of the lateral palatal shelves secondary to hypoplasia of the primary palate, ± central mega incisor.	The palate is normally composed of the primary palate bone anterior to the incisive fossa and the two lateral palatal shelves that extend medially from the maxillae. The primary palate is derived from the medial nasal embryonic prominences that originate from the first pair of pharyngeal arches at 4–8 weeks of gestation. Abnormal hypoplastic development of the anterior portion of the primary palate results in narrowing of the anterior nasal cavity. Nasal aperture stenosis is an uncommon cause of nasal obstruction in neonates.

(continued on page 276)

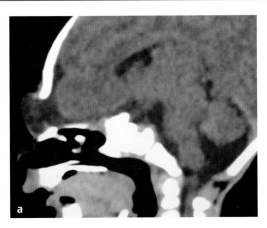
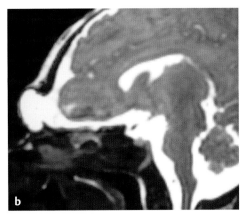

Fig. 3.6 A 2-day-old male neonate with a frontonasal cephalocele. **(a)** Sagittal CT and **(b)** sagittal T2-weighted imaging show an osseous defect between the lower frontal bone and nasal bones that is traversed by a meningocele.

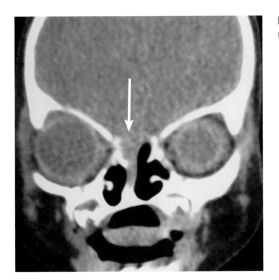

Fig. 3.7 Fronto-ethmoidal cephalocele. Coronal CT image shows a defect at the right cribiform plate with inferior extension of brain and meninges (*arrow*).

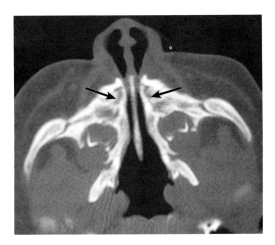

Fig. 3.8 A 1-month-old male with congenital nasal aperture stenosis (*arrows*) seen on axial CT.

Table 3.1 *(cont.)*   Congenital and developmental abnormalities

	Imaging Findings	Comments
Cleft lip with or without cleft palate **(Fig. 3.9)**	*CT and MRI:* Cleft lip with or without associated cleft palate and/or defect through the maxillary alveolar arch between the lateral incisor and adjacent bicuspid tooth.	Cleft lip is the most common maxillofacial malformation; it results from failure of fusion between the embryonic medial nasal and maxillary nasal prominences derived from the first pair of pharyngeal arches at 4–8 weeks of gestation. May occur in isolation or may be associated with cleft palate, which results from incomplete fusion of the primary palate with the secondary palate.
Nasopalatine duct cyst **(Fig. 3.10)**	*CT:* Circumscribed ovoid or spheroid radiolucent zone within the incisive canal, often with a thin sclerotic rim. Usually located superior to the roots of the maxillary incisors. Average cyst diameter is 1.5 cm. *MRI:* Circumscribed ovoid or spheroid zone with low signal on T1-weighted imaging and high signal on T2-weighted imaging, with thin peripheral rim of gadolinium contrast enhancement.	Non-odontogenic developmental fissural cyst that arises from epithelial remnants within the incisive canal (embryologic nasopalatine duct) near the anterior palatine papilla. Cyst walls are lined by stratified squamous epithelium ± pseudostratifed columnar epithelium and simple columnar epithelium. Patients range from 30 to 60 years old (mean age = 49 years). Cyst is usually asymptomatic, occasionally associated with palatine swelling, ± mucus drainage, pain. Most frequent non-odontogenic cyst of the mandible and accounts for up to 11% of jaw cysts. Treatment is surgical resection.
Nasolabial cyst **(Fig. 3.11)**	*CT:* Circumscribed spheroid or ovoid structure with low attenuation in the nasal fossa in the nasolabial sulcus anterior to the maxilla. *MRI:* Circumscribed ovoid or spheroid structure with low signal on T1-weighted imaging and high signal on T2-weighted imaging. Usually no gadolinium contrast enhancement unless there is superimposed infection.	Rare, non-odontogenic developmental cyst located within the skin adjacent to the ala of the nose near the upper portion of the nasolabial crease, and superficial to the alveolar process above the maxillary incisors. These cysts are slow growing and often measure between 1.5 and 3.0 cm. Cysts are lined by various cells types, such as squamous epithelium and pseudostratified columnar epithelium, ± fibrous connective tissue. Treatment is surgical excision.
Dacrocystocele **(Fig. 3.12)**	*CT:* Spheroid zone with low attenuation usually at the medial canthus, ± expanded lacrimal duct, with thinned bone margins. *MRI:* Spheroid zone with low signal on T1-weighted imaging and high signal on T2-weighted imaging that is commonly located at the medial canthus. Usually no gadolinium contrast enhancement unless there is superimposed infection.	The nasolacrimal duct develops from progressive canalization of ectodermal tissue along the nasolacrimal groove in the second month of gestation. Obstruction of the lacrimal ductal system results in accumulation of secretions in a focal lesion with thin walls. The proximal obstruction is often at the level of Rosenmüller's valve (junction of the upper portion of the canal with the lacrimal sac). The distal obstruction often occurs at the junction of the canal with the inferior meatus from lack of involution of the Hasner membrane.

(continued on page 278)

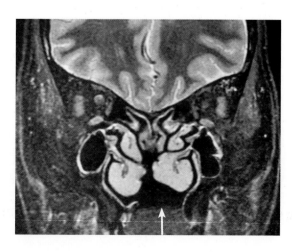

Fig. 3.9   Coronal STIR shows a defect in the hard palate representing a cleft palate (*arrow*).

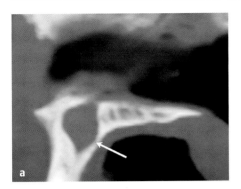
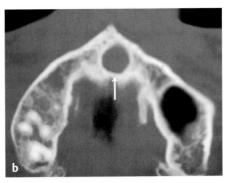
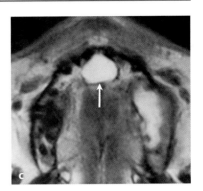
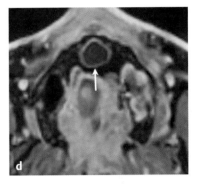

Fig. 3.10 Nasopalatine duct cyst. A circumscribed radiolucent zone (*arrows*) is seen within the incisive canal on **(a)** sagittal (*arrow*) and **(b)** axial CT (*arrow*). **(c)** The lesion has high signal (*arrow*) on axial T2-weighted imaging and **(d)** low signal centrally surrounded by a thin peripheral rim of gadolinium contrast enhancement (*arrow*) on axial fat-suppressed T1-weighted imaging.

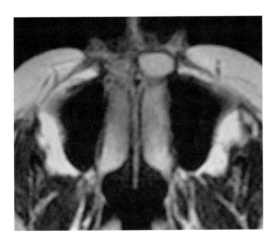

Fig. 3.11 A 55-year-old woman with a nasolabial cyst on the left that has high signal on axial T2-weighted imaging.

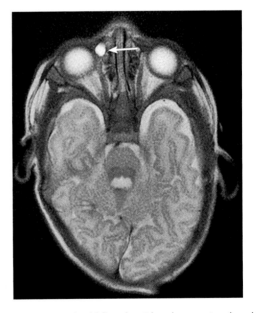

Fig. 3.12 A 4-month-old female with a dacrocystocele, which is seen as a small spheroid zone with high signal on axial T2-weighted imaging located at the medial canthus (*arrow*).

Table 3.1 *(cont.)*   Congenital and developmental abnormalities

	Imaging Findings	Comments
Choanal atresia and stenosis (**Fig. 3.13**, **Fig. 3.14**, and **Fig. 3.15**)	*CT:* Soft tissue or bony septum narrowing or occluding the channels (choanae) between the posterior nasal cavity and nasopharynx, with the posterior choanal opening < 0.34 cm in infants < 2 years old, ± medial bowing of the posterior maxilla, thickening of the vomer. *MRI:* Soft tissue or bony septum narrowing or occluding the channels (choanae) between the posterior nasal cavity and nasopharynx.	The choanae are bony channels between the nasal cavity and nasopharynx. Choanal atresia/stenosis is the most common cause of neonatal nasal obstruction, which occurs in ~ 1 in 5,000 neonates. Results from lack of normal embryonic involution of the oronasal membrane separating the nasal cavity and posterior oral cavity at 6 weeks of gestation (osseous atresia, 85% of cases) or lack of involution of nasal epithelial plugs filling the choanae (membranous choanal atresia, 15% of cases). Can be uni- or bilateral. Up to 50% are associated with disorders like the CHARGE or Treacher Collins syndromes. Surgical reconstruction or endoscopic perforation is used for neonates with respiratory distress.
Nasal septum: deviation, perforation, and osteophyes (**Fig. 3.16** and **Fig. 3.17**)	*CT and MRI:* Deviation of the nasal septum from the midline varies in degree. Can be associated with nasal septal osteophytes, which can be in close proximity to the nasal turbinates, resulting in a barrier to endoscopy.	The nasal septum separates the two nasal cavities. The anterior portion of the nasal septum is composed of the septal cartilage, which is attached posteriorly and superiorly to the perpendicular plate of the ethmoid bone, and to the vomer bone posteriorly and inferiorly. The floor of the nasal cavity is composed of the medial projections from the maxillae anteriorly and palatine bone posteriorly. Small vertical projections (crests) extend from these bones to attach to the septum. The inferior and dorsal margins of the septal cartilage fit into a groove along the upper edge of the vomer. Deviation of the nasal septum occurs in up to 80% of patients. Perforations of the nasal septum can result from trauma, surgery, inflammatory diseases, developmental anomalies (cleft palate, etc.), and drug use (cocaine). Nasal septal osteophytes can occur at the junction of the vomer with the perpendicular plate of the ethmoid bone.
Concha bullosa (**Fig. 3.18**)	Concha bullosa can be unilateral or bilateral and small or large. Large concha bullosa can be a barrier to endoscopy, as well as be associated with nasal septal deviation and narrowing of the infundibula of the ostiomeatal units.	Developmental pneumatization of the middle turbinates and rarely the inferior and superior turbinates. Results from the posterior ethmoid air cells extending to pneumatize the middle turbinates. Occurs in 40% of patients, with equal unilateral and bilateral frequency.

(continued on page 280)

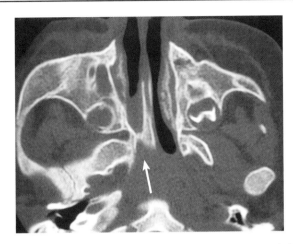

Fig. 3.13 Axial CT of an 8-month-old male shows unilateral choanal atresia on the right (*arrow*), with a bony septum occluding the channel between the posterior right nasal cavity and nasopharynx.

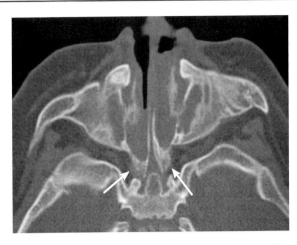

Fig. 3.14 Axial CT of 9-month-old male shows bilateral choanal atresia with bony septa (*arrows*) occluding the channels between the posterior nasal cavities and nasopharynx.

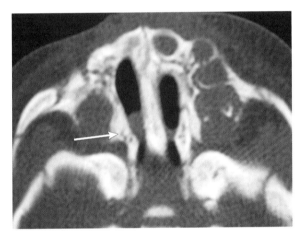

Fig. 3.15 Axial CT of 1-day-old female shows bilateral choanal atresia with soft tissue septa occluding the channels between the posterior nasal cavities and nasopharynx, thicker on the right (*arrow*) than on the left.

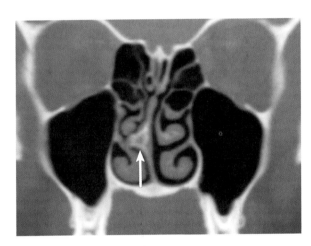

Fig. 3.16 Coronal CT shows mild deviation of the nasal septum to the right as well as an osteophyte at the right side of the nasal septum (*arrow*) that is in contact with the base of the right inferior turbinate.

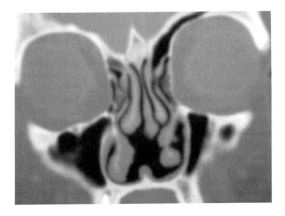

Fig. 3.17 Coronal CT shows a defect in the nasal septum (nasal septal perforation).

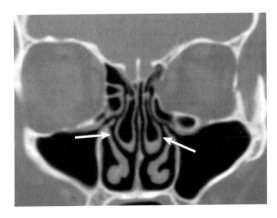

Fig. 3.18 Coronal CT shows bilateral concha bullosa (*arrows*). Also seen are infraorbital air cells on the left.

Table 3.1 *(cont.)* Congenital and developmental abnormalities

	Imaging Findings	Comments
Paranasal Sinuses		
Sphenoid cephalocele (**Fig. 3.19** and **Fig. 3.20**)	*CT and MRI:* Defect in the skull through which there is herniation of either meninges and CSF (meningocele) or meninges, CSF, and brain tissue (meningoencephaloceles).	Congenital malformation involving lack of separation of neuroectoderm from surface ectoderm, with resultant localized failure of bone formation. Can involve the sphenoid bone with extension into the sella, sphenoid bone and sinus, and nasopharynx. Incidence of transsphenoidal meningoencephaloceles is 1 per 700,000 live births. Clinical findings include difficulty in feeding and nasal obstruction in the first year, and potential for CSF leaks and meningitis. Cephaloceles can also result from trauma or surgery.
Apert syndrome (**Fig. 3.21**)	Irregular craniosynostosis (bilateral involvement of coronal sutures is most common), hypertelorism, midface hypoplasia/ underdevelopment, and symmetric complex syndactyly involving hands and feet.	Most common syndromic craniosynostosis, caused by autosomal dominant mutation of gene for fibroblast growth factor receptor 2 *(FGFR2)* at 10q26.13. Incidence is 1/55,000 live births. Features include irregular craniosynostosis, midface hypoplasia, and syndactyly of fingers and toes. Mental function impairment occurs in 70% of cases and is often severe. High association with brain anomalies (abnormal olfactory bulbs/tracts; malformations of the hippocampi/amygdala-limbic system, septum pellucidum, and corpus callosum; gray matter heterotopias; and ventriculomegaly). Patients present with headaches, seizures, and conductive hearing loss.
Crouzon syndrome (**Fig. 3.22**)	Premature ossification and closure of the coronal and lambdoid sutures, causing brachycephaly, followed by early closure of the other sutures. Shallow orbits, hypertelorism, maxillary hypoplasia, enlarged jaw, ± acanthosis nigricans (with *FGFR3* mutation), and Chiari I malformation.	Crouzon syndrome, also known as craniofacial dysostosis, is an autosomal dominant syndrome caused by mutation of the *FGFR2* gene at 10q26.13 or the *FGFR3* gene at 4p16.3. Craniosynostosis and often fusion of the synchondroses at the skull base are evident at birth. Also, maxillary hypoplasia, shallow orbits with proptosis, and bifid uvula, ± cleft palate. Up to 70% have Chiari I malformation. Progressive hydrocephalus in 50%.
Hemifacial microsomia (Goldenhar syndrome, oculoauriculovertebral spectrum) (**Fig. 3.23**)	Findings include facial asymmetry from unilateral and/or bilateral hypoplasia of the mandible, maxilla, and zygomatic arches; atresia or stenosis of the external auditory canals; hypoplasia of the middle ear; malformations and/or fusion of the ossicles; oval window atresia; and abnormal position of CN VII.	Asymmetric abnormal development of the first and second branchial arches related to autosomal dominant mutation of the *TCOF1* gene on chromosome 5q32-q33.1. Results in deafness/hearing loss and airway narrowing.

(continued on page 282)

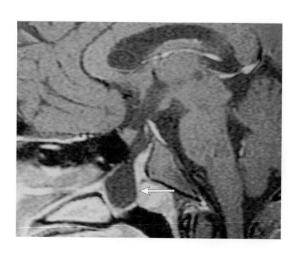

Fig. 3.19 A 17-year-old female with a meningocele (*arrow*) extending inferiorly into the nasopharynx through an osseous defect in the sphenoid bone located posterior to the pituitary gland, as seen on sagittal T1-weighted imaging.

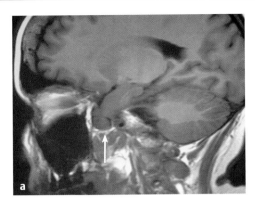
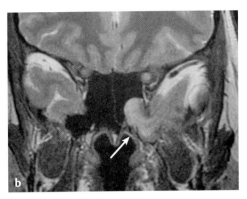

Fig. 3.20   **(a)** Sagittal T1-weighted imaging and **(b)** coronal T2-weighted imaging show an osseous defect at the left lower sphenoid bone through which a meningoencephalocele (*arrows*) protrudes into the sphenoid sinus.

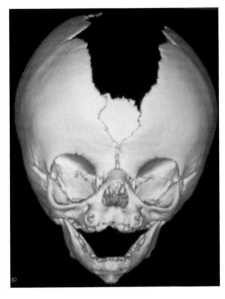

Fig. 3.21   Apert syndrome. Coronal volume-rendered CT shows craniosynostosis consisting of premature closure of the coronal suture, resulting in a widened sagittal suture as well as midface hypoplasia.

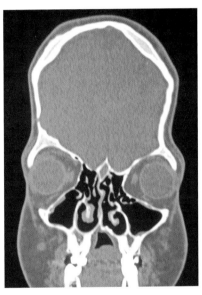

Fig. 3.22   A 15-year-old male with Crouzon syndrome. Coronal CT shows shallow orbits, hypertelorism, and mild maxillary hypoplasia.

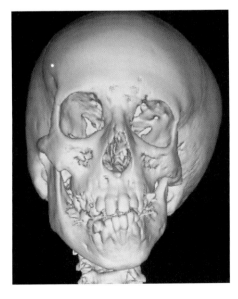

Fig. 3.23   A 12-year-old male with hemifacial microsomia (Goldenhar syndrome, oculoauriculovertebral spectrum). Coronal 3D/volume-rendered CT shows facial asymmetry from unilateral hypoplasia of the left maxilla and left maxillary sinus, left mandible, and left zygomatic arch.

Table 3.1 *(cont.)*   Congenital and developmental abnormalities

	Imaging Findings	Comments
Treacher Collins syndrome (**Fig. 3.24**)	Bilateral symmetric hypoplasia of the mandible (± absence of the mandibular rami—retrognathia), maxillae, and zygomatic arches, ± cleft palate, atresia of the external auditory canals, ossicular hypoplasia, deformed pinnae, and colobomas.	Autosomal dominant mutation of *TCOF1* gene on chromosome 5q32, which results in impaired function of the gene product treacle-protein. Deficiency of treacle protein causes apoptosis of embryonic neural crest cells, leading to bilateral symmetric hypoplasia of first branchial arch structures, such as the maxillae, mandibles, and zygomatic arches.
Silent sinus syndrome (**Fig. 3.25** and **Fig. 3.26**)	Small maxillary sinus with retained secretions, inward deviation of thinned bony walls and orbital floor, and nasal septal deviation toward the atelectatic maxillary sinus. Downward deviation of the orbital floor causes an increase in orbital volume, resulting in enophthalmos (posterior positioning of the eye within the orbit), and hypoglobus (inferior postioning of the eye in the orbit).	Uncommon subclinical inflammatory sinus disorder consisting of a unilateral atelectatic maxillary sinus resulting from hypoventilation of the maxillary sinus secondary to obstruction of the ostiomeatal complex. Hypoventilation leads to resorption of gases into the capillaries of the closed sinus, with resulting negative pressure, accumulation of secretions, and wall collapse, including the orbital floor. Collapse of the orbital floor causes posterior and inferior positioning of the eye (enophthalmos and hypoglobus, respectively) within the orbit secondary to increased orbital volume, resulting in facial/orbital asymmetry with a "sunken eye" appearance. Usually presents in the third to fifth decades. Treatment includes sinus surgery with orbital floor reconstruction.

(continued on page 284)

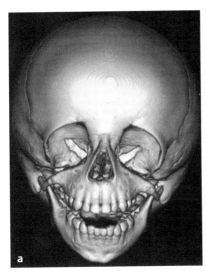
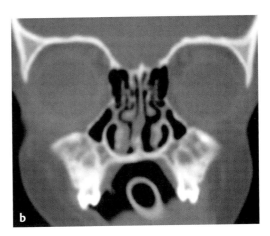

Fig. 3.24 A 3-year-old male with Treacher Collins syndrome. **(a)** Coronal volume-rendered CT and **(b)** coronal CT show bilateral symmetric hypoplasia of the maxillae, zygomatic arches, and mandible.

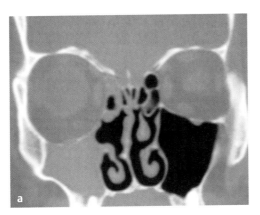
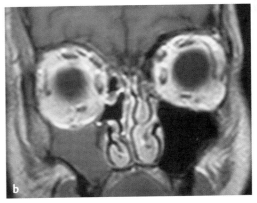

Fig. 3.25 A 48-year-old woman with silent sinus syndrome. **(a)** Coronal CT and **(b)** coronal T1-weighted imaging show a small right maxillary sinus with retained secretions, inward deviation of bony walls and orbital floor, and nasal septal deviation toward the atelectatic maxillary sinus. Downward deviation of the orbital floor causes an increase in orbital volume, resulting in enophthalmos.

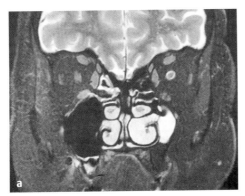
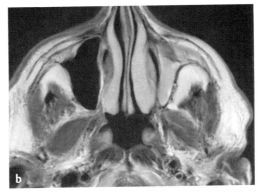

Fig. 3.26 A 69-year-old man with silent sinus syndrome. **(a)** Coronal fat-suppressed T2-weighted imaging and **(b)** axial T2-weighted imaging show a small left maxillary sinus with retained secretions and inward deviation of bony walls and orbital floor.

Table 3.1 *(cont.)*   Congenital and developmental abnormalities

	Imaging Findings	Comments
Infraorbital air cells (Haller cells) (**Fig. 3.27**)	Single or multiple ethmoid air cells that extend inferomedially under the orbit. Can be unilateral or bilateral. May be aerated or filled with retained secretions. Can result in narrowing the infundibulum of the ostiomeatal complex.	Ethmoid air cells that extend below the floor of the orbit and are located medial and inferior to the ethmoid bulla. Can narrow the infundibulum of the ostiomeatal complex.
Agger nasi cells (**Fig. 3.28**)	Single or multiple air cells in the lacrimal bone and/or frontal process of the maxilla, which are located anterior to the frontal recess, usually anterior or medial to the nasolacrimal canal.	Agger nasi is Latin for nasal mound. Agger nasi cells are air cells that occur within the lacrimal bone and/or frontal process of the maxilla, which are located anterior to the ethmoid bulla and vertical attachment of the middle turbinate to the skull base. Forms the anterior and inferior margins of the frontal recess. If enlarged, agger nasi cells can narrow the frontal recess, predisposing to obstruction of mucus drainage from the frontal sinus, with resultant sinusitis.
Frontoethmoidal (Kuhn) cells	*Type 1:* Single anterior ethmoid cell that extends only above an agger nasi cell into the frontal recess *Type 2:* Two or more anterior ethmoid air cells that extend above the agger nasi cells. *Type 3:* Single anterior ethmoid air cell above the agger nasi that extends above and anterior to the frontoethmoidal recess into the frontal sinus. *Type 4:* Isolated air cell within the anterior lower portion of the frontal sinus.	Accessory air cells located in the anterior portion of the frontoethmoidal recess superior to the agger nasi cells. Can result in narrowing of the frontoethmoidal recess predisposing to obstruction and sinus infections. Relevant for endoscopic surgical planning.
Onodi cell (**Fig. 3.29**)	Ethmoid air cell that extends posterolaterally above the sphenoid sinus and adjacent to the optic nerve canal.	Posterior ethmoid air cell that pneumatizes posterolateral and superior to the sphenoid sinus and adjacent to the optic nerve canal. Prevalence of 8–14%. Can extend around the optic canal, possibly causing confusion about the location of the optic canal relative to the sphenoid sinus during surgery. Inflammation of the Onodi cell (sinusitis) can cause optic neuropathy. Mucoceles involving the Onodi cell rarely occur.

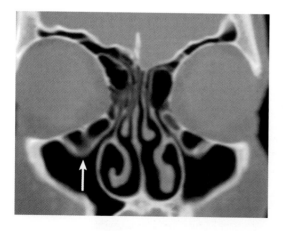

Fig. 3.27   Coronal CT shows bilateral infraorbital air cells (Haller cells), larger on the right (*arrow*) than on the left, which result in narrowing of the infundibula of both ostiomeatal complexes.

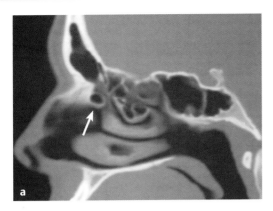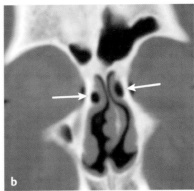

Fig. 3.28 **(a)** Sagittal and **(b)** coronal CT scans show agger nasi cells (*arrows*) in two different patients.

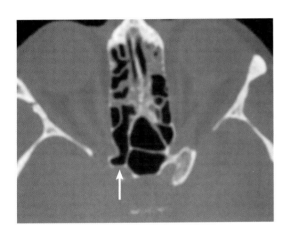

Fig. 3.29 A 31-year-old woman with an Onodi cell on the right (*arrow*) representing a posterior ethmoid air cell that extends posterolaterally above the sphenoid sinus and adjacent to the optic nerve canal.

Table 3.2 Solitary lesions involving the paranasal sinuses and nasal cavity

- Neoplasms—Benign
  - Osteoma
  - Ossifying fibroma
  - Inverted papilloma
  - Juvenile nasopharyngeal angiofibroma
  - Schwannoma
  - Minor salivary gland tumor
  - Hemangioma
  - Invasive pituitary adenoma
  - Odontogenic radicular (periapical) cyst
  - Odontogenic follicular (dentigerous) cyst
  - Keratocystic odontogenic tumor (odontogenic keratocyst)
  - Ameloblastoma
  - Odontogenic intraosseous myxoma
- Neoplasms—Malignant
  - Squamous cell carcinoma
  - Sinonasal undifferentiated carcinoma
  - Esthesioneuroblastoma
  - Adenoid cystic carcinoma
  - Adenocarcinoma and mucoepidermoid carcinoma
  - Melanoma
  - Lymphoma
  - Metastatic lesions
  - Myeloma
  - Osteosarcoma
  - Chordoma
  - Chondrosarcoma
  - Ewing's sarcoma
  - Rhabdomyosarcoma
  - Invasive pituitary carcinoma
- Tumorlike Lesions
  - Fibrous dysplasia
  - Paget disease
- Inflammatory Lesions
  - Mucous retention cyst/solitary polyp
  - Mucocele
  - Pyocele
  - Pott's puffy tumor
  - Rhinolith
  - Langerhans' cell histiocytosis

Table 3.2 Solitary lesions involving the paranasal sinuses and nasal cavity

Lesion	Imaging Findings	Comments
Neoplasms—Benign		
Osteoma (**Fig. 3.30**)	*CT:* Well-circumscribed lesions in the skull with high attenuation. *MRI:* Well-circumscribed lesions in the skull with low-intermediate signal on T1- and T2-weighted imaging, typically with no significant gadolinium contrast enhancement.	Benign primary bone tumor composed of dense lamellar, woven, and/or compact cortical bone usually located at the surface of the skull or paranasal sinuses (frontal (80%) > ethmoid > maxillary > sphenoid). Most common benign sinonasal tumor. Found in 3% of CT exams of the paranasal sinuses. Account for less than 1% of primary benign bone tumors. Present in patients 16 to 74 years old, most frequently in the sixth decade.
Ossifying fibroma (**Fig. 3.31** and **Fig. 3.32**)	*CT:* Expansile, well-circumscribed lesions in bone containing varying proportions of low, intermediate, and/or high attenuation based on the composition of fibrous, calcified, and ossified contents. *MRI:* Expansile, well-circumscribed osseous lesions that often have low-intermediate signal on T1-weighted imaging and mixed low, intermediate, and/or slightly high to high signal on T2-weighted imaging. Usually show heterogeneous gadolinium contrast enhancement.	Benign, rare, slow-growing fibro-osseous tumor composed of proliferating fibroblasts within fibrous stroma with varying amounts of woven and lamellar bone and cementumlike material replacing normal bone. Most commonly occur in the mandible, followed by the maxilla and paranasal sinuses. Female to male ratio of 2–9 to 1, age range 7 to 55 years, most commonly diagnosed in second to fourth decades. Two juvenile subtypes (trabecular and psammomatoid types) occur in children < 15 years old, have cell-rich fibrous stroma, and can show more rapid growth. The psammomatoid type contains small uniform ossicles, and the trabecular type contains trabeculae and osteoid and woven bone. Treatment is surgical excision or curettage, with recurrence rates of 8 to 28%.
Inverted papilloma (**Fig. 3.33**)	*CT:* Unilateral opacification of the nasal cavity, maxillary sinus, and ethmoid air cells, ± medial bulging of the nasal septum, remodeling and/or erosion of adjacent bone. *MRI:* Well-circumscribed lobulated or ovoid lesions at the lateral nasal wall that often extend medially to the nasal septum and laterally into the maxillary sinus via the infundibulum of the ostiomeatal complex. Tumors often have low-intermediate signal on T1-weighted imaging and intermediate to slightly high signal on T2-weighted imaging (T2WI). Striated linear zones with low signal may occur in the tumor on T2WI from high cellularity epithelial cells compared with the higher signal from the stroma resulting in a "cerebriform pattern." Tumors show heterogeneous gadolinium contrast enhancement, often in a cerebriform pattern.	Most common of three types of ectodermally derived papillary tumors arising from the ciliated respiratory mucosa lining the paranasal sinuses and nasal cavity (Schneiderian membrane). Usually occurs in patients from 40 to 70 years old and is more common in men than in women. Accounts for up to 4.7% of sinonasal tumors. Fifty times less common than inflammatory polyps. Tumors consist of ribbons of basement membrane enclosing multilayered epithelial cells that extend endophytically into stroma. Epithelial cell layers consist of ciliated columnar cells overlying nonkeratinizing squamous or transitional epithelial cells. Eighty-five percent are benign; 15% are malignant. May be associated with infection by human papillomavirus or Epstein-Barr virus. Immunoreactive to CD44; decreased immunoreactivity is associated with malignancy. Treatment is lateral rhinotomy and medial maxillectomy. Other types of Schneiderian papillomas include oncocytic and exophytic papillomas.

(continued on page 288)

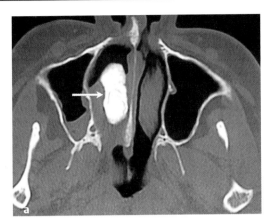
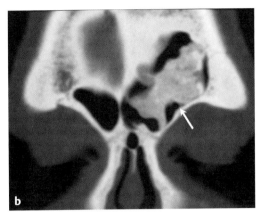

Fig. 3.30 **(a)** Axial CT of a 26-year-old woman and **(b)** coronal CT of a 70-year-old man shows osteomas (*arrows*) with high attenuation similar to cortical bone in the nasal cavity and left frontal sinus, respectively.

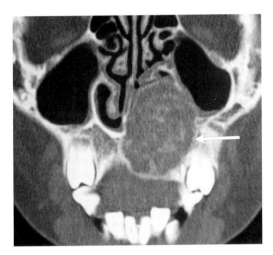

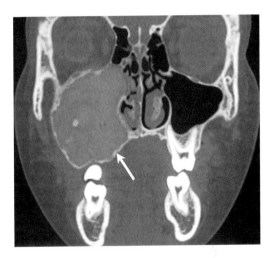

Fig. 3.31 Coronal CT of a 10-year-old male shows an ossifying fibroma (*arrow*) in the left maxilla that contains mixed low, intermediate, and high attenuation.

Fig. 3.32 Coronal CT of an 11-year-old female shows an ossifying fibroma (psammomatoid type) filling the right maxillary sinus (*arrow*), with mixed intermediate and slightly high attenuation as well as several small calcifications. The lesion is associated with expansion of the sinus, with thinned osseous margins.

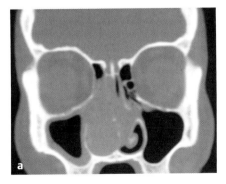
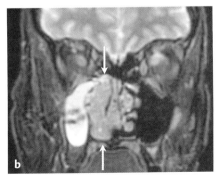
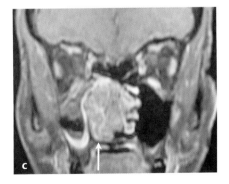

Fig. 3.33 A 44-year-old woman with an inverted papilloma. **(a)** Coronal CT shows opacification of the right nasal cavity and several right anterior ethmoid air cells. Also seen is medial bulging of the nasal septum with erosion of adjacent bone. **(b)** Coronal STIR shows a lesion with intermediate to slightly high signal at the lateral right nasal wall that extends medially to the nasal septum and laterally into the infundibulum of the right ostiomeatal complex (*arrows*). **(c)** The tumor shows heterogeneous gadolinium contrast enhancement in a cerebriform pattern on coronal fat-suppressed T1-weighted imaging (*arrow*).

Table 3.2 *(cont.)* Solitary lesions involving the paranasal sinuses and nasal cavity

Lesion	Imaging Findings	Comments
Juvenile nasopharyngeal angiofibroma (**Fig. 3.34**)	*CT:* Lesions often have intermediate attenuation, ± hemorrhage, erosion, and/or remodeling of adjacent bone, such as widening of the pterygopalatine/ pterygomaxillary fossae and/or sphenopalatine foramina and vidian canals. *MRI:* Origin of lesion is the pterygopalatine fossa. The lesions grow medially into the nasal cavity and nasopharynx via the sphenopalatine foramen, laterally into the pterygomaxillary fissure, and superiorly via the inferior orbital fissure into the orbital apex, ± middle cranial fossa via the superior orbital fissure. Lesions often have intermediate signal on T1-weighted imaging and slightly high to high signal on T2-weighted imaging, ± flow voids and prominent gadolinium contrast enhancement.	Benign cellular and vascularized mesenchymal lesion/ malformation that occurs in the posterolateral nasal wall or nasopharynx from testosterone-sensitive cells, associated with high propensity to hemorrhage. Composed of thin-walled slitlike or dilated vessels of varying sizes lined by endothelial cells within fibrous stroma containing spindle, round, or stellate cells and varying amounts of collagen. Immunoreactive to platelet-derived growth factor B, insulinlike growth factor type II, vimentin, and smooth muscle actin. Typically occurs in males, with peak age at presentation in the second decade, and incidence of 1 in 5,000–60,000. Exhibits locally aggressive growth, with erosion and/or remodeling of adjacent bone, and can spread through skull base foramina. Treatment can include embolization or hormonal treatment and, if necessary, surgical resection.
Schwannoma (**Fig. 3.35**)	*CT:* Circumscribed spheroid or ovoid lesions with intermediate attenuation, + contrast enhancement. *MRI:* Circumscribed spheroid or ovoid lesions with low-intermediate signal on T1-weighted imaging and high signal on T2-weighted imaging (T2WI) and fat-suppressed T2WI, and usually with prominent gadolinium (Gd) contrast enhancement. High signal on T2WI and Gd contrast enhancement can be heterogeneous in large lesions due to cystic degeneration and/or hemorrhage.	Schwannomas are benign encapsulated tumors that contain differentiated neoplastic Schwann cells. Can arise from ophthalmic or maxillary branches of the trigeminal nerve, branches of the olfactory nerve (filia olfactoria), or autonomic nerves. Multiple schwannomas are often associated with neurofibromatosis type 2 (NF2), which is an autosomal dominant disease involving a gene mutation at chromosome 22q12. In addition to schwannomas, patients with NF2 can also have multiple meningiomas and ependymomas. The incidence of NF2 is 1/37,000 to 1/50,000 newborns. Age at presentation is 22 to 72 years (mean age = 46 years). Peak incidence is in the fourth to sixth decades. Many patients with NF2 present in the third decade with bilateral vestibular schwannomas.
Minor salivary gland tumor (**Fig. 3.36**)	*CT:* Circumscribed or lobulated lesions with intermediate attenuation, + contrast enhancement. *MRI:* Circumscribed lesions with low-intermediate signal on T1-weighted imaging and slightly high signal on T2-weighted imaging (T2WI) and fat-suppressed T2WI, usually with gadolinium contrast enhancement.	This category includes benign glandular tumors of the sinonasal tract. Most common type is the pleomorphic adenoma composed of modified myoepithelial cells associated with sparse stromal elements. Most arise from the submucosa of the nasal septum or lateral sinus wall. Usually occur in patients between 20 and 60 years old. Other rare types of adenomas include myoepithelioma and oncocytoma.

(continued on page 290)

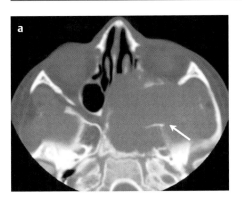
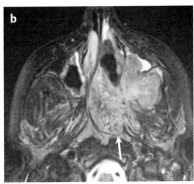
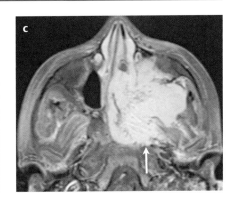

Fig. 3.34 An 11-year-old male with a juvenile nasopharyngeal angiofibroma. **(a)** Axial CT shows a large lesion with intermediate attenuation in the left nasopharynx associated with erosion and remodeling of adjacent bone (*arrow*). The lesion extends into the left nasal cavity and laterally into the pterygomaxillary fissure. **(b)** The lesion has heterogeneous slightly high to high signal on axial fat-suppressed T2-weighted imaging with flow voids (*arrow*) and **(c)** shows prominent gadolinium contrast enhancement on axial fat-suppressed T1-weighted imaging (*arrow*).

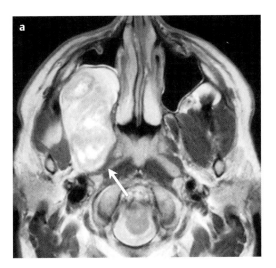
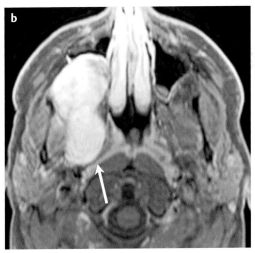

Fig. 3.35 A 30-year-old man with a trigeminal schwannoma that extends into the right maxillary sinus. **(a)** The lesion has circumscribed margins and heterogeneous mostly high signal on axial T2-weighted imaging (*arrow*), and **(b)** shows gadolinium contrast enhancement on axial fat-suppressed T1-weighted imaging (*arrow*).

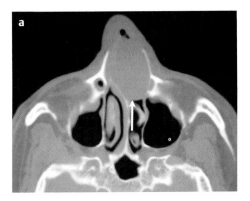
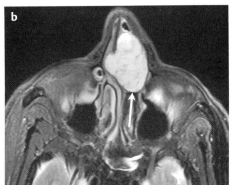
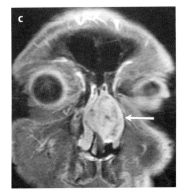

Fig. 3.36 A 46-year-old man with a pleomorphic adenoma involving the nasal septum that has **(a)** intermediate attenuation on axial CT (*arrow*), **(b)** heterogeneous high signal on axial fat-suppressed T2-weighted imaging (*arrow*), and **(c)** heterogeneous gadolinium contrast enhancement on coronal fat-suppressed T1-weighted imaging (*arrow*).

Table 3.2 *(cont.)*   Solitary lesions involving the paranasal sinuses and nasal cavity

Lesion	Imaging Findings	Comments
Hemangioma **(Fig. 3.37)**	*CT:* Expansile bony lesions with a radiating pattern of bony trabeculae oriented toward the center. Hemangiomas in soft tissue have mostly intermediate attenuation, ± zones of fat attenuation. *MRI:* Circumscribed or poorly marginated structures (< 4 cm in diameter) in bone marrow or soft tissue with intermediate-high signal on T1-weighted imaging (often isointense to marrow fat) and high signal on T2-weighted imaging (T2WI) and fat-suppressed T2WI, and typically gadolinium contrast enhancement, ± expansion of bone.	Benign lesions of bone or soft tissue composed of capillary, cavernous, and/or malformed venous vessels. Considered to be a hamartomatous disorder. Hemangiomas occur in patients 1 to 84 years old (median age = 33 years).
Invasive pituitary adenoma	*CT:* Often has intermediate attenuation, ± necrosis, ± cyst, ± hemorrhage, usually with contrast enhancement, extension into suprasellar cistern with waist at diaphragma sella, ± extension into cavernous sinus, and can invade the skull base. *MRI:* Often has intermediate signal on T1- and T2-weighted imaging, often similar to gray matter, ± necrosis, ± cyst, ± hemorrhage, usually with prominent gadolinium contrast enhancement, extension into suprasellar cistern with waist at diaphragma sella, ± extension into cavernous sinus, and occasionally invasion of skull base.	Histologically benign pituitary macroadenomas can occasionally have an invasive growth pattern, with extension into the sphenoid bone, clivus, ethmoid sinus, orbits, and/or interpeduncular cistern.
Odontogenic radicular (periapical) cyst **(Fig. 3.38)**	*CT:* Circumscribed zone of decreased attenuation at the apex of a tooth and adjacent maxilla, ± thin rim of sclerotic bone, ± cortical expansion from the cyst, ± resorption of tooth apex and adjacent teeth, ± displacement of adjacent teeth and mandibular canal. *MRI:* Cyst contents have variable signal on T1-weighted imaging related to protein concentration and usually have slightly high to high signal on T2-weighted imaging. A thin peripheral rim of gadolinium contrast enhancement is often present.	Most common type of odontogenic cyst. Results from trauma, dental caries, and chronic infection of a tooth causing periapical periodontitis, periapical abscess, and/or periapical granuloma. Borders can consist of a thin rim of cortical bone lined by squamous epithelium. Usually occurs in adults between 30 and 50 years old. Treatment includes tooth extraction and periodontal therapy.
Odontogenic follicular (dentigerous) cyst **(Fig. 3.39)**	*CT:* Well-circumscribed radiolucent lesion adjacent to the crown of an un-erupted tooth, ± thin sclerotic margin. The roots of the affected tooth are usually outside the lesion. Can become large adjacent to the roots of other teeth. Cortical bone margins are usually intact, except in large lesions. *MRI:* Circumscribed lesions with high signal on T2-weighted imaging (T2WI), ± zones of low signal on T2WI. Thin peripheral gadolinium contrast enhancement is seen along the walls of the lesion. The un-erupted tooth has low signal on T1- and T2WI.	Common maxillary cyst of odontogenic cell origin associated with un-erupted teeth. Fluid collects between the epithelium and tooth enamel. Often presents in patients between 30 and 40 years old. Usually occur as solitary lesions; multiple lesions can be seen with mucopolysaccharidoses and cleidocranial dysplasia. Treatment includes enucleation for small lesions and surgical drainage with marsupialization for large lesions.

(continued on page 292)

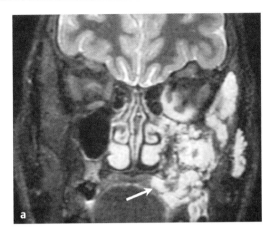
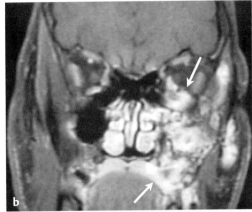

Fig. 3.37 A 19-year-old man with a hemangioma involving the soft tissues of the left face, left palate, left maxilla, left maxillary sinus, left orbit, and left temporalis muscle. **(a)** The infiltrative lesion has high signal on coronal fat-suppressed T2-weighted imaging (*arrow*) and **(b)** shows gadolinium contrast enhancement on coronal fat-suppressed T1-weighted imaging (*arrows*).

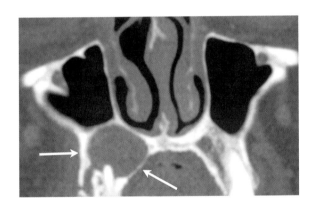

Fig. 3.38 Coronal CT shows a radicular cyst (*arrows*) that is seen as a circumscribed zone of decreased attenuation at the apex of a tooth and adjacent maxilla and is associated with cortical expansion toward the right maxillary sinus and hard palate.

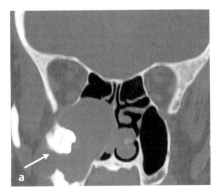
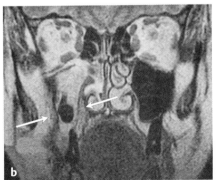
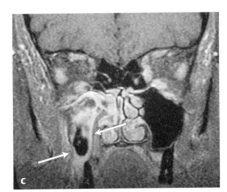

Fig. 3.39 Odontogenic dentigerous/follicular cyst. **(a)** Coronal CT shows a well-circumscribed radiolucent lesion adjacent to the crown of an un-erupted tooth (*arrow*) in the right maxillary sinus with expanded, thinned, bony margins. **(b)** The right maxillary sinus is filled with high-signal material on coronal T2-weighted imaging (*arrows*). **(c)** Irregular peripheral gadolinium contrast enhancement is seen in the right maxillary sinus on coronal fat-suppressed T1-weighted imaging (*arrows*). The un-erupted tooth has low signal on T2-weighted imaging **(b)**, and on fat-suppressed T1-weighted imaging **(c)**.

Table 3.2 *(cont.)*   Solitary lesions involving the paranasal sinuses and nasal cavity

Lesion	Imaging Findings	Comments
Keratocystic odontogenic tumor (odontogenic keratocyst) **(Fig. 3.40)**	*CT:* Well-circumscribed unilocular or multilocular radiolucent lesions in the maxilla, ± thin sclerotic margins, ± associated impacted tooth, ± thinning and expansion of cortical bone. *MRI:* Circumscribed lesions with intermediate signal on T1-weighted imaging and intermediate to high signal on T2-weighted imaging related to variable protein content. Thin peripheral gadolinium contrast enhancement is seen along the walls of the lesion.	Benign, locally aggressive tumors derived from the stratified keratinizing squamous epithelium of the dental lamina and overlying alveolar mucosa. Account for up to 17% of jaw cysts. Often present in patients beween the second and fourth decades. Can be either solitary or multiple in association with the basal cell nevus syndrome (Gorlin-Goltz syndrome).
Ameloblastoma **(Fig. 3.41)**	*CT:* Lesions are often radiolucent, with associated bone expansion and cortical thinning, ± hyperostotic margins. *MRI:* Tumors often have circumscribed margins and can have mixed low, intermediate, and/or high signal on T1-weighted imaging, T2-weighted imaging (T2WI), and fat-suppressed T2WI. Cystic portions have high signal on T2WI. Lesions can show heterogeneous irregular gadolinium contrast enhancement.	The most common odontogenic tumor, ameloblastomas are slow-growing, benign, locally aggressive epithelial tumors that contain epithelioid cells (basaloid and/or squamous types) associated with regions of spindle cells and fibrous stroma. These odontogenic tumors fail to form calcified tooth enamel or dentin. Five subtypes: unicystic, solid and multicystic, desmoplastic, peripheral, and malignant. Eighty percent of these tumors occur in the mandible, and they typically lack metastatic potential except for the malignant subtype.
Odontogenic intraosseous myxoma **(Fig. 3.42)**	*CT:* Lesions occur as unilocular or multilocular radiolucent zones with associated bone expansion and cortical scalloping and thinning, ± cortical interruption, ± fine bony trabeculae, ± extension into adjacent structures, such as the nasal or oral cavities, paranasal sinuses, or orbits. In the maxilla, lesions often occur in the premolar, molar, and tuberosity areas. In the mandible, lesions often occur in the body and ramus. *MRI:* Tumors often have circumscribed margins and can have mixed low and intermediate signal on T1-weighted imaging and heterogeneous intermediate, slightly high, and/or high signal on T2-weighted imaging (T2WI). Myxoid portions have high signal on T2WI. Lesions show heterogeneous, irregular gadolinium contrast enhancement.	Rare, benign, locally invasive, non-encapsulated tumor that arises from the odontogenic ectomesenchyme of a developing tooth or undifferentiated mesenchymal cells in the periodontal ligament. Tumors contain loosely arranged spindle, round, and/or stellate cells within myxoid stroma. Account for 3 to 9% of odontogenic tumors, and typically occur in patients between 10 and 40 years old (mean age = 31 years), with a female/male predominance of 2/1. The tumors occur in the maxilla and mandible and only rarely in other bones. Treatment is surgical excision and reconstruction.

(continued on page 294)

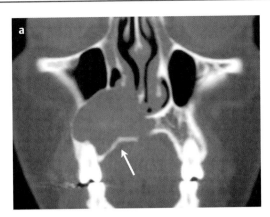
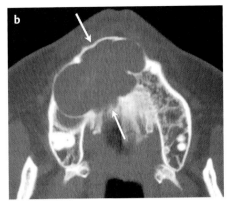

Fig. 3.40 Keratocystic odontogenic tumor. **(a)** Coronal CT of a 16-year-old male and **(b)** axial CT of a 22-year-old male show well-circumscribed unilocular radiolucent lesion involving the right maxilla, with expanded, thin, sclerotic margins (*arrows*).

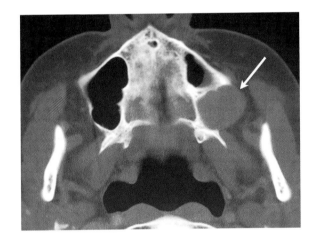

Fig. 3.41 Ameloblastoma. Axial CT shows a radiolucent lesion in the left maxilla with soft tissue attenuation (*arrow*).

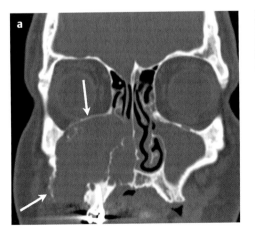
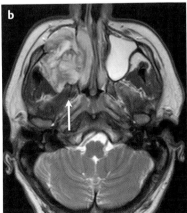
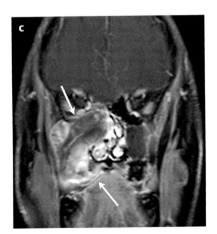

Fig. 3.42 A 32-year-old man with an odontogenic myxoma. **(a)** Coronal CT shows a lesion (*arrows*) with soft tissue attenuation in the right maxillary sinus associated with expansion of thinned and interrupted cortical margins and extension into the right nasal cavity. **(b)** The lesion has mixed low, intermediate, slightly high, and high signal on axial T2-weighted imaging (*arrow*) and **(c)** shows heterogeneous irregular gadolinium contrast enhancement on coronal fat-suppressed T1-weighted imaging (*arrows*).

Table 3.2 *(cont.)* Solitary lesions involving the paranasal sinuses and nasal cavity

Lesion	Imaging Findings	Comments
Neoplasms—Malignant		
Squamous cell carcinoma **(Fig. 3.43)**	*CT:* Tumors have intermediate attenuation and mild contrast enhancement, and can be large lesions (± necrosis and/or hemorrhage). *MRI:* Lesions in the nasal cavity, paranasal sinuses, nasopharynx, ± intracranial extension via bone destruction or perineural spread. Tumors have intermediate signal on T1-weighted imaging, intermediate to slightly high signal on T2-weighted imaging, and mild gadolinium contrast enhancement. Can be large lesions (± necrosis and/or hemorrhage).	Malignant epithelial tumors originating from the mucosal epithelium of the paranasal sinuses (maxillary, 60%; ethmoid, 14%; sphenoid and frontal sinuses, 1%) and nasal cavity (25%). Include both keratinizing and nonkeratinizing types. Account for 80% of malignant sinonasal tumors and 3% of malignant tumors of the head and neck. Occur in adults usually > 55 years old, and occur in males more than in females. Associated with occupational or other exposure to tobacco smoke, nickel, chlorophenols, chromium, mustard gas, radium, and material in the manufacture of wood products.
Sinonasal undifferentiated carcinoma **(Fig. 3.44)**	*CT:* Tumors have intermediate attenuation and variable mild, moderate, or prominent contrast enhancement. *MRI:* Locally destructive lesions usually larger than 4 cm, with low-intermediate signal on T1-weighted imaging and intermediate-high signal on T2-weighted imaging, + prominent gadolinium contrast enhancement. Locations: superior nasal cavity and ethmoid air cells, with occasional extension into the other paranasal sinuses, orbits, anterior cranial fossa, and cavernous sinuses.	Malignant tumor composed of pleomorphic neoplastic cells with medium to large nuclei, prominent single nucleoli, and small amounts of eosinophilic cytoplasm. Mitotic activity is typically high and necrosis is common. Immunoreactive to CK7, CK8, and CK19, ± to p53, epithelial membrane antigen, and neuron-specific enolase. Poor prognosis, with 5-year survival of less than 20%.
Esthesioneuroblastoma **(Fig. 3.45)**	*CT:* Tumors have intermediate attenuation and variable mild, moderate, or prominent contrast enhancement. *MRI:* Locally destructive lesions with low-intermediate signal on T1-weighted imaging and intermediate-high signal on T2-weighted imaging, + prominent gadolinium contrast enhancement, ± tumoral cysts. Locations: superior nasal cavity and ethmoid air cells, with occasional extension into the other paranasal sinuses, orbits, anterior cranial fossa, and cavernous sinuses.	Also referred to as olfactory neuroblastoma, these malignant neoplasms of neuroectodermal origin arise from olfactory epithelium in the upper nasal cavity and cribriform region. Tumors consist of immature neuroblasts with variable nuclear pleomorphism, mitoses, and necrosis. Tumor cells occur in a neurofibrillary intercellular matrix. Bimodal occurrence in adolescents (11–20 years old) and adults (50–60 years old), and occur in males more than in females.

(continued on page 296)

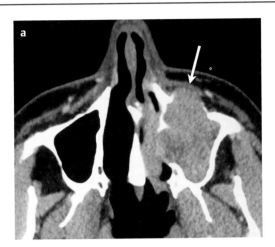
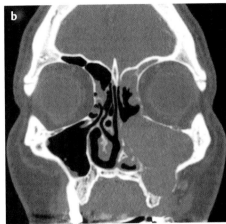

Fig. 3.43 **(a)** Axial and **(b)** coronal CT of a 65-year-old woman shows a squamous cell carcinoma in the left maxillary sinus that has soft tissue attenuation and extends anteriorly (*arrow*), medially and inferiorly through sites of bone destruction.

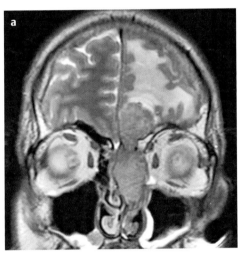
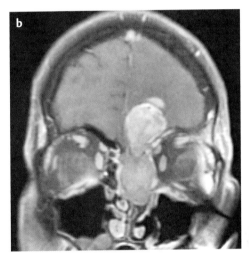

Fig. 3.44 A 47-year-old woman with a sinonasal undifferentiated carcinoma in the left ethmoid sinus that extends intracranially and inferiorly into the left nasal cavity through sites of bone destruction. **(a)** The tumor has intermediate to slightly high signal on coronal T2-weighted imaging and **(b)** shows gadolinium contrast enhancement on coronal fat-suppressed T1-weighted imaging.

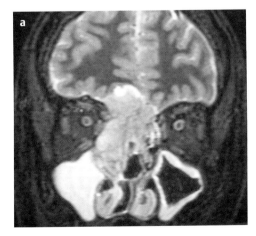
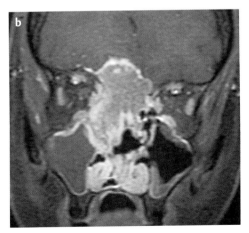

Fig. 3.45 A 30-year-old woman with an esthesioneuroblastoma in the right ethmoid sinus that is associated with bone destruction and tumor extension intracranially, inferiorly into the right nasal cavity, medially into the left ethmoid sinus, and laterally into the right orbit. **(a)** The tumor has slightly high signal on coronal fat-suppressed T2-weighted imaging and **(b)** shows gadolinium contrast enhancement on coronal fat-suppressed T1-weighted imaging.

Table 3.2 *(cont.)*   Solitary lesions involving the paranasal sinuses and nasal cavity

Lesion	Imaging Findings	Comments
Adenoid cystic carcinoma (**Fig. 3.46**)	*CT:* Tumors have intermediate attenuation and variable mild, moderate, or prominent contrast enhancement. Destruction of adjacent bone is commonly seen. *MRI:* Lesions in the nasal cavity or sinuses with intracranial extension via bone destruction or perineural spread, intermediate signal on T1-weighted imaging and intermediate-high signal on T2-weighted imaging, and variable mild, moderate, or prominent gadolinium contrast enhancement.	Basaloid tumor composed of neoplastic epithelial and myoepithelial cells. Morphologic tumor patterns include tubular, cribriform, and solid. Most common sinonasal malignancy of salivary gland origin. Accounts for 10% of epithelial salivary neoplasms. Most commonly involves the parotid, submandibular, and minor salivary glands (palate, tongue, buccal mucosa, and floor of the mouth, other locations). Perineural tumor spread common, ± facial nerve paralysis. Usually occurs in adults > 30 years old. Solid type has the worst prognosis. Up to 90% of patients die 10–15 years after diagnosis.
Adenocarcinoma and mucoepidermoid carcinoma	*CT:* Tumors have intermediate attenuation and variable mild, moderate, or prominent contrast enhancement. Destruction of adjacent bone is commonly seen. *MRI:* Lesions in the nasal cavity or paranasal sinuses with intracranial extension via bone destruction or perineural spread, intermediate signal on T1-weighted imaging, intermediate-high signal on T2-weighted imaging, and variable mild, moderate, or prominent gadolinium contrast enhancement.	Second and third most common malignant sinonasal tumors derived from salivary glands. Adenocarcinomas contain small to medium-sized neoplastic cells with oval nuclei, typically immunoreactive to cytokeratin, vimentin, and S-100 protein. Mucoepidermoid carcinomas often have solid portions with basaloid or cuboidal neoplastic cells, and cystic portions containing sialomucin lined by mucous cells with peripheral nuclei within pale cytoplasm. Most commonly occur in the maxillary sinus and nasal cavity. Tumors usually are intermediate to high grade, and often are advanced at presentation, ± metastases, ± perineural tumor spread.
Melanoma (**Fig. 3.47** and **Fig. 3.48**)	*CT:* Tumors have intermediate attenuation and variable mild, moderate, or prominent contrast enhancement. Destruction of adjacent bone is commonly seen. *MRI:* Tumors can have well-defined or irregular margins, and usually have intermediate or slightly high signal on T1-weighted imaging, depending on the melanin content, and low-intermediate to slightly high signal on T2-weighted imaging (T2WI) and fat-suppressed T2WI. Tumors usually show gadolinium contrast enhancement, ± destruction of adjacent bone.	Rare malignant tumors with melanocytic differentiation (immunoreactive to S-100 protein, HMB45) that occur in patients between 10 and 50 years old. Primary sinonasal melanoma accounts for less than 2.5% of all melanomas. Commonly occurs in the nasal septum, lateral nasal wall, and turbinates. Forty percent have lymph node metastases at presentation, and local recurrence occurs in up to 65% of cases.

(continued on page 298)

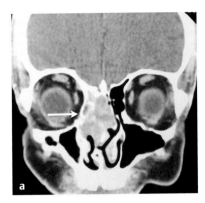
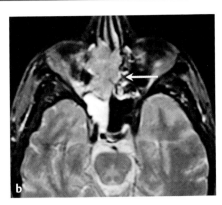
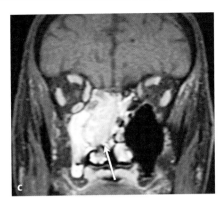

Fig. 3.46 A 55-year-old man with an adenoid cystic carcinoma in the right ethmoid sinus that is associated with bone destruction and tumor extension medially into the left ethmoid sinus and inferiorly into the right nasal cavity. **(a)** The tumor has intermediate to slightly high attenuation on coronal CT (*arrow*), **(b)** intermediate to slightly high signal on axial fat-suppressed T2-weighted imaging, and **(c)** shows gadolinium contrast enhancement on coronal fat-suppressed T1-weighted imaging (*arrow*).

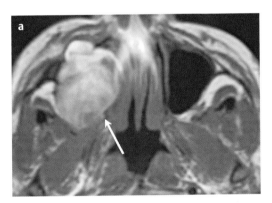
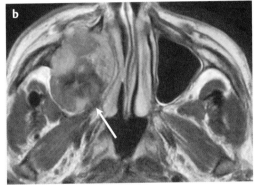

Fig. 3.47 **(a)** A 90-year-old woman with a melanoma in the right maxillary sinus that has heterogeneous high and slightly high signal on axial T1-weighted imaging (*arrow*) and **(b)** mixed low, intermediate, and slightly high signal on axial T2-weighted imaging (*arrow*).

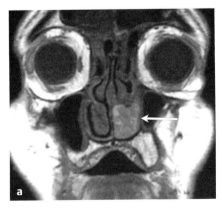
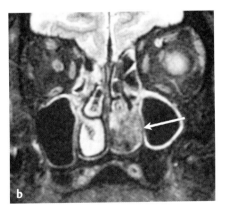
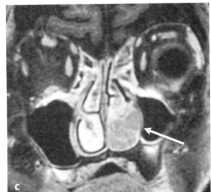

Fig. 3.48 **(a)** A 77-year-old man with a melanoma involving the left inferior turbinate. The tumor has slightly high signal on coronal T1-weighted imaging (*arrow*), **(b)** mixed low, intermediate, and slightly high signal on coronal STIR (*arrow*), and **(c)** gadolinium contrast enhancement on coronal fat-suppressed T1-weighted imaging (*arrow*).

Table 3.2 *(cont.)*   Solitary lesions involving the paranasal sinuses and nasal cavity

Lesion	Imaging Findings	Comments
Lymphoma **(Fig. 3.49)**	*CT:* Lesions have low-intermediate attenuation and may show contrast enhancement, ± bone destruction. *MRI:* Lesions have low-intermediate signal on T1-weighted imaging and intermediate to slightly high signal on T2-weighted imaging, ± restricted diffusion, + gadolinium contrast enhancement. Lesions are locally invasive, associated with bone erosion/destruction, and can have intracranial extension with meningeal involvement (up to 5%). B-cell non-Hodgkin lymphoma (NHL) often occurs in the maxillary sinuses, whereas T-cell NHL frequently occurs in the midline, including the septum.	Lymphoma represents a group of malignancies whose neoplastic cells typically arise within lymphoid tissue (lymph nodes and reticuloendothelial organs). Most lymphomas in the nasopharynx, nasal cavity, and paranasal sinuses are non-Hodgkin lymphomas (B-cell types more common than T-cell types), and are more commonly disseminated disease than primary sinonasal tumors. Sinonasal lymphoma has a poor prognosis, with 5-year survival of less than 65%.
Metastatic lesions **(Fig. 3.50)**	Single or multiple well-circumscribed or poorly defined lesions. *CT:* Intraosseous lesions are usually radiolucent, may also be sclerotic, ± extraosseous tumor extension, usually + contrast enhancement, ± compression of neural tissue or vessels. *MRI:* Single or multiple well-circumscribed or poorly defined lesions involving the craniofacial bones with low-intermediate signal on T1-weighted imaging and intermediate-high signal on T2-weighted imaging, usually showing gadolinium contrast enhancement, ± bone destruction, ± compression of neural tissue or vessels.	Metastatic lesions represent proliferating neoplastic cells that are located in sites or organs separated or distant from their origins. Metastatic carcinoma is the most frequent malignant tumor involving bone. In adults, metastatic lesions to bone occur most frequently from carcinomas of the lung, breast, prostate, kidney, and thyroid, as well as from sarcomas. Primary malignancies of the lung, breast, and prostate account for 80% of bone metastases. Metastatic tumor may cause variable destructive or infiltrative changes in single or multiple sites of involvement.
Myeloma **(Fig. 3.51)**	Multiple myeloma or single plasmacytoma are well-circumscribed or poorly defined lesions involving the craniofacial bones. *CT:* Lesions have low-intermediate attenuation, usually + contrast enhancement, + bone destruction. *MRI:* Well-circumscribed or poorly defined lesions involving the skull and dura with low-intermediate signal on T1-weighted imaging and intermediate-high signal on T2-weighted imaging, usually with gadolinium contrast enhancement, + bone destruction.	Multiple myeloma are malignant tumors composed of proliferating antibody-secreting plasma cells derived from single clones. Multiple myeloma is primarily located in bone marrow. A solitary myeloma or plasmacytoma is an infrequent variant in which a neoplastic mass of plasma cells occurs at a single site in bone or soft tissues. In the United States, 14,600 new cases occur per year. Multiple myeloma is the most common primary neoplasm of bone in adults. Median age at presentation = 60 years. Most patients are more than 40 years old. Tumors occur in the vertebrae > ribs > femur > iliac bone > humerus > craniofacial bones > sacrum > clavicle > sternum > pubic bone > tibia.

(continued on page 300)

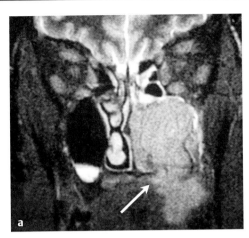
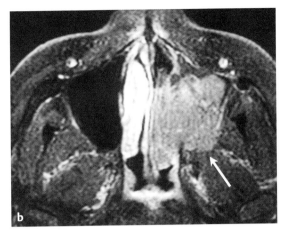

Fig. 3.49 A 59-year-old man with non-Hodgkin lymphoma in the left maxillary sinus that is associated with bone destruction and tumor extension medially into the left nasal cavity, laterally and inferiorly. **(a)** The tumor has slightly high to high signal on coronal fat-suppressed T2-weighted imaging (*arrow*) and **(b)** shows gadolinium contrast enhancement on axial fat-suppressed T1-weighted imaging (*arrow*).

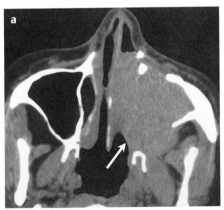
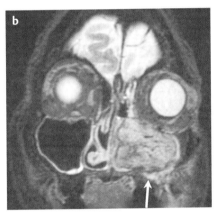
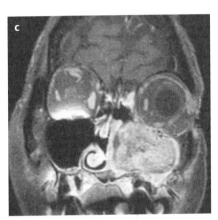

Fig. 3.50 **(a)** A 70-year-old woman with renal cell carcinoma and a metastatic lesion involving the left maxillary sinus that is associated with bone destruction and tumor extension medially into the left nasal cavity anteriorly, posteriorly, and inferiorly. The tumor has intermediate attenuation on axial CT (*arrow*), **(b)** slightly high to high signal on coronal fat-suppressed T2-weighted imaging (*arrow*), and **(c)** gadolinium contrast enhancement on coronal fat-suppressed T1-weighted imaging.

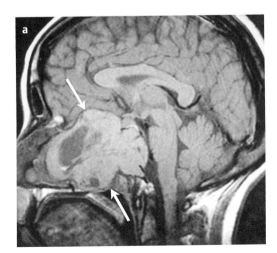
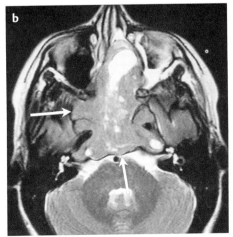

Fig. 3.51 A 28-year-old woman with a large plasmacytoma in the nasal cavity, nasopharynx, ethmoid and sphenoid sinuses, clivus, and sella on **(a)** sagittal T1-weighted imaging (*arrows*) and **(b)** axial T2-weighted imaging (*arrows*).

Table 3.2 *(cont.)*   Solitary lesions involving the paranasal sinuses and nasal cavity

Lesion	Imaging Findings	Comments
Osteosarcoma (**Fig. 3.52**)	*CT:* Tumors have low-intermediate attenuation, usually with matrix mineralization/ossification, + bone destruction, and often show contrast enhancement (usually heterogeneous). *MRI:* Tumors often have poorly defined margins and commonly extend from the marrow through destroyed bone cortex into adjacent soft tissues. Tumors usually have low-intermediate signal on T1-weighted imaging. Zones of low signal often correspond to areas of tumor calcification/mineralization and/or necrosis. Zones of necrosis typically have high signal on T2-weighted imaging (T2WI), whereas mineralized zones usually have low signal on T2WI. Tumors can have variable signal on T2WI and fat-suppressed (FS) T2WI depending upon the relative amounts of calcified/mineralized osteoid, chondroid, fibroid, hemorrhagic, and necrotic components. Tumors may have low, low-intermediate, and intermediate to high signal on T2WI and FS T2WI. After gadolinium contrast administration, osteosarcomas typically show prominent enhancement in nonmineralized/calcified portions.	Osteosarcomas are malignant tumors composed of proliferating neoplastic spindle cells, which produce osteoid and/or immature tumoral bone. Osteosarcomas occur in children as primary tumors and in adults they are associated with Paget disease, irradiated bone, chronic osteomyelitis, osteoblastoma, giant cell tumor, and fibrous dysplasia.
Chordoma (**Fig. 3.53**)	Well-circumscribed, lobulated lesions along dorsal surface of clivus, vertebral bodies, or sacrum, + localized bone destruction. *CT:* Lesions have low-intermediate attenuation, ± calcifications from destroyed bone carried away by tumor, + contrast enhancement. *MRI:* Lesions have low-intermediate signal on T1-weighted images and high signal on T2-weighted imaging, + gadolinium contrast enhancement (usually heterogeneous). Lesions are locally invasive and are associated with bone erosion/destruction and encasement of vessels (usually without arterial narrowing) and nerves. Skull base-clivus is a common location, usually in the midline for conventional chordomas, which account for 80% of skull base chordomas. Chondroid chordomas tend to be located off midline near skull base synchondroses..	Rare, locally aggressive, slow-growing, low to intermediate grade malignant tumors derived from ectopic notochordal remnants along the axial skeleton. Chondroid chondromas (5–15% of all chordomas) have both chordomatous and chondromatous differentiation. Chordomas that contain sarcomatous components (5% of all chordomas) are referred to as dedifferentiated or sarcomatoid chordomas. Chordomas account for 2–4% of primary malignant bone tumors, 1–3% of all primary bone tumors, and less than 1% of intracranial tumors. The annual incidence has been reported to be 0.18 to 0.3 per million. Dedifferentiated or sarcomatoid chordomas account for less than 5% of all chordomas. For cranial chordomas, patients' mean age = 37 to 40 years.
Chondrosarcoma (**Fig. 3.54**)	Lobulated lesions with bone destruction at synchondroses. *CT:* Lesions have low-intermediate attenuation associated with localized bone destruction, ± chondroid matrix calcifications, + contrast enhancement. *MRI:* Lesions have low- intermediate signal on T1-weighted imaging, high signal on T2-weighted imaging (T2WI), ± matrix mineralization with low signal on T2WI, + gadolinium contrast enhancement (usually heterogeneous). Tumors are locally invasive and are associated with bone erosion/destruction and encasement of vessels and nerves. Commonly located at the skull base in petro-occipital synchondrosis, usually off midline.	Chondrosarcomas are malignant tumors containing cartilage formed within sarcomatous stroma. Chondrosarcomas can contain areas of calcification/mineralization, myxoid material, and/or ossification. Chondrosarcomas rarely arise within synovium. Chondrosarcomas represent 12–21% of malignant bone lesions, 21–26% of primary sarcomas of bone, 9–14% of all bone tumors, 6% of skull-base tumors, and 0.15% of all intracranial tumors.

(continued on page 302)

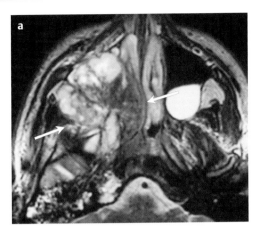
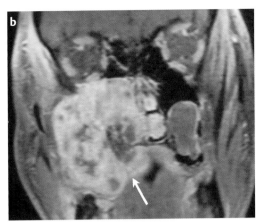

Fig. 3.52 A 27-year-old man with an osteosarcoma involving the right maxillary sinus that is associated with bone destruction and tumor extension medially into the right nasal cavity anteriorly, laterally, posteriorly, and inferiorly. **(a)** The tumor has mixed low, intermediate, and high signal on axial T2-weighted imaging (*arrows*) and **(b)** gadolinium contrast enhancement on coronal fat-suppressed T1-weighted imaging (*arrow*).

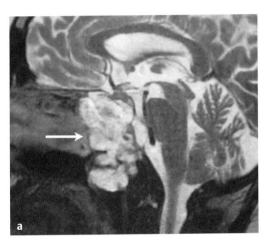
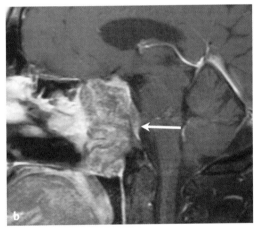

Fig. 3.53 A 77-year-old woman with a clival chordoma that is associated with bone destruction and tumor extension anteriorly into the sella, sphenoid sinus, and nasopharynx. The tumor also destroys the clivus and extends intracranially into the prepontine cistern. **(a)** The tumor has heterogeneous, mostly high signal on sagittal fat-suppressed T2-weighted imaging (*arrow*) and **(b)** gadolinium contrast enhancement on sagittal fat-suppressed T1-weighted imaging (*arrow*).

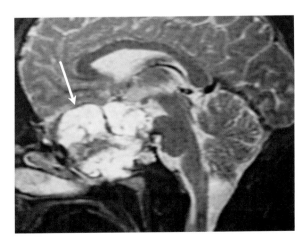

Fig. 3.54 A 24-year-old man with a chondrosarcoma (*arrow*) that involves the ethmoid and sphenoid sinuses and that is associated with bone destruction and tumor extension intracranially as well as into the nasopharynx, nasal cavity, and sella. The tumor has heterogeneous, mostly high signal on sagittal fat-suppressed T2-weighted imaging, as well as irregular zones with low signal.

Table 3.2 *(cont.)* Solitary lesions involving the paranasal sinuses and nasal cavity

Lesion	Imaging Findings	Comments
Ewing's sarcoma (**Fig. 3.55**)	*CT:* Destructive lesions that involve the skull base, with low-intermediate attenuation, and that can show contrast enhancement (usually heterogeneous). *MRI:* Destructive lesions involving the craniofacial bones, with low-intermediate signal on T1-weighted imaging and mixed low, intermediate, and high signal on T2-weighted imaging, + gadolinium contrast enhancement (usually heterogeneous).	Malignant primitive tumor of bone composed of undifferentiated small cells with round nuclei. Accounts for 6–11% of primary malignant bone tumors and 5–7% of primary bone tumors. Ewing's sarcomas commonly have translocations involving chromosomes 11 and 22: t(11;22) (q24:q12), which results in fusion of the FL1-1 gene at 11q24 to the EWS gene at 22q12. Usually occurs in patients between 5 and 30 years old, and in males more than in females. Rare lesions involving the skull base that are locally invasive, with high metastatic potential.
Rhabdomyosarcoma (**Fig. 3.56**)	*CT:* Soft tissue lesions that usually can have circumscribed or irregular margins. Calcifications are uncommon. Tumors can have mixed attenuation, with solid zones of soft tissue attenuation, cystic appearing and/or necrotic zones, and occasional foci of hemorrhage, ± bone invasion and destruction. *MRI:* Tumors can have circumscribed and/or poorly defined margins, and typically have low-intermediate signal on T1-weighted imaging and heterogeneous signal (various combinations of intermediate, slightly high, and/or high signal) on T2-weighted imaging (T2WI) and fat-suppressed T2WI. Tumors show variable degrees of gadolinium contrast enhancement, ± bone destruction and invasion.	Malignant mesenchymal tumors with rhabdomyoblastic differentiation that occur primarily in soft tissue and only very rarely in bone. There are three subgroups of rhabdomyosarcoma (embryonal, 50 to 70%; alveolar, 18 to 45%; and pleomorphic, 5 to 10%). Embryonal and alveolar rhabdomyosarcomas occur primarily in children < 10 years old, and pleomorphic rhabdomyosarcomas occur mostly in adults. Pleomorphic rhabdomyosarcomas typically occur in adults (median age = sixth decade). Alveolar and pleomorphic rhabdomyosarcomas occur frequently in the extremities. Embryonal rhabdomyosarcomas occur mostly in the head and neck.
Invasive pituitary carcinoma	*CT:* These tumors often have intermediate attenuation, ± necrosis, ± cyst, ± hemorrhage, and usually show contrast enhancement. They can extend into the suprasellar cistern with waist at diaphragma sella, ± extension into cavernous sinus, and they can invade the skull base. *MRI:* Often have intermediate signal on T1- and T2-weighted imaging, often similar to gray matter, ± necrosis, ± cyst, ± hemorrhage, and usually show prominent gadolinium contrast enhancement. Can extend into suprasellar cistern with waist at diaphragma sella, ± extension into cavernous sinus, and occasionally invade the skull base.	Pituitary carcinomas can occasionally have an invasive growth pattern with extension into the sphenoid bone, clivus, ethmoid sinus, orbits, and/or interpeduncular cistern.

(continued on page 304)

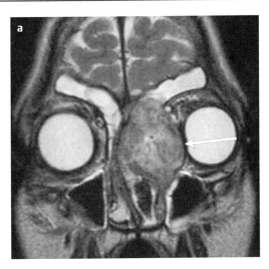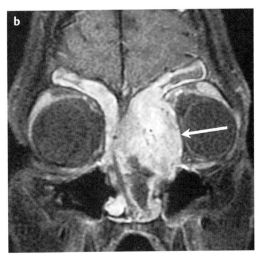

Fig. 3.55 A 12-year-old female with a Ewing's sarcoma in the left ethmoid sinus that is associated with bone destruction and tumor extension medially into the right ethmoid sinus, inferiorly into the left nasal cavity and left maxillary sinus, laterally into the left orbit, and superiorly into the left frontal sinus, causing obstruction of mucus outflow, with retained secretions filling both frontal sinuses. **(a)** The tumor has heterogeneous intermediate and slightly high signal on coronal T2-weighted imaging (*arrow*) and **(b)** gadolinium contrast enhancement on coronal fat-suppressed T1-weighted imaging (*arrow*).

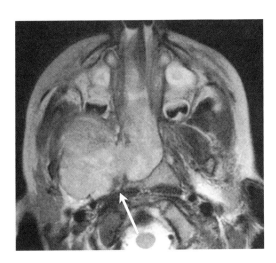

Fig. 3.56 A 5-year-old male with a rhabdomyosarcoma (*arrow*) in the right nasopharynx, right nasal cavity, and right parapharyngeal and masticator spaces that has heterogeneous slightly high and high signal on axial T2-weighted imaging.

Table 3.2 *(cont.)*   Solitary lesions involving the paranasal sinuses and nasal cavity

Lesion	Imaging Findings	Comments
Tumorlike Lesions		
Fibrous dysplasia **(Fig. 3.57)**	*CT:* Lesions in the skull are often associated with bone expansion. Lesions have variable density and attenuation on radiographs and CT, respectively, depending on the degree of mineralization and number of bony spicules. Attenuation coefficients can range from 70 to 400 Hounsfield units. Lesions in fibrous dysplasia can have a "ground glass" radiographic appearance secondary to the mineralized spicules of immature woven bone. Sclerotic borders of varying thickness can be seen surrounding parts or all of the lesions. *MRI:* Features depend on the proportions of bony spicules, collagen, fibroblastic spindle cells, and hemorrhagic and/or cystic changes. Lesions are usually well circumscribed and have low or low-intermediate signal on T1-weighted imaging. On T2-weighted imaging, lesions have variable mixtures of low, intermediate, and/or high signal, often surrounded by a low-signal rim of variable thickness. Internal septations and cystic changes are seen in a minority of lesions. Bone expansion is commonly seen. All or portions of the lesions can show gadolinium contrast enhancement in a heterogeneous, diffuse, or peripheral pattern.	Benign medullary fibro-osseous lesion of bone, most often sporadic involving a single site, referred to as monostotic (80 to 85%), or in multiple locations (polyostotic fibrous dysplasia). Results from developmental failure in the normal process of remodeling primitive bone to mature lamellar bone, with resultant zone or zones of immature trabeculae within dysplastic fibrous tissue. The lesions do not mineralize normally and can result in cranial neuropathies from neuroforaminal narrowing, facial deformities, sinonasal drainage disorders, and sinusitis. McCune-Albright syndrome accounts for 3% of polyostotic fibrous dysplasia.
Paget disease	*CT:* Lesions often have mixed intermediate to high attenuation, with irregular/indistinct borders between marrow and inner margins of the outer and inner tables of the skull. *MRI:* Most cases involving the craniofacial bones are in the late or inactive phases. Findings include osseous expansion and cortical thickening with low signal on T1-weighted imaging (T1WI) and T2-weighted imaging (T2WI). The inner margins of the thickened cortex can be irregular and indistinct. Zones of low signal on T1- and T2WI can be seen in the marrow secondary to thickened bony trabeculae. Marrow in the late or inactive phases of Paget disease can: (1) have signal similar to normal marrow, (2) contain focal areas of fat signal, (3) have low signal on T1- and T2WI secondary to regions of sclerosis, and (4) have areas of high signal on fat-suppressed T2WI from edema or persistent fibrovascular tissue.	Paget disease is a chronic skeletal disease in which there is disordered bone resorption and woven bone formation, resulting in osseous deformity. A paramyxovirus may be an etiologic agent. Paget disease is polyostotic in up to 66% of patients. Paget disease is associated with a risk of less than 1% for developing secondary sarcomatous changes. Occurs in 2.5 to 5% of Caucasians more than 55 years old, and 10% of those over the age of 85 years. Can result in narrowing of neuroforamina, with cranial nerve compression and basilar impression, ± compression of brainstem.
Inflammatory Lesions		
Mucous retention cyst/ solitary polyp **(Fig. 3.58, Fig. 3.59, Fig. 3.60**, and **Fig. 3.61)**	*CT:* Circumscribed soft tissue structures with low to intermediate attenuation depending on the proportions of protein and water. *MRI:* Circumscribed lesion that often has low signal on T1-weighted imaging (T1WI) and high signal on T2-weighted imaging (T2WI), ± thin peripheral gadolinium contrast enhancement. In mucous retention cysts or polyps with inspissated secretions and elevated protein concentration, the signal can vary from intermediate to high on T1WI and low, intermediate, to slightly high on T2WI.	Mucous retention cysts arise from obstruction of a seromucinous gland. Serous retention cysts occur from accumulation of fluid in the submucosal layer. Polyps are defined as collections of fluid within the mucosa that also contain eosinophils. Retention cysts and polyps occur as a complication of inflammatory sinus disease and have similar imaging features. They can occur as sporadic solitary or multiple lesions and are clinically insignificant unless there is obstruction of sinus ostia. Most commonly occur in the maxillary sinuses. Sinochoanal polyps are polyps that occur within, or grow into, sinus ostia and extend to the choanae. The antrochoanal polyp is the most common type; it extends from the maxillary sinus and can be fibrotic.

(continued on page 306)

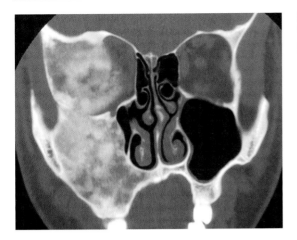

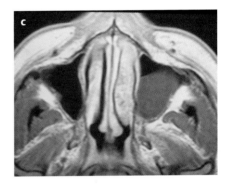

Fig. 3.57 A 19-year-old man with fibrous dysplasia involving the right maxilla and right sphenoid bone, resulting in narrowing of the dimensions of the pneumatized portion of the right maxillary sinus and right orbit on coronal CT.

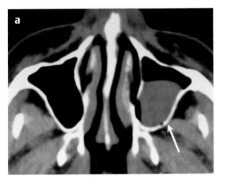

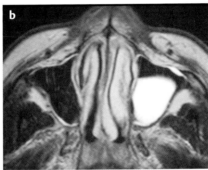

Fig. 3.58 **(a)** A 44-year-old woman with a mucous retention cyst that has fluid attenuation on axial CT (*arrow*), **(b)** high signal on axial T2-weighted imaging, and **(c)** low signal without contrast enhancement on postcontrast axial T1-weighted imaging.

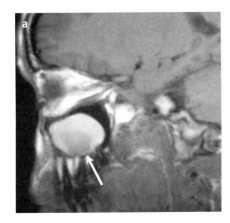

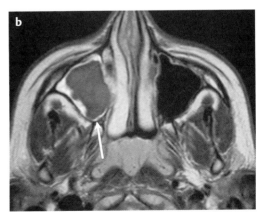

Fig. 3.59 **(a)** Mucous retention cyst with high protein concentration (inspissated secretions) in the right maxillary sinus that has high signal on sagittal T1-weighted imaging (*arrow*) and **(b)** low signal centrally surrounded by a thin zone of high signal on axial T2-weighted imaging (*arrow*).

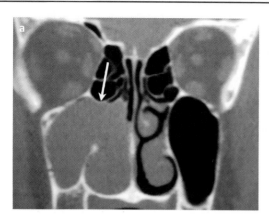
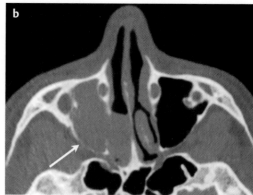

Fig. 3.60 (a) Coronal and (b) axial CT images show an antrochoanal polyp (*arrows*) within the right maxillary sinus and sinus ostium and extending to the choana.

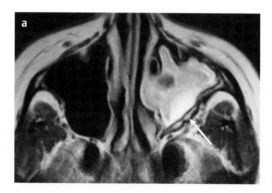
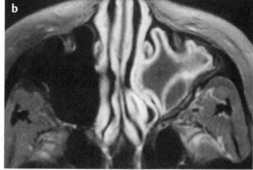

Fig. 3.61 (a) Polyp within the infundibulum of the left ostiomeatal unit that extends medially into the right nasal cavity and laterally into the left maxillary sinus. The polyp has high signal on axial T2-weighted imaging (*arrow*) and (b) thin peripheral gadolinium contrast enhancement on axial fat-suppressed T1-weighted imaging.

Table 3.2 *(cont.)* Solitary lesions involving the paranasal sinuses and nasal cavity

Lesion	Imaging Findings	Comments
Mucocele (**Fig. 3.62** and **Fig. 3.63**)	*CT:* Airless expanded sinuses containing mucus (10–18 HU). *MRI:* Expanded sinuses with contents that have low signal on T1-weighted imaging (T1WI) and high signal on T2-weighted imaging (T2WI); and that can have high signal on T1WI and low signal on T2WI with inspissated secretions that have high protein content or superimposed infection (pyocele).	Inflammation/infection of paranasal sinuses can cause obstruction of the sinus ostium, resulting in accumulation of mucus and desquamated epithelium. Progressive remodeling and expansion of sinus bone walls into orbits and cranial compartments can occur. Involves frontal sinuses (65%), ethmoid air cells (25%), and maxillary sinuses (10%).
Pyocele (**Fig. 3.64**)	*CT:* Airless expanded sinus with contents of low and/or intermediate attenuation, + erosion of expanded and thinned bone, ± abnormal attenuation in structures adjacent to the pyocele from extension of infection. *MRI:* Lesion with low-intermediate signal on T1-weighted imaging and low, intermediate, and/or high signal on T2-weighted imaging. Irregular peripheral gadolinium contrast enhancement can be seen.	Infection of a mucocele with erosion of remodeled, expanded bone walls, ± extension of infection into orbits and cranial compartments.

(continued on page 308)

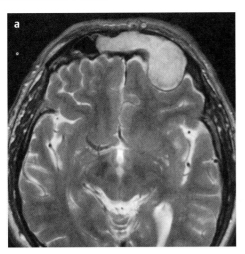

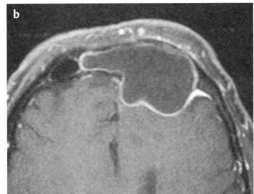

Fig. 3.62 **(a)** Mucocele in the left frontal sinus has mostly high signal on axial T2-weighted imaging and **(b)** has thin peripheral gadolinium contrast enhancement on axial fat-suppressed T1-weighted imaging. The sinus walls are thinned and expanded.

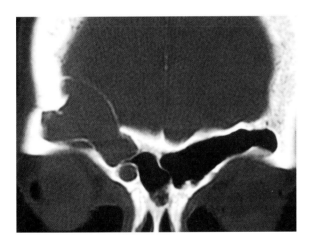

Fig. 3.63 Coronal CT shows a mucocele in the right frontal sinus that has thinned and expanded bony margins. The involved sinus is filled with retained secretions.

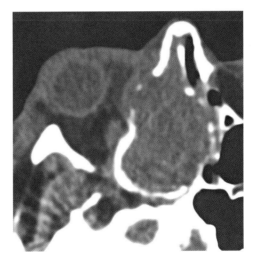

Fig. 3.64 Axial CT of a pyocele shows an airless expanded right ethmoid sinus filled with mixed low and intermediate attenuation associated with sites of cortical disruption laterally and extension of the inflammatory disease into the medial portion of the right orbit.

Table 3.2 *(cont.)* Solitary lesions involving the paranasal sinuses and nasal cavity

Lesion	Imaging Findings	Comments
Pott's puffy tumor (**Fig. 3.65**)	*CT:* Airless expanded sinus with contents of low and/or intermediate attenuation, + erosion of expanded and thinned bone, ± abnormal low- attenuation collection and edema in the overlying scalp from extension of infection. *MRI:* The frontal sinus usually contains low-intermediate signal on T1-weighted imaging and slightly high and/or high signal on T2-weighted imaging (T2WI). Irregular peripheral gadolinium (Gd) contrast enhancement can be seen. Superificial to the involved frontal bone, there is a collection with high signal on T2WI surrounded by peripheral Gd contrast enhancement representing the subperiosteal abscess and cellulitis.	Complication of frontal sinusitis, with erosion and perforation of the anterior table of the frontal bone resulting in subperiosteal abscess, cellulitis, granulation tissue, and edema of the adjacent scalp (Pott's puffy tumor). Sinusitis resulting in perforation of the posterior table can lead to formation of an epidural abscecess or subdural empyema. In children, microorganisms commonly involved include *Streptococcus, Haemophilus influenzae, Fusobacterium, Bacteroides, Staphylococcus aureus,* and *Enterococcus.* Treatment includes surgical debridement and intravenous antibiotics.
Rhinolith (**Fig. 3.66**)	*CT:* irregular zone of calcification within the nasal cavity or in a maxillary sinus, ± associated mucosal thickening and/or retained secretions, ± adjacent osseous erosion.	Dense, hard, calcified mass in the nasal cavity or maxillary sinus (antrolith) that results from deposition of calcium salts around bacteria, leukocytes, mucus, blood clots, or foreign bodies. More common in the nasal cavity than maxillary sinus.
Langerhans' cell histiocytosis (**Fig. 3.67**)	Single or multiple circumscribed soft tissue lesions in the marrow of the skull and craniofacial bones associated with focal bony destruction/erosion and with extension extra- or intracranially or both. *CT:* Lesions usually have low-intermediate attenuation, + contrast enhancement, ± enhancement of the adjacent dura. *MRI:* Lesions typically have low-intermediate signal on T1-weighted imaging and heterogeneous slightly high to high signal on T2-weighted imaging (T2WI) and fat-suppressed (FS) T2WI. Poorly defined zones of high signal on T2WI and FS T2WI are usually seen in the marrow and soft tissues peripheral to the lesions secondary to inflammatory changes. Lesions typically show prominent gadolinium contrast enhancement in marrow and extraosseous soft tissue portions.	Disorder of reticuloendothelial system in which bone marrow–derived dendritic Langerhans' cells infiltrate various organs as focal lesions or in diffuse patterns. Langerhans' cells have eccentrically located ovoid or convoluted nuclei with pale to eosinophilic cytoplasm. Lesions often consist of Langerhans' cells, macrophages, plasma cells, and eosinophils. Lesions are immunoreactive to S-100, CD1a, CD-207, HLA-DR, and β_2-microglobulin. Prevalence of 2 per 100,000 children < 15 years old; only a third of lesions occur in adults. Localized lesions (eosinophilic granuloma) can be single or multiple in the skull, usually at the skull base. Single lesions are commonly seen in males more than in females, in patients < 20 years old, with proliferation of histiocytes in medullary bone resulting in localized destruction of cortical bone and with extension into adjacent soft tissues. Multiple lesions are associated with Letterer-Siwe disease (lymphadenopathy and hepatosplenomegaly) in children < 2 years old and Hand-Schüller-Christian disease (lymphadenopathy, exophthalmos, and diabetes insipidus) in children 5–10 years old.

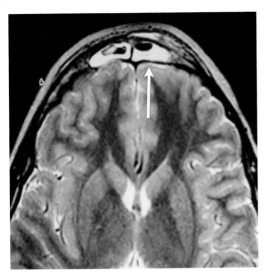

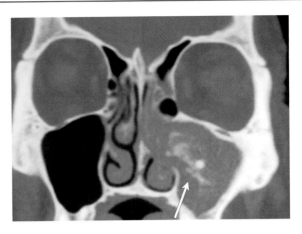

Fig. 3.66 Coronal CT of a 66-year-old man shows retained secretions filling the left maxillary sinus, which contains an irregular zone of calcification (*arrow*) representing a rhinolith.

Fig. 3.65 Pott's puffy tumor. The frontal sinus is almost completely filled with high signal in association air–fluid levels on axial T2-weighted imaging (*arrow*). Superficial to the involved frontal bone, the collection with high signal represents a subperiosteal abscess and cellulitis.

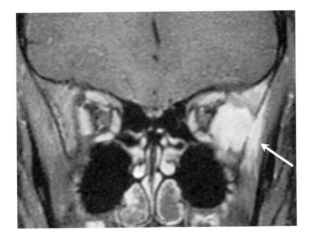

Fig. 3.67 Coronal fat-suppressed T1-weighted imaging shows a gadolinium-enhancing eosinophilic granuloma (*arrow*) destroying the osseous lateral margin of the left orbit, with medial extension of the lesion into the orbit and lateral extension involving the left temporalis muscle.

Table 3.3 Multifocal or diffuse sinonasal disease

- Acute and subacute rhinosinusitis
- Chronic rhinosinusitis
- Sinonasal polyposis
- Mucoceles
- Fungal sinusitis, noninvasive type
- Fungal sinusitis, active invasive type

- Chronic invasive fungal disease of the paranasal sinuses
- Granulomatosis with polyangiitis (Wegener's granulomatosis)
- Churg-Strauss syndrome
- Sarcoidosis
- Sjögren's syndrome
- Polyostotic fibrous dysplasia
- Craniofacial fractures
- Cerebrospinal fluid leaks

Table 3.3 Multifocal or diffuse sinonasal disease

Disease/Disorder	Findings	Comments
Acute and subacute rhinosinusitis (**Fig. 3.68** and **Fig. 3.69**)	*CT:* Air–fluid levels, mucosal thickening in involved sinus and nasal cavity, ± orbital involvement from ethmoid disease, ± subperiosteal abscess, meningitis from frontal sinusitis. *MRI:* Air–fluid levels with fluid having low signal on T1-weighted imaging and high signal on T2-weighted imaging, and with mucosal thickening showing gadolinium contrast enhancement; ± complications, such as pre- or postseptal orbital cellulitis, and/or meningitis, epidural or subdural empyema, cerebritis, and brain abscess.	Inflammation of the mucosal lining of the nasal cavity or paranasal sinuses. Can be caused by viral infection, bacteria, fungi, dental caries/abscesses, allergens, or environmental irritants. Symptoms include facial pain or pressure, nasal congestion, mucopurulent nasal discharge, hyposmia, anosmia, and/or dental pain. Infection can spread directly into the orbit or via small valveless venous connections between the sinuses and orbits. Intracranial spread of infection can result in meningitis, epidural or subdural empyema, cerebritis, and/or brain abscess. *Acute rhinosinusitis* is the clinical diagnosis when symptoms have lasted < 4 weeks. *Subacute rhinosinusitis* is defined as duration of symptoms from 4 weeks to 12 weeks. Treatment of acute/subacute rhinosinusitis includes saline irrigation, nasal corticosteroids, and decongestants.

(continued on page 312)

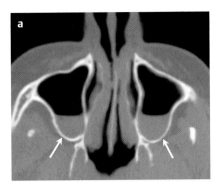
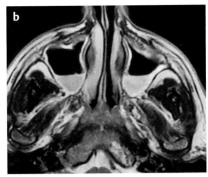
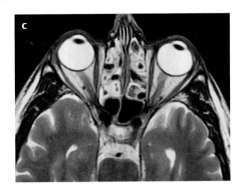

Fig. 3.68 Acute rhinosinusitis. **(a)** Axial CT (*arrows*) and **(b)** axial T2-weighted imaging show air–fluid levels in both maxillary sinuses. **(c)** Extensive mucosal thickening is also seen in the ethmoid sinuses on axial T2-weighted imaging.

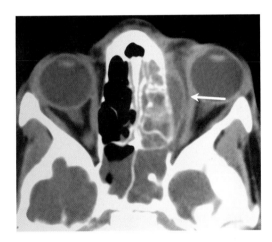

Fig. 3.69 Axial CT in an 11-year-old female with left ethmoid and sphenoid sub-acute sinusitis shows a subperiosteal abscess (*arrow*) and postseptal cellulitis in the left orbit.

Table 3.3 *(cont.)* Multifocal or diffuse sinonasal disease

Disease/Disorder	Findings	Comments
Chronic rhinosinusitis (**Fig. 3.70**, **Fig. 3.71**, and **Fig. 3.72**)	*CT:* Sinus secretions can have low, intermediate, and/ or slightly high attenuation related to protein content, superimposed bacterial or fungal infection, ± air–fluid levels, mucosal thickening in involved sinus and nasal cavity, ± reactive bone thickening (osteitis). *MRI:* Sinus secretions can have low, intermediate, and/ or slightly high signal on T1-weighted imaging (T1WI) and T2-weighted imaging (T2WI) related to protein content. With protein content over 25%, retained secretions can have slightly high to high signal on T1WI and low signal on T2WI, ± air–fluid levels and mucosal thickening, as well as show gadolinium contrast enhancement. *CT and MRI:* Findings of superimposed fungal infection in chronic rhinosinusitis can vary based on the presence of calcium, iron, and manganese in hyphae. Bacteria contain iron/Fe^{3+}-binding siderophores, which can result in sinus contents with intermediate to high signal on T1WI and low signal on T2WI.	Inflammation of the mucosal lining of the nasal cavity or paranasal sinuses for more than 12 weeks. Can result from anatomic variants with narrowed ostia, nasal allergy, iatrogenic causes (nasogastric tubes, mechanical ventilation, nasal packing), or postoperative scarring. Systemic diseases that predispose to chronic rhinosinusitis include cystic fibrosis, primary ciliary dyskinesia, aspirin-exacerbated respiratory disease, and antibody immunodeficiency. Superimposed fungal and bacterial infection can occur. Cystic fibrosis is caused by an autosomal recessive mutation involving the cystic fibrosis transmembrane regulator *(CFTR)* gene, which results in defective chloride ion channels in epithelial cell membranes, causing increased viscosity of mucous secretions by exocrine glands. Results in impaired clearance of viscous mucus, leading to bacterial colonization and chronic rhinosinusitis in most patients. Primary ciliary dyskinesia is a rare, heterogeneous, autosomal recessive disease associated with defective function of motile cilia, resulting in chronic rhinosinusitis, bronchitis, pneumonia, bronchiectasis, otitis media, male infertility, and situs inversus (Kartagener syndrome) in 50% of cases. Aspirin-exacerbated respiratory disease is an adult-onset disorder with rhinosinusitis, nasal polyposis, and asthma (Samter's triad) that occurs after use of aspirin or other NSAIDs. Treatment of chronic rhinosinusitis includes saline irrigation, nasal and/or oral corticosteroids, decongestants, and surgery.

(continued on page 314)

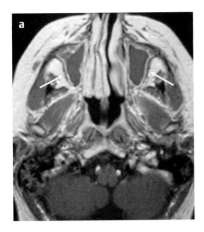
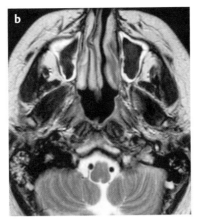
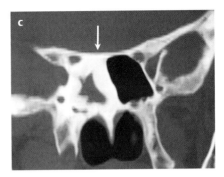

Fig. 3.70 Chronic rhinosinusitis. MRI shows both maxillary sinuses filled with mucus that has elevated protein content and that has **(a)** low-intermediate signal on axial postcontrast T1-weighted imaging (*arrows*), with thin peripheral gadolinium contrast enhancement of the mucosa, and **(b)** low signal centrally on axial T2-weighted imaging. **(c)** Coronal CT shows retained secretions filling the right side of the sphenoid sinus (*arrow*) surrounded by reactive bone thickening (osteitis).

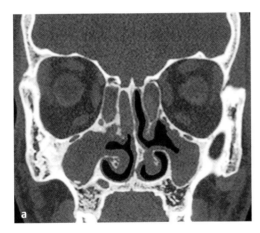
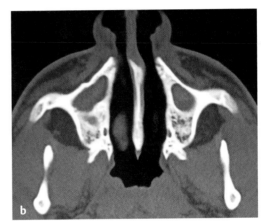

Fig. 3.71 An 18-year-old man with cystic fibrosis and chronic rhinosinusitis. **(a)** Coronal and **(b)** axial CT images show hypoplasia of the maxillary sinuses. Mucosal thickening and retained secretions with mixed intermediate and slightly high attenuation are seen filling the maxillary and ethmoid sinuses.

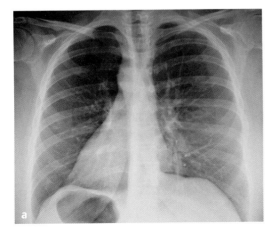
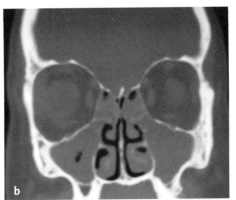

Fig. 3.72 A 35-year-old woman with Kartagener syndrome. **(a)** PA radiograph of the chest shows situs inversus and dextrocardia. **(b)** Coronal CT shows chronic inflammatory sinus disease with mucosal thickening and retained secretions filling the ethmoid and maxillary sinuses.

Table 3.3 *(cont.)* Multifocal or diffuse sinonasal disease

Disease/Disorder	Findings	Comments
Sinonasal polyposis (**Fig. 3.73**)	*CT:* Circumscribed soft tissue structures with low to intermediate attenuation depending on the proportions of protein and water. *MRI:* Circumscribed lesions that have low signal on T1-weighted imaging (T1WI) and high signal on T2-weighted imaging (T2WI). In polyps with inspissated secretions and elevated protein concentration, the signal can vary from intermediate to high on T1WI and from low to intermediate to slightly high on T2WI, ± thin peripheral gadolinium contrast enhancement.	Polyps are defined as collections of fluid within the mucosa that also contain eosinophils. Polyps occur as a complication of allergic or infective sinus disease and have imaging features similar to mucous retention cysts. Polyps can occur as multiple lesions and are clinically insignificant unless there is obstruction of sinus ostia. Most commonly occur in the ethmoid and maxillary sinuses. Sinochoanal polyps are polyps that occur within, or grow into, sinus ostia and extend to the choanae. The antrochoanal polyp is the most common type, extends from the maxillary sinus, and can be fibrotic. Superimposed fungal colonization can occur, with hyphae containing calcium and paramagnetic elements such as manganese and iron.
Mucoceles (**Fig. 3.74** and **Fig. 3.75**)	*CT:* Airless expanded sinuses containing mucus (10–18 HU). *MRI:* Expanded sinuses with contents that have low signal on T1-weighted imaging (T1WI) and high signal on T2-weighted imaging (T2WI) and that can have high signal on T1WI and low signal on T2WI with inspissated secretions that have high protein content or superimposed infection (pyocele).	Inflammation/infection of paranasal sinuses can cause obstruction of the sinus ostia, resulting in accumulation of mucus and desquamated epithelium. Progressive remodeling and expansion of sinus bone walls into orbits and cranial compartments can occur. Mucoceles are found in frontal sinuses (65%), ethmoid air cells (25%), and maxillary sinuses (10%). Can be multiple.

(continued on page 316)

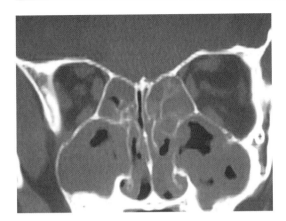

Fig. 3.73 Sinonasal polyposis. Coronal CT shows lobulated soft tissue structures representing polyps in the maxillary sinuses and nasal cavity. Mucosal thickening and retained secretions fill the ethmoid sinuses.

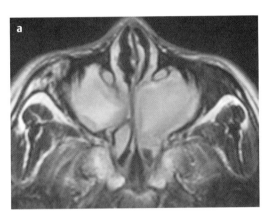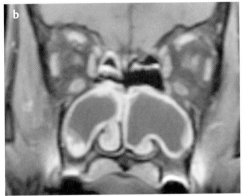

Fig. 3.74 A 30-year-old man with mucoceles in both maxillary sinuses. The expanded maxillary sinuses are filled with retained secretions that have **(a)** high signal on axial T2-weighted imaging and **(b)** low signal on postcontrast coronal fat-suppressed T1-weighted imaging with peripheral enhancement of the mucosa.

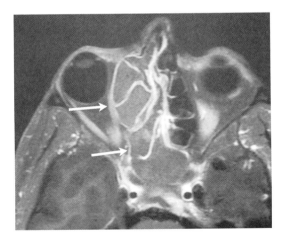

Fig. 3.75 A 33-year-old man with mucoceles (*arrows*) involving multiple right ethmoid air cells, as seen on axial postcontrast fat-suppressed T1-weighted imaging.

Table 3.3 *(cont.)* Multifocal or diffuse sinonasal disease

Disease/Disorder	Findings	Comments
Fungal sinusitis, noninvasive type (**Fig. 3.76**)	*CT:* Sinus secretions can have low, intermediate, and/ or slightly high attenuation related to protein and fungal content, ± air–fluid levels, mucosal thickening in involved sinus and nasal cavity, ± reactive bone thickening (osteitis) and/or expansion of sinus walls. Fungus balls within sinuses contain central zones with high attenuation (100–200 HU), with calcifications occurring in up to 67%. Unilateral involvement is more common than bilateral. *MRI:* Sinus secretions can have low, intermediate, and/ or slightly high signal on T1-weighted imaging (T1WI) and T2-weighted imaging (T2WI) related to protein and fungal content. With protein content over 25%, retained secretions can have slightly high to high signal on T1WI and low signal on T2WI, ± air–fluid levels, mucosal thickening, and gadolinium (Gd) contrast enhancement. Fungus balls often have low signal on T1WI and T2WI from paramagnetic metals and calcification and typically show no Gd contrast enhancement. *CT and MRI:* Findings of superimposed fungal infection in chronic rhinosinusitis can vary based on the presence of calcium, iron, and manganese in hyphae.	Fungal colonization of the nasal cavity and/or paranasal sinuses in immunocompetent patients, which can occur as localized colonization with hyphae growing saprophytically within mucus and mucous crusts, as a fungus ball (mycetoma) consisting of dense accumulations of hyphae (often *Aspergillus* species) without transmucosal invasion, or as allergic fungal rhinosinusitis (AFR), which is a hypersensitivity reaction to fungal antigens in atopic patients. Clinical diagnostic criteria for AFR are: nasal polyposis, presence of fungi seen on microscopy, eosinophilic mucin without transmucosal invasion, type 1 hypersensitivity to fungi via skin testing, and CT findings of sinus opacification. Treatment of localized fungal colonization includes mechanical removal and sinus rinses. Treatment of fungus balls is endoscopic removal. Treatment of AFR includes nasal saline irrigation, topical steroids, short courses of systemic corticosteroids, antibiotics, and functional endoscopic sinus surgery for refractory cases.
Fungal sinusitis, active invasive type (**Fig. 3.77** and **Fig. 3.78**)	*CT:* Sinus secretions can have low, intermediate, and/ or slightly high attenuation related to protein and fungal content, ± air–fluid levels, mucosal thickening in involved sinus and nasal cavity, + osseous erosion/ destruction. *MRI:* Sinus secretions can have low, intermediate, and/or slightly high signal on T1- and T2-weighted imaging related to protein and fungal content. Mucosal thickening can show gadolinium (Gd) contrast enhancement. Abnormal signal and contrast enhancement are seen in adjacent tissue at sites of erosion/destruction of bony walls of sinus. Arterial/venous occlusion by fungal invasion can result in necrosis of tissue, with lack of Gd contrast enhancement.	Aggressive fungal rhinosinusitis of less than 4 weeks duration that occurs in immunocompromised or poorly controlled diabetic patients. Life-threatening disease in which insufficient immune response allows fungi to invade mucosa, bone, and blood vessels and to spread rapidly into the orbits, cavernous sinuses, and/or CNS. Fungi commonly involved include *Aspergillus* spp. and members of the order Mucorales (*Rhizopus* and *Mucor* spp.). Treatment includes immune reconstitution, systemic antifungal therapy, and surgical debridement.
Chronic invasive fungal disease of the paranasal sinuses	*CT:* Sinus secretions can have intermediate and/or slightly high to high attenuation related to protein and fungal content, + osseous erosion/destruction, ± mottled radiolucent osseous changes in sinus walls. *MRI:* Sinus secretions can have low, intermediate, and/or slightly high signal on T1- and T2-weighted imaging related to protein and fungal content. Mucosal thickening shows gadolinium contrast enhancement. Abnormal signal and contrast enhancement can be seen in adjacent tissue at sites of erosion/destruction of bony walls of sinus.	Slowly progressing fungal rhinosinusitis of more than 12 weeks duration that often occurs in immunocompetent patients. Histologic findings include noncaseating granulomas with vasculitis, perivascular fibrosis, and/or vascular proliferation. Patients can present with chronic sinusitis, facial soft tissue swelling, ocular symptoms, and/or neurologic deficits.

(continued on page 318)

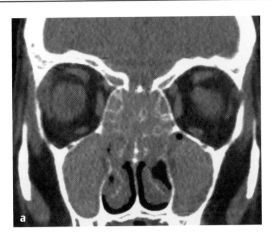
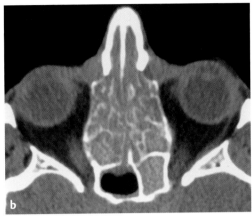

Fig. 3.76 A 59-year-old woman with noninvasive fungal sinusitis. **(a)** Coronal and **(b)** axial CT images show retained secretions that fill the maxillary and ethmoid sinuses as well as the left side of the sphenoid sinus and that have low, intermediate, and/or slightly high attenuation related to protein and fungal content.

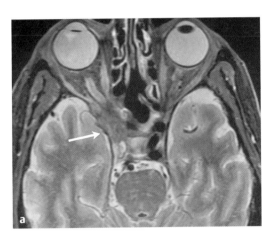
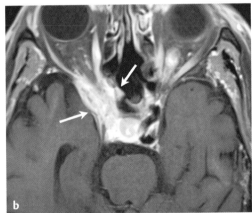

Fig. 3.77 An 84-year-old man with aspergillosis and invasive fungal sinusitis. **(a)** Poorly defined zones with abnormal slightly high signal on axial fat-suppressed T2-weighted imaging (*arrow*) and **(b)** gadolinium contrast enhancement on axial fat-suppressed T1-weighted imaging (*arrows*) are seen in the right side of the sphenoid sinus, right orbital apex, right cavernous sinus, and anteromedial portion of the right middle cranial fossa.

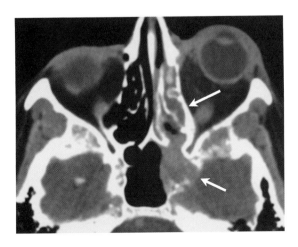

Fig. 3.78 A 58-year-old man with invasive fungal sinusitis caused by *Mucor*. Axial CT shows irregular zones with low and intermediate attenuation involving the left ethmoid air cells and left side of the sphenoid sinus (*arrows*) associated with adjacent osseous erosion.

Table 3.3 *(cont.)*   Multifocal or diffuse sinonasal disease

Disease/Disorder	Findings	Comments
Granulomatosis with polyangiitis (Wegener's granulomatosis) (**Fig. 3.79**)	*CT:* Zones with soft tissue attenuation, ± bone destruction. *MRI:* Poorly defined zones of soft tissue thickening with low-intermediate signal on T1-weighted imaging, slightly high to high signal on T2-weighted imaging, and gadolinium contrast enhancement within the nasal cavity, paranasal sinuses, orbits, infratemporal fossa, and external auditory canal, ± invasion and destruction of bone and nasal septum, ± extension into the skull base with involvement of the dura, leptomeninges, brain, or venous sinuses.	Multisystem autoimmune disease with necrotizing granulomas in the respiratory tract, focal necrotizing angiitis of small arteries and veins of various tissues, and glomerulonephritis. Can involve the paranasal sinuses, orbits, skull base, dura, leptomeninges, and occasionally the temporal bone. Typically, positive immunoreactivity to cytoplasmic antineutrophil cytoplasmic antibody (c-ANCA). Treatment includes corticosteroids, cyclophosphamide, and anti-TNF agents.
Churg-Strauss syndrome (**Fig. 3.80**)	*CT:* Multifocal mucosal thickening in the nasal cavity and paranasal sinuses. *MRI:* Poorly defined zones of mucosal soft tissue thickening in the nasal cavity and paranasal sinuses, with low-intermediate signal on T1-weighted imaging, slightly high to high signal on T2-weighted imaging, and gadolinium contrast enhancement.	Granulomatous angiitis associated with asthma, eosinophilia (> 10% in peripheral blood), paranasal sinusitis, transient pulmonary infiltrates, mononeuritis or polyneuropathy, and immunoreactivity to perinuclear antineutrophil cytoplasmic antibody (p-ANCA). Treatment includes corticosteroids, cyclophosphamide, and leukotriene receptor agonists.
Sarcoidosis	*CT:* Multifocal mucosal thickening in the nasal cavity and paranasal sinuses. Intraosseous lesions are associated with localized bony destruction and can extend into the sinuses. Lesions have soft tissue attenuation. Intraosseous sarcoid lesions usually appear as intramedullary radiolucent zones, rarely with sclerotic/high attenuation. *MRI:* Poorly defined zones of mucosal soft tissue thickening in the nasal cavity and paranasal sinuses, with low-intermediate signal on T1-weighted imaging (T1WI), slightly high to high signal on T2-weighted imaging (T2WI), and gadolinium (Gd) contrast enhancement. Intraosseous lesions often have low to intermediate signal on T1WI and slightly high signal on T2WI and fat-suppressed T2WI. After Gd contrast administration, lesions typically show Gd contrast enhancement. Extension of intraosseous sarcoid into the sinuses can occur.	Sarcoidosis is a multisystem, noncaseating, granulomatous disease of uncertain cause that can involve the CNS in 5– 15%. Sinonasal involvement is uncommon and occurs in 2 to 10% of patients with sarcoid. Submucosal sarcoid granulomas can be seen on biopsies of the nasal septum and turbinates. Up to 60% of patients with sarcoid have an elevated serum level of angiotensin-converting enzyme (ACE). Sarcoid within bone can also extend into the adjacent extraosseous structures, including the paranasal sinuses. Treatment of sinonasal sarcoid includes nasal and oral corticosteroids, methotrexate, anti-TNF-a agents, and surgical debulking.
Sjögren's syndrome (**Fig. 3.81**)	*CT:* Mucosal thickening in multiple sinuses. *MRI:* Mucosal thickening with low-intermediate signal on T1-weighted imaging, high signal on T2-weighted imaging (T2WI) and fat-suppressed T2WI, and gadolinium contrast enhancement.	Common autoimmune disease in which a mononuclear lymphocytic infiltration can occur in one or more exocrine glands (lacrimal, parotid, submandibular, and minor salivary glands), resulting in acinar cell destruction and impaired gland function. Can be a primary disorder or a secondary form associated with other autoimmune diseases, such as rheumatoid arthritis and systemic lupus erythematosus. Patients present with decreased lacrimal and salivary gland function, xerostomia, keratoconjunctivitis sicca, and chronic rhinosinusitis.

(continued on page 320)

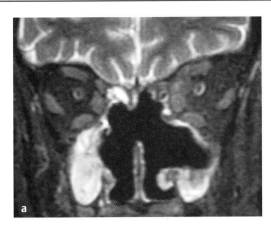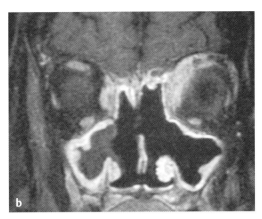

Fig. 3.79 A 65-year-old woman with granulomatosis with polyangiitis (Wegener's granulomatosis). **(a)** Irregular zones of mucosal thickening with high signal on coronal fat-suppressed T2-weighted imaging and **(b)** gadolinium contrast enhancement on coronal fat-suppressed T1-weighted imaging are seen within the nasal cavity and maxillary and ethmoid sinuses and are associated with destruction of bone and portions of the nasal septum. Inflammatory involvement of the medial portion of the left orbit is also seen.

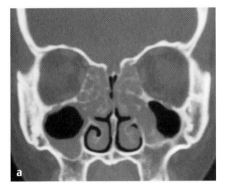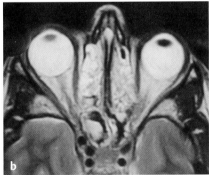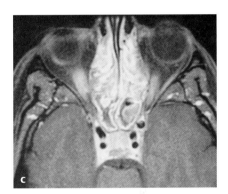

Fig. 3.80 A 42-year-old woman with Churg-Strauss syndrome. **(a)** Coronal CT, **(b)** axial T2-weighted imaging, and **(c)** postcontrast axial fat-suppressed T1-weighted imaging show mucosal thickening in the maxillary sinuses and filling of the ethmoid and sphenoid sinuses with retained secretions and mucosal thickening.

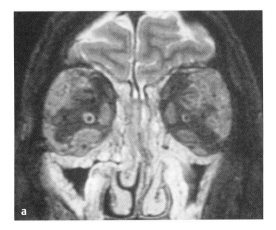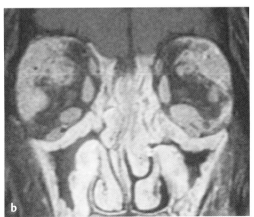

Fig. 3.81 A 58-year-old man with Sjögren's syndrome who has extensive mucosal thickening in the maxillary and sphenoid sinuses, as seen on **(a)** coronal STIR and **(b)** coronal postcontrast fat-suppressed T1-weighted imaging. Irregular contrast-enhancing soft tissue with ill-defined margins is seen within both orbits.

Table 3.3 *(cont.)* Multifocal or diffuse sinonasal disease

Disease/Disorder	Findings	Comments
Polyostotic fibrous dysplasia (**Fig. 3.82**)	*CT:* Lesions involving the craniofacial bones are often associated with osseous expansion. Lesions have variable density and attenuation on radiographs and CT, respectively, depending on the degree of mineralization and the number of bony spicules in the lesions. Attenuation coefficients can range from 70 to 400 Hounsfield units. Lesions can have a "ground glass" radiographic appearance secondary to the mineralized spicules of immature woven bone. Sclerotic borders of varying thickness can be seen surrounding parts or all of the lesions. *MRI:* Features depend on the proportions of bony spicules, collagen, fibroblastic spindle cells, and hemorrhagic and/or cystic changes. Lesions are usually well circumscribed and have low or low-intermediate signal on T1-weighted imaging. On T2-weighted imaging, lesions have variable mixtures of low, intermediate, and/or high signal, often surrounded by a low-signal rim of variable thickness. Bone expansion is commonly seen. All or portions of the lesions can show gadolinium contrast enhancement in a heterogeneous, diffuse, or peripheral pattern.	Benign medullary fibro-osseous lesion of bone, most often sporadic, involving a single site (referred to as monostotic fibrous dysplasia; 80 to 85% of cases) or in multiple locations (polyostotic fibrous dysplasia). Results from developmental failure in the normal process of remodeling primitive bone to mature lamellar bone, with resultant zone or zones of immature trabeculae within dysplastic fibrous tissue. The lesions do not mineralize normally and can result in cranial neuropathies from neuroforaminal narrowing, facial deformities, sinonasal drainage disorders, and sinusitis. McCune-Albright syndrome accounts for 3% of polyostotic fibrous dysplasia. The syndrome may include the presence of pigmented cutaneous macules (sometimes referred to as café-au-lait spots) with irregular indented borders that are ipsilateral to bone lesions, precocious puberty, and/or other endocrine disorders, such as acromegaly, hyperthyroidism, hyperparathyroidism, and Cushing's syndrome. *Leontiasis ossea* is a rare form of polyostotic fibrous dyplasia that involves the craniofacial bones and results in facial enlargement and deformity. Age at presentation ranges from < 1 year to 76 years; 75% occur before the age of 30 years. Median age for monostotic fibrous dysplasia = 21 years; mean and median ages for polyostotic fibrous dysplasia are between 8 and 17 years. Most cases are diagnosed in patients between 3 and 20 years old.

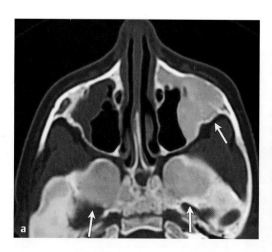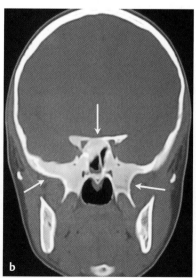

Fig. 3.82 A 5-year-old female with polyostotic fibrous dysplasia who has multiple expansile bone lesions in the maxilla and sphenoid bone that have a "ground glass" appearance on **(a)** axial (*arrows*) and **(b)** coronal CT (*arrows*).

Disease/Disorder	Findings	Comments
Craniofacial fractures (**Fig. 3.83**, **Fig. 3.84**, **Fig. 3.85**, and **Fig. 3.86**) Simple isolated fractures Complex fractures	*CT:* Cortical bone discontinuities with or without displaced bone fragments. In orbital floor fractures, herniation of orbital fat and inferior rectus muscle can occur through the fracture into the maxillary sinus. Fractures involving the orbital roof and frontal bone can result in intracranial complications, such as hemorrhage, CSF leakage, and/or infection. *Nasoethmoid orbital fractures* involve the nasal bone and ethmoid bone (lamina papyracea) or lacrimal bone. *Zygomaticomaxillary complex fractures* result in separation of the zygoma due to fractures involving all four buttresses (zygomaticofrontal, zygomaticomaxillary, infraorbital rim, and zygomatic arch). The *LeFort I hemifracture* consists of a comminuted fracture of the maxillary sinus (medial and lateral buttresses) and ipsilateral pterygoid plate; it can be unilateral or bilateral. The *LeFort II hemifracture* consists of fractures through the nasoethmoid orbital region extending through the orbital floor, inferior orbital rim, and zygomaticomaxillary buttress and posteriorly through the ipsilateral pterygoid plate; it can be unilateral or bilateral. The *LeFort III hemifracture* consists of fractures involving the nasoethmoid orbital region and extending through the orbital floor, zygomaticosphenoid articulation, lateral orbital wall, zygomaticofrontal buttress, zygomatic arch, and unilateral pterygoid plate; it can be unilateral or bilateral.	Traumatic osseous fractures involving the paranasal sinuses can occur in isolation or in combination with other craniofacial fractures. *Simple isolated fractures* involve the frontal sinus, orbital roof, orbital floor, zygomatic arch, maxilla, and palate. Fractures involving the orbital floor or medial wall usually result from blunt trauma that causes an abrupt increase in orbital pressure. Fractures involving the orbital roof result from direct blunt trauma. *Complex fractures* involving multiple bones often result from high-impact and/or high-velocity forces and include the nasoethmoid orbital fractures, zygomaticomaxillary complex fractures, and pterygofacial LeFort types I, II, and III fractures. Complications of sinus wall fractures include epidural hematoma, subdural hematoma, subarachnoid hemorrhage, CSF leakage (rhinorrhea/otorrhea), and diplopia.

(continued on page 323)

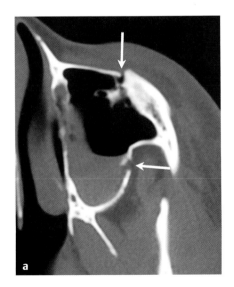 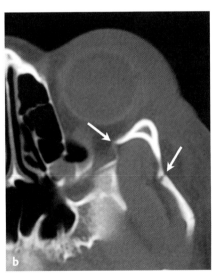 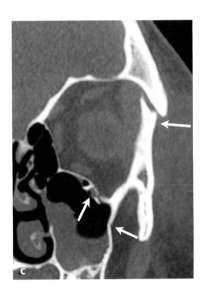

Fig. 3.83 Tripod fracture. **(a,b)** Axial and **(c)** coronal images show fractures involving all four buttresses (zygomaticofrontal, zygomaticomaxillary, infraorbital rim, and zygomatic arch) of the zygomaticomaxillary complex (*arrows*).

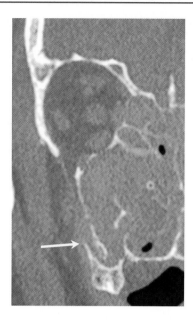

Fig. 3.84 Coronal CT shows a LeFort I hemifracture consisting of a comminuted right maxillary sinus fracture (medial and lateral buttresses) and fracture of the ipsilateral pterygoid plate (*arrow*).

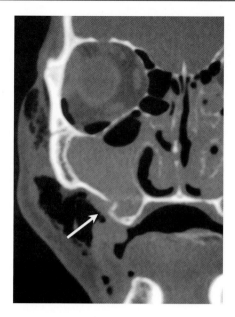

Fig. 3.85 Coronal CT shows a LeFort II hemifracture consisting of fractures through the nasoethmoid orbital region and extending through the orbital floor, inferior orbital rim with resultant orbital emphysema, and zygomaticomaxillary buttress (*arrow*). The fracture also involved the ipsilateral pterygoid plate (not shown).

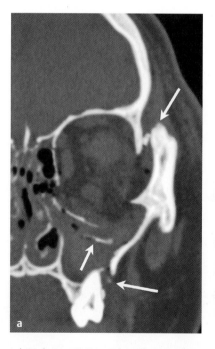
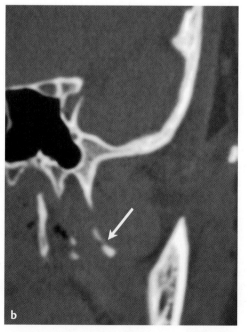

Fig. 3.86 **(a,b)** Coronal CT shows a LeFort III hemifracture (*arrows*) with fractures involving the left nasoethmoid-orbital region and extending through the orbital floor, lateral orbital wall, zygomaticofrontal buttress, lateral maxillary buttress, and left pterygoid plate (*arrow* in **b**).

Table 3.3 *(cont.)* Multifocal or diffuse sinonasal disease

Disease/Disorder	Findings	Comments
Cerebrospinal fluid leaks **(Fig. 3.87)**	*CT:* Thin-section CT shows an osseous defect at the skull base associated with fluid in the adjacent paranasal sinus. For CSF leaks involving the temporal bone, fluid in the middle ear is associated with a defect of the tegmen tympani or fracture involving the inner ear. Accuracy of thin-section CT for CSF leaks is reported to be up to 92%. *CT cisternography:* Ten mL of iodinated contrast administered into the CSF via lumbar puncture is used to opacify the basal cisterns by Trendelenburg positioning. CSF defects can be seen as localized skull defects with intervals of increased attenuation of fluid within the adjacent paranasal sinus or middle ear cavity. *MRI:* Osseous defect at the skull base associated with fluid with high signal on T2-weighted imaging in the adjacent paranasal sinus. For CSF leaks involving the temporal bone, fluid in the middle ear is associated with a defect of the tegmen tympani or fracture involving the inner ear. MRI is useful in distinguishing fluid from brain herniation (encephalocele) through a skull-base defect. Thin-section MRI with fat-suppressed long TR/long TE fast spin echo images (MR cisternography) has been used to identify the CSF fistula tract from the subarachnoid space to the extracranial locations. *Nuclear medicine:* Radionuclide cisternography using technetium 99m–labeled or indium 111– labeled diethylene triaminepentaacetic acid placed in the lumbar CSF indicates a CSF leak when tracer is detected in rhinorrhea samples on nasal pledgets.	CSF leaks occur due to osseous or dural defects at the skull base, with communication of the intracranial subarachnoid space with the paranasal sinuses, nasal cavity (rhinorrhea), or middle ear (otorrhea). Up to 90% of CSF leaks result from trauma and surgical or other procedural complications. Traumatic fracture involving the anterior skull base resulting in CSF rhinorrhea accounts for up to 80% of cases, and otorrhea accounts for the majority of the remainder. Nontraumatic etiologies of CSF leak include: neoplasms involving the skull base, intracranial hypertension, infection, congenital abnormalities, radiation treatment, or chemotherapy. Diagnostic testing of patient samples of more than 10 μL for β_2-transferrin (β_2-trf) or 200 μL for β-trace protein (β-TP) is a reliable noninvasive method to detect CSF leaks. Some posttraumatic CSF leaks resolve with conservative treatment. Persistent CSF leaks can be treated with intracranial surgical repair or extracranial endoscopic repair.

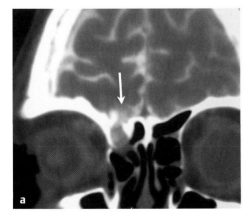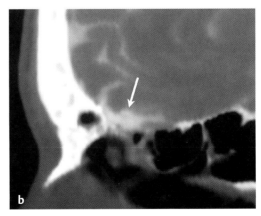

Fig. 3.87 **(a)** Coronal and **(b)** sagittal CT cisternographic images show a localized skull defect (*arrows*) with CSF-containing contrast extending inferiorly into the right ethmoid air cells, representing a CSF leak.

References

Anatomic Variants of the Nasal Cavity and Paranasal Sinuses

1. Baxter DJG, Shroff MM. Developmental maxillofacial anomalies. Semin Ultrasound CT MR 2011;32(6):555–568
2. Beale TJ, Madani G, Morley SJ. Imaging of the paranasal sinuses and nasal cavity: normal anatomy and clinically relevant anatomical variants. Semin Ultrasound CT MR 2009;30(1):2–16
3. Cashman EC, Macmahon PJ, Smyth D. Computed tomography scans of paranasal sinuses before functional endoscopic sinus surgery. World J Radiol 2011;3(8):199–204
4. Goodacre T, Swan MC. Cleft lip and palate: current management. Paediatr Child Health 2008;18:283–292
5. Hoang JK, Eastwood JD, Tebbit CL, Glastonbury CM. Multiplanar sinus CT: a systematic approach to imaging before functional endoscopic sinus surgery. AJR Am J Roentgenol 2010;194(6):W527–W536
6. Jog M, McGarry GW. How frequent are accessory sinus ostia? J Laryngol Otol 2003;117(4):270–272
7. Johnson JM, Moonis G, Green GE, Carmody R, Burbank HN. Syndromes of the first and second branchial arches, part 1: embryology and characteristic defects. AJNR Am J Neuroradiol 2011;32(1):14–19
8. Johnson JM, Moonis G, Green GE, Carmody R, Burbank HN. Syndromes of the first and second branchial arches, part 2: syndromes. AJNR Am J Neuroradiol 2011;32(2):230–237
9. Kantarci M, Karasen RM, Alper F, Onbas O, Okur A, Karaman A. Remarkable anatomic variations in paranasal sinus region and their clinical importance. Eur J Radiol 2004;50(3):296–302
10. Mann WJ, Tóth M, Gouveris H, Amedee RG. The drainage system of the paranasal sinuses: a review with possible implications for balloon catheter dilation. Am J Rhinol Allergy 2011;25(4):245–248
11. Mossa-Basha M, Blitz AM. Imaging of the paranasal sinuses. Semin Roentgenol 2013;48(1):14–34
12. Mossey PA, Little J, Munger RG, Dixon MJ, Shaw WC. Cleft lip and palate. Lancet 2009;374(9703):1773–1785
13. Senggen E, Laswed T, Meuwly JY, et al. First and second branchial arch syndromes: multimodality approach. Pediatr Radiol 2011;41(5):549–561
14. Shin JH, Kim SW, Hong YK, et al. The Onodi cell: an obstacle to sellar lesions with a transsphenoidal approach. Otolaryngol Head Neck Surg 2011;145(6):1040–1042
15. Wormald PJ. The agger nasi cell: the key to understanding the anatomy of the frontal recess. Otolaryngol Head Neck Surg 2003;129(5):497–507

Arhinia

16. Brusati R, Donati V, Marelli S, Ferrari M. Management of a case of arhinia. J Plast Reconstr Aesthet Surg 2009;62(7):e206–e210
17. Sato D, Shimokawa O, Harada N, et al. Congenital arhinia: molecular-genetic analysis of five patients. Am J Med Genet A 2007;143A(6):546–552
18. Zhang MM, Hu YH, He W, Hu KK. Congenital arhinia: A rare case. Am J Case Rep 2014;15:115–118

Cerebrospinal Fluid Leaks

19. Lin DT, Lin AC. Surgical treatment of traumatic injuries of the cranial base. Otolaryngol Clin North Am 2013;46(5):749–757
20. Lloyd KM, DelGaudio JM, Hudgins PA. Imaging of skull base cerebrospinal fluid leaks in adults. Radiology 2008;248(3):725–736
21. Mantur M, Łukaszewicz-Zając M, Mroczko B, et al. Cerebrospinal fluid leakage—reliable diagnostic methods. Clin Chim Acta 2011;412(11-12):837–840
22. Mokri B. Radioisotope cisternography in spontaneous CSF leaks: interpretations and misinterpretations. Headache 2014;54(8):1358–1368
23. Psaltis AJ, Schlosser RJ, Banks CA, Yawn J, Soler ZM. A systematic review of the endoscopic repair of cerebrospinal fluid leaks. Otolaryngol Head Neck Surg 2012;147(2):196–203

Chronic Rhinosinusitis

24. Babinski D, Trawinska-Bartnicka M. Rhinosinusitis in cystic fibrosis: not a simple story. Int J Pediatr Otorhinolaryngol 2008;72(5):619–624
25. Crockett DJ, Wilson KF, Meier JD. Perioperative strategies to improve sinus surgery outcomes in patients with cystic fibrosis: a systematic review. Otolaryngol Head Neck Surg 2013;149(1):30–39

26. Eggesbø HB, Dølvik S, Stiris M, Søvik S, Storrøsten OT, Kolmannskog F. Complementary role of MR imaging of ethmomaxillary sinus disease depicted at CT in cystic fibrosis. Acta Radiol 2001;42(2):144–150
27. Knowles MR, Daniels LA, Davis SD, Zariwala MA, Leigh MW. Primary ciliary dyskinesia. Recent advances in diagnostics, genetics, and characterization of clinical disease. Am J Respir Crit Care Med 2013;188(8):913–922
28. Liang J, Higgins TS, Ishman SL, Boss EF, Benke JR, Lin SY. Surgical management of chronic rhinosinusitis in cystic fibrosis: a systematic review. Int Forum Allergy Rhinol 2013;3(10):814–822
29. Robertson JM, Friedman EM, Rubin BK. Nasal and sinus disease in cystic fibrosis. Paediatr Respir Rev 2008;9(3):213–219
30. Ryan MW. Diseases associated with chronic rhinosinusitis: what is the significance? Curr Opin Otolaryngol Head Neck Surg 2008;16(3):231–236
31. Zariwala MA, Omran H, Ferkol TW. The emerging genetics of primary ciliary dyskinesia. Proc Am Thorac Soc 2011;8(5):430–433

Craniofacial Fractures

32. Balakrishnan K, Ebenezer V, Dakir A, Kumar S, Prakash D. Management of tripod fractures (zygomaticomaxillary complex) 1 point and 2 point fixations: a 5-year review. J Pharm Bioallied Sci 2015;7(Suppl 1):S242–S247
33. Buchanan EP, Hopper RA, Suver DW, Hayes AG, Gruss JS, Birgfeld CB. Zygomaticomaxillary complex fractures and their association with naso-orbito-ethmoid fractures: a 5-year review. Plast Reconstr Surg 2012;130(6):1296–1304
34. Follmar KE, Baccarani A, Das RR, Erdmann D, Marcus JR, Mukundan S. A clinically applicable reporting system for the diagnosis of facial fractures. Int J Oral Maxillofac Surg 2007;36(7):593–600
35. Fraioli RE, Branstetter BF IV, Deleyiannis FWB. Facial fractures: beyond Le Fort. Otolaryngol Clin North Am 2008;41(1):51–76, vi
36. Zimmermann CE, Troulis MJ, Kaban LB. Pediatric facial fractures: recent advances in prevention, diagnosis and management. Int J Oral Maxillofac Surg 2006;35(1):2–13

Cystic Fibrosis

37. Fundakowski C, Ojo R, Younis R. Rhinosinusitis in the pediatric patient with cystic fibrosis. Curr Pediatr Rev 2014;10(3):198–201
38. Kang SH, Dalcin PdeT, Piltcher OB, Migliavacca RdeO. Chronic rhinosinusitis and nasal polyposis in cystic fibrosis: update on diagnosis and treatment. J Bras Pneumol 2015;41(1):65–76
39. Magit A. Pediatric rhinosinusitis. Otolaryngol Clin North Am 2014;47(5):733–746

Development of the Nasal Cavity and Paranasal Sinuses

40. Pohunek P. Development, structure and function of the upper airways. Paediatr Respir Rev 2004;5(1):2–8
41. Som PM, Lawson W, Fatterpkar GM, Zinreich SJ. Embryology, anatomy, physiology, and imaging of the sinonasal cavities. Head and Neck Imaging. 5th ed. St. Louis, MO: Elsevier-Mosby; 2011:99–166

Fungal Rhinosinusitis

42. Callejas CA, Douglas RG. Fungal rhinosinusitis: what every allergist should know. Clin Exp Allergy 2013;43(8):835–849
43. Ilica AT, Mossa-Basha M, Maluf F, Izbudak I, Aygun N. Clinical and radiologic features of fungal diseases of the paranasal sinuses. J Comput Assist Tomogr 2012;36(5):570–576
44. Mossa-Basha M, Blitz AM. Imaging of the paranasal sinuses. Semin Roentgenol 2013;48(1):14–34
45. Mossa-Basha M, Ilica AT, Maluf F, Karakoç Ö, Izbudak I, Aygün N. The many faces of fungal disease of the paranasal sinuses: CT and MRI findings. Diagn Interv Radiol 2013;19(3):195–200
46. Seo YJ, Kim J, Kim K, Lee JG, Kim CH, Yoon JH. Radiologic characteristics of sinonasal fungus ball: an analysis of 119 cases. Acta Radiol 2011;52(7):790–795

Granulomatous Sinus Disease

47. Guillevin L, Pagnoux C, Mouthon L. Churg-Strauss syndrome. Semin Respir Crit Care Med 2004;25(5):535–545
48. Fuchs HA, Tanner SB. Granulomatous disorders of the nose and paranasal sinuses. Curr Opin Otolaryngol Head Neck Surg 2009;17(1):23–27
49. Greco A, Rizzo MI, De Virgilio A, et al. Churg-Strauss syndrome. Autoimmun Rev 2015;14(4):341–348

50. Kohanski MA, Reh DD. Chapter 11: Granulomatous diseases and chronic sinusitis. Am J Rhinol Allergy 2013;27(Suppl 1):S39–S41
51. Tami TA. Granulomatous diseases and chronic rhinosinusitis. Otolaryngol Clin North Am 2005;38(6):1267–1278, x
52. Trimarchi M, Sinico RA, Teggi R, Bussi M, Specks U, Meroni PL. Otorhinolaryngological manifestations in granulomatosis with polyangiitis (Wegener's). Autoimmun Rev 2013;12(4):501–505

Inflammatory Sinus Disease

53. Brook I. Acute sinusitis in children. Pediatr Clin North Am 2013;60(2):409–424
54. Eggesbø HB. Radiological imaging of inflammatory lesions in the nasal cavity and paranasal sinuses. Eur Radiol 2006;16(4):872–888
55. Maroldi R, Ravanelli M, Borghesi A, Farina D. Paranasal sinus imaging. Eur J Radiol 2008;66(3):372–386

Mucous Retention Cysts and Polyps

56. Kim YK, Kim HJ, Kim J, et al. Nasal polyps with metaplastic ossification: CT and MR imaging findings. Neuroradiology 2010;52(12):1179–1184
57. Maroldi R, Ravanelli M, Borghesi A, Farina D. Paranasal sinus imaging. Eur J Radiol 2008;66(3):372–386
58. Momeni AK, Roberts CC, Chew FS. Imaging of chronic and exotic sinonasal disease: review. AJR Am J Roentgenol 2007;189(6, Suppl):S35–S45

Nasal Septum

59. Kim SW, Rhee CS. Nasal septal perforation repair: predictive factors and systematic review of the literature. Curr Opin Otolaryngol Head Neck Surg 2012;20(1):58–65
60. Orlandi RR. A systematic analysis of septal deviation associated with rhinosinusitis. Laryngoscope 2010;120(8):1687–1695

Nasolabial Cyst

61. Kajla P, Lata J, Agrawal R. Nasolabial cyst: review of literature and a case report. J Maxillofac Oral Surg 2014;13(2):227–230
62. Perez AJ, Castle JT. Nasolabial cyst. Head Neck Pathol 2013;7(2):155–158
63. Sumer AP, Celenk P, Sumer M, Telcioglu NT, Gunhan O. Nasolabial cyst: case report with CT and MRI findings. Oral Surg Oral Med Oral Pathol Oral Radiol Endod 2010;109(2):e92–e94

Nasopalatine Duct Cyst

64. Cecchetti F, Ottria L, Bartuli F, Bramanti NE, Arcuri C. Prevalence, distribution, and differential diagnosis of nasopalatine duct cysts. Oral Implantol (Rome) 2012;5(2-3):47–53
65. Escoda Francolí J, Almendros Marqués N, Berini Aytés L, Gay Escoda C. Nasopalatine duct cyst: report of 22 cases and review of the literature. Med Oral Patol Oral Cir Bucal 2008;13(7):E438–E443
66. Nelson BL, Linfesty RL. Nasopalatine duct cyst. Head Neck Pathol 2010;4(2):121–122

Neuroglial Heterotopia

67. Hagiwara A, Nagai N, Ogawa Y, Suzuki M. A case of nasal glial heterotopia in an adult. Case Reports Otolaryngol 2014; doi.org/10.1155/2014/354672.
68. Husein OF, Collins M, Kang DR. Neuroglial heterotopia causing neonatal airway obstruction: presentation, management, and literature review. Eur J Pediatr 2008;167(12):1351–1355

Odontogenic Myxoma

69. Gupta S, Grover N, Kadam A, Gupta S, Sah K, Sunitha JD. Odontogenic myxoma. Natl J Maxillofac Surg 2013;4(1):81–83
70. Kheir E, Stephen L, Nortje C, van Rensburg LJ, Titinchi F. The imaging characteristics of odontogenic myxoma and a comparison of three different imaging modalities. Oral Surg Oral Med Oral Pathol Oral Radiol 2013;116(4):492–502
71. Kleiber GM, Skapek SX, Lingen M, Reid RR. Odontogenic myxoma of the face: mimicry of cherubism. J Oral Maxillofac Surg 2014;72(11):2186–2191
72. Manjunath SM, Gupta AA, Swetha P, Moon NJ, et al. Report of a rare case of an odontogenic myxoma of the maxilla and review of the literature. Ann Med Health Sci Res 2014;4:45–48

73. Noffke CE, Raubenheimer EJ, Chabikuli NJ, Bouckaert MMR. Odontogenic myxoma: review of the literature and report of 30 cases from South Africa. Oral Surg Oral Med Oral Pathol Oral Radiol Endod 2007;104(1):101–109

Ossifying Fibroma

74. Hara M, Matsuzaki H, Katase N, et al. Ossifying fibroma of the maxilla: a case report including its imaging features and dynamic magnetic resonance imaging findings. Oral Surg Oral Med Oral Pathol Oral Radiol 2012;114(4):e139–e146
75. Sarode SC, Sarode GS, Waknis P, Patil A, Jashika M. Juvenile psammomatoid ossifying fibroma: a review. Oral Oncol 2011;47(12):1110–1116
76. Triantafillidou K, Venetis G, Karakinaris G, Iordanidis F. Ossifying fibroma of the jaws: a clinical study of 14 cases and review of the literature. Oral Surg Oral Med Oral Pathol Oral Radiol 2012;114(2):193–199
77. Yang BT, Wang YZ, Wang XY, Wang ZC. Imaging study of ossifying fibroma with associated aneurysmal bone cyst in the paranasal sinus. Eur J Radiol 2012;81(11):3450–3455

Pediatric Midline Nasofrontal Mass

78. Kadom N, Sze RW. Radiological reasoning: pediatric midline nasofrontal mass. AJR Am J Roentgenol 2010;194(3, Suppl):WS10–WS13

Pott's Puffy Tumor

79. Haider HR, Mayatepek E, Schaper J, Vogel M. Pott's puffy tumor: a forgotten differential diagnosis of frontal swelling of the forehead. J Pediatr Surg 2012;47(10):1919–1921
80. Kombogiorgas D, Solanki GA. The Pott puffy tumor revisited: neurosurgical implications of this forgotten entity. J Neurosurg 2006;105:143–149
81. Parida PK, Surianarayanan G, Ganeshan S, Saxena SK. Pott's puffy tumor in pediatric age group: a retrospective study. Int J Pediatr Otorhinolaryngol 2012;76(9):1274–1277

Primary Ciliary Dyskinesia/Kartagener Syndrome

82. Leigh MW, Pittman JE, Carson JL, et al. Clinical and genetic aspects of primary ciliary dyskinesia/Kartagener syndrome. Genet Med 2009;11(7):473–487
83. Mener DJ, Lin SY, Ishman SL, Boss EF. Treatment and outcomes of chronic rhinosinusitis in children with primary ciliary dyskinesia: where is the evidence? A qualitative systematic review. Int Forum Allergy Rhinol 2013;3(12):986–991

Rhinolith

84. Barros CA, Martins RR, Silva JB, et al. Rhinolith: a radiographic finding in a dental clinic. Oral Surg Oral Med Oral Pathol Oral Radiol Endod 2005;100(4):486–490
85. Shenoy V, Maller V, Maller V. Maxillary antrolith: a rare cause of recurrent sinusitis. Case Rep Otolaryngol 2013;2013:527152

Silent Sinus Syndrome

86. Annino DJ Jr, Goguen LA. Silent sinus syndrome. Curr Opin Otolaryngol Head Neck Surg 2008;16(1):22–25
87. Hourany R, Aygun N, Della Santina CC, Zinreich SJ. Silent sinus syndrome: an acquired condition. AJNR Am J Neuroradiol 2005;26(9):2390–2392
88. Liss JA, Patel RD, Stefko ST. A case of bilateral silent sinus syndrome presenting with chronic ocular surface disease. Ophthal Plast Reconstr Surg 2011;27(6):e158–e160

Sinonasal Neoplasms

89. Barnes L, Tse LLY, Hunt JL. Schneiderian papillomas. In: Barnes L, Eveson JW, Reichart P, Sidransky D, eds. World Health Organization Classification of Tumours. Pathology and Genetics of Head and Neck Tumours. Lyon: IARC Press; 2005:28–32
90. Boo H, Hogg JP. Nasal cavity neoplasms: a pictorial review. Curr Probl Diagn Radiol 2010;39(2):54–61
91. Eggesbø HB. Imaging of sinonasal tumours. Cancer Imaging 2012;12:136–152
92. El-naggar AK, Huvos AG. Adenoid cystic carcinoma. In: Barnes L, Eveson JW, Reichart P, Sidransky D, eds. World Health Organization Classification of Tumours. Pathology and Genetics of Head and Neck Tumours. Lyon: IARC Press; 2005:221–222

93. Eveson JW. Salivary gland-type adenomas. In: Barnes L, Eveson JW, Reichart P, Sidransky D, eds. World Health Organization Classification of Tumours. Pathology and Genetics of Head and Neck Tumours. Lyon: IARC Press; 2005:34

94. Goode RK, El-Naggar AK. Mucoepidermoid carcinoma. In: Barnes L, Eveson JW, Reichart P, Sidransky D, eds. World Health Organization Classification of Tumours. Pathology and Genetics of Head and Neck Tumours. Lyon: IARC Press; 2005:219–220

95. Kim YK, Kim HJ, Kim J, et al. Nasal polyps with metaplastic ossification: CT and MR imaging findings. Neuroradiology 2010; 52(12):1179–1184

96. Madani G, Beale TJ, Lund VJ. Imaging of sinonasal tumors. Semin Ultrasound CT MR 2009;30(1):25–38

97. Melroy CT, Senior BA. Benign sinonasal neoplasms: a focus on inverting papilloma. Otolaryngol Clin North Am 2006;39(3):601–617, x

98. Momeni AK, Roberts CC, Chew FS. Imaging of chronic and exotic sinonasal disease: review. review AJR Am J Roentgenol 2007;189(6, Suppl):S35–S45

99. Raghavan P, Phillips CD. Magnetic resonance imaging of sinonasal malignancies. Top Magn Reson Imaging 2007;18(4):259–267

100. Thompson LDR, Fanburg-Smith JC. Nasopharyngeal angiofibroma. In: Barnes L, Eveson JW, Reichart P, Sidransky D, eds. World Health Organization Classification of Tumours. Pathology and Genetics of Head and Neck Tumours. Lyon: IARC Press; 2005:102–103

Sinonasal Sarcoidosis

101. Braun JJ, Gentine A, Pauli G. Sinonasal sarcoidosis: review and report of fifteen cases. Laryngoscope 2004;114(11):1960–1963

102. Kirsten AM, Watz H, Kirsten D. Sarcoidosis with involvement of the paranasal sinuses—a retrospective analysis of 12 biopsy-proven cases. BMC Pulm Med 2013;13:59

Sinusitis

103. Brook I. Acute sinusitis in children. Pediatr Clin North Am 2013; 60(2):409–424

104. Callejas CA, Douglas RG. Fungal rhinosinusitis: what every allergist should know. Clin Exp Allergy 2013;43(8):835–849

105. Eggesbø HB. Radiological imaging of inflammatory lesions in the nasal cavity and paranasal sinuses. Eur Radiol 2006;16(4):872–888

106. Fuchs HA, Tanner SB. Granulomatous disorders of the nose and paranasal sinuses. Curr Opin Otolaryngol Head Neck Surg 2009;17(1):23–27

107. Kombogiorgas D, Solanki GA. The Pott puffy tumor revisited: neurosurgical implications of this unforgotten entity. Case report and review of the literature. J Neurosurg 2006; 105(2, Suppl):143–149

108. Han JK. Subclassification of chronic rhinosinusitis. Laryngoscope 2013;123(Suppl 2):S15–S27

109. Madani G, Beale TJ. Sinonasal inflammatory disease. Semin Ultrasound CT MR 2009;30(1):17–24

110. Madani G, Beale TJ. Differential diagnosis in sinonasal disease. Semin Ultrasound CT MR 2009;30(1):39–45

111. Masterson L, Leong P. Pott's puffy tumour: a forgotten complication of frontal sinus disease. Oral Maxillofac Surg 2009;13(2):115–117

112. Mossa-Basha M, Ilica AT, Maluf F, Karakoç Ö, Izbudak I, Aygün N. The many faces of fungal disease of the paranasal sinuses: CT and MRI findings. Diagn Interv Radiol 2013;19(3):195–200

113. Reddy CEE, Gupta AK, Singh P, Mann SBS. Imaging of granulomatous and chronic invasive fungal sinusitis: comparison with allergic fungal sinusitis. Otolaryngol Head Neck Surg 2010;143(2):294–300

Sinus Polyps

114. Kim YK, Kim HJ, Kim J, et al. Nasal polyps with metaplastic ossification: CT and MR imaging findings. Neuroradiology 2010; 52(12):1179–1184

Chapter 4
Suprahyoid Neck

4

4 Suprahyoid Neck

Table 4.1	Pharyngeal mucosal space lesions
Table 4.2	Lesions of the prestyloid parapharyngeal space
Table 4.3	Lesions of the retrostyloid parapharyngeal space
Table 4.4	Retropharyngeal space lesions
Table 4.5	Lesions of the parotid space
Table 4.6	Lesions involving the masticator space
Table 4.7	Temporomandibular joint abnormalities
Table 4.8	Lesions involving the oropharynx, oral cavity, and floor of the mouth
Table 4.9	Submandibular space lesions
Table 4.10	Buccal space lesions

Introduction

Development of the Neck

Many structures of the head and neck develop via the transient embryonic branchial apparatus that forms between the fourth and seventh weeks of gestation. The branchial apparatus consists of branchial arches, pharyngeal pouches, and branchial grooves and membranes.

The branchial apparatus consists of four major and two rudimentary arches of mesoderm lined by ectoderm externally and endoderm internally within pouches that form at the end of the fourth week of gestation (**Fig. 4.1**). The mesoderm contains a dominant artery, nerve, cartilage, and muscle. The four major arches are separated by grooves (clefts). Each arch develops into a defined neck structure, with eventual obliteration of the branchial clefts. The first arch forms the external auditory canal, eustachian tube, most of the middle ear ossicles, mastoid air cells, muscles of mastication, mandible, external carotid artery, sensory nerves of the trigeminal nerve, and motor fibers of the oculomotor nerve. The second arch develops into the neck of the malleus, styloid process, stapedius muscle, motor fibers of the facial nerve, sensory fibers from the tongue, hyoid bone and adjacent muscles, and tonsillar and supratonsillar fossae. The third arch forms the inferior parathyroid glands, thymus, lower portion of the hyoid bone, proximal internal carotid artery, upper common carotid artery, motor fibers of CN IX to the pharynx, and sensory fibers from the posterior third of the tongue. The fourth arch develops into the superior parathyroid glands, epiglottis, thyroid cartilage, laryngeal muscles, superior laryngeal nerve from the vagus nerve, aortic arch, and proximal right subclavian artery. The fifth arch is not visible on the surface and forms the cricoid, arytenoid, and corniculate cartilages of the larynx, the laryngeal muscles, the recurrent laryngeal nerves from the vagus nerve, and the proximal pulmonary arteries and ductus arteriosus. The sixth arch forms the branch nerves from CN X and CN XI, which merge into the recurrent laryngeal nerve and innervate the intrinsic muscles of the larynx, and the striated muscle of the upper cervical esophagus.

The first branchial cleft forms the epithelium of the external auditory canal. The other branchial clefts progressively involute.

4.1 Pharyngeal Mucosal Space Lesions

The pharyngeal mucosal space (PMS) is the portion of the nasopharynx and oropharynx along the upper airway that is bordered by the buccopharyngeal fascia (middle layer of the deep cervical fascia), which separates the PMS from the parapharyngeal space laterally and the retropharyngeal space dorsally (**Fig. 4.2**). The PMS includes mucous membranes, submucosa/minor salivary glands, lymphoid tissue (Waldeyer's ring: adenoids and palatine and lingual tonsils), the superior constrictor muscle of the pharynx, pharyngobasilar fascia (aponeurosis that connects the superior constrictor muscle to the skull base), the cartilaginous portion of the eustachian tube, the levator palatini muscle, and the outer margin of the buccopharyngeal fascia. The upper margin of the PMS is at the sphenoid and occipital bones. The inferior border is located at the level of the glossoepiglottic and pharyngoepiglottic folds of the hypopharynx.

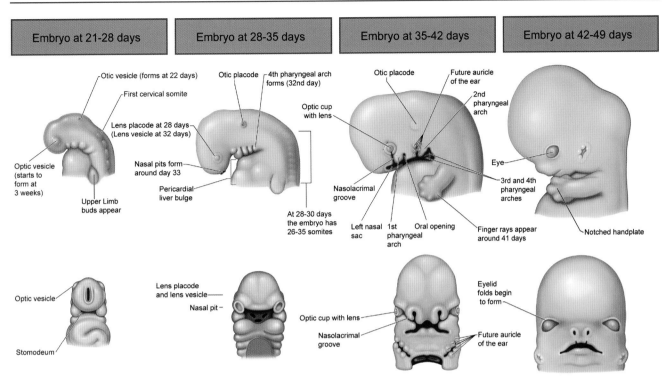

| Embryo at 21-28 days | Embryo at 28-35 days | Embryo at 35-42 days | Embryo at 42-49 days |

Fig. 4.1   Diagram shows progressive embryonic development of the pharyngeal (branchial) arches from 3 to 7 weeks of gestation.

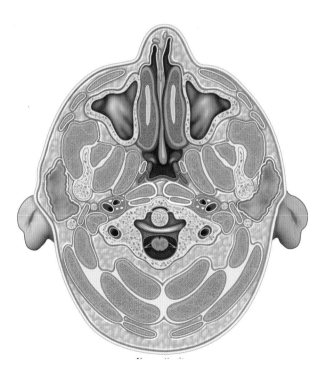

Fig. 4.2   Axial diagram shows the pharyngeal mucosal space in color.

Table 4.1   Pharyngeal mucosal space lesions

- Benign Neoplasms
  - Juvenile angiofibroma
  - Minor salivary gland tumor
  - Hemangioma
- Malignant Tumors
  - Squamous cell carcinoma
  - Sinonasal undifferentiated carcinoma
  - Adenoid cystic carcinoma
  - Adenocarcinoma and mucoepidermoid carcinoma
  - Non-Hodgkin lymphoma (NHL)
  - Rhabdomyosarcoma
- Tumorlike Lesions
  - Tornwaldt cyst
  - Nasopharyngeal mucous retention cyst
  - Lymphoid hyperplasia
  - Cephalocele (meningocele or meningoencephalocele)
  - Neuroglial heterotopia
- Inflammatory Lesions
  - Tonsillitis/peritonsillar abscess
  - Granulomatosis with polyangiitis (Wegener's granulomatosis)

Table 4.1 Pharyngeal mucosal space lesions

Lesion	Imaging Findings	Comments
Benign Neoplasms		
Juvenile angiofibroma (**Fig. 4.3**; see **Fig. 3.34**)	*MRI:* Origin of lesion is the pterygopalatine fossa. These lesions grow medially into the nasal cavity and nasopharynx via the sphenopalatine foramen, laterally into the pterygomaxillary fissure, superiorly via the inferior orbital fissure into the orbital apex, ± middle cranial fossa via the superior orbital fissure. Lesions often have intermediate signal on T1-weighted imaging and slightly high to high signal on T2-weighted imaging, ± flow voids, and prominent gadolinium contrast enhancement. *CT:* Lesions often have intermediate attenuation, ± hemorrhage, as well as erosion and/or remodeling of adjacent bone, such as widening of the pterygopalatine/pterygomaxillary fossae and/or sphenopalatine foramina and vidian canals.	Benign, cellular, and vascularized mesenchymal lesion/ malformation that occurs in the posterolateral nasal wall or nasopharynx from testosterone-sensitive cells and that is associated with high propensity to hemorrhage. Composed of thin-walled slitlike or dilated vessels of varying sizes lined by endothelial cells within fibrous stroma containing spindle, round, or stellate cells and varying amounts of collagen. Immunoreactive to platelet-derived growth factor B, insulin-like growth factor type II, vimentin, and smooth muscle actin. Typically occurs in males, with peak incidence in the second decade and overall incidence of 1 in 5,000–60,000. The lesion exhibits locally aggressive growth with erosion and/ or remodeling of adjacent bone and can spread through skull base foramina. Treatment can include embolization or hormonal therapy and, if necessary, surgical resection.
Minor salivary gland tumor (**Fig. 4.4**)	*MRI:* Circumscribed lesions with low-intermediate signal on T1-weighted imaging and slightly high signal on T2-weighted imaging (T2WI) and fat-suppressed T2WI, usually with gadolinium contrast enhancement. *CT:* Circumscribed or lobulated lesions with intermediate attenuation, + contrast enhancement.	This category includes benign glandular tumors of the sinonasal tract. Most common type is the pleomorphic adenoma, composed of modified myoepithelial cells associated with sparse stromal elements. Most arise from the submucosa of the nasal septum or lateral sinus wall. Usually occur in patients between 20 and 60 years old. Other, rare types of adenomas include myoepithelioma and oncocytoma.
Hemangioma (**Fig. 4.5**)	*MRI:* Circumscribed or poorly marginated structures (< 4 cm in diameter) in bone marrow or soft tissue with intermediate-high signal on T1-weighted imaging (often containing portions that are isointense to marrow fat) and high signal on T2-weighted imaging (T2WI) and fat-suppressed T2WI, typically with gadolinium contrast enhancement, ± expansion of bone. *CT:* Expansile bone lesions with a radiating pattern of bony trabeculae oriented toward the center. Hemangiomas in soft tissue have mostly intermediate attenuation, ± zones of fat attenuation.	Benign lesions of bone or soft tissue composed of capillary, cavernous, and/or malformed venous vessels. Considered to be a hamartomatous disorder. Occur in patients 1 to 84 years old (median age = 33 years).

(continued on page 332)

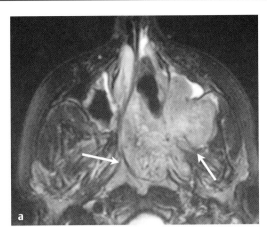
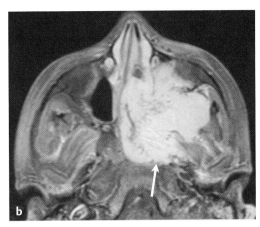

Fig. 4.3 **(a)** An 11-year-old male with a juvenile nasopharyngeal angiofibroma in the left nasopharynx with extension into the left nasal cavity and laterally into the pterygomaxillary fissure. The lesion has heterogeneous slightly high to high signal on axial fat-suppressed T2-weighted imaging with flow voids (*arrows*), and **(b)** shows prominent gadolinium contrast enhancement on axial fat-suppressed T1-weighted imaging (*arrow*).

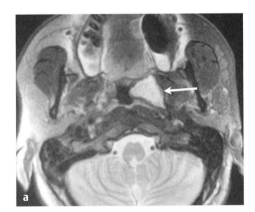
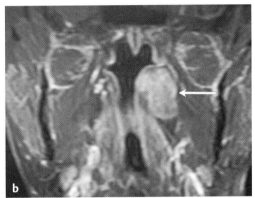

Fig. 4.4 **(a)** A 51-year-old man with a pleomorphic adenoma of a minor salivary gland involving the pharyngeal mucosal space of the left nasopharynx, which has high signal on axial T2-weighted imaging (*arrow*) and **(b)** shows gadolinium contrast enhancement on coronal fat-suppressed T1-weighted imaging (*arrow*).

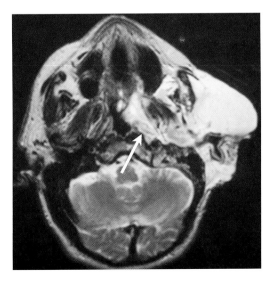

Fig. 4.5 A 65-year-old man with a large hemangioma involving the soft tissues of the left face, left parotid, and left masticator spaces, as well as the pharyngeal mucosal space of the left nasopharynx (*arrow*), with high signal on axial T2-weighted imaging.

Table 4.1 *(cont.)*   Pharyngeal mucosal space lesions

Lesion	Imaging Findings	Comments
Malignant Tumors		
Squamous cell carcinoma (**Fig. 4.6** and **Fig. 4.7**)	*MRI:* Lesions in the nasal cavity, paranasal sinuses, and nasopharynx, ± intracranial extension via bone destruction or perineural spread. Lesions have intermediate signal on T1-weighted imaging, intermediate-slightly high signal on T2-weighted imaging, and mild gadolinium contrast enhancement. Can be large lesions (± necrosis and/or hemorrhage). *CT:* Tumors have intermediate attenuation and mild contrast enhancement and can be large lesions (± necrosis and/or hemorrhage).	Malignant epithelial tumors originating from the mucosal epithelium of the paranasal sinuses (maxillary, 60%; ethmoid, 14%; sphenoid and frontal sinuses, 1%) and nasal cavity (25%). Include both keratinizing and nonkeratinizing types. Account for 80% of malignant sinonasal tumors and 3% of malignant tumors of the head and neck. Occurs in adults (usually more than 55 years old) and in males more than in females. Associated with occupational or other exposure to tobacco smoke, nickel, chlorophenols, chromium, mustard gas, radium, and material in the manufacture of wood products.
Sinonasal undifferentiated carcinoma (**Fig. 4.8**)	*MRI:* Locally destructive lesions, usually larger than 4 cm, with low-intermediate signal on T1-weighted imaging and intermediate to high signal on T2-weighted imaging, + prominent gadolinium contrast enhancement. Locations: superior nasal cavity, ethmoid air cells with occasional extension into the other paranasal sinuses, orbits, anterior cranial fossa, and cavernous sinuses. *CT:* Tumors have intermediate attenuation and variable mild, moderate, or prominent contrast enhancement.	Malignant tumor composed of pleomorphic neoplastic cells with medium to large nuclei, prominent single nucleoli, and small amounts of eosinophilic cytoplasm. Mitotic activity is typically high and necrosis is common. Immunoreactive to CK7, CK8, CK19, ± to p53, epithelial membrane antigen, and neuron-specific enolase. Poor prognosis, with 5-year survival less than 20%.

(continued on page 334)

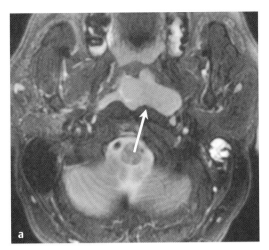
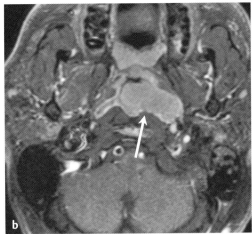

Fig. 4.6 **(a)** A 47-year-old man with a squamous cell carcinoma in the pharyngeal mucosal space of the posterior nasopharynx that has slightly high signal on axial fat-suppressed T2-weighted imaging (*arrow*) and **(b)** shows gadolinium contrast enhancement on axial fat-suppressed T1-weighted imaging (*arrow*).

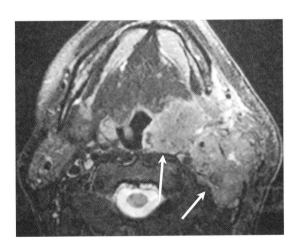

Fig. 4.7 A 57-year-old man with a squamous cell carcinoma (T2M2B) in the pharyngeal mucosal space that invades the adjacent soft tissues. The large tumor (*arrows*) has ill-defined margins and has heterogeneous slightly high signal on axial fat-suppressed T2-weighted imaging.

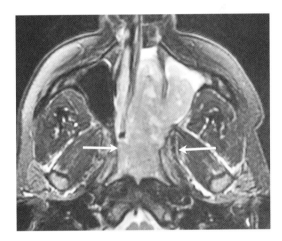

Fig. 4.8 A 41-year-old woman with a sinonasal undifferentiated carcinoma in the nasopharynx that extends into the nasal cavity and left maxillary sinus. The tumor has heterogeneous high signal on axial fat-suppressed T2-weighted imaging (*arrows*).

Table 4.1 *(cont.)*   Pharyngeal mucosal space lesions

Lesion	Imaging Findings	Comments
Adenoid cystic carcinoma (**Fig. 4.9** and **Fig. 4.10**; see **Fig. 3.46**)	*MRI:* Lesions in the nasal cavity or sinuses with intracranial extension via bone destruction or perineural spread. Lesions have intermediate signal on T1-weighted imaging, intermediate to high signal on T2-weighted imaging, and variable mild, moderate, or prominent gadolinium contrast enhancement. *CT:* Tumors have intermediate attenuation and variable mild, moderate, or prominent contrast enhancement. Destruction of adjacent bone is commonly seen.	Basaloid tumor comprised of neoplastic epithelial and myoepithelial cells. Morphologic tumor patterns include tubular, cribriform, and solid. Most common sinonasal malignancy of salivary gland origin. Accounts for 10% of epithelial salivary neoplasms. Most commonly involves the parotid, submandibular, and minor salivary glands (palate, tongue, buccal mucosa, floor of the mouth, and other locations). Perineural tumor spread is common, ± facial nerve paralysis. Usually occurs in adults > 30 years old. Solid type has the worst prognosis. Up to 90% of patients die within 10–15 years of diagnosis.
Adenocarcinoma and mucoepidermoid carcinoma (**Fig. 4.11** and **Fig. 4.12**)	*MRI:* Lesions in the nasal cavity or paranasal sinuses with intracranial extension via bone destruction or perineural spread. Lesions have intermediate signal on T1-weighted imaging intermediate to high signal on T2-weighted imaging, and variable mild, moderate, or prominent gadolinium contrast enhancement. *CT:* Tumors have intermediate attenuation and variable mild, moderate, or prominent contrast enhancement. Destruction of adjacent bone is commonly seen.	Second and third most common malignant sinonasal tumors derived from salivary glands. Adenocarcinomas contain small to medium-size neoplastic cells with oval nuclei, typically immunoreactive to cytokeratin, vimentin, and S-100 protein. Mucoepidermoid carcinomas often have solid portions with basaloid or cuboidal neoplastic cells and cystic portions containing sialomucin lined by mucous cells with peripheral nuclei within pale cytoplasm. Most commonly occur in the maxillary sinus and nasal cavity. Tumors usually are intermediate to high grade and often are advanced at presentation, ± metastases, ± perineural tumor spread.

(continued on page 336)

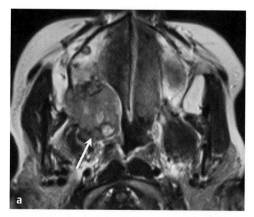 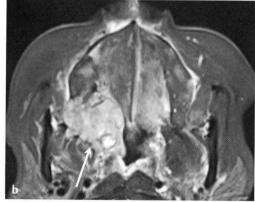

Fig. 4.9 **(a)** A 57-year-old woman with an adenoid cystic carcinoma in the pharyngeal mucosal space of the right nasopharynx that extends laterally into the right parapharyngeal and masticator spaces and anteriorly into the right nasal cavity with invasion of the maxilla. The tumor has heterogeneous intermediate to slightly high signal on axial T2-weighted imaging (*arrow*) and **(b)** shows gadolinium contrast enhancement on axial fat-suppressed T1-weighted imaging (*arrow*).

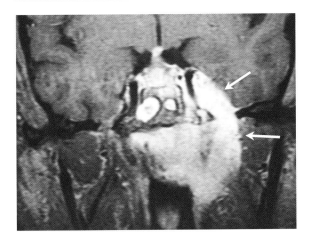

Fig. 4.10 Coronal fat-suppressed T1-weighted imaging shows a gadolinium-enhancing adenoid cystic carcinoma (*arrows*) in the pharyngeal mucosal space of the left nasopharynx that extends intracranially through a widened left foramen ovale.

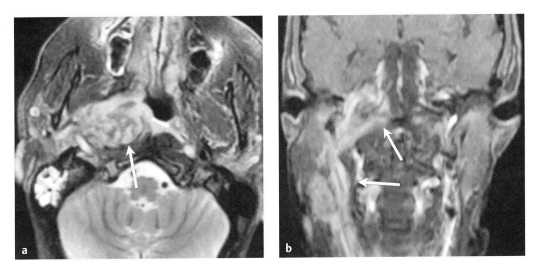

Fig. 4.11 **(a)** Axial fat-suppressed T2-weighted imaging shows a mucoepidermoid carcinoma in the posterior right nasopharynx that invades the retropharyngeal space posteriorly and parapharyngeal space laterally (*arrow*). **(b)** The tumor (*arrows*) shows gadolinium contrast enhancement and perineural neoplastic spread along the right CN V through the foramen ovale and along CN VII (*lower arrow*).

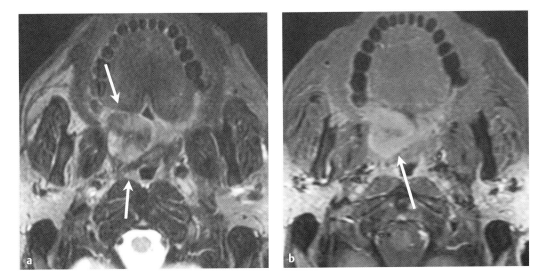

Fig. 4.12 **(a)** Axial T2-weighted imaging shows an adenocarcinoma in the pharyngeal mucosal space at the right side of the nasopharynx that has mixed intermediate, low, and slightly high signal on axial T2-weighted imaging (*arrows*) and **(b)** shows mild gadolinium contrast enhancement on axial fat-suppressed T1-weighted imaging (*arrow*).

Table 4.1 *(cont.)* Pharyngeal mucosal space lesions

Lesion	Imaging Findings	Comments
Non-Hodgkin lymphoma (NHL) (**Fig. 4.13** and **Fig. 4.14**)	*MRI:* Lesions have low-intermediate signal on T1-weighted imaging and intermediate to slightly high signal on T2-weighted imaging, + gadolinium contrast enhancement. Can be locally invasive and associated with bone erosion/destruction, intracranial extension with meningeal involvement (up to 5%). B-cell NHL often occurs in the maxillary sinuses, whereas T-cell NHL frequently occurs in the midline, including the septum. *CT:* Lesions have low-intermediate attenuation and may show contrast enhancement, ± bone destruction.	Lymphomas are a group of tumors whose neoplastic cells typically arise within lymphoid tissue (lymph nodes and reticuloendothelial organs). Most lymphomas in the nasopharynx, nasal cavity, and paranasal sinuses are NHL (B-cell NHL is more common than T-cell NHL) and more commonly are related to disseminated disease than to primary sinonasal tumors. Sinonasal lymphoma has a poor prognosis, with 5-year survival of less than 65%.
Rhabdomyosarcoma (**Fig. 4.15**)	*MRI:* Tumors can have circumscribed and/or poorly defined margins and typically have low-intermediate signal on T1-weighted imaging and heterogeneous signal (various combinations of intermediate, slightly high, and/or high signal) on T2-weighted imaging (T2WI) and fat-suppressed T2WI. Tumors show variable degrees of gadolinium contrast enhancement, ± bone destruction and invasion. *CT:* Soft tissue lesions that can have circumscribed or irregular margins. Calcifications are uncommon. Tumors can have mixed CT attenuation, with solid zones of soft tissue attenuation, cystic appearing and/or necrotic zones, and occasional foci of hemorrhage, ± bone invasion and destruction.	Malignant mesenchymal tumors with rhabdomyoblastic differentiation that occur primarily in soft tissue, and only very rarely in bone. There are three subgroups of rhabdomyosarcoma: embryonal (50–70%), alveolar (18–45%), and pleomorphic (5–10%). Embryonal and alveolar rhabdomyosarcomas occur primarily in children < 10 years old, and pleomorphic rhabdomyosarcomas occur mostly in adults. (median age in the sixth decade). Alveolar and pleomorphic rhabdomyosarcomas occur frequently in the extremities. Embryonal rhabdomyosarcomas occur mostly in the head and neck.

(continued on page 338)

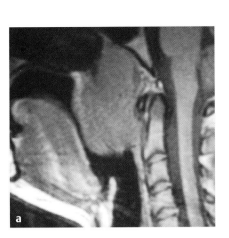
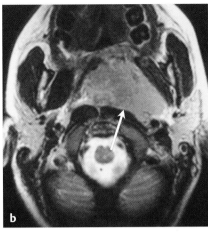
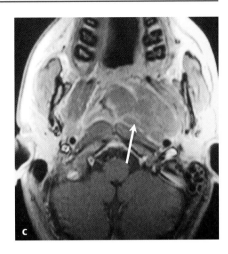

Fig. 4.13 **(a)** A 16-year-old female with non-Hodgkin lymphoma in the pharyngeal mucosal space of the nasopharynx that has intermediate signal on sagittal T1-weighted imaging, **(b)** intermediate to slightly high signal on axial T2-weighted imaging (*arrow*), and **(c)** mild gadolinium contrast enhancement on axial T1-weighted imaging (*arrow*).

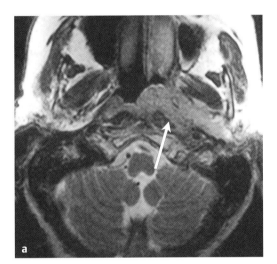
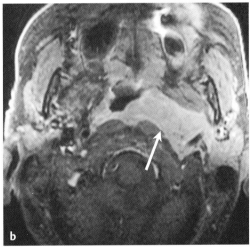

Fig. 4.14 **(a)** A 78-year-old woman with non-Hodgkin lymphoma in the left side of the pharyngeal mucosal space at the nasopharynx that invades the retropharyngeal space posteriorly and left parapharyngeal space laterally. The neoplasm has intermediate signal on axial T2-weighted imaging (*arrow*) and **(b)** shows gadolinium contrast enhancement on axial fat-suppressed T1-weighted imaging (*arrow*).

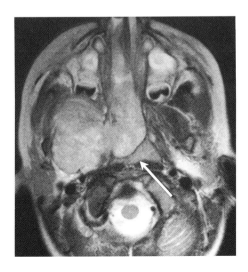

Fig. 4.15 A 5-year-old male with a rhabdomyosarcoma (*arrow*) in the right nasopharynx (pharyngeal mucosal space), right nasal cavity, and right parapharyngeal and masticator spaces that has heterogeneous slightly high and high signal on axial T2-weighted imaging.

Table 4.1 *(cont.)*   Pharyngeal mucosal space lesions

Lesion	Imaging Findings	Comments
Tumorlike Lesions		
Tornwaldt cyst (**Fig. 4.16** and **Fig. 4.17**)	*MRI:* Circumscribed lesion in the dorsal nasopharynx, in the midline, which often has low-intermediate signal on T1-weighted imaging (T1WI) and high signal on T2-weighted imaging (T2WI). High signal on FLAIR is seen in 65%. Approximately one-third of Tornwaldt cysts have elevated protein concentration, and the signal can vary from intermediate to high on T1WI and low, intermediate, to slightly high on T2WI, ± thin peripheral gadolinium contrast enhancement. *CT:* Circumscribed soft tissue structures in the dorsal nasopharynx, in the midline, measuring < 1.6 cm, with low to intermediate attenuation depending on the proportions of protein and water.	Common benign cystic lesion in the posterior wall of the nasopharynx, in the midline (98%) or parasagittal location (2%). Prevalence of 6%, with age of peak prevalence between 51 and 60 years. Arises from outpouching of the pharyngeal mucosa related to retraction of notochord. Measures up to 16 mm. Typically asymptomatic unless complicated by infection. Cyst-wall linings contain columnar epithelial cells.
Nasopharyngeal mucous retention cyst (**Fig. 4.18**)	*MRI:* Circumscribed lesion that often has low signal on T1-weighted imaging (T1WI) and high signal on T2-weighted imaging (T2WI). Mucous retention cysts or polyps can have inspissated secretions and elevated protein concentration, and the signal can vary from intermediate to high on T1WI, and low, intermediate, to slightly high on T2WI, ± thin peripheral gadolinium contrast enhancement. *CT:* Circumscribed, soft tissue structures with low to intermediate attenuation depending on the proportions of protein and water.	Mucous retention cysts arise from obstruction of seromucinous glands. Serous retention cysts occur from accumulation of fluid in the submucosal layer. Mucous retention cysts contain a rim of granulation tissue, inflammatory cells, residual lymphoid tissue, and mucus with varying concentrations of protein. Measure up to 16 mm. Prevalence of up to 10% in adult patients. Occur in parasagittal locations (54%), laterally (40%), and in the midline (7%). Can occur as solitary or multiple lesions (up to 60%) and are usually asymptomatic.

(continued on page 340)

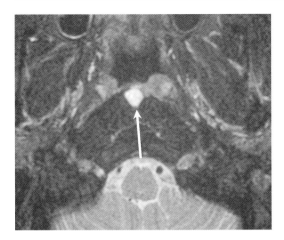

Fig. 4.16 A 44-year-old man with a Tornwaldt cyst (*arrow*) that is seen as a small circumscribed lesion in the dorsal nasopharynx in the midline and that has high signal on axial fat-suppressed T2-weighted imaging.

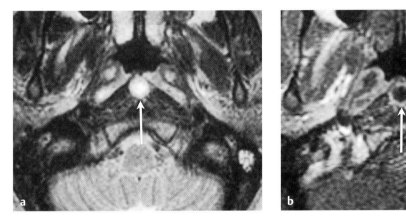

Fig. 4.17 **(a)** A 35-year-old woman with a Tornwaldt cyst that is seen as a small circumscribed lesion in the dorsal nasopharynx in the midline and that has high signal on axial T2-weighted imaging (*arrow*) and **(b)** low signal centrally with thin peripheral gadolinium contrast enhancement on axial T1-weighted imaging (*arrow*).

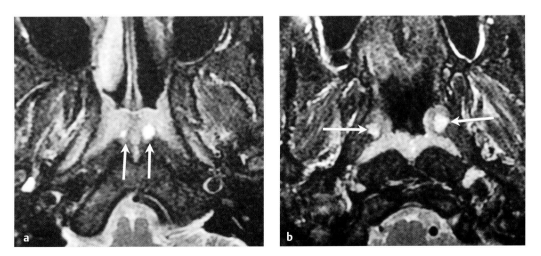

Fig. 4.18 **(a,b)** A 37-year-old man with nasopharyngeal mucous retention cysts (*arrows*) in the pharyngeal mucosal space that have high signal on axial fat-suppressed T2-weighted imaging.

Table 4.1 *(cont.)* Pharyngeal mucosal space lesions

Lesion	Imaging Findings	Comments
Lymphoid hyperplasia (**Fig. 4.19**)	*MRI:* In adults, median nasopharyngeal mucosal thickness of the posterior and lateral walls is 3–4 mm, and thickness of the roof ranges from 7 to 12 mm. With lymphoid hyperplasia, there is typically symmetric thickening in the nasopharyngeal roof and/or posterior and lateral walls of the nasopharynx. Enlarged adenoids from lymphoid hyperplasia can have vertically aligned thin bands of gadolinium contrast with intervening hypo-enhancing thin bands. Nonenhancing small mucous retention cysts occur in up 41% of nasopharyngeal mucosa. Collapse of the nasopharyngeal recess from lymphoid hyperplasia can also be seen. *CT:* Symmetric thickening of the walls of the nasopharynx, including the adenoids and palatine and/or lingual tonsils.	Nasopharyngeal mucosa has variable amounts of lymphoid tissue in the upper posterior portion (adenoids). Adenoids progressively enlarge in children up to 7 years old, followed by gradual regression. Benign lymphoid hyperplasia involving the adenoids and lingual and palatine tonsils can occur from environmental irritants and infection. In up to 95% of cases, the nasopharyngeal wall thickening is symmetric. Adenoid thickening up to 15 mm can occur in elderly patients from lymphoid hyperplasia. Biopsies typically show lymphoid follicles.
Cephalocele (meningocele or meningoencephalocele) (**Fig. 4.20**)	CT and *MRI:* Defect in skull through which there is herniation of either meninges and CSF (meningocele) or meninges, CSF, and brain tissue (meningoencephalocele).	Congenital malformation involving lack of separation of neuroectoderm from surface ectoderm, with resultant localized failure of bone formation. Can involve the sphenoid bone with extension into the sella, sphenoid bone and sinus, and nasopharynx. Incidence of transsphenoidal meningoencephaloceles is 1 per 700,000 live births. Clinical findings include difficulty in feeding and nasal obstruction in the first year, as well as potential for CSF leaks and meningitis.
Neuroglial heterotopia (**Fig. 4.21**)	*MRI:* Lesions usually have circumscribed margins and can contain various combinations and proportions of zones with low and/or intermediate signal on T1-weighted imaging and intermediate, high, and/or low signal on T2-weighted imaging (T2WI) and fat-suppressed T2WI. Lesions usually show no gadolinium contrast enhancement unless traumatized or infected. *CT:* Can contain zones with low and intermediate attenuation.	Rare congenital lesions that result from encephaloceles that become sequestered on the extracranial side of the skull base and that contain mature neuroglial elements. Can occur in the nasal cavity or nasopharynx, with or without neonatal airway obstruction. Can be associated with an osseous defect at the skull base. Typically there is no communication with the intracranial subarachnoid space.

(continued on page 342)

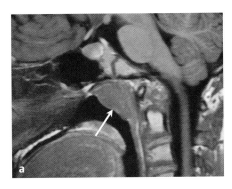
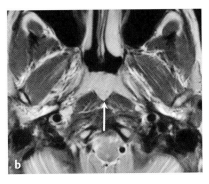
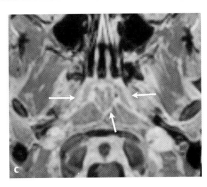

Fig. 4.19   (a) A 17-year-old male with adenoidal lymphoid hyperplasia that has intermediate signal on sagittal T1-weighted imaging (*arrow*). **(b)** Symmetric thickening of lymphoid tissue in the posterior nasopharynx (*arrow*) has slightly high signal on axial T2-weighted imaging and **(c)** has vertically aligned thin bands of gadolinium contrast with intervening hypo-enhancing thin bands on axial T1-weighted imaging (*arrows*).

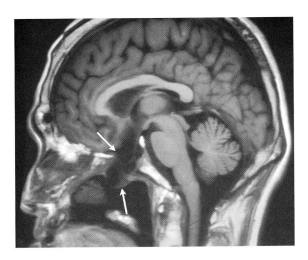

Fig. 4.20   Sagittal T1-weighted imaging of a 40-year-old man shows a meningocele (*arrows*) extending into the nasopharynx through a skull defect involving the anterior sella and planum sphenoidale.

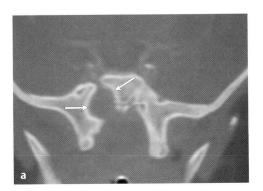
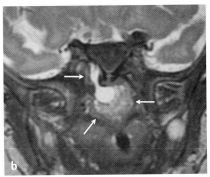
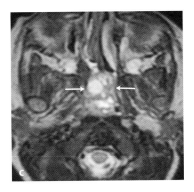

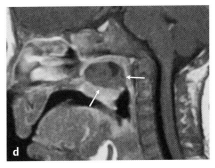

Fig. 4.21   (a) Coronal CT of an 8-week-old female shows a defect at the right side of the sphenoid bone (*arrows*) associated with a nasopharyngeal lesion that has mixed intermediate and high signal on **(b)** coronal and **(c)** axial T2-weighted imaging (*arrows*). **(d)** The nasopharyngeal lesion shows no gadolinium contrast enhancement on sagittal T1-weighted imaging (*arrows*). The pathologic diagnosis of the resected lesion was neuroglial heterotopia.

Table 4.1 *(cont.)* Pharyngeal mucosal space lesions

Lesion	Imaging Findings	Comments
Inflammatory Lesions		
Tonsillitis/ peritonsillar abscess **(Fig. 4.22)**	*MRI:* Soft tissue thickening at the palatine tonsil and adjacent lateral soft tissue with poorly defined, slightly high signal on T2-weighted imaging (T2WI) and fat-suppressed T2WI. Peritonsillar abscesses are collections with high signal on T2WI surrounded by a peripheral rim of gadolinium contrast enhancement. Soft tissue thickening with slightly high to high signal on T2WI lateral to the tonsil without a rim-enhancing collection can represent a phlegmon. *CT:* Soft tissue thickening at the palatine tonsil with adjacent lateral rim-enhancing fluid collection. Soft tissue thickening lateral to the tonsil without a rim-enhancing collection can represent a phlegmon.	Infection of the palatine tonsils (acute tonsillitis) is a clinical diagnosis and is typically treated with antibiotics. Tonsillar abscesses rarely occur. Extension of tonsillitis beyond the fibrous tonsillar capsule into the peritonsillar space (potential space between the palatine tonsil and the superior constrictor muscle) can result in peritonsillar cellulitis and peritonsillar abscess. Peritonsillar abscess is the most common infection involving the head and neck. Occurs in young children and adults, often during times with the highest incidence of streptococcal pharyngitis and exudative tonsillitis (November–December, and April–May). Treatment of a peritonsillar phlegmon can be with antibiotics, whereas a peritonsillar abscess requires drainage. If not treated appropriately, the infection can extend into the adjacent parapharyngeal, masticator, and/or submandibular spaces.
Granulomatosis with polyangiitis (Wegener's granulomatosis) **(Fig. 4.23)**	*MRI:* Poorly defined zones of soft tissue thickening with low-intermediate signal on T1-weighted imaging, slightly high to high signal on T2-weighted imaging, and gadolinium contrast enhancement within the nasal cavity, paranasal sinuses, orbits, infratemporal fossa, and external auditory canal, ± invasion and destruction of bone and nasal septum, ± extension into the skull base with involvement of the dura, leptomeninges, brain, or venous sinuses. *CT:* Zones with soft tissue attenuation, ± bone destruction.	Multisystem autoimmune disease with necrotizing granulomas in the respiratory tract, focal necrotizing angiitis of small arteries and veins of various tissues, and glomerulonephritis. Can involve the paranasal sinuses, orbits, skull base, dura, leptomeninges, and occasionally the temporal bone. Typically, positive immunoreactivity to cytoplasmic antineutrophil cytoplasmic antibody (c-ANCA). Treatment includes corticosteroids, cyclophosphamide, and anti-TNF agents.

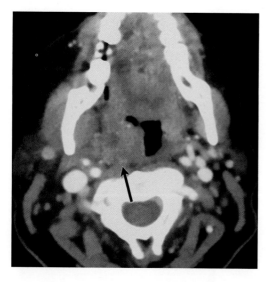

Fig. 4.22 A 57-year-old man with tonsillitis and a right peritonsillar abscess. Axial CT shows soft tissue thickening at the right palatine tonsil (*arrow*) with an adjacent lateral fluid collection.

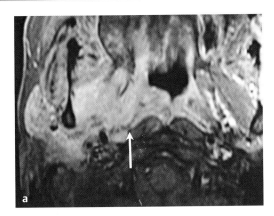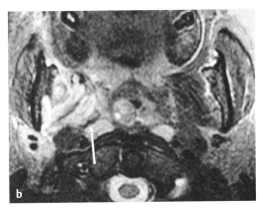

Fig. 4.23 A 46-year-old woman who has granulomatosis with polyangiitis. **(a)** Poorly defined zones with abnormal high signal on axial fat-suppressed T2-weighted imaging (*arrow*) and **(b)** gadolinium contrast enhancement on axial fat-suppressed T1-weighted imaging (*arrow*) are seen from granulomatous disease involving the pharyngeal mucosal space of the right posterior nasopharynx as well as the retropharyngeal, right parapharyngeal, and masticator spaces.

4.2 Lesions of the Prestyloid Parapharyngeal Space

The parapharyngeal space (PPS) is a region in the upper neck located lateral to the pharynx, deep to the pterygoid muscles and parotid glands, and anterior to the prevertebral muscles. The upper border of the PPS is the skull base and the lower border is the hyoid bone. It is separated from the pharyngeal mucosal space medially by the buccopharyngeal fascia (middle layer of the deep cervical fascia), anterolaterally from the masticator space by the superficial layer of the deep cervical fascia, and posteromedially from the prevertebral muscles by the deep layer of the deep cervical fascia. These fascial layers result in relative barriers to spread of disease to and from the PPS. Posterolaterally, there is a lack of continuous fascia separating the PPS from the deep portion of the parotid gland and anteroinferiorly from the sublingual and submandibular spaces. As a result, lesions are readily able to pass between the PPS and these spaces.

The PPS is divided into an anterolateral portion (prestyloid parapharyngeal space; PPPS) and posterolateral portion (poststyloid or retrostyloid parapharyngeal space; RPPS), which are separated by the fascia that extends from the styloid process to the tensor veli palatine muscle (**Fig. 4.24**). The PPPS contains fat, connective tissue, second-division branches of the trigeminal nerve, internal maxillary artery and ascending pharyngeal artery from the external carotid artery, veins, lymph nodes, and minor salivary glands. The RPPS is the suprahyoid extension of the carotid space and contains the internal carotid artery, internal jugular vein, cranial nerves IX, X, XI, and XII, and sympathetic plexus (**Fig. 4.25**).

Mass lesions within the PPPS displace the lateral wall of the pharyngeal mucosal space medially, the internal carotid artery and other RPPS contents posteriorly, and the deep portion of the parotid gland laterally. A mass lesion in the RPPS (suprahyoid carotid space) displaces the fat of the PPPS fat anteriorly and the parotid space contents laterally. Lesions within the RPPS can displace the internal carotid artery anteriorly. Paragangliomas in the RPPS, such as carotid body tumors, can splay apart the internal and external carotid arteries within this space.

Lesions adjacent to the PPPS can result in patterns of displacement of the fat in the PPPS. Lesions in the masticator space displace the PPPS fat posteromedially, lesions in the pharyngeal mucosal space displace the PPPS fat laterally, lesions in the parotid space displace the PPPS fat medially, lesions in the RPPS displace the PPPS fat anteriorly, and lesions in the retropharyngeal space displace the PPPS fat anterolaterally.

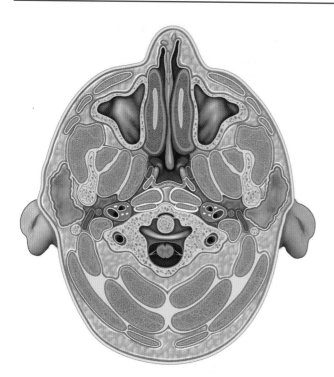

Fig. 4.24 Axial view diagram shows the prestyloid parapharyngeal space in color.

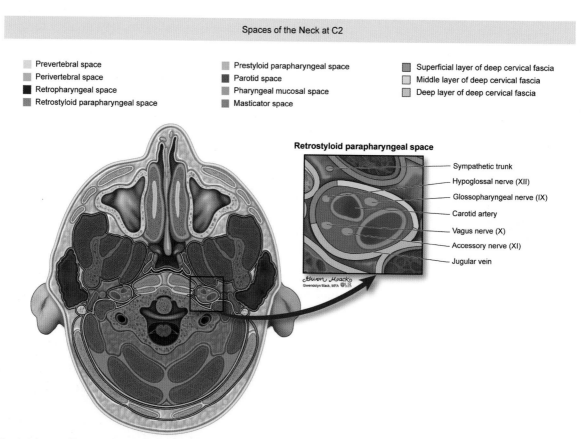

Fig. 4.25 Axial view diagram shows the retrostyloid parapharyngeal space in relation to the other suprahyoid spaces and layers of the deep cervical fascia.

Table 4.2 Lesions of the prestyloid parapharyngeal space

- Benign Neoplasms
  - Pleomorphic adenoma
  - Lipoma
  - Hemangioma
  - Schwannoma
- Malignant Tumors
  - Squamous cell carcinoma
  - Sinonasal undifferentiated carcinoma
  - Adenoid cystic carcinoma
  - Adenocarcinoma and mucoepidermoid carcinoma

- Non-Hodgkin lymphoma (NHL)
- Metastatic malignancies
- Rhabdomyosarcoma
- Hemangioendothelioma
- Teratoma
- Tumorlike Lesions
  - Branchial cleft cyst
- Inflammatory Lesions
  - Spread of infection from peritonsillar or retropharyngeal phlegmon and/or abscess
  - Granulomatosis with polyangiitis (Wegener's granulomatosis)

Table 4.2 Lesions of the prestyloid parapharyngeal space

Lesion	Imaging Findings	Comments
Benign Neoplasms		
Pleomorphic adenoma (**Fig. 4.26** and **Fig. 4.27**)	*MRI:* Circumscribed lesions with low-intermediate signal on T1-weighted imaging, slightly high signal on T2-weighted imaging (T2WI) and fat-suppressed T2WI, and usually gadolinium contrast enhancement. *CT:* Circumscribed or lobulated lesions with intermediate attenuation, + contrast enhancement.	Pleomorphic adenomas arise from the deep portion of the parotid gland or from minor salivary gland rests in the parapharyngeal space. They are composed of modified myoepithelial cells associated with sparse stromal elements. Usually occur in patients between 20 and 60 years old. Other, rare types of minor salivary gland adenomas include myoepithelioma and oncocytoma.

(continued on page 346)

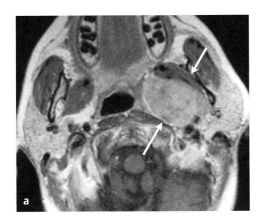
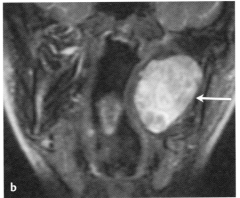

Fig. 4.26 **(a)** A 35-year-old woman with a pleomorphic adenoma in the left parapharyngeal space that has intermediate signal on axial T1-weighted imaging (*arrows*) and **(b)** heterogeneous high signal on coronal fat-suppressed T2-weighted imaging (*arrow*).

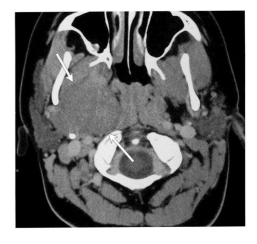

Fig. 4.27 Pleomorphic adenoma (*arrows*) in the right parapharyngeal space that has intermediate attenuation on axial CT.

Table 4.2 *(cont.)*   Lesions of the prestyloid parapharyngeal space

Lesion	Imaging Findings	Comments
Lipoma (**Fig. 4.28**)	*MRI:* Lipomas have MRI signal isointense to subcutaneous fat on T1-weighted imaging (high signal). On T2-weighted imaging, signal suppression occurs with frequency-selective fat saturation techniques or with a short time to inversion recovery (STIR) method. Typically there is no gadolinium contrast enhancement or peripheral edema. *CT:* Lipomas have CT attenuation similar to subcutaneous fat and typically no contrast enhancement or peripheral edema.	Common benign hamartomas composed of mature white adipose tissue without cellular atypia. Most common soft tissue tumor, representing 16% of all soft tissue tumors.
Hemangioma	*MRI:* Circumscribed or poorly marginated structures (< 4 cm in diameter) in bone marrow or soft tissue with intermediate-high signal on T1-weighted imaging (often with portions that are isointense to marrow fat) and high signal on T2-weighted imaging (T2WI) and fat-suppressed T2WI, typically with gadolinium contrast enhancement, ± expansion of bone. *CT:* Expansile bone lesions with a radiating pattern of bony trabeculae oriented toward the center. Hemangiomas in soft tissue have mostly intermediate attenuation, ± zones of fat attenuation.	Benign lesions of bone or soft tissue composed of capillary, cavernous, and/or malformed venous vessels. Considered to be a hamartomatous disorder. Occur in patients 1 to 84 years old (median age = 33 years).
Schwannoma (**Fig. 4.29**)	*MRI:* Circumscribed spheroid or ovoid lesions with low-intermediate signal on T1-weighted imaging, high signal on T2-weighted imaging (T2WI) and fat-suppressed T2WI, and usually prominent gadolinium (Gd) contrast enhancement. High signal on T2WI and Gd contrast enhancement can be heterogeneous in large lesions due to cystic degeneration and/or hemorrhage. *CT:* Circumscribed spheroid or ovoid lesions with intermediate attenuation, + contrast enhancement. Large lesions can have cystic degeneration and/or hemorrhage.	Schwannomas are benign encapsulated tumors that contain differentiated neoplastic Schwann cells. They most commonly occur as solitary, sporadic lesions. Multiple schwannomas are often associated with neurofibromatosis type 2 (NF2), which is an autosomal dominant disease involving a gene at chromosome 22q12. In addition to schwannomas, patients with NF2 can also have multiple meningiomas and ependymomas. The incidence of NF2 is 1/37,000 to 1/50,000 newborns. Age at presentation is 22 to 72 years (mean age = 46 years). Peak incidence is in the fourth to sixth decades. Many patients with NF2 present in the third decade with bilateral vestibular schwannomas.
Malignant Tumors		
Squamous cell carcinoma	*MRI:* Lesions in the nasal cavity, paranasal sinuses, and nasopharynx, ± intracranial extension via bone destruction or perineural spread. Lesions have intermediate signal on T1-weighted imaging, intermediate to slightly high signal on T2-weighted imaging, and mild gadolinium contrast enhancement. Can be large lesions (± necrosis and/or hemorrhage). *CT:* Tumors have intermediate attenuation and mild contrast enhancement and can be large lesions (± necrosis and/or hemorrhage).	Malignant epithelial tumors originating from the mucosal epithelium of the paranasal sinuses and nasal cavity can extend into the prestyloid parapharyngeal space. Include both keratinizing and nonkeratinizing types. Account for 80% of malignant sinonasal tumors and 3% of malignant tumors of the head and neck. Occur in adults, usually > 55 years old, and in males more than in females. Associated with occupational or other exposure to tobacco smoke, nickel, chlorophenols, chromium, mustard gas, radium, and material in the manufacture of wood products.
Sinonasal undifferentiated carcinoma	*MRI:* Locally destructive lesions, usually larger than 4 cm, with low-intermediate signal on T1-weighted imaging and intermediate to high signal on T2-weighted imaging, + prominent gadolinium contrast enhancement. Locations: superior nasal cavity, ethmoid air cells with occasional extension into the other paranasal sinuses, orbits, anterior cranial fossa, and cavernous sinuses. *CT:* Tumors have intermediate attenuation and variable mild, moderate, or prominent contrast enhancement.	Malignant tumor composed of pleomorphic neoplastic cells with medium to large nuclei, prominent single nucleoli, and small amounts of eosinophilic cytoplasm. Mitotic activity is typically high and necrosis is common. Immunoreactive to CK7, CK8, CK19, ± to p53, epithelial membrane antigen, and neuron-specific enolase. Poor prognosis, with 5-year survival less than 20%.

(continued on page 348)

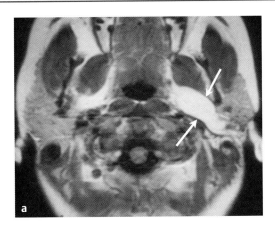 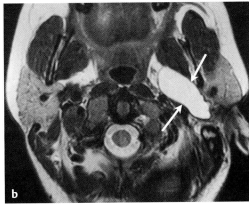

Fig. 4.28 **(a)** A 37-year-old woman with a lipoma in the left parapharyngeal space that has high signal on axial T1-weighted imaging (*arrows*) and **(b)** axial T2-weighted imaging (*arrows*).

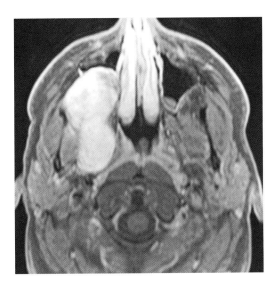

Fig. 4.29 A 30-year-old man with a right trigeminal schwannoma in the right parapharyngeal space and extending into the right maxillary sinus that shows gadolinium contrast enhancement on axial fat-suppressed T1-weighted imaging.

Table 4.2 *(cont.)*   Lesions of the prestyloid parapharyngeal space

Lesion	Imaging Findings	Comments
Adenoid cystic carcinoma (**Fig. 4.30**; see **Fig. 3.46**)	*MRI:* Lesions in the nasal cavity or sinuses with intracranial extension via bone destruction or perineural spread. Lesions have intermediate signal on T1-weighted imaging, intermediate to high signal on T2-weighted imaging, and variable mild, moderate, or prominent gadolinium contrast enhancement. *CT:* Tumors have intermediate attenuation and variable mild, moderate, or prominent contrast enhancement. Destruction of adjacent bone is commonly seen.	Basaloid tumor composed of neoplastic epithelial and myoepithelial cells. Morphologic tumor patterns include tubular, cribriform, and solid. Most common sinonasal malignancy of salivary gland origin. Accounts for 10% of epithelial salivary neoplasms. Most commonly involves the parotid, submandibular, and minor salivary glands (palate, tongue, buccal mucosa, and floor of the mouth, other locations). Perineural tumor spread common, ± facial nerve paralysis. Usually occurs in adults > 30 years old. Solid type has the worst prognosis. Up to 90% of patients die within 10–15 years of diagnosis.
Adenocarcinoma and mucoepidermoid carcinoma (**Fig. 4.31**)	*MRI:* Lesions in the nasal cavity or paranasal sinuses, ± intracranial extension via bone destruction or perineural spread. Lesions have intermediate signal on T1-weighted imaging intermediate to high signal on T2-weighted imaging, and variable mild, moderate, or prominent gadolinium contrast enhancement. *CT:* Tumors have intermediate attenuation and variable mild, moderate, or prominent contrast enhancement. Destruction of adjacent bone is commonly seen.	Second and third most common malignant sinonasal tumors derived from salivary glands. Adenocarcinomas contain small to medium-size neoplastic cells with oval nuclei, typically immunoreactive to cytokeratin, vimentin, and S-100 protein. Mucoepidermoid carcinomas often have solid portions with basaloid or cuboidal neoplastic cells and cystic portions containing sialomucin lined by mucous cells with peripheral nuclei within pale cytoplasm. Most commonly occur in the maxillary sinus and nasal cavity. Tumors usually are intermediate to high grade and often are advanced at presentation, ± metastases, ± perineural tumor spread.
Non-Hodgkin lymphoma (NHL) (**Fig. 4.32**)	*MRI:* Lesions have low-intermediate signal on T1-weighted imaging and intermediate to slightly high signal on T2-weighted imaging, + gadolinium contrast enhancement. Can be locally invasive and associated with bone erosion/destruction, intracranial extension with meningeal involvement (up to 5%). B-cell NHL often occurs in the maxillary sinuses, whereas T-cell NHL frequently occurs in the midline, including the septum. *CT:* Lesions have low-intermediate attenuation and may show contrast enhancement, ± bone destruction.	Lymphomas are a group of tumors whose neoplastic cells typically arise within lymphoid tissue (lymph nodes and reticuloendothelial organs). Most lymphomas in the nasopharynx, nasal cavity, and paranasal sinuses are NHL (B-cell NHL is more common than T-cell NHL) and more commonly are related to disseminated disease than to primary sinonasal tumors. Sinonasal lymphoma has a poor prognosis, with 5-year survival of less than 65%.
Metastatic malignancies	*MRI:* Circumscribed spheroid lesions that often have low-intermediate signal on T1-weighted imaging and intermediate-high signal on T2-weighted imaging, ± hemorrhage, calcifications, and cysts. Variable gadolinium contrast enhancement. *CT:* Lesions usually have low-intermediate attenuation, ± hemorrhage, calcifications, and cysts. Variable contrast enhancement, ± bone destruction, ± compression of neural tissue or vessels.	Primary extracranial tumor source: lung > breast > GI > GU > melanoma. Can occur as single or multiple well-circumscribed or poorly defined lesions. Metastatic tumors may cause variable destructive or infiltrative changes in single or multiple sites.

(continued on page 350)

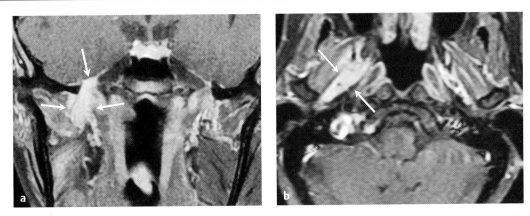

Fig. 4.30 **(a)** Coronal and **(b)** axial fat-suppressed T1-weighted images of 57-year-old woman show a gadolinium-enhancing adenoid cystic carcinoma (*arrows*) in the right parapharyngeal space with perineural spread superiorly along the right trigeminal nerve into the right foramen ovale.

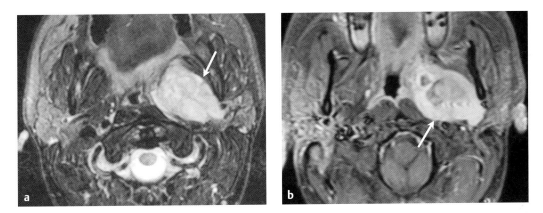

Fig. 4.31 **(a)** A 26-year-old man with an adenocarcinoma in the left parapharyngeal space that has heterogeneous high signal on axial fat-suppressed T2-weighted imaging (*arrow*) and **(b)** shows heterogeneous gadolinium contrast enhancement with slightly irregular margins on axial fat-suppressed T1-weighted imaging (*arrow*).

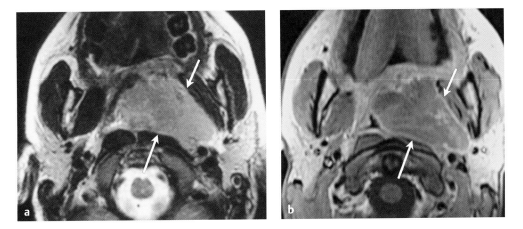

Fig. 4.32 **(a)** Non-Hodgkin lymphoma (*arrows*) is seen in the left parapharyngeal space, with extension into the retropharyngeal and pharyngeal mucosal spaces, that has intermediate to slightly high signal on axial T2-weighted imaging (*arrows*) and **(b)** heterogeneous gadolinium contrast enhancement on axial T1-weighted imaging (*arrows*).

Table 4.2 *(cont.)* Lesions of the prestyloid parapharyngeal space

Lesion	Imaging Findings	Comments
Rhabdomyosarcoma **(Fig. 4.33)**	*MRI:* Tumors can have circumscribed and/or poorly defined margins and typically have low-intermediate signal on T1-weighted imaging and heterogeneous signal (various combinations of intermediate, slightly high, and/or high signal) on T2-weighted imaging (T2WI) and fat-suppressed T2WI. Tumors show variable degrees of gadolinium contrast enhancement, ± bone destruction and invasion. *CT:* Soft tissue lesions that usually can have circumscribed or irregular margins. Calcifications are uncommon. Tumors can have mixed CT attenuation, with solid zones of soft tissue attenuation, cystic appearing and/or necrotic zones, and occasional foci of hemorrhage, ± bone invasion and destruction.	Malignant mesenchymal tumors with rhabdomyoblastic differentiation that occur primarily in soft tissue, and only very rarely in bone. There are three subgroups of rhabdomyosarcoma: embryonal (50–70%), alveolar (18–45%), and pleomorphic (5–10%). Embryonal and alveolar rhabdomyosarcomas occur primarily in children < 10 years old, and pleomorphic rhabdomyosarcomas occur mostly in adults (median age in the sixth decade). Alveolar and pleomorphic rhabdomyosarcomas occur frequently in the extremities. Embryonal rhabdomyosarcomas occur mostly in the head and neck.
Hemangioendothelioma (See **Fig. 6.26**)	*MRI:* Tumors have lobulated, well-defined or irregular margins and have intermediate signal on T1-weighted imaging and heterogeneous predominantly high signal on T2-weighted imaging, with or without internal low-signal septations. Flow voids may be seen with the lesions. Tumors show heterogeneous gadolinium contrast enhancement. *CT:* Can have circumscribed or irregular margins, ± bone invasion and destruction.	Low-grade malignant neoplasms composed of vasoformative/endothelial elements that occur in soft tissues and bone. These tumors are locally aggressive and rarely metastasize, compared with the high-grade endothelial tumors like angiosarcoma. Account for < 1% of malignant and all soft tissue tumors. Patients range in age from 17 to 60 years (mean age = 40 years).
Teratoma **(Fig. 4.34)**	*MRI:* Lesions usually have circumscribed margins and can contain various combinations and proportions of zones with low, intermediate, and/or high signal on T1-weighted imaging (T1WI), T2-weighted imaging (T2WI), and fat-suppressed (FS) T2WI. Can contain teeth and zones of bone formation, as well as amorphous, clumplike, and/or curvilinear calcifications with low signal on T1WI, T2WI, and FS T2WI. Fluid–fluid and fat–fluid levels may be seen within teratomas. Gadolinium contrast enhancement is usually seen in solid portions and septa. Invasion of adjacent tissue and bone destruction, as well as metastases, are findings associated with malignant teratomas. *CT:* Can contain zones with low and intermediate attenuation, with or without calcifications	Teratomas arise from displaced embryonic germ cells (multipotent germinal cells) and contain various combinations of cells and tissues derived from more than one germ layer (endoderm, mesoderm, ectoderm). Teratomas are the second most common type of germ cell tumors; occur in children; occur in males more than in females; and have benign or malignant types, composed of derivatives of ectoderm, mesoderm, and/or endoderm. *Mature teratomas* have differentiated cells from ectoderm (brain, skin, and/or choroid plexus), mesoderm (cartilage, bone, muscle, and/or fat); and endoderm (cysts with enteric or respiratory epithelia). *Immature teratomas* contain partially differentiated ectodermal, mesodermal, or endodermal cells.

(continued on page 352)

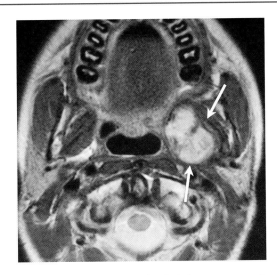

Fig. 4.33 A 14-year-old male with a rhabdomyosarcoma (*arrows*) in the left parapharyngeal space that has irregular margins and heterogeneous high signal on axial T2-weighted imaging.

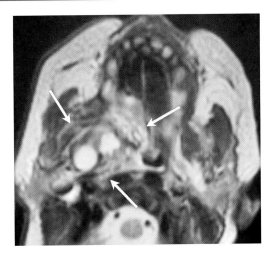

Fig. 4.34 Teratoma in the right parapharyngeal space with involvement of the pharyngeal mucosal, retropharyngeal, and masticator spaces. The lesion has ill-defined margins and contains zones with intermediate, slightly high, and high signal on axial T2-weighted imaging (*arrows*).

Table 4.2 *(cont.)*   Lesions of the prestyloid parapharyngeal space

Lesion	Imaging Findings	Comments
Tumorlike Lesions		
Branchial cleft cyst (**Fig. 4.35**)	*MRI:* Circumscribed lesion that often has low-intermediate signal on T1-weighted imaging and high signal on T2-weighted imaging. Usually there is no gadolinium contrast enhancement unless there is superimposed infection. *CT:* Circumscribed, cystic lesion with low to intermediate attenuation depending on the proportions of protein and water. *First branchial cleft cysts* can be located adjacent to the external auditory canal (type 1 first branchial cleft cyst) or superficial portion of the parotid gland, ± extension into the parapharyngeal space, posterior to the submandibular gland, and/or up to the external auditory canal (type 2). *Second branchial cleft cysts* can be anterior to the sternocleidomastoid muscle (SCM) and medial to the carotid arteries (type 1), anteromedial to the SCM with or without extension posterior to the carotid sheath (type 2), or extend into the parapharyngeal space and between the internal and external carotid arteries (type 3). *Third branchial cleft cysts* are located at the lower anterior margin of the SCM at the level of the upper thyroid lobe, ± extension into the sinus tract posterior to the carotid artery and glossopharyngeal nerve, passing through the thyroid membrane above the level of the internal branch of the superior laryngeal nerve into base of the piriform sinus. *Fourth branchial cleft cysts* occur in the lower third of the neck laterally and anterior to the lower SCM and level of the aortic arch, ± visible connecting sinus tract on the right below the subclavian artery or on the left below the aortic arch that extends superiorly and dorsal to the carotid artery up to the level of the hypoglossal nerve and then downward along the SCM to the piriform sinus.	Branchial cleft cysts are developmental anomalies involving the branchial apparatus. The branchial apparatus consists of four major and two rudimentary arches of mesoderm lined by ectoderm externally and endoderm internally within pouches that form at the end of the fourth week of gestation. The mesoderm contains a dominant artery, nerve, cartilage, and muscle. The four major arches are separated by clefts. Each arch develops into a defined neck structure, with eventual obliteration of the branchial clefts. The first arch forms the external auditory canal, eustachian tube, middle ear, and mastoid air cells. The second arch develops into the hyoid bone and tonsillar and supratonsillar fossae. The third and fourth arches develop into the pharynx below the hyoid bone. Branchial anomalies include cysts, sinuses, and fistulae. Second branchial cleft cysts account for up to 90% of all branchial cleft malformations. Cysts are lined by squamous epithelium (90%), ciliated columnar epithelium (8%), or both types (2%). Sebaceous glands, salivary tissue, lymphoid tissue, and cholesterol crystals in mucoid fluid can also occur. There are four types of second branchial cleft cysts. Type 1 is located anterior to the SCM and deep to the platysma muscle. type 2 (the most common type) is located at the anteromedial surface of the SCM, lateral to the retrostyloid parapharyngeal space and posterior to the submandibular gland. Type 3 is located lateral to pharyngeal wall and medial to the carotid arteries, ± extension between the external and internal carotid arteries (*beak sign*). Type 4 is located between the medial aspect of the carotid sheath and pharynx at the level of the tonsillar fossa and can extend superiorly to the skull base. Typically, branchial cleft cysts are asymptomatic unless complicated by infection.

(continued on page 354)

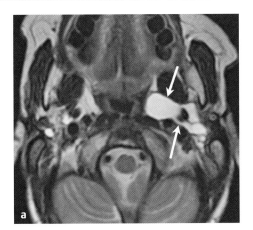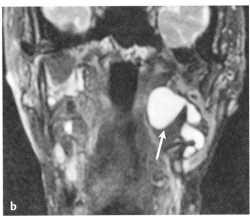

Fig. 4.35 An 81-year-old woman with a second branchial cleft cyst that has circumscribed serpinginous and lobulated margins and contents with high signal (*arrows*) on **(a)** axial and **(b)** coronal fat-suppressed T2-weighted imaging. This type 3 second branchial cleft cyst extends into the left parapharyngeal space between the internal and external carortid arteries (*arrow*).

Table 4.2 *(cont.)*   Lesions of the prestyloid parapharyngeal space

Lesion	Imaging Findings	Comments
Inflammatory Lesions		
Spread of infection from peritonsillar or retropharyngeal phlegmon and/or abscess (**Fig. 4.36, Fig. 4.37**, and **Fig. 4.38**)	*MRI:* Soft tissue thickening at the palatine tonsil and adjacent lateral soft tissue, with poorly defined, slightly high signal on T2-weighted imaging (T2WI) and fat-suppressed T2WI. Peritonsillar abscesses are collections with high signal on T2WI surrounded by a peripheral rim of gadolinium contrast enhancement. Soft tissue thickening with slightly high to high signal on T2WI lateral to the tonsil without a rim-enhancing collection can represent a phlegmon. *CT:* Soft tissue thickening at the palatine tonsil with adjacent lateral rim-enhancing fluid collection. Soft tissue thickening lateral to the tonsil without a rim-enhancing collection can represent a phlegmon.	Infection of the palatine tonsils (acute tonsillitis) is a clinical diagnosis and is typically treated with antibiotics. Tonsillar abscesses rarely occur. Extension of tonsillitis beyond the fibrous tonsillar capsule into the peritonsillar space (potential space between the palatine tonsil and the superior constrictor muscle) can result in peritonsillar cellulitis and peritonsillar abscess. Peritonsillar abscess is the most common infection in the head and neck, and it occurs in young children and adults, often during times with highest incidence of streptococcal pharyngitis and exudative tonsillitis (November–December, and April–May). Treatment of a peritonsillar phlegmon can be with antibiotics, whereas a peritonsillar abscess requires drainage. If not treated appropriately, the infection can extend into the adjacent parapharyngeal, masticator, and/or submandibular spaces.
Granulomatosis with polyangiitis (Wegener's granulomatosis) (**Fig. 4.39**)	*MRI:* Poorly defined zones of soft tissue thickening with low-intermediate signal on T1-weighted imaging, slightly high to high signal on T2-weighted imaging, and gadolinium contrast enhancement within the nasal cavity, paranasal sinuses, orbits, infratemporal fossa, and external auditory canal, ± invasion and destruction of bone and nasal septum, ± extension into the skull base with involvement of the dura, leptomeninges, brain, or venous sinuses. *CT:* Zones with soft tissue attenuation, ± bone destruction.	Multisystem autoimmune disease with necrotizing granulomas in the respiratory tract, focal necrotizing angiitis of small arteries and veins of various tissues, and glomerulonephritis. Can involve the paranasal sinuses, orbits, skull base, dura, leptomeninges, and occasionally the temporal bone. Typically, positive immunoreactivity to cytoplasmic antineutrophil cytoplasmic antibody (c-ANCA). Treatment includes corticosteroids, cyclophosphamide, and anti-TNF agents.

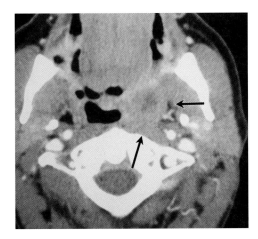

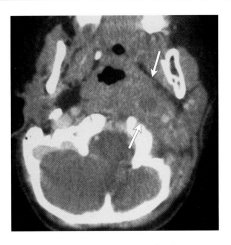

Fig. 4.36 A 35-year-old woman with a left peritonsillar abscess extending into the left prestyloid parapharyngeal space that is seen as soft tissue thickening at the left palatine tonsil with adjacent lateral rim-enhancing fluid collection (*arrows*) on axial CT.

Fig. 4.37 Axial CT of a 2-year-old female shows a retropharyngeal abscess with extension of infection into the left prestyloid parapharyngeal space (*arrows*).

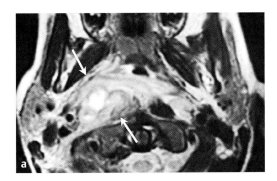

Fig. 4.38 A 6-year-old male with a retropharyngeal abscess with extension of infection into the right prestyloid parapharyngeal and prevertebral spaces. **(a)** Poorly defined zones with abnormal high signal and a fluid collection are seen on axial T2-weighted imaging (*arrows*), with **(b)** corresponding poorly defined gadolinium contrast enhancement at the sites of infection on axial fat-suppressed T1-weighted imaging (*arrow*).

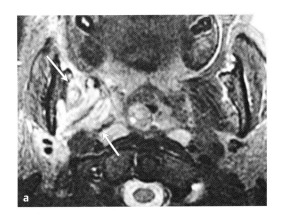

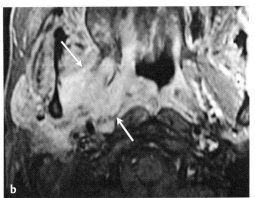

Fig. 4.39 A 46-year-old woman who has granulomatosis with polyangiitis. **(a)** Poorly defined zones with abnormal high signal on axial fat-suppressed T2-weighted imaging (*arrows*) and **(b)** gadolinium contrast enhancement on axial fat-suppressed T1-weighted imaging (*arrows*) are due to granulomatous disease in the right posterior nasopharynx as well as the retropharyngeal, right parapharyngeal, and masticator spaces.

4.3 Lesions of the Retrostyloid Parapharyngeal Space

The retrostyloid parapharyngeal space (RPPS) is the suprahyoid extension of the carotid space above the hyoid bone that contains the internal carotid artery, internal jugular vein, cranial nerves IX, X, XI, and XII, sympathetic plexus, and deep cervical lymph nodes (**Fig. 4.40**). The carotid space and RPPS are located lateral to the pharyngeal mucosal space, anterior to the prevertebral space, and posteromedial to the sternocleidomastoid muscles. The carotid space is enclosed by the carotid sheath, which is composed of portions from the three layers (superficial, middle, and deep) of the deep cervical fascia. The RPPS is separated from the prestyloid parapharyngeal space by a fascial layer that extends from the styloid process to the tensor veli palatini muscle. Within the carotid sheath, the carotid artery (CA) is located medial to the internal jugular vein (IJV), and the vagus nerve is located dorsal to both the CA and IJV. The cervical sympathetic plexus is located in the posterior portion of the carotid sheath. The ansa cervicalis is a loop of nerves of the cervical plexus arising from the ventral rami of the first three to four cervical nerves that innervates the infrahyoid, sternothyroid, sternohyoid, and omohyoid muscles. The ansa cervicalis is located in the anterior portion of the carotid sheath.

Table 4.3 Lesions of the retrostyloid parapharyngeal space

- Benign Neoplasms
  - Paraganglioma
  - Schwannoma
  - Neurofibroma
  - Meningioma extending into the jugular foramen
  - Lipoma
  - Hemangioma
- Malignant Tumors
  - Direct extension from squamous cell carcinoma or malignant salivary gland tumor
  - Rhabdomyosarcoma
  - Metastatic malignancies
  - Non-Hodgkin lymphoma (NHL)
  - Hemangioendothelioma
- Tumorlike Lesions
  - Branchial cleft cyst
- Inflammatory Lesions
  - Spread of infection from peritonsillar or retropharyngeal phlegmon and/or abscess
  - Granulomatosis with polyangiitis
- Vascular Abnormality
  - Ectasia and tortuosity of the carotid artery
  - Aneurysm of the carotid artery
  - Arterial dissection
  - Vasculitis
  - Thrombosis and/or thrombophlebitis of the internal jugular veins
  - Venolymphatic malformation

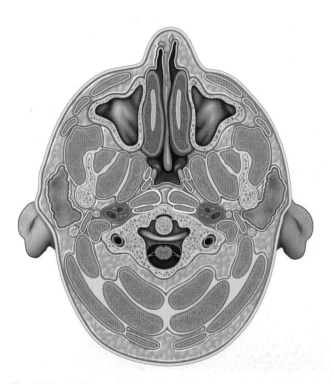

Fig. 4.40 Axial view diagram shows the retrostyloid parapharyngeal space in color.

Table 4.3 Lesions of the retrostyloid parapharyngeal space

Lesion	Imaging Findings	Comments
Benign Neoplasms		
Paragangliomas (**Fig. 4.41, Fig. 4.42**, and **Fig. 4.43**)	Ovoid or fusiform lesions with low-intermediate attenuation. *MRI:* Spheroid or lobulated lesions with intermediate signal on T1-weighted imaging (T1WI), intermediate to high signal on T2-weighted imaging (T2WI) and fat-suppressed T2WI, ± tubular zones of flow voids, usually prominent gadolinium contrast enhancement, ± foci of high signal on T1WI from mucin or hemorrhage, ± peripheral rim of low signal (hemosiderin) on T2WI. *CT:* Lesions can show contrast enhancement. Often erode adjacent bone.	Benign encapsulated neuroendocrine tumors that arise from neural crest cells associated with autonomic ganglia (paraganglia) throughout the body. These lesions, also referred to as chemodectomas, are named according to location (glomus jugulare, tympanicum, vagale). Paragangliomas represent 0.6% of tumors of the head and neck, and 0.03% of all neoplasms.

(continued on page 359)

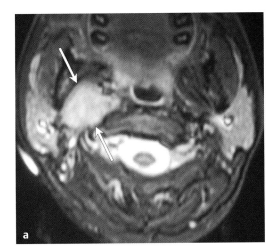 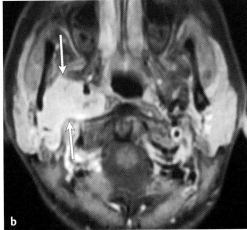

Fig. 4.41 **(a)** Paraganglioma in the right retrostyloid parapharyngeal space has slightly high to high signal on axial fat-suppressed T2-weighted imaging (*arrows*) and **(b)** shows gadolinium contrast enhancement on axial fat-suppressed T1-weighted imaging (*arrows*). The tumor displaces the right carotid artery anteriorly.

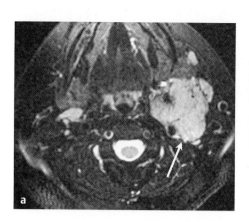
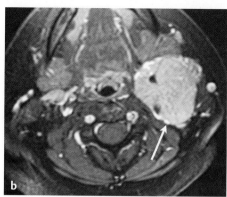
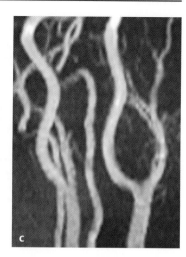

Fig. 4.42 **(a)** A 27-year-old woman with a paraganglioma located between the left external and internal carotid arteries that has heterogeneous high signal on axial fat-suppressed T2-weighted imaging (*arrow*) and **(b)** shows gadolinium contrast enhancement on axial fat-suppressed T1-weighted imaging (*arrow*). **(c)** The tumor splays apart the left internal and external carotid arteries on oblique coronal MRA.

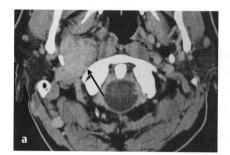
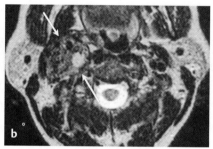
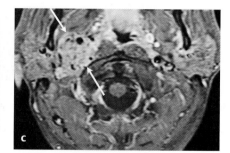

Fig. 4.43 **(a)** Axial CT shows a paraganglioma with intermediate attenuation in the retrostyloid parapharyngeal space (*arrow*). **(b)** The lesion has mixed low, intermediate, and slightly high signal on axial T2-weighted imaging (*arrows*) and **(c)** shows heterogeneous gadolinium contrast enhancement on axial fat-suppressed T1-weighted imaging (*arrows*). The lesion displaces the right carotid artery anteriorly.

Table 4.3 *(cont.)* Lesions of the retrostyloid parapharyngeal space

Lesion	Imaging Findings	Comments
Schwannoma (**Fig. 4.44** and **Fig. 4.45**)	*MRI:* Circumscribed spheroid or ovoid lesions with low-intermediate signal on T1-weighted imaging, high signal on T2-weighted imaging (T2WI) and fat-suppressed T2WI, and usually prominent gadolinium (Gd) contrast enhancement. High signal on T2WI and Gd contrast enhancement can be heterogeneous in large lesions due to cystic degeneration and/or hemorrhage. *CT:* Circumscribed spheroid or ovoid lesions with intermediate attenuation, + contrast enhancement. Large lesions can have cystic degeneration and/or hemorrhage.	Schwannomas are benign encapsulated tumors that contain differentiated neoplastic Schwann cells. They most commonly occur as solitary, sporadic lesions. Multiple schwannomas are often associated with neurofibromatosis type 2 (NF2), which is an autosomal dominant disease involving a gene mutation at chromosome 22q12. In addition to schwannomas, patients with NF2 can also have multiple meningiomas and ependymomas. The incidence of NF2 is 1/37,000 to 1/50,000 newborns. Age at presentation is 22 to 72 years (mean age = 46 years). Peak incidence is in the fourth to sixth decades. Many patients with NF2 present in the third decade with bilateral vestibular schwannomas.

(continued on page 360)

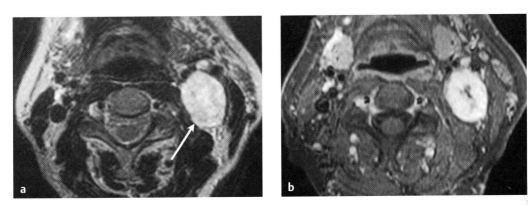

Fig. 4.44 A 46-year-old woman with a schwannoma of the left vagus nerve that displaces the left carotid artery and jugular vein anteriorly. **(a)** The schwannoma has high signal on axial T2-weighted imaging (*arrow*) and **(b)** shows gadolinium contrast enhancement on axial fat-suppressed T1-weighted imaging.

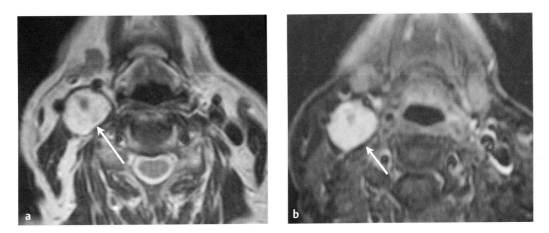

Fig. 4.45 A 52-year-old woman with a schwannoma that displaces the right internal and external carotid arteries anteriorly. **(a)** The schwannoma has high signal on axial T2-weighted imaging (*arrow*) and **(b)** shows gadolinium contrast enhancement on axial fat-suppressed T1-weighted imaging (*arrow*).

Table 4.3 *(cont.)* Lesions of the retrostyloid parapharyngeal space

Lesion	Imaging Findings	Comments
Neurofibroma (**Fig. 4.46** and **Fig. 4.47**)	*MRI:* Solitary neurofibromas are circumscribed spheroid, ovoid, or lobulated extra-axial lesions with low-intermediate signal on T1-weighted imaging (T1WI), intermediate-high signal on T2-weighted imaging (T2WI), and prominent gadolinium (Gd) contrast enhancement. High signal on T2WI and Gd contrast enhancement can be heterogeneous in large lesions. Plexiform neurofibromas appear as curvilinear and multinodular lesions involving multiple nerve branches and have low to intermediate signal on T1WI and intermediate or slightly high to high signal on T2WI and fat-suppressed T2WI, with or without bands or strands of low signal. Lesions usually show Gd contrast enhancement. *CT:* Ovoid or fusiform lesions with low-intermediate attenuation. Lesions can show contrast enhancement. Often erode adjacent bone.	Neurofibromas are benign nerve sheath tumors that contain mixtures of Schwann cells, perineural-like cells, and interlacing fascicles of fibroblasts associated with abundant collagen. Unlike schwannomas, neurofibromas lack Antoni A and B regions and cannot be separated pathologically from the underlying nerve. Neurofibromas most frequently occur as sporadic, localized, solitary lesions, less frequently as diffuse or plexiform lesions. Multiple neurofibromas are typically seen in neurofibromatosis type 1 (NF1), which is an autosomal dominant disorder (1/2,500 births) caused by mutations of the neurofibromin gene on chromosome 17q11.2. NF1 is the most common type of neurocutaneous syndrome and is associated with neoplasms of the central and peripheral nervous systems (optic gliomas, astrocytomas, plexiform and solitary neurofibromas) and skin lesions (café-au-lait spots, axillary and inguinal freckling). Also associated with meningeal and skull dysplasias, as well as hamartomas of the iris (Lisch nodules).
Meningioma extending into the jugular foramen	Extra-axial dura-based lesions that are well circumscribed. Locations are: supra- > infratentorial, parasagittal > convexity > sphenoid ridge > parasellar > posterior fossa > optic nerve sheath > intraventricular. *MRI:* Tumors often have intermediate signal on T1-weighted imaging and intermediate to slightly high signal on T2-weighted imaging, and typically show prominent gadolinium contrast enhancement, ± calcifications, ± hyperostosis and/or invasion of adjacent skull. Can extend through foramina at the skull base. Some meningiomas have high signal on diffusion-weighted imaging. *CT:* Tumors have intermediate attenuation and usually prominent contrast enhancement, ± calcifications, ± hyperostosis of adjacent bone.	Benign, slow-growing tumors involving cranial and/or spinal dura that are composed of neoplastic meningothelial (arachnoidal or arachnoid cap) cells. Usually solitary and sporadic but can also occur as multiple lesions in patients with neurofibromatosis type 2. Most are benign, although ~ 5% have atypical histologic features. Anaplastic meningiomas are rare and account for < 3% of meningiomas. Meningiomas account for up to 26% of primary intracranial tumors. Annual incidence is 6 per 100,000. Typically occur in adults (> 40 years old) and in women more than in men. Can result in compression of adjacent brain parenchyma, encasement of arteries, and compression of dural venous sinuses. Rarely, invasive/malignant types occur.
Lipoma (**Fig. 4.48**)	*MRI:* Lipomas have MRI signal isointense to subcutaneous fat on T1-weighted imaging (high signal). On T2-weighted imaging, signal suppression occurs with frequency-selective fat saturation techniques or with a short time to inversion recovery (STIR) method. Typically there is no gadolinium contrast enhancement or peripheral edema. *CT:* Lipomas have CT attenuation similar to subcutaneous fat and typically no contrast enhancement or peripheral edema.	Common benign hamartomas composed of mature white adipose tissue without cellular atypia. Most common soft tissue tumor, representing 16% of all soft tissue tumors. May contain calcifications and/or traversing blood vessels.
Hemangioma (**Fig. 4.49**)	*MRI:* Circumscribed or poorly marginated structures (< 4 cm in diameter) in bone marrow or soft tissue with intermediate-high signal on T1-weighted imaging and high signal on T2-weighted imaging (T2WI) and fat-suppressed T2WI, typically with gadolinium contrast enhancement, ± expansion of bone. *CT:* Expansile bone lesions with a radiating pattern of bony trabeculae oriented toward the center. Hemangiomas in soft tissue have mostly intermediate attenuation, ± zones of fat attenuation.	Benign lesions of bone or soft tissue composed of capillary, cavernous, and/or malformed venous vessels. Considered to be a hamartomatous disorder. Occur in patients 1 to 84 years old (median age = 33 years).

(continued on page 362)

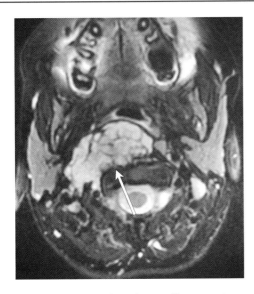

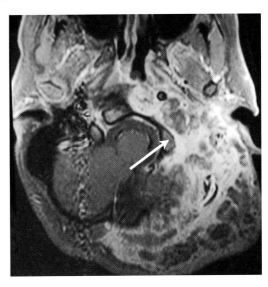

Fig. 4.46 A 10-year-old male with neurofibromatosis type 1 who has a conglomeration of neurofibromas with high signal on axial fat-suppressed T2-weighted imaging (*arrow*) in the retrostyloid parapharyngeal space that displace the adjacent right carotid arteries posteriorly.

Fig. 4.47 A 19-year-old woman with neurofibromatosis type 1 and a gadolinium-enhancing plexiform neurofibroma in the superficial soft tissues that is associated with erosion and remodeling of the left occipital and temporal bones and with extension into the left retrostyloid parapharyngeal, retropharyngeal, and prevertebral spaces on axial fat-suppressed T1-weighted imaging (*arrow*).

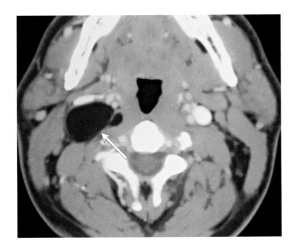

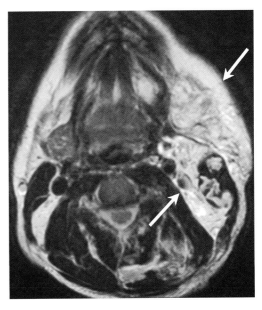

Fig. 4.48 Axial CT of 42-year-old man shows a lipoma (*arrow*) with low attenuation in the right retrostyloid parapharyngeal space. The lipoma displaces the right carotid arteries and jugular vein anteriorly.

Fig. 4.49 A 22-year-old woman with an infiltrative hemangioma (*arrows*) in the soft tissues of the lower left face, left submandibular space, and left poststyloid parapharyngeal space, where it partially surrounds the left carotid artery. The lesion has high signal on axial T2-weighted imaging.

Table 4.3 *(cont.)*   Lesions of the retrostyloid parapharyngeal space

Lesion	Imaging Findings	Comments
Malignant Tumors		
Direct extension from squamous cell carcinoma or malignant salivary gland tumor (**Fig. 4.50** and **Fig. 4.51**)	*MRI:* Malignant lesions from the nasopharynx, oropharynx, prestyloid parapharyngeal space (PPPS), and deep portion of the parotid gland can invade the retrostyloid parapharyngeal space (RPPS). Tumors often have intermediate signal on T1-weighted imaging, intermediate to slightly high signal on T2-weighted imaging, and mild gadolinium contrast enhancement. Can be large lesions (± necrosis and/or hemorrhage). *CT:* Tumors have intermediate attenuation and mild contrast enhancement. Can be large lesions (± necrosis and/or hemorrhage).	Malignant tumors from the nasopharynx and deep portion of the parotid gland can invade the RPPS. *Squamous cell carcinomas* are malignant epithelial tumors originating from the mucosal epithelium of the paranasal sinuses and nasal cavity that can extend into the PPPS and RPPS. They include both keratinizing and nonkeratinizing types, and account for 80% of malignant sinonasal tumors and 3% of malignant tumors of the head and neck. Occur in adults, usually more than 55 years old, and in males more than in females. *Malignant salivary gland tumors* include adenoid cystic carcinoma, adenocarcinoma, and mucoepidermoid carcinoma.
Rhabdomyosarcoma (**Fig. 4.52**)	*MRI:* Tumors can have circumscribed and/or poorly defined margins and typically have low-intermediate signal on T1-weighted imaging and heterogeneous signal (various combinations of intermediate, slightly high, and/or high signal) on T2-weighted imaging (T2WI) and fat-suppressed T2WI. Tumors show variable degrees of gadolinium contrast enhancement, ± bone destruction and invasion. *CT:* Soft tissue lesions that usually can have circumscribed or irregular margins. Calcifications are uncommon. Tumors can have mixed CT attenuation, with solid zones of soft tissue attenuation, cystic appearing and/or necrotic zones, and occasional foci of hemorrhage, ± bone invasion and destruction.	Malignant mesenchymal tumors with rhabdomyoblastic differentiation that occur primarily in soft tissue, and only very rarely in bone. There are three subgroups of rhabdomyosarcoma: embryonal (50–70%), alveolar (18–45%), and pleomorphic (5–10%). Embryonal and alveolar rhabdomyosarcomas occur primarily in children < 10 years old, and pleomorphic rhabdomyosarcomas occur mostly in adults (median age in the sixth decade). Alveolar and pleomorphic rhabdomyosarcomas occur frequently in the extremities. Embryonal rhabdomyosarcomas occur mostly in the head and neck.
Metastatic malignancies	*MRI:* Circumscribed spheroid lesions that often have low-intermediate signal on T1-weighted imaging and intermediate to high signal on T2-weighted imaging, ± irregular margins, ± hemorrhage, ± calcifications, ± cysts, and variable gadolinium contrast enhancement. *CT:* Lesions usually have low-intermediate attenuation, ± hemorrhage, ± calcifications, ± cysts, variable contrast enhancement, ± bone destruction, ± compression of neural tissue or vessels.	Primary extracranial tumor source: lung > breast > GI > GU > melanoma. Can occur as single or multiple well-circumscribed or poorly defined lesions. Metastatic tumors may cause variable destructive or infiltrative changes in single or multiple sites.
Non-Hodgkin lymphoma (NHL) (**Fig. 4.53**)	*MRI:* Lesions have low-intermediate signal on T1-weighted imaging and intermediate to slightly high signal on T2-weighted imaging, + gadolinium contrast enhancement. Can be locally invasive and associated with bone erosion/destruction, intracranial extension with meningeal involvement (up to 5%). B-cell NHL often occurs in the maxillary sinuses, whereas T-cell NHL frequently occurs in the midline, including the septum. *CT:* Lesions have low-intermediate attenuation and may show contrast enhancement, ± bone destruction.	In lymphoma, neoplastic cells typically arise within lymphoid tissue (lymph nodes and reticuloendothelial organs). Most lymphomas in the nasopharynx, nasal cavity, and paranasal sinuses are NHL (B-cell NHL is more common than T-cell NHL) and more commonly are related to disseminated disease than to primary sinonasal tumors. Sinonasal lymphoma has a poor prognosis, with 5-year survival of less than 65%.

(continued on page 364)

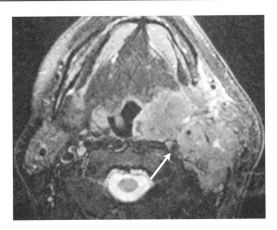

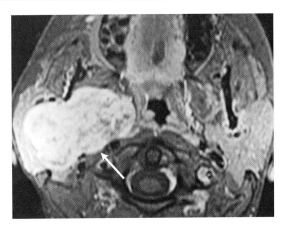

Fig. 4.50 Axial fat-suppressed T2-weighted imaging shows an invasive squamous cell carcinoma (*arrow*) with slightly high signal and poorly defined margins that involves the left nasopharynx, prestyloid and retrostyloid parapharyngeal spaces, parotid space, and superficial soft tissues.

Fig. 4.51 A 32-year-old woman with an adenoid cystic carcinoma involving the right parotid gland and that extends medially to involve the right parapharyngeal space immediately anterior to the right carotid artery. The large tumor shows heterogeneous gadolinium contrast enhancement on axial fat-suppressed T1-weighted imaging (*arrow*) and indents and displaces the right pterygoid muscles.

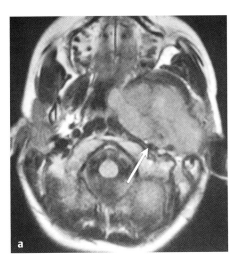

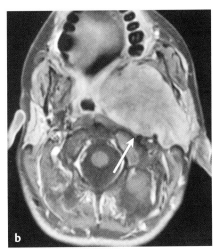

Fig. 4.52 A 13-year-old male with a rhabdomyosarcoma involving the left parotid, left prestyloid, and retrostyloid parapharyngeal spaces. **(a)** The tumor has heterogeneous slightly high signal on axial T2-weighted imaging (*arrow*) and **(b)** shows gadolinium contrast enhancement on axial fat-suppressed T1-weighted imaging (*arrow*).

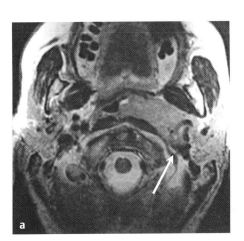

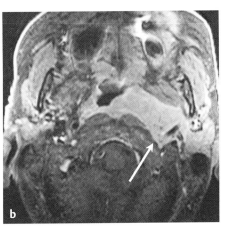

Fig. 4.53 **(a)** A 78-year-old woman with non-Hodgkin lymphoma involving the prestyloid and retrostyloid parapharyngeal spaces that has intermediate signal on axial T2-weighted imaging (*arrow*) and **(b)** shows gadolinium contrast enhancement on axial fat-suppressed T1-weighted imaging (*arrow*).

Table 4.3 *(cont.)*   Lesions of the retrostyloid parapharyngeal space

Lesion	Imaging Findings	Comments
Hemangioendothelioma (**Fig. 4.54**)	*MRI:* Tumors have irregular or well-defined margins and often have intermediate signal on T1-weighted imaging and heterogeneous predominantly high signal on T2-weighted imaging, with or without internal low-signal septations. Flow voids may be seen in the lesions. Tumors show heterogeneous gadolinium contrast enhancement. *CT:* Hemangioendotheliomas have low-intermediate attenuation and usually show contrast enhancement, ± contrast-enhancing vessels within the lesions.	Low-grade malignant neoplasms composed of vasoformative/endothelial elements that occur in soft tissues and bone. The tumors are locally aggressive and rarely metastasize, compared with the high-grade endothelial tumors like angiosarcoma. Account for < 1% of malignant and all soft tissue tumors. Patients range in age from 17 to 60 years (mean age = 40 years).
Tumorlike Lesions		
Branchial cleft cyst (**Fig. 4.55**)	*MRI:* Circumscribed lesion that often has low-intermediate signal on T1-weighted imaging and high signal on T2-weighted imaging. Usually there is no gadolinium contrast enhancement unless there is superimposed infection. *CT:* Circumscribed, cystic lesion with low to intermediate attenuation depending on the proportions of protein and water. *First branchial cleft cysts* can be located adjacent to the external auditory canal (type 1 first branchial cleft cyst) or superficial portion of the parotid gland, ± extension into the parapharyngeal space, posterior to the submandibular gland, and/or up to the external auditory canal (type 2). *Second branchial cleft cysts* can be anterior to the sternocleidomastoid muscle (SCM) and medial to the carotid arteries (type 1), anteromedial to the SCM with or without extension posterior to the carotid sheath (type 2), or extend into the parapharyngeal space and between the internal and external carotid arteries (type 3). *Third branchial cleft cysts* are located at the lower anterior margin of the SCM at the level of the upper thyroid lobe, ± extension into the sinus tract posterior to the carotid artery and glossopharyngeal nerve, passing through the thyroid membrane above the level of the internal branch of the superior laryngeal nerve into base of the piriform sinus. *Fourth branchial cleft cysts* occur in the lower third of the neck laterally and anterior to the lower SCM and level of the aortic arch, ± visible connecting sinus tract on the right below the subclavian artery or on the left below the aortic arch that extends superiorly and dorsal to the carotid artery up to the level of the hypoglossal nerve and then downward along the SCM to the piriform sinus.	Branchial cleft cysts are developmental anomalies involving the branchial apparatus. The branchial apparatus consists of four major and two rudimetary arches of mesoderm lined by ectoderm externally and endoderm internally within pouches that form at the end of the fourth week of gestation. The mesoderm contains a dominant artery, nerve, cartilage, and muscle. The major four arches are separated by clefts. Each arch develops into a defined neck structure with eventual obliteration of the branchial clefts. The first arch forms the external auditory canal, eustachian tube, middle ear, and mastoid air cells. The second arch develops into the hyoid bone and tonsillar and supratonsillar fossae. The third and fourth arches develop into the pharynx below the hyoid bone. Branchial anomalies include cysts, sinuses, and fistulae. Second branchial cleft cysts account for up to 90% of all branchial cleft malformations. Cysts are lined by squamous epithelium (90%), ciliated columnar epithelium (8%), or both types (2%). Sebaceous glands, salivary tissue, lymphoid tissue, and cholesterol crystals in mucoid fluid can also occur. There are four types of second branchial cleft cysts. Type 1 is located anterior to the SCM and deep to the platysma muscle. Type 2 (the most common type) is located at the anteromedial surface of the SCM, lateral to the carotid space and posterior to the submandibular gland. Type 3 is located lateral to pharyngeal wall and medial to the carotid arteries, ± extension between the external and internal carotid arteries (*beak sign*). Type 4 is located between the medial aspect of the carotid sheath and pharynx at the level of the tonsillar fossa, and it can extend superiorly to the skull base. The cysts are typically asymptomatic unless complicated by infection.

(continued on page 366)

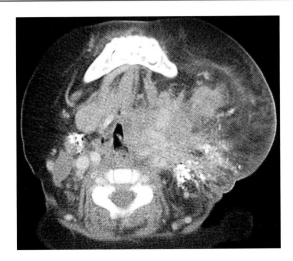

Fig. 4.54 Axial CT of a 1-day-old neonate with a hemangioendothelioma involving the soft tissues of the face on the left, with involvement of the prestyloid and retrostyloid parapharyngeal spaces. The tumor has ill-defined margins and has mostly intermediate attenuation with irregular calcifications.

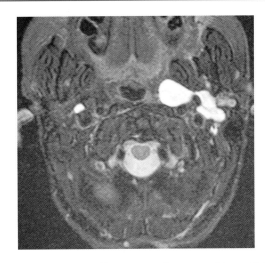

Fig. 4.55 An 81-year-old woman with a second branchial cleft cyst that has circumscribed serpinginous and lobulated margins and contents with high signal on axial fat-suppressed T2-weighted imaging. This type 3 second branchial cleft cyst extends into the left parapharyngeal space between the internal and external carotid arteries.

Table 4.3 *(cont.)*   Lesions of the retrostyloid parapharyngeal space

Lesion	Imaging Findings	Comments
Inflammatory Lesions		
Spread of infection from peritonsillar or retropharyngeal phlegmon and/or abscess (**Fig. 4.56**)	*MRI:* Soft tissue thickening at the palatine tonsil and adjacent soft tissue laterally that has poorly-defined slightly high to high signal on T2-weighted imaging (T2WI) and fat-suppressed T2WI. Peritonsillar abscesses are collections with high signal on T2WI surrounded by a peripheral rim of Gd-contrast enhancement. Soft tissue thickening with slightly high to high signal on T2WI lateral to the tonsil without a rim-enhancing collection can represent a phlegmon. *CT:* Soft tissue thickening at the palatine tonsil with adjacent lateral rim-enhancing fluid collection. Soft tissue thickening lateral to the tonsil without a rim-enhancing collection can represent a phlegmon.	Infection of the palatine tonsils (acute tonsillitis) is a clinical diagnosis and is typically treated with antibiotics. Tonsillar abscesses rarely occur. Extension of tonsillitis beyond the fibrous tonsillar capsule into the peritonsillar space (potential space between the palatine tonsil and the superior constrictor muscle) can result in peritonsillar cellulitis and peritonsillar abscess. Peritonsillar abscess is the most common infection in the head and neck and occurs in young children and adults, often during times with highest incidence of streptococcal pharyngitis and exudative tonsillitis (November–December, and April–May). Treatment of a peritonsillar phlegmon can be with antibiotics, whereas a peritonsillar abscess requires drainage. If not treated appropriately, the infection can extend into the adjacent parapharyngeal, masticator, and/or submandibular spaces.
Granulomatosis with polyangiitis (**Fig. 4.57**)	*MRI:* Poorly defined zones of soft tissue thickening with low-intermediate signal on T1-weighted imaging, slightly high to high signal on T2-weighted imaging, gadolinium contrast enhancement within the nasal cavity, paranasal sinuses, orbits, infratemporal fossa, external auditory canal, ± invasion and destruction of bone and nasal septum, ± extension into the parapharyngeal space, and into the skull base with involvement of the dura, leptomeninges, brain, or venous sinuses. *CT:* Zones with soft tissue attenuation, ± bone destruction.	Multisystem autoimmune disease with necrotizing granulomas in the respiratory tract, focal necrotizing angiitis of small arteries and veins of various tissues, and glomerulonephritis. Can involve the paranasal sinuses, nasopharynx with extension into the parapharyngeal space, orbits, skull base, dura, leptomeninges, and occasionally the temporal bone. Typically has positive immunoreactivity to cytoplasmic antineutrophil cytoplasmic antibody (c-ANCA). Treatment includes corticosteroids, cyclophosphamide, and anti-TNF agents.
Vascular Abnormality		
Ectasia and tortuosity of the carotid artery (**Fig. 4.58**)	*CTA and MRA* show medial deviation of the course of the common and/or internal carotid arteries in the upper neck.	The internal and upper common carotid arteries can be ectatic and tortuous, and they may course medially, resulting in a pulsatile retropharyngeal or retrotonsillar mass. Identification of this arterial position is important for surgical planning and for avoiding unnecessary biopsies.

(continued on page 368)

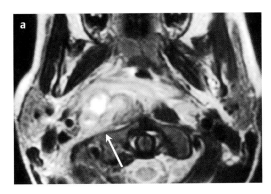
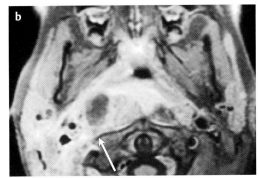

Fig. 4.56 **(a)** Axial T2-weighted imaging of a 6-year-old male shows poorly defined zones (*arrow*) with abnormal high signal and **(b)** corresponding gadolinium contrast enhancement on axial fat-suppressed T1-weighted imaging (*arrow*) from spread of infection from retropharyngeal phlegmon and abscess that involves the right prestyloid and retrostyloid parapharyngeal spaces.

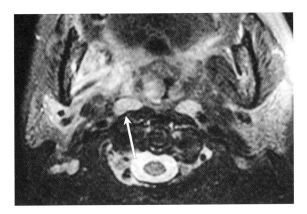

Fig. 4.57 Granulomatosis with polyangiitis. Poorly defined zones with high signal on axial fat-suppressed T2-weighted imaging are seen involving the right parapharyngeal, right parotid, and right masticator spaces (*arrow*).

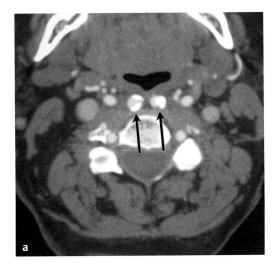
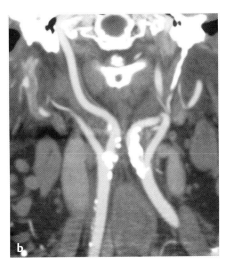

Fig. 4.58 A 76-year-old woman with tortuous and medially positioned carotid arteries as seen on **(a)** axial (*arrows*) and **(b)** coronal CTA.

Table 4.3 *(cont.)*   Lesions of the retrostyloid parapharyngeal space

Lesion	Imaging Findings	Comments
Aneurysm of the carotid artery (**Fig. 4.59**)	A *saccular aneurysm* is a focal well-circumscribed zone of contrast enhancement seen on conventional arteriography, CTA, and MRA. It can also be seen on noncontrast MRI and CT. A *fusiform aneurysm* is a tubular dilatation of the involved artery. With *dissecting aneurysms* (intramural hematoma), initially the involved arterial wall is thickened in a circumferential or semilunar configuration and has intermediate attenuation with luminal narrowing. Evolution of the intramural hematoma can lead to focal dilatation of the arterial wall hematoma. *Giant aneurysms* are saccular aneuryms that are more than 2.5 cm in diameter. They often contain mural thrombus that has layers with intermediate to high attenuation on NCECT and intermediate to high signal on T1- and T2-weighted imaging. The patent portion of the aneurysm shows contrast enhancement on CT, CTA, MRI, and MRA. *CT:* Saccular aneurysms are focal circumscribed outpouches of an artery and can have low-intermediate and/or high attenuation. Fusiform aneurysms represent diffuse abnormal dilatation of an artery.	Abnormal fusiform or focal saccular dilatation of artery secondary to acquired/degenerative etiology, polycystic disease, connective tissue disease, atherosclerosis, trauma, infection (mycotic), oncotic, arteriovenous malformation, vasculitis, and drugs. Focal aneurysms, also referred to as saccular aneurysms, typically occur at arterial bifurcations and are multiple in 20% of cases. The chance of rupture of a saccular aneurysm is related to the size of the aneurysm. Saccular aneurysms > 2.5 cm in diameter are referred to as giant aneurysms. Fusiform aneurysms are often related to atherosclerosis or collagen vascular disease (Marfan syndrome, Ehlers-Danlos syndrome, etc.). In dissecting aneurysms, hemorrhage occurs in the arterial wall from incidental or significant trauma.
Arterial dissection (**Fig. 4.60** and **Fig. 4.61**)	*MRI:* Crescentic zone with high signal on proton density-weighted imaging and fat-suppressed T1-weighted imaging involving the wall of a cervical carotid artery and resulting in narrowing of the intraluminal flow void. The intramural hematoma can progress and fill to occlude the lumen, obliterating the flow void of the artery. *CT:* The involved arterial wall is thickened in a circumferential or semilunar configuration and has intermediate attenuation. Lumen may be narrowed or occluded.	Arterial dissections can be related to trauma, collagen vascular disease (Marfan syndrome, Ehlers-Danlos syndrome, etc.), or fibromuscular dysplasia, or they can be idiopathic. Hemorrhage occurs in the arterial wall and can cause stenosis, occlusion, and stroke.
Vasculitis	*MRI/MRA:* Zones of arterial occlusion and/or foci of stenosis and poststenotic dilatation can be seen involving small or medium-size intracranial and extracranial arteries. With acute active vasculitis, Gd-contrast enhancement can be seen in the involved arterial wall. Can result in narrowing of artery leading to cerebral or cerebellar infarcts. Dilatation of involved artery can be a late effect of vasculitis. *CT/CTA:* Asymmetric or symmetric arterial wall thickening ± luminal narrowing. Can be associated with cerebral and cerebellar infarcts. Dilatation of involved artery can be a late effect of vasculitis. *Conventional arteriography* shows zones of arterial occlusion and/or foci of stenosis and poststenotic dilatation. May involve large, medium, or small intracranial and extracranial arteries.	Uncommon mixed group of inflammatory diseases/disorders involving the walls of cerebral blood vessels. Can involve small arteries (CNS vasculitis), small and medium-size arteries (polyarteritis nodosa, Kawasaki disease), or large arteries with diameters of 7 to 35 mm, such as the aorta and its main branches (Takayasu arteritis, giant cell arteritis). Vasculitis can be a primary disease in which biopsies show transmural vascular inflammation. Vasculitis can occur as a secondary disease in association with other disorders, such as systemic disease (polyarteritis nodosa, granulomatosis with polyangiitis, giant cell arteritis, Takayasu arteritis, sarcoid, Behçet's disease, systemic lupus erythematosus, Sjögren's syndrome, dermatomyositis, mixed connective tissue disease), drug use (amphetamine, ephedrine, phenylpropaline, cocaine), or viral, bacterial, fungal, or parasitic infections.

(continued on page 370)

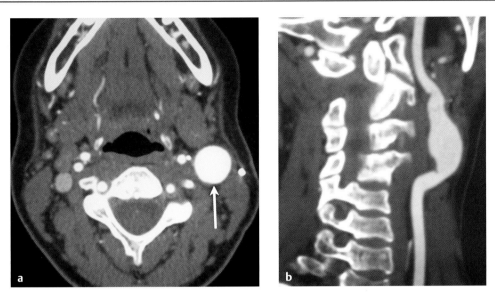

Fig. 4.59   A 27-year-old woman with an aneurysm of the left internal carotid artery on **(a)** axial (*arrow*) and **(b)** oblique sagittal CTA.

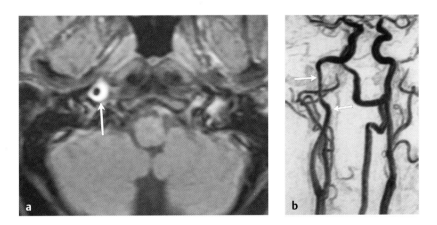

Fig. 4.60   **(a)** A 45-year-old man with dissection of the right internal carotid artery that is seen as a circumferential zone of high signal on axial fat-suppressed T1-weighted imaging surrounding a narrowed arterial flow void (*arrow*). **(b)** Oblique coronal MRA shows narrowed flow signal (*arrows*) involving the right internal carotid artery secondary to the intramural hematoma (arterial dissection).

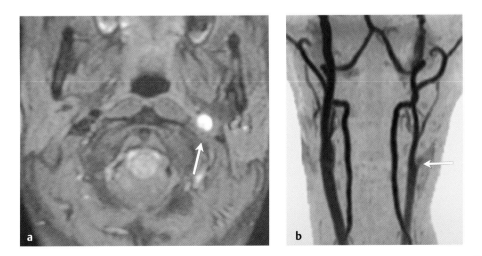

Fig. 4.61   **(a)** Dissection of the left internal carotid artery causing complete arterial occlusion, which is seen as a zone of high signal on axial fat-suppressed T1-weighted imaging filling the lumen (*arrow*). **(b)** Coronal MRA shows abrupt tapering of the left internal carotid artery (*arrow*) secondary to the intramural hematoma (arterial dissection).

Table 4.3 *(cont.)*   Lesions of the retrostyloid parapharyngeal space

Lesion	Imaging Findings	Comments
Thrombosis and/or thrombophlebitis of the internal jugular veins (**Fig. 4.62** and **Fig. 4.63**)	*MRI:* Acute thrombus can have high signal on T2-weighted imaging (T2WI), whereas subacute thrombus can have low signal on T2WI. With Lemierre syndrome, poorly defined zones with high signal on T2WI and gadolinium contrast enhancement are seen in the adjacent soft tissues of the retrostyloid parapharyngeal space and retropharyngeal space. *Contrast-enhanced CT and CTA:* Tubular intraluminal zone with low-intermediate attenuation and reduced or absent contrast enhancement, ± peripheral contrast enhancement of the vaso vasorum of the vessel wall. *Ultrasound:* Dilated and incompressible vein with lack of blood flow on Doppler.	Internal jugular vein (IJV) thrombosis can result from surgical or procedural complications, trauma, polycythemia, coagulopathies, malignancies, IV drug abuse, and compression from adjacent lymphadenopathy. IJV thrombosis can also result from adjacent inflammation and/or infection. Extension of odontogenic and/or oropharyngeal infections can cause IJV thrombophlebitis (Lemierre syndrome). Lemierre syndrome often occurs in healthy young adults from oropharyngeal spread of infection from the usually commensal bacteria *Fusobacterium necrophorum* secondary to an altered host-defense mechanism with damage to the mucosa (trauma or bacterial or viral pharyngitis). Complications include septic embolization and bacteremia. Treatment of Lemierre syndrome is with broad-spectrum antibiotics ± anticoagulation.
Venolymphatic malformation	Can be circumscribed lesions or may occur in an infiltrative pattern with extension into soft tissue and between muscles. *MRI:* Often contain single or multiple cystic zones that can be large (macrocystic type) or small (microcystic type), which have predominantly low signal on T1-weighted imaging (T1WI) and high signal on T2-weighted imaging (T2WI) and fat-suppressed T2WI. Fluid–fluid levels and zones with high signal on T1WI and variable signal on T2WI may result from cysts containing hemorrhage, high protein concentration, and/or necrotic debris. Septa between the cystic zones can vary in thickness and gadolinium (Gd) contrast enhancement. Nodular zones within the lesions can have variable degrees of Gd contrast enhancement. Microcystic types typically show more Gd contrast enhancement than the macrocystic type. *CT:* The macrocystic lesions are usually low-attenuation cystic lesions (10–25 HU) separated by thin walls, ± intermediate or high attenuation resulting from hemorrhage or infection, ± fluid–fluid levels.	Benign vascular anomalies (also referred to as lymphangioma or cystic hygroma) that primarily result from abnormal lymphangiogenesis. Up to 75% occur in the head and neck. Can be observed in utero with MRI or sonography, at birth (50–65%) or within the first 5 years, and ~ 85% are detected by age 2. Lesions are composed of endothelium-lined lymphatic ± venous channels interspersed within connective tissue stroma. Account for less than 1% of benign soft tissue tumors and 5.6% of all benign lesions of infancy and childhood. Can occur in association with Turner syndrome and Proteus syndrome.

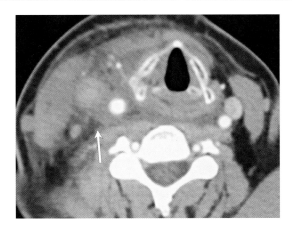

Fig. 4.62 On axial CT, thrombosis of the right internal jugular vein is seen as intermediate attenuation in the right internal jugular vein and lack of contrast enhancement (*arrow*).

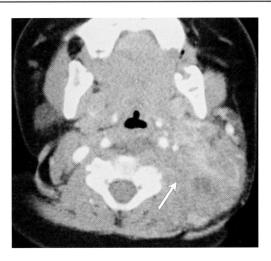

Fig. 4.63 Infection with thrombophlebitis resulting in occlusion of the left internal jugular vein is seen on axial CT as an irregular, poorly defined zone of inflammatory soft tissue attenuation in the left neck, including the retrostyloid parapharyngeal space (*arrow*), and with lack of contrast enhancement of the left internal jugular vein.

4.4 Retropharyngeal Space Lesions

The retropharyngeal space (RPS) is a small potential space that is located between the pharyngeal mucosal space anteriorly, the prevertebral space posteriorly, the retrostyloid parapharyngeal space (RPPS) laterally, and the skull base superiorly (**Fig. 4.64** and **Fig. 4.65**). The anterior border is the buccopharyngeal fascia (middle layer of the deep cervical fascia). The lateral border is the cloison sagittale, which are bilateral thin bands of fascia that extend dorsally from the buccopharyngeal fascia to the prevertebral fascia (deep layer of the deep cervical fascia) near the transverse processes of the cervical vertebrae. The cloison sagittale separates the RPS from the RPPS. The posterior border of the RPS is the alar fascia, which is a subdivision of the deep cervical fascia that extends from the skull base to the upper thoracic levels, where it fuses with the visceral fascia (infrahyoid extension of the buccopharyngeal fascia–middle layer of the deep cervical fascia). The inferior border of the RPS (where the alar fascia fuses with the visceral fascia is commonly at the C7–T1 level, although can vary from the T1 to T6 levels. The alar fascia is located anterior to the prevertebral fascia (deep layer of the deep cervical fascia). Between the alar fascia and the prevertebral fascia is the potential danger space, which consists of loose areolar tissue. Typically below the T2 level, the danger space continues inferiorly to the level of the diaphragm between the prevertebral fascia posteriorly and fused alar fascia and visceral fascia anteriorly. Infections or neoplasms that extend into the danger space can spread between the skull base and mediastinum. The prevertebral fascia extends from the skull base to the coccyx, although it fuses with the anterior longitudinal ligament at the T3 level, resulting in restriction of neoplasm or infection below the T3 level.

The RPS contains fat and lateral and medial retropharyngeal lymph nodes. The lateral retropharyngeal nodes (LRP nodes; Rouvier lymph nodes) drain lymph from the nasopharynx, oropharynx, paranasal sinuses, nasal cavity, and middle ear. In children, the LRP nodes can measure up to 2 cm, whereas in adults they usually measure less than 1 cm. Metastatic lymphadenopathy in the RPS nodes occurs from nasopharyngeal carcinomas, squamous cell carcinomas, salivary gland neoplasms, thyroid carcinomas, and melanoma. Direct spread to the RPS through the buccopharyngeal fascia can occur from nasopharyngeal carcinomas, squamous cell carcinomas, sinonasal undifferentiated carcinomas, malignant salivary gland neoplasms, and esthesioneuroblastomas. Invasion of the RPS can also occur from neoplasms extending from the prevertebral space, such as metastatic vertebral disease, myeloma, chordomas, and chondrosarcomas, or from infections, such as vertebral osteomyelitis. Primary tumors of the RPS are uncommon. Included in this category are lipomas, liposarcomas, nerve sheath tumors, lymphoma, hemangiomas, and other mesenchymal neoplasms.

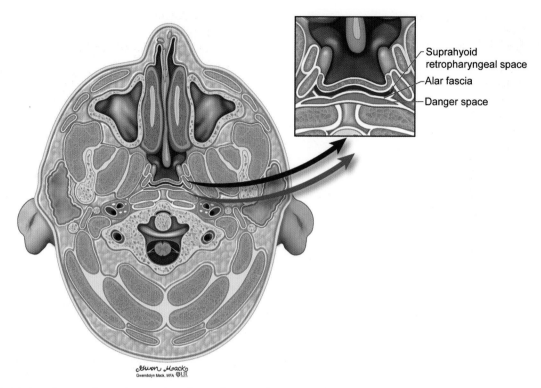

Fig. 4.64 Axial view diagram shows the suprahyoid retropharyngeal space in color.

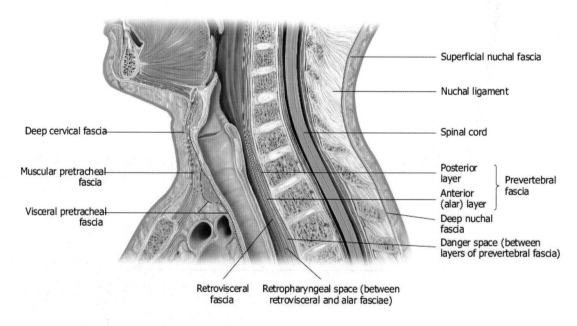

Fig. 4.65 Sagittal view diagram shows the retropharyngeal and danger spaces in relation to adjacent structures. From THIEME Atlas of Anatomy: Head and Neuroanatomy, © Thieme 2007, Illustration by Karl Wesker.

Table 4.4   Retropharyngeal space lesions

- – Malignant lymphadenopathy
- – Malignant neoplasms
- Inflammatory Lesions
  - – Lymphadenitis (presuppurative and suppurative)
  - – Retropharyngeal abscess
  - – Infection extending into the retropharyngeal space
  - – Granulomatosis with polyangiitis
- Vascular Abnormality
  - – Ectasia and tortuosity of the carotid artery
  - – Thrombophlebitis of the internal jugular vein
- Benign Lesions
  - – Lipoma
  - – Thyroid—multinodular goiter
  - – Hemangioma
  - – Venolymphatic malformation
- Congenital/Developmental Abnormality
  - – Branchial cleft cyst
  - – Neurenteric cyst

Table 4.4   Retropharyngeal space lesions

Lesions	Imaging Findings	Comments
Malignant lymphadenopathy (**Fig. 4.66**)	*CT and MRI:* In adults, features of retropharyngeal nodal metastases include enlarged nodes larger than 6 mm in the short axis, more than two enlarged lymph nodes on one side, ill-defined margins, and nodal necrosis.	Malignant neoplasms involving the pharyngeal wall, such as nasopharyngeal carcinoma and squamous cell carcinomas from the sinuses, oral cavity, pharynx, and larynx, can metastasize to the retropharyngeal nodes. Other neoplasms associated with retropharyngeal nodal metastasis are esthesioneurblastoma, sinonasal undifferentiated carcinoma, malignant salivary gland tumors, thyroid carcinoma, and melanoma. Leukemia and non-Hodgkin lymphoma can also involve the retropharyngeal nodes. Unilateral or bilateral retropharyngeal metastases are associated with increased risk for other nodal and distant metastases, as well as a poor prognosis.

(continued on page 374)

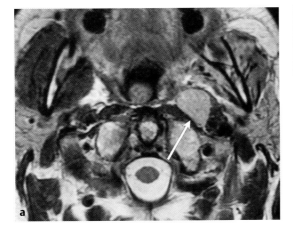 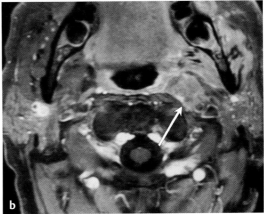

Fig. 4.66   **(a)** A 72-year-old woman with history of a squamous cell carcinoma who has an abnormally enlarged, malignant lateral retropharyngeal lymph node on the left that has slightly high signal on axial T2-weighted imaging (*arrow*) and **(b)** shows mild heterogeneous gadolinium contrast enhancement on axial fat-suppressed T1-weighted imaging (*arrow*).

Table 4.4 *(cont.)*   Retropharyngeal space lesions

Lesions	Imaging Findings	Comments
Malignant neoplasms (**Fig. 4.67**, **Fig. 4.68**, **Fig. 4.69**, and **Fig. 4.70**)	*MRI:* Malignant lesions from the nasopharynx, oropharynx, prestyloid parapharyngeal space, retrostyloid parapharyngeal space, deep portion of the parotid gland, and prevertebral space can invade the retropharyngeal space (RPS). Tumors often have intermediate signal on T1-weighted imaging, intermediate to slightly high signal on T2-weighted imaging, and mild gadolinium contrast enhancement. Can be large lesions (± necrosis and/or hemorrhage). *CT:* Tumors have intermediate attenuation; mild contrast-enhancement; large lesions (± necrosis and/or hemorrhage).	Direct spread to the RPS through the buccopharyngeal fascia can occur from nasopharyngeal carcinomas, squamous cell carcinomas, sinonasal undifferentiated carcinomas, malignant salivary gland neoplasms, esthesioneuroblastomas, rhabdomyosarcomas, and non-Hodgkin lymphoma. Invasion of the RPS posteriorly from lesions penetrating the prevertebral fascia can occur from metastatic vertebral disease, myeloma, chordomas, chondrosarcomas, and infections, such as vertebral osteomyelitis. Rare primary tumors that involve the RPS include liposarcomas and malignant nerve sheath tumors.
Inflammatory Lesions		
Lymphadenitis (presuppurative and suppurative) (**Fig. 4.71** and **Fig. 4.72**)	*MRI:* Enlarged presuppurative retropharyngeal nodes have intermediate signal on T1-weighted imaging (T1WI) and slightly high signal on T2-weighted imaging (T2WI), and show gadolinium (Gd) contrast enhancement. Suppurative retropharyngeal nodes have low-intermediate signal on T1WI, slightly high to high signal on T2WI, and rim Gd contrast enhancement. Irregular increased signal on T2WI and Gd contrast enhancement are typically seen in the adjacent soft tissue. *CT:* Presuppurative enlarged lymph nodes are associated with loss of the fatty hilum, slightly decreased attenuation, increased contrast enhancement, and reticulation of adjacent fat. Suppurative lymph nodes are typically enlarged and have low attenuation centrally surrounded by a rim of contrast enhancement.	The lymph nodes of the retropharyngeal space (RPS) drain the nasal cavity, paranasal sinuses, nasopharynx, oropharynx, and middle ear. Infections in the nasopharynx or oropharynx can spread to the retropharyngeal lymph nodes through capillary lymphatic channels, resulting in enlarged retropharyngeal nodes (presuppurative adenitis). Most presuppurative lymph nodes measure < 1.2 cm. The involved enlarged lymph nodes can undergo liquefactive necrosis, causing suppurative adenitis (purulent lymph nodes). In children, lymphadenitis can result from upper respiratory viral infections, as well as from bacteria, such as *Staphylococcus aureus* and *Streptococcus pyogenes*. Purulent lymph nodes measure up to 4.5 cm. Treatment with IV antibiotics is usually effective when the volume of the suppurative low-attenuation nodes measures less than 2 cm. Larger suppurative lymph nodes usually require surgical drainage, especially when the airway is compromised. In young adults, generalized lymphadenopathy in the RPS can be caused by mononucleosis and HIV. In adults, suppurative adenitis often results from trauma and procedural or surgical complications. Gram-positive cocci are common pathogens for suppurative adenitis in adults.

(continued on page 377)

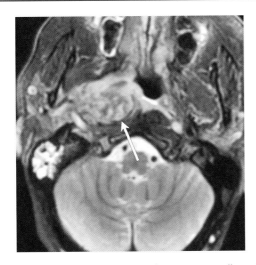

Fig. 4.67 A 60-year-old woman with squamous cell carcinoma in the right nasopharynx and parapharyngeal space that has ill-defind margins and heterogeneous low-intermediate and slightly high signal on axial fat-suppressed T2-weighted imaging (*arrow*). The tumor extends posteriorly to involve the retropharyngeal space and occludes the right eustachian tube, resulting in retained fluid filling the right mastoid air cells.

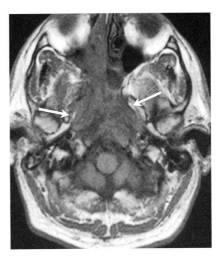

Fig. 4.68 Squamous cell carcinoma in the posterior nasopharynx has ill-defined margins and intermediate signal on axial T1-weighted imaging (*arrows*). The tumor invades the retropharyngeal and prevertebral spaces as well as the bone marrow of the lower clivus.

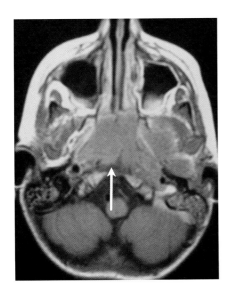

Fig. 4.69 A 6-year-old male with a large lesion in the posterior nasopharynx from non-Hodgkin lymphoma. The lesion shows mild gadolinium contrast enhancement on axial T1-weighted imaging and involves the pharyngeal mucosal space, the left parapharyngal space, and the retropharyngeal space (*arrow*).

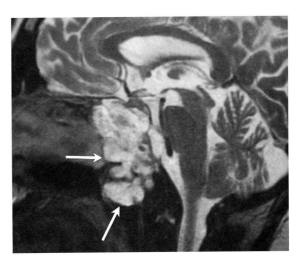

Fig. 4.70 Sagittal fat-suppressed T2-weighted imaging of a 77-year-old woman shows a chordoma with mostly high signal that involves the clivus associated with bone destruction and extension into the sphenoid and ethmoid sinuses and nasopharynx, including the retropharyngeal space (*arrows*).

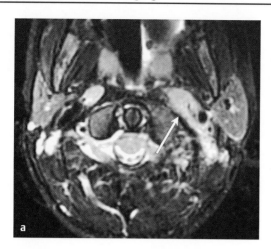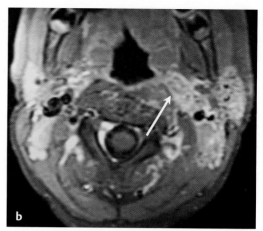

Fig. 4.71 A 1-year-old male with an abnormally enlarged left retropharyngeal lymph node representing presuppurative lymphadenitis from methicillin-resistant *Staphylococcus aureus* (MRSA). **(a)** The lymph node has slightly high to high signal on axial fat-suppressed T2-weighted imaging (*arrow*) and **(b)** shows heterogeneous gadolinium contrast enhancement on axial fat-suppressed T1-weighted imaging (*arrow*).

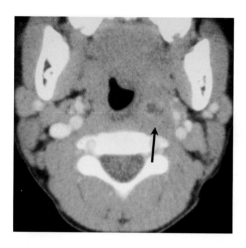

Fig. 4.72 Axial postcontrast CT of a 5-year-old male shows a left peritonsillar suppurative lymph node (*arrow*) that has low attenuation centrally surrounded by a rim of contrast enhancement. Infection extends posteriorly to involve the retropharyngeal space and is associated with lateral displacement of the left carotid arteries.

Table 4.4 (cont.) Retropharyngeal space lesions

Lesions	Imaging Findings	Comments
Retropharyngeal abscess (**Fig. 4.73, Fig. 4.74**, and **Fig. 4.75**)	*MRI:* Retropharyngeal space (RPS) abscesses have low-intermediate signal on T1-weighted imaging and slightly high to high signal on T2-weighted imaging (T2WI), as well as rim gadolinium (Gd) contrast enhancement. Irregular increased signal on T2WI and Gd contrast enhancement are typically seen in the adjacent soft tissue. *CT:* Asymmetric low-attenuation fluid collection in the RPS with anterior displacement of the posterior wall of the nasopharynx and/or oropharynx from the prevertebral space. Irregular, thin peripheral contrast enhancement with scalloped/lobulated margins can be seen.	Retropharyngeal abscesses can result from inadequately treated suppurative lymphadenitis, trauma, foreign bodies, or extension of infection from adjacent structures. A trial of IV antibiotics may be successful for small abscesses, whereas larger abscesses (> 2 cm) associated with narrowing of the airway are usually treated with surgical drainage in addition to IV antibiotics.

(continued on page 378)

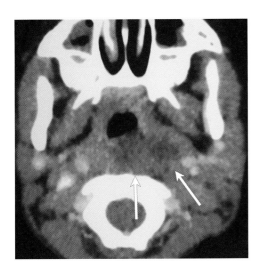

Fig. 4.73 Axial postcontrast CT of a 5-year-old male shows suppurative lymphadenitis with abscess formation in the retropharyngeal space (*arrows*).

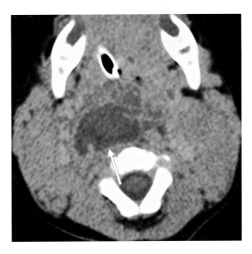

Fig. 4.74 Axial CT of a 7-month-old female with a retropharyngeal abscess (*arrow*), which is seen as an asymmetric low-attenuation fluid collection in the retropharyngeal space with anterior displacement of the posterior wall of the oropharynx from the prevertebral space. The abscess has irregular peripheral contrast enhancement with lobulated margins.

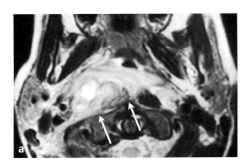 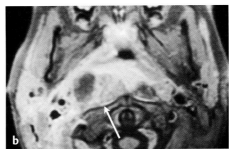 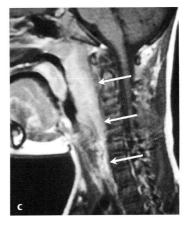

Fig. 4.75 **(a)** Axial T2-weighted imaging of a 6-year-old male shows poorly defined zones (*arrows*) with abnormal high signal and **(b)** corresponding gadolinium contrast enhancement on axial fat-suppressed T1-weighted imaging from retropharyngeal phlegmon and abscess that involves the right prestyloid and retrostyloid parapharyngeal spaces, as well as the retropharyngeal space (*arrow*). **(c)** Sagittal T1-weighted imaging shows abnormal gadolinium contrast enhancement from the infection extending inferiorly within the danger space (*arrows*).

Table 4.4 *(cont.)* Retropharyngeal space lesions

Lesions	Imaging Findings	Comments
Infection extending into the retropharyngeal space (**Fig. 4.76** and **Fig. 4.77**)	*MRI:* Irregular soft tissue thickening with poorly defined, slightly high signal on T2-weighted imaging (T2WI) and fat-suppressed T2WI (phlegmon). Abscesses are collections with high signal on T2WI surrounded by a peripheral rim of gadolinium (Gd) contrast enhancement. Soft tissue thickening with slightly high to high signal on T2WI is typically seen adjacent to the abscess. Inferior extension of infection with high signal abnormality on T2WI and Gd contrast enhancement can occur with involvement of both the retropharyngeal space (RPS) and danger space, although extension below the T4 level is typical for infection involving the danger space. *CT:* Irregular soft tissue thickening with ill-defined margins (phlegmon), ± rim-enhancing fluid collection (abscess). Suppurative lymphadentitis can appear as enlarged paramedian nodes with slightly low attenuation centrally surrounded by a contrast-enhancing rim. Lesions can be unilateral.	Peritonsillar abscess is the most common infection involving the head and neck. Occurs in young children and adults, often during times with highest incidence of streptococcal pharyngitis and exudative tonsillitis. Treatment of a peritonsillar phlegmon can be with antibiotics, whereas a peritonsillar abscess requires drainage. If not treated appropriately, the infection can extend into the adjacent parapharyngeal, retropharyngeal, danger, masticator, and/or submandibular spaces. Pharyngitis and sinusitis in young children and adults can result in suppurative lymphadenitis in the retropharyngeal nodes, which can result in abscess formation if not treated promptly with antibiotics. Other etiologies for RPS infection include complications from intubation, nasogastric tubes, surgery, foreign bodies, and necrotizing otitis externa. Infection involving the RPS and danger space can extend inferiorly into the mediastinum, causing mediastinitis. Infection and abscess formation in the RPS can also result from extension of pyogenic or tuberculous vertebral osteomyelitis through the prevertebral fascia. Patients with infection in the RPS and danger space often present with odynophagia, dysphagia, stiff neck, backward head tilt, and dyspnea.
Granulomatosis with polyangiitis (**Fig. 4.78**)	*MRI:* Poorly defined zones of mucosal soft tissue thickening with low-intermediate signal on T1-weighted imaging, slightly high to high signal on T2-weighted imaging, and gadolinium contrast enhancement within the nasal cavity, paranasal sinuses, retropharyngeal space, orbits, infratemporal fossa, and external auditory canal, ± invasion and destruction of bone and nasal septum, ± extension into the skull base with involvement of the dura, leptomeninges, brain, or venous sinuses. *CT:* Zones with soft tissue attenuation, ± bone destruction.	Multisystem autoimmune disease with necrotizing granulomas in the respiratory tract, focal necrotizing angiitis of small arteries and veins of various tissues, and glomerulonephritis. Can involve the paranasal sinuses, nasopharynx, oropharynx, orbits, skull base, dura, leptomeninges, and occasionally the temporal bone. Typically has positive immunoreactivity to cytoplasmic antineutrophil cytoplasmic antibody (c-ANCA). Treatment includes corticosteroids, cyclophosphamide, and anti-TNF agents.

(continued on page 380)

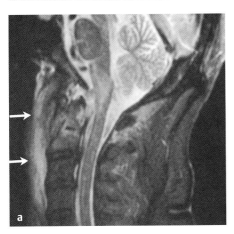
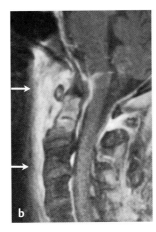
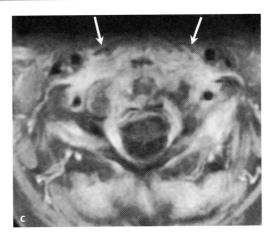

Fig. 4.76 **(a)** A 59-year-old man with vertebral osteomyelitis from methicillin-resistant *Staphylococcus aureus* (MRSA) that is seen as abnormal high signal (*arrows*) on sagittal fat-suppressed T2-weighted imaging and corresponding gadolinium contrast enhancement on **(b)** sagittal (*arrows*) and **(c)** axial (*arrows*) fat-suppressed T1-weighted imaging. The osteomyelitis involves the marrow of the C2 vertebra and prevertebral and retropharyngeal spaces, and it is associated with bone destruction and epidural abscess at the C1–2 level.

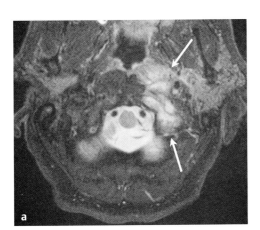
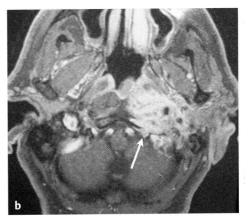

Fig. 4.77 **(a)** A 72-year-old man with necrotizing otitis externa extending inferiorly to involve the left parapharyngeal space and left retropharyngeal and prevertebral spaces, seen as poorly defined zones of abnormal high signal on axial fat-suppressed T2-weighted imaging (*arrows*) and **(b)** as gadolinium contrast enhancement on axial fat-suppressed T1-weighted imaging (*arrow*). Abnormal signal and gadolinium contrast enhancement are also seen at the left skull base, representing osteomyelitis.

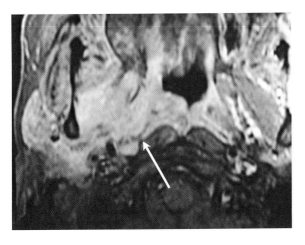

Fig. 4.78 A 46-year-old woman who has granulomatosis with polyangiitis. Poorly defined zones with gadolinium contrast enhancement are seen in the right parapharyngeal, right parotid, right retropharyngeal (*arrow*), and right masticator spaces.

Table 4.4 *(cont.)* Retropharyngeal space lesions

Lesions	Imaging Findings	Comments
Vascular Abnormality		
Ectasia and tortuosity of the carotid artery (**Fig. 4.79**; see **Fig. 4.58**)	*CTA and MRA* show medial deviation of the course of the common and/or internal carotid arteries in the upper neck, including the retropharyngeal space.	The internal and upper common carotid arteries can be ectatic and tortuous. May course medially, resulting in a pulsatile retropharyngeal or retrotonsillar mass. Identification of the arterial position is important for surgical planning and avoiding unnecessary biopsies.
Thrombophlebitis of the internal jugular vein (**Fig. 4.80**)	*MRI:* Acute thrombus can have high signal on T2-weighted imaging (T2WI), whereas subacute thrombus can have low signal on T2WI. Poorly defined zones with high signal on T2WI and gadolinium contrast enhancement are seen in the adjacent soft tissues of the retrostyloid parapharyngeal space (RPPS) and retropharyngeal space (RPS). *Contrast-enhanced CT and CTA:* Tubular intraluminal zone with low-intermediate attenuation lacking contrast enhancement, ± peripheral contrast enhancement of the vaso vasorum of the vessel wall. *Ultrasound:* Dilated and incompressible vein with lack of blood flow on Doppler.	Internal jugular vein (IJV) thrombosis can result from adjacent inflammation and/or infection in the RPPS and RPS. Extension of odontogenic and/or oropharyngeal infections can cause IJV thrombophlebitis (Lemierre syndrome). Lemierre syndrome often occurs in healthy young adults from oropharyngeal spread of infection from the usually commensal bacteria *Fusobacterium necrophorum* secondary to an altered host-defense mechanism with damage to the mucosa (trauma, bacterial or viral pharyngitis). Complications include septic embolization and bacteremia. Treatment of Lemierre syndrome is with broad-spectrum antibiotics, ± anticoagulation.
Benign Lesions		
Lipoma (See **Fig. 4.48**)	*MRI:* Lipomas have MRI signal isointense to subcutaneous fat on T1-weighted imaging (high signal). On T2-weighted imaging, signal suppression occurs with frequency-selective fat saturation techniques or with a short time to inversion recovery (STIR) method. Typically there is no gadolinium contrast enhancement or peripheral edema. *CT:* Lipomas have CT attenuation similar to subcutaneous fat and typically no contrast enhancement or peripheral edema.	Common benign hamartomas composed of mature white adipose tissue without cellular atypia. Most common soft tissue tumor, representing 16% of all soft tissue tumors. May contain calcifications and/or traversing blood vessels.

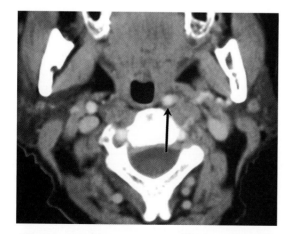

Fig. 4.79 Axial postcontrast CT shows medial position of left internal carotid artery (*arrow*).

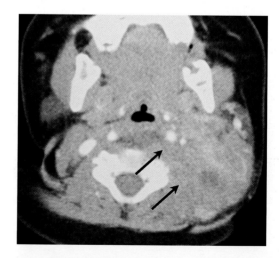

Fig. 4.80 Infection with thrombophlebitis resulting in occlusion of the left internal jugular vein is seen on axial CT as an irregular, poorly defined zone of inflammatory soft tissue attenuation in the left neck, including the retropharyngeal and retrostyloid parapharyngeal spaces (*arrows*), with lack of contrast enhancement of the left internal jugular vein.

Lesions	Imaging Findings	Comments
Thyroid—multinodular goiter (**Fig. 4.81**)	*MRI:* Simple goiters show diffuse enlargement of the thyroid gland. Multinodular goiters have circumscribed margins and contain multiple nodules. Nodules can have low, intermediate, or high signal on T1-weighted imaging (T1WI) and T2-weighted imaging (T2WI). High signal on T1WI can be secondary to cysts with colloid or hemorrhage. Low signal foci on T1WI and T2WI can occur from calcifications. Can displace and/ or compress the trachea and/or esophagus, ± extend inferiorly into the mediastinum. *CT:* Simple goiters appear as diffuse enlargement of the thyroid gland. Multinodular goiters have multiple nodules that often have low attenuation, ± cystic zones and calcifications. Margins are usually well circumscribed. Can displace and/or compress the trachea and/or esophagus, ± extension inferiorly into the mediastinum. *Ultrasound:* Simple goiters are associated with diffuse enlargement of the thyroid gland that has uniform or heterogeneous echogenicity. Multinodular goiters can have heterogeneous echogenicity with multiple hypoechoic nodules, ± cystic or necrotic zones, ± calcifications, ± hemorrhage. Toxic nodules chow increased systolic velocities on color Doppler sonography. *Nuclear scintigraphy:* Iodine 123, iodine 131, or technetium 99m pertechnetate uptake often occurs in multiple nodules.	Goiter is an enlargement of the thyroid gland without or with multiple nodules (multinodular goiter). Simple diffuse goiters result from inadequate output of thyroid hormone, which causes compensatory hypertrophy of follicular thyroid epithelium. The simple, diffuse, nontoxic goiters usually have an initial phase of follicular cell growth with hyperemia. Patients with simple diffuse goiters are usually euthyroid. Endemic goiters occur in areas when dietary iodine is insufficient. Another type is the simple sporadic goiter, which usually occurs in females with onset around puberty. Eventually, there is often colloid involution that progresses to nodule formation within the goiter (multinodular goiter). Toxic multinodular goiters are associated with hyperthyroidism and have one or more autofunctioning nodules (Plummer disease). Most toxic goiters occur in patients who initially had nontoxic goiters. Patients present with a neck mass and neck discomfort. Goiters can extend into the mediastinum and lower neck without or with displacement and compression of the trachea and esophagus, resulting in shortness of breath and dysphagia. Multinodular goiters contain various-sized nodules that contain follicles distended by colloid, papillary hyperplasia, cystic and/or hemorrhagic zones, cholesterol clefts, dystrophic calcifications, ossifications, and necrosis. Multinodular goiter is found in up to 5% of the population, with a 2–4:1 female:male predominance. Rapid increase in the size of multinodular goiter can be associated with anaplastic thyroid carcinoma (5% risk).

(continued on page 382)

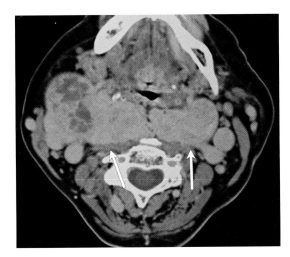

Fig. 4.81 Axial CT shows cephalad extension of a large mulitnodular goiter (*arrows*) into the retropharyngeal space bilaterally.

Table 4.4 *(cont.)*　Retropharyngeal space lesions

Lesions	Imaging Findings	Comments
Hemangioma (See **Fig. 4.49**)	*MRI:* Circumscribed or poorly marginated structures (< 4 cm in diameter) in bone marrow or soft tissue with intermediate-high signal on T1-weighted imaging (often isointense to marrow fat) and high signal on T2-weighted imaging (T2WI) and fat-suppressed T2WI, typically with gadolinium contrast enhancement, ± expansion of bone. *CT:* Expansile bone lesions with a radiating pattern of bony trabeculae oriented toward the center. Hemangiomas in soft tissue have mostly intermediate attenuation, ± zones of fat attenuation.	Benign lesions of bone or soft tissue composed of capillary, cavernous, and/or malformed venous vessels. Considered to be a hamartomatous disorder. Occur in patients 1 to 84 years old (median age = 33 years).
Venolymphatic malformation	Can be circumscribed lesions or occur in an infiltrative pattern with extension within soft tissue and between muscles. *MRI:* Often contain single or multiple cystic zones that can be large (macrocystic type) or small (microcystic type), and that have predominantly low signal on T1-weighted imaging (T1WI) and high signal on T2-weighted imaging (T2WI) and fat-suppressed T2WI. Fluid–fluid levels and zones with high signal on T1WI and variable signal on T2WI may result from cysts containing hemorrhage, high protein concentration, and/or necrotic debris. Septa between the cystic zones can vary in thickness and gadolinium (Gd) contrast enhancement. Nodular zones within the lesions can have variable degrees of Gd contrast enhancement. Microcystic types typically show more Gd contrast enhancement than the macrocystic type. *CT:* Macrocystic lesions are usually low-attenuation cystic lesions (10–25 HU) separated by thin walls, ± intermediate or high attenuation that can result from hemorrhage or infection; ± fluid–fluid levels.	Benign vascular anomalies (also referred to as lymphangioma or cystic hygroma) that primarily result from abnormal lymphangiogenesis. Up to 75% occur in the head and neck. Can be observed in utero with MRI or sonography, at birth (50–65%), or within the first 5 years, and ~ 85% are detected by age 2. Lesions are composed of endothelium-lined lymphatic ± venous channels interspersed within connective tissue stroma.

Lesions	Imaging Findings	Comments
Congenital/Developmental Abnormality		
Branchial cleft cyst (See **Fig. 4.55**)	*MRI:* Circumscribed lesion that often has low-intermediate signal on T1-weighted imaging and high signal on T2-weighted imaging. Usually there is no gadolinium contrast enhancement unless there is superimposed infection. *CT:* Circumscribed, cystic lesion with low to intermediate attenuation depending on the proportions of protein and water. *First branchial cleft cysts* can be located adjacent to the external auditory canal (type 1 first branchial cleft cyst) or superficial portion of the parotid gland, ± extension into the parapharyngeal space, posterior to the submandibular gland, and/or up to the external auditory canal (type 2). *Second branchial cleft cysts* can be anterior to the sternocleidomastoid muscle (SCM) and medial to the carotid arteries (type 1), anteromedial to the SCM with or without extension posterior to the carotid sheath (type 2), or extend into the parapharyngeal space and between the internal and external carotid arteries (type 3). *Third branchial cleft cysts* are located at the lower anterior margin of the SCM at the level of the upper thyroid lobe, ± extension into the sinus tract posterior to the carotid artery and glossopharyngeal nerve, passing through the thyroid membrane above the level of the internal branch of the superior laryngeal nerve into the base of the piriform sinus. *Fourth branchial cleft cysts* occur in the lower third of the neck laterally and anterior to the lower SCM and level of the aortic arch, ± visible connecting sinus tract on the right below the subclavian artery or on the left below the aortic arch that extends superiorly and dorsal to the carotid artery up to the level of the hypoglossal nerve and then downward along the SCM to the piriform sinus.	Represent developmental anomalies involving the branchial apparatus. The branchial apparatus consists of four major and two rudimetary arches of mesoderm lined by ectoderm externally and endoderm internally within pouches that form at the end of the fourth week of gestation. The mesoderm contains a dominant artery, nerve, cartilage, and muscle. The four major arches are separated by clefts. Each arch develops into a defined neck structure, with eventual obliteration of the branchial clefts. The first arch forms the external auditory canal, eustachian tube, middle ear, and mastoid air cells. The second arch develops into the hyoid bone and tonsillar and supratonsillar fossae. The third and fourth arches develop into the pharynx below the hyoid bone. Branchial anomalies include cysts, sinuses, and fistulae. Second branchial cleft cysts account for up to 90% of all branchial cleft malformations. Cysts are lined by squamous epithelium (90%), ciliated columnar epithelium (8%), or both types (2%). Sebaceous glands, salivary tissue, lymphoid tissue, and cholesterol crystals in mucoid fluid can also occur. There are four types of second branchial cleft cysts. Type 1 is located anterior to the sternocleidomastoid muscle (SCM) and deep to the platysma muscle. Type 2 (the most common type) is located at the anteromedial surface of the SCM, lateral to the carotid space and posterior to the submandibular gland. Type 3 is located lateral to the pharyngeal wall and medial to the carotid arteries, ± extension between the external and internal carotid arteries (*beak sign*). Type 4 is located between the medial aspect of the carotid sheath and pharynx at the level of the tonsillar fossa and can extend superiorly to the skull base. Typically asymptomatic unless complicated by infection.
Neurenteric cyst	*MRI:* Well-circumscribed spheroid intradural extra-axial lesions, with low, intermediate, or high signal on T1- and T2-weighted imaging and usually no gadolinium contrast enhancement. *CT:* Circumscribed intradural extra-axial structures with low-intermediate attenuation. Usually no contrast enhancement.	Neurenteric cysts are malformations in which there is a persistent communication between the ventrally located endoderm and the dorsally located ectoderm secondary to developmental failure of separation the notochord and foregut. Obliteration of portions of a dorsal enteric sinus can result in cysts lined by endothelium, fibrous cords, or sinuses. Observed in patients < 40 years old. Locations are thoracic > cervical > posterior cranial fossa > craniovertebral junction > lumbar. Cysts are usually midline in position and often ventral to the spinal cord or brainstem. Associated with anomalies of the adjacent vertebrae and clivus.

4.5 Parotid Space

The parotid space extends from the external auditory canal and mastoid tip to the angle of the mandible and is enclosed within the superficial layers of the deep cervical fascia (**Fig. 4.82**). The parotid space is located posterior to the masticator space and lateral to the prestyloid and retrostyloid parapharyngeal spaces. The parotid space contains the parotid gland, proximal parotid duct (Stensen's duct), intra- and extraparotid lymph nodes, the retromandibular vein, branches of the external carotid artery, and extracranial portions of the facial nerve. The parotid gland is the first major salivary gland to develop and begins to form at 4 to 6 weeks of gestation. The parotid gland becomes encapsulated after development of the lymphatic system and normally contains lymph nodes, unlike the other major salivary glands. The parotid gland contains secretory ectodermal-derived epithelial cells, glandular structures (oral epithelial derivation), and stroma (mesenchymal derivation). The parotid gland has two major portions (deep and superficial). The deep and superficial portions are separated by the position of the retromandibular vein. The deep portion is located medial to the retromandibular vein, and the superficial portion is located laterally. The retromandibular vein is an important landmark for surgical planning because the extracranial portion of the facial nerve is located just lateral to the retromandibular vein. The deep portion of the parotid gland extends medially between the styloid process and posterior margin of the mandible (stylomandibular tunnel), which is contiguous with the prestyloid parapharyngeal space.

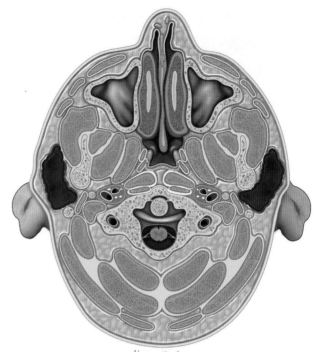

Fig. 4.82 Axial view diagram shows the parotid space in color.

Table 4.5 Lesions of the parotid space

- Benign Neoplasms
  - Pleomorphic adenoma (benign mixed tumor)
  - Warthin tumor (papillary cystadenoma lymphomatosum)
  - Lipoma
  - Schwannoma
  - Neurofibroma
- Malignant Tumors
  - Mucoepidermoid carcinoma
  - Adenoid cystic carcinoma
  - Acinic cell carcinoma
  - Squamous cell carcinoma
  - Malignant mixed tumor (carcinoma ex pleomorphic adenoma)
  - Non-Hodgkin lymphoma (NHL)
  - Metastatic malignancies
  - Melanoma

- Tumorlike Lesions
  - Epidermoid cyst
- Inflammatory Disease
  - Parotiditis/sialadenitis
  - Sialolithiasis and sialadenitis
  - Reactive adenopathy
  - Juvenile recurrent parotiditis
  - Benign lymphoepithelial lesions (HIV, AIDS)
  - Sjögren's syndrome
  - Sarcoidosis
  - Kimura disease
- Congenital/Developmental
  - First branchial cleft cyst
  - Hemangioma
  - Venolymphatic malformation

Table 4.5 Lesions of the parotid space

Lesions	Imaging Findings	Comments
Benign Neoplasms		
Pleomorphic adenoma (benign mixed tumor) (**Fig. 4.83, Fig. 4.84,** and **Fig. 4.85**)	*MRI:* Circumscribed lesions, ± lobulated margins, with low-intermediate signal on T1-weighted imaging, slightly high or high signal on T2-weighted imaging (T2WI) and fat-suppressed T2WI, and usually gadolinium contrast enhancement, which is often homogeneous for small lesions and heterogeneous for large lesions. *CT:* Circumscribed or lobulated lesions with intermediate attenuation, + contrast enhancement.	Most common benign tumor of the major salivary glands, accounting for up to 60% of all salivary gland tumors. Eighty percent of pleomorphic adenomas occur in the parotid glands, 10% in the submandibular glands, and 10% in the minor salivary glands. Incidence of 3 per 100,000 (mean age = 46 years). These slow-growing, encapsulated tumors are morphologically diverse and are composed of epithelial cells with low mitotic activity arranged in glandular, ductal, and/or solid patterns associated with sparse stromal elements. Lesions also contain modified myoepithelial cells that can contain chondroid or fibromyxoid zones, ± zones of hemorrhage, necrosis, and/or calcification. Immunoreactive to cytokeratin, vimentin, and p63. Most tumors have abnormal karyotypes and mutations involving the *PLAG1* gene on chromosome 8q12. Usually occur in patients between 20 and 60 years old. Other, rare types of minor salivary gland adenomas include myoepithelioma and oncocytoma. Local tumor recurrence rate of 7% after 10 years.

(continued on page 387)

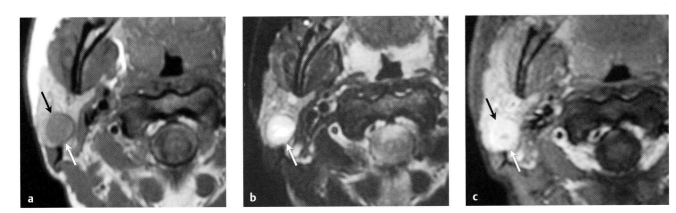

Fig. 4.83 **(a)** A 16-year-old female with a pleomorphic adenoma (benign mixed tumor) in the right parotid gland that has intermediate signal on axial T1-weighted imaging (*arrows*), **(b)** heterogeneous high signal on axial T2-weighted imaging (*arrow*), and **(c)** gadolinium contrast enhancement on axial fat-suppressed T1-weighted imaging (*arrows*).

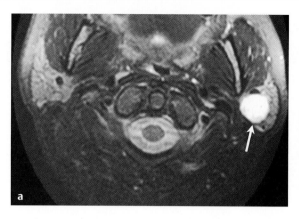
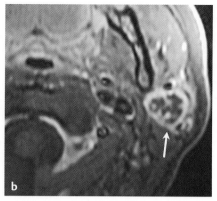

Fig. 4.84 **(a)** A 42-year-old man with a pleomorphic adenoma in the left parotid gland dorsal to the retromandibular vein that has high signal on axial T2-weighted imaging (*arrow*) and **(b)** shows heterogeneous gadolinium contrast enhancement on axial fat-suppressed T1-weighted imaging (*arrow*).

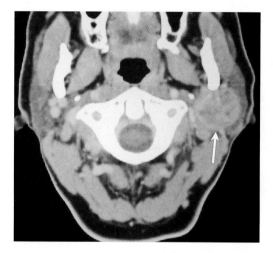

Fig. 4.85 A 43-year-old woman with a pleomorphic adenoma in the left parotid gland (*arrow*) that has intermediate attenuation and small zones with low attenuation on axial CT.

Table 4.5 *(cont.)* Lesions of the parotid space

Lesions	Imaging Findings	Comments
Warthin tumor (papillary cystadenoma lymphomatosum) (**Fig. 4.86, Fig. 4.87**, and **Fig. 4.88**)	*MRI:* Circumscribed ovoid lesions, ± lobulated margins, often located in the lower superficial portions of the parotid glands. Can be bilateral. Lesions have low-intermediate signal on T1-weighted imaging, slightly high or high signal on T2-weighted imaging (T2WI) and fat-suppressed T2WI, ± cystic zones with high signal on T2WI, ± gadolinium contrast enhancement of solid portions. *CT:* Circumscribed or lobulated lesions with intermediate attenuation, + contrast enhancement.	Second most common benign tumor of the parotid gland composed of lymphoid stroma and epithelial cells within a capsule. The epithelial cells can be arranged as papillary projections into cystic spaces. The epithelial cells are bilayered, with a layer of columnar eosinophilic or palisading oncocytic cells, and adjacent cuboidal cells. The stroma contains lymphoid tissue, ± germinal centers, mast cells, and plasma cells. Slow-growing lesions that account for up to 10% of parotid tumors. Most common bilateral parotid lesion (25% are synchronous, 75% are metachronous). Treatment is surgical resection, and there is a very low recurrence rate.

(continued on page 388)

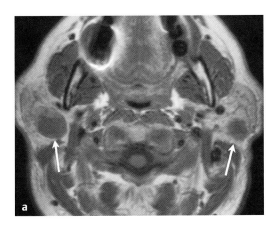
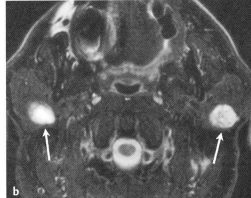

Fig. 4.86 **(a)** A 55-year-old man with bilateral Warthin tumors that have low signal on axial T1-weighted imaging (*arrows*) and **(b)** slightly heterogeneous high signal on axial fat-suppressed T2-weighted imaging (*arrows*).

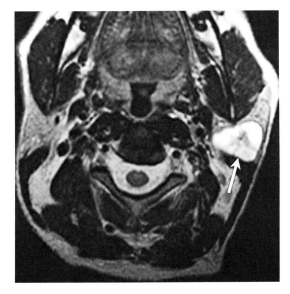

Fig. 4.87 A 45-year-old man with a Warthin tumor (*arrow*) in the left parotid gland that has slightly heterogeneous high signal on axial T2-weighted imaging.

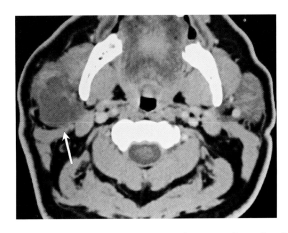

Fig. 4.88 A 52-year-old man with a Warthin tumor (*arrow*) in the right parotid gland that has mostly low attenuation on axial CT.

Table 4.5 *(cont.)* Lesions of the parotid space

Lesions	Imaging Findings	Comments
Lipoma (**Fig. 4.89**)	*MRI:* Lipomas have MRI signal isointense to subcutaneous fat on T1-weighted imaging (high signal). On T2-weighted imaging, signal suppression occurs with frequency-selective fat saturation techniques or with a short time to inversion recovery (STIR) method. Typically there is no gadolinium contrast enhancement or peripheral edema. *CT:* Lipomas have CT attenuation similar to subcutaneous fat and typically no contrast enhancement or peripheral edema.	Common benign hamartomas composed of mature white adipose tissue without cellular atypia. Most common soft tissue tumor, representing 16% of all soft tissue tumors.
Schwannoma (**Fig. 4.90** and **Fig. 4.91**)	*MRI:* Circumscribed spheroid or ovoid lesions with low-intermediate signal on T1-weighted imaging, high signal on T2-weighted imaging (T2WI) and fat-suppressed T2WI, and usually prominent gadolinium (Gd) contrast enhancement. High signal on T2WI and Gd contrast enhancement can be heterogeneous in large lesions due to cystic degeneration and/or hemorrhage. *CT:* Circumscribed spheroid or ovoid lesions with intermediate attenuation, + contrast enhancement. Large lesions can have cystic degeneration and/or hemorrhage.	Schwannomas are benign encapsulated tumors that contain differentiated neoplastic Schwann cells. They most commonly occur as solitary, sporadic lesions. Multiple schwannomas are often associated with neurofibromatosis type 2 (NF2), which is an autosomal dominant disease involving a gene mutation at chromosome 22q12. In addition to schwannomas, patients with NF2 can also have multiple meningiomas and ependymomas. The incidence of NF2 is 1/37,000 to 1/50,000 newborns. Age at presentation is 22 to 72 years (mean age = 46 years). Peak incidence is in the fourth to sixth decades. Many patients with NF2 present in the third decade with bilateral vestibular schwannomas.
Neurofibroma	*MRI:* *Solitary neurofibromas* are circumscribed spheroid, ovoid, or lobulated extra-axial lesions with low-intermediate signal on T1-weighted imaging (T1WI), intermediate-high signal on T2-weighted imaging (T2WI), and prominent gadolinium (Gd) contrast enhancement. High signal on T2WI and Gd contrast enhancement can be heterogeneous in large lesions. *Plexiform neurofibromas* appear as curvilinear and multinodular lesions involving multiple nerve branches and have low to intermediate signal on T1WI and intermediate or slightly high to high signal on T2WI and fat-suppressed T2WI, with or without bands or strands of low signal. Lesions usually show Gd contrast enhancement. *CT:* Ovoid or fusiform lesions with low-intermediate attenuation. Lesions can show contrast enhancement. Often erode adjacent bone.	Neurofibromas are benign nerve sheath tumors that contain mixtures of Schwann cells, perineural-like cells, and interlacing fascicles of fibroblasts associated with abundant collagen. Unlike schwannomas, neurofibromas lack Antoni A and B regions and cannot be separated pathologically from the underlying nerve. Neurofibromas most frequently occur as sporadic, localized, solitary lesions, less frequently as diffuse or plexiform lesions. Multiple neurofibromas are typically seen in neurofibromatosis type 1 (NF1), which is an autosomal dominant disorder (1/2,500 births) caused by mutations of the neurofibromin gene on chromosome 17q11.2. NF1 is the most common type of neurocutaneous syndrome and is associated with neoplasms of the central and peripheral nervous systems (optic gliomas, astrocytomas, plexiform and solitary neurofibromas) and skin (café-au-lait spots, axillary and inguinal freckling). Also associated with meningeal and skull dysplasias, as well as hamartomas of the iris (Lisch nodules).

(continued on page 390)

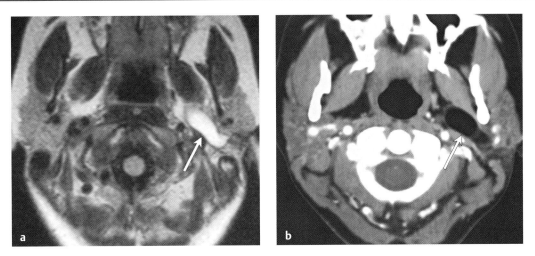

Fig. 4.89 **(a)** A 27-year-old woman with a lipoma involving the deep portion of the left parotid gland that has high signal on axial T1-weighted imaging (*arrow*) and **(b)** low attenuation on axial CT (*arrow*).

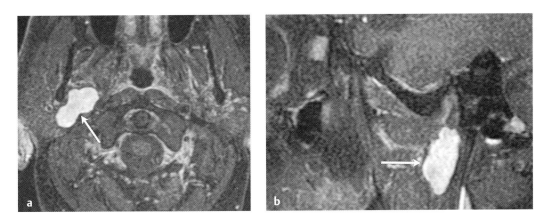

Fig. 4.90 A 69-year-old woman with a schwannoma of the right facial nerve located in the deep portion of the right parotid gland. The schwannoma has circumscribed margins and has high signal on **(a)** axial (*arrow*) and **(b)** sagittal (*arrow*) fat-suppressed T2-weighted imaging.

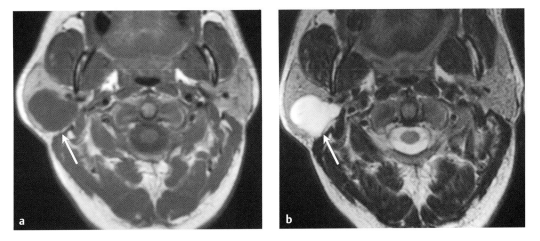

Fig. 4.91 A 44-year-old man with a schwannoma in the right parotid gland that has **(a)** low-intermediate signal on axial T1-weighted imaging (*arrow*) and **(b)** high signal on axial T2-weighted imaging (*arrow*).

Table 4.5 *(cont.)* Lesions of the parotid space

Lesions	Imaging Findings	Comments
Malignant Tumors		
Mucoepidermoid carcinoma **(Fig. 4.92)**	*MRI:* Nodular lesions with ill-defined or well-defined margins. Higher-grade tumors often have poorly defined margins. Tumors have intermediate signal on T1-weighted imaging, intermediate to high signal on T2-weighted imaging, and variable mild, moderate, or prominent gadolinium contrast enhancement. *CT:* Tumors have intermediate attenuation and variable mild, moderate, or prominent contrast enhancement. Destruction of adjacent bone is commonly seen.	Mucoepidermoid carcinomas are malignant glandular epithelial tumors that occur in children and adults, most often between the ages of 35 and 65 years (mean age = 45 years). Often have irregular margins. Tumors contain solid portions with intermediate to high-grade neoplastic squamoid mucus-producing cells and cystic portions containing sialomucin lined by basaloid or cuboidal neoplastic mucous cells with peripheral nuclei within pale cytoplasm. Most common malignant tumor of the parotid gland and a common tumor of the submandibular gland. Accounts for up to 15% of all salivary gland tumors, and 53% involve the major salivary glands (45%, parotid glands; 7%, submandibular glands; and 1%, sublingual glands). Tumors often are advanced at presentation, ± metastases to lymph nodes, bone, and lung, ± perineural tumor spread. Tumors can spread to adjacent preauricular lymph nodes and submandibular nodes. Prognosis is worse with MIB index of > 10%.
Adenoid cystic carcinoma **(Fig. 4.93)**	*MRI:* Nodular lesions with ill-defined or well-defined margins. Higher-grade tumors often have poorly defined margins. Lesions have intermediate signal on T1-weighted imaging, intermediate to high signal on T2-weighted imaging, and variable mild, moderate, or prominent gadolinium contrast enhancement. *CT:* Tumors have intermediate attenuation and variable mild, moderate, or prominent contrast enhancement. Destruction of adjacent bone is commonly seen.	Basaloid tumor composed of neoplastic epithelial and myoepithelial cells. Morphologic tumor patterns include tubular, cribriform, and solid. Second most common major salivary gland malignancy and most common malignant tumor of the submandibular gland. Accounts for 6% of malignant tumors of the parotid gland, 10% of epithelial salivary neoplasms, and 30% of epithelial tumors of minor salivary glands. Most commonly occurs in the parotid, submandibular, and minor salivary glands (palate, tongue, buccal mucosa, floor of the mouth, and other locations). Perineural tumor spread is common, ± facial nerve paralysis. Usually occurs in adults > 30 years old, most commonly between the ages of 55 and 75 years. Solid type has the worst prognosis. Up to 90% of patients die within 10–15 years of diagnosis.

(continued on page 392)

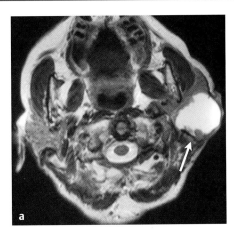 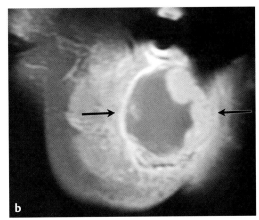

Fig. 4.92 (a) A 66-year-old woman with a mucoepidermoid carcinoma involving the left parotid gland that has irregular margins and high signal centrally on axial T2-weighted imaging (*arrow*) and (b) has irregular peripheral gadolinium contrast enhancement with ill-defined margins on sagittal fat-suppressed T1-weighted imaging (*arrows*).

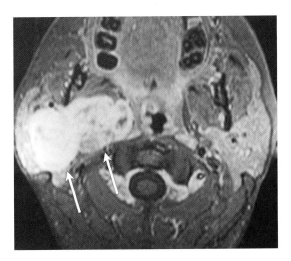

Fig. 4.93 A 32-year-old woman with an adenoid cystic carcinoma (*arrows*) involving the deep and superficial portions of the right parotid gland that has heterogeneous gadolinium contrast enhancement on axial fat-suppressed T1-weighted imaging.

Table 4.5 *(cont.)*   Lesions of the parotid space

Lesions	Imaging Findings	Comments
Acinic cell carcinoma (**Fig. 4.94** and **Fig. 4.95**)	*MRI:* Lesions can be solid or solid and cystic. Tumors range in size from 1 to 5 cm (mean = 3 cm). Tumors have low or intermediate signal on T1-weighted imaging and intermediate to high signal on T2-weighted imaging, ± cystic and/or hemorrhagic zones. Tumors show variable mild or moderate heterogeneous gadolinium contrast enhancement. *CT:* Tumors have intermediate attenuation and variable mild, moderate, or prominent contrast enhancement. Destruction of adjacent bone is commonly seen.	Malignant epithelial tumor in salivary glands composed of tumor cells showing differentiation toward serous acinar cells. The large neoplastic acinar cells are polygonal, with round eccentric nuclei within basophilic granular cytoplasm containing PAS-positive zymogenlike granules. Immunoreactive to cytokeratin, transferrin, lactoferrin, α_1-antitrypsin, IgA, and amylase. Occurs in children and in adults more than 20 years old (usually between 38 and 46 years). Accounts for 3% of all salivary gland tumors: 80% occur in the parotid gland, 17% involve the minor salivary glands, 4% occur in the submandibular gland, and 1% involve the sublingual gland. Can be bilateral. Local recurrence rate of 35%. Prognosis is poor for Ki-67 indices > 10%.
Squamous cell carcinoma	*MRI:* Lesions in the nasal cavity, paranasal sinuses, and nasopharynx, ± intracranial extension via bone destruction or perineural spread. Lesions have intermediate signal on T1-weighted imaging, intermediate to slightly high signal on T2-weighted imaging, and mild gadolinium contrast enhancement. Can be large lesions (± necrosis and/or hemorrhage). *CT:* Tumors have intermediate attenuation and mild contrast enhancement and can be large lesions (± necrosis and/or hemorrhage).	Malignant epithelial tumors originating from the mucosal epithelium of the paranasal sinuses. Include both keratinizing and nonkeratinizing types. Account for 80% of malignant sinonasal tumors and 3% of malignant tumors of the head and neck. Occur in adults, usually more than 55 years old, and in males more than in females. Associated with occupational or other exposure to tobacco smoke, nickel, chlorophenols, chromium, mustard gas, radium, and material in the manufacture of wood products. Can involve the parotid gland due to extension from adjacent tissue or squamous metaplasia within the parotid gland from chronic inflammation.
Malignant mixed tumor (carcinoma ex pleomorphic adenoma) (**Fig. 4.96**)	*MRI:* Nodular lesions with ill-defined and/or well-defined margins. Higher-grade tumors often have mostly poorly defined margins. Lesions have intermediate signal on T1-weighted imaging and intermediate to high signal on T2-weighted imaging, ± areas of hemorrhage or necrosis. Variable mild, moderate, or prominent gadolinium contrast enhancement. *CT:* Tumors have intermediate attenuation and variable mild, moderate, or prominent contrast enhancement.	Malignant tumor associated with a pleomorphic adenoma or history of resected pleomorphic adenoma. Malignant changes can occur in up to 10% of pleomorphic adenomas. Related to genetic instability of pleomorphic adenoma. Accounts for 3% of salivary gland tumors and 12% of salivary gland malignancies. Typically is adenocarcinoma. Patient ages are often between 50 and 70 years. Clinical finding is often rapid enlargement of a long-standing (> 3 years) nodular parotid lesion.

(continued on page 394)

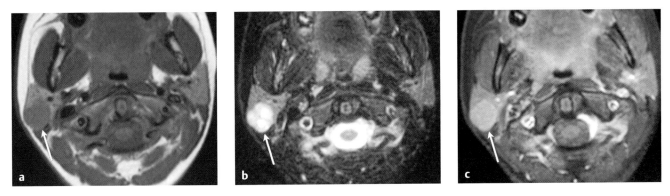

Fig. 4.94 An 11-year-old female with an acinic cell carcinoma in the superficial portion of the right parotid gland that has **(a)** low-intermediate signal on axial T1-weighted imaging (*arrow*), **(b)** heterogeneous high signal on axial fat-suppressed T2-weighted imaging (*arrow*), and **(c)** gadolinium contrast enhancement on axial fat-suppressed T1-weighted imaging (*arrow*).

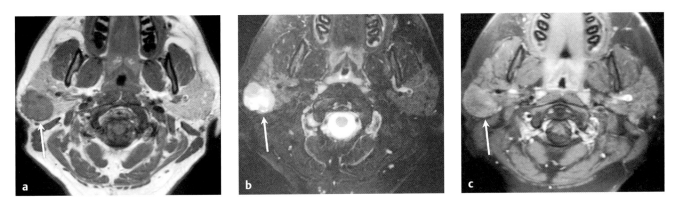

Fig. 4.95 An 18-year-old man with acinic cell carcinoma in the superficial portion of the right parotid gland that has **(a)** low-intermediate signal on axial T1-weighted imaging (*arrow*), **(b)** heterogeneous slightly high and high signal on axial fat-suppressed T2-weighted imaging (*arrow*), and **(c)** mild gadolinium contrast enhancement on axial fat-suppressed T1-weighted imaging (*arrow*).

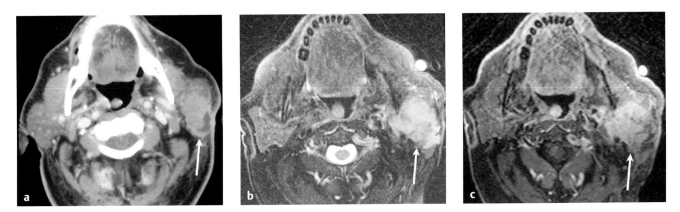

Fig. 4.96 A 79-year-old man with a malignant mixed tumor (carcinoma ex pleomorphic adenoma) in the left parotid gland that has **(a)** ill-defined margins and mixed intermediate and low attenuation on axial CT (*arrow*), **(b)** slightly high signal on axial fat-suppressed T2-weighted imaging (*arrow*), and **(c)** heterogeneous gadolinium contrast enhancement on axial fat-suppressed T1-weighted imaging (*arrow*).

Table 4.5 *(cont.)*   Lesions of the parotid space

Lesions	Imaging Findings	Comments
Non-Hodgkin lymphoma (NHL) **(Fig. 4.97)**	*MRI:* Lesions have low-intermediate signal on T1-weighted imaging and intermediate to slightly high signal on T2-weighted imaging, + gadolinium contrast enhancement. Can be locally invasive and can be associated with bone erosion/destruction. *CT:* Lesions have low-intermediate attenuation and may show contrast enhancement, ± bone destruction.	In lymphoma, neoplastic cells typically arise within lymphoid tissue (lymph nodes and reticuloendothelial organs). Most lymphomas in the nasopharynx, nasal cavity, paranasal sinuses, and parotid gland are NHL (B-cell NHL is more common than T-cell NHL), and more commonly are related to disseminated disease than to primary tumors. Secondary salivary gland lymphomas are seen in up to 8% of patients with systemic lymphoma, with the parotid gland being the most common site of salivary gland involvement. Primary parotid lymphoma (mucosa-associated lymphoma, MALT) can occur with autoimmune diseases, such as Sjögren's syndrome and rheumatoid disease treated with immunosuppressants.
Metastatic malignancies **(Fig. 4.98)**	*MRI:* Circumscribed or poorly marginated spheroid lesions that often have low-intermediate signal on T1-weighted imaging and intermediate to high signal on T2-weighted imaging, ± hemorrhage, calcifications, and cysts. Variable gadolinium contrast enhancement. *CT:* Lesions usually have low-intermediate attenuation, ± hemorrhage, calcifications, and cysts. Variable contrast enhancement, ± bone destruction, ± compression of neural tissue or vessels.	Nodal metastases seen in the parotid gland are related to lymph drainage from primary tumors located in the anterior face, lateral scalp, and external auditory canal. Most common metastatic malignancies are squamous cell carcinoma, melanoma, and basal cell carcinoma. Can occur as single or multiple well-circumscribed or poorly defined nodal lesions. Metastatic nodal tumor may cause variable locally destructive or infiltrative changes.
Melanoma	*MRI:* Tumors can have well-defined or irregular margins, and usually have intermediate or slightly high signal on T1-weighted imaging, depending on the melanin content, and low-intermediate to slightly high signal on T2-weighted imaging (T2WI) and fat-suppressed T2WI. Tumors usually show gadolinium contrast enhancement, ± destruction of adjacent bone. *CT:* Tumors have intermediate attenuation and variable mild, moderate, or prominent contrast enhancement. Destruction of adjacent bone is commonly seen.	Malignancy with melanocytic differentiation (immunoreactive to S-100 protein and HMB45) involving the parotid gland that occurs from extension of tumors in the skin or external auditory canal. Typically occurs in patients between 10 and 50 years old. Forty percent of melanomas involving the skin have lymph node metastases at presentation. Local recurrence occurs in up to 65%.
Tumorlike Lesions		
Epidermoid cyst **(Fig. 4.99)**	*MRI:* Well-circumscribed spheroid or multilobulated extra-axial ectodermal-inclusion cystic lesions with low-intermediate signal on T1-weighted imaging and high signal on T2-weighted imaging and diffusion-weighted imaging. Mixed low, intermediate, or high signal on FLAIR images, and no gadolinium contrast enhancement. *CT:* Well-circumscribed spheroid or multilobulated extra-axial ectodermal-inclusion cystic lesions with low-intermediate attenuation. Can be associated with bone.	Nonneoplastic congenital or acquired ectodermal inclusion cysts filled with desquamated cells and keratin debris, usually with mild mass effect on adjacent orbital structures, ± related clinical symptoms. Occur in males and females equally frequently.

(continued on page 396)

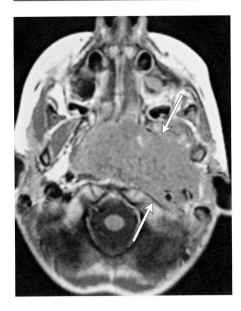

Fig. 4.97 A 6-year-old male with non-Hodgkin lymphoma (*arrows*) in the nasopharynx with extension into the left parapharyngeal, retropharyngeal, and parotid spaces. The neoplasm shows mild gadolinium contrast enhancement on axial T1-weighted imaging.

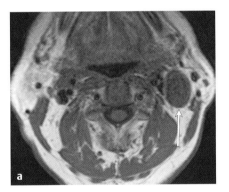
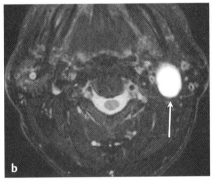
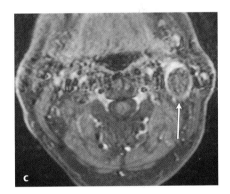

Fig. 4.98 A 57-year-old man with human papilloma virus–associated squamous cell carcinoma and a metastatic lesion in the left parotid space that has **(a)** circumscribed margins and low-intermediate signal on axial T1-weighted imaging (*arrow*), **(b)** high signal on axial fat-suppressed T2-weighted imaging (*arrow*), and **(c)** a peripheral rim pattern of gadolinium contrast enhancement on axial fat-suppressed T1-weighted imaging (*arrow*).

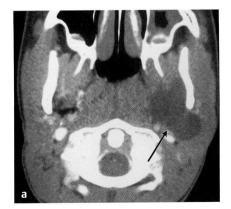
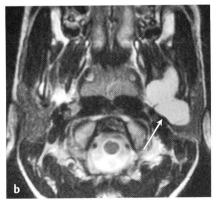
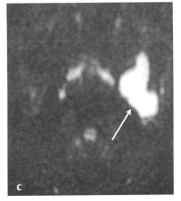

Fig. 4.99 An 11-year-old male with an epidermoid in the left parotid space that has **(a)** low attenuation on axial CT (*arrow*), **(b)** high signal on axial T2-weighted imaging (*arrow*), and **(c)** restricted diffusion on axial diffusion-weighted imaging (*arrow*).

Table 4.5 *(cont.)* Lesions of the parotid space

Lesions	Imaging Findings	Comments
Inflammatory Disease		
Parotiditis/sialadenitis (**Fig. 4.100, Fig. 4.101,** and **Fig. 4.102**) Acute parotiditis Chronic parotiditis	*Parotiditis/sialadenitis* *MRI:* Diffuse enlargement of parotid gland, with or without ill-defined margins. Involved glands typically show increased signal on T2-weighted imaging (T2WI) and fat-suppressed T2WI, and increased gadolinium (Gd) contrast enhancement compared with the contralateral normal gland, ± intraparotid ductal dilatation related to sialoliths, ± progression to abscess formation. *CT:* Diffuse enlargement of parotid gland, with or without ill-defined margins. Involved glands typically show increased attenuation relative to contralateral normal gland, ± sialolith(s), ± intraparotid ductal dilatation, ± abscess. *Chronic parotiditis* *MRI:* Chronic disease from obstruction (sialoliths or ductal stenosis), with increased size of gland, ± increased heterogeneous signal on T2WI, ductal ectasia, ± Gd contrast enhancement. *CT:* Chronic disease from obstruction (sialoliths or ductal stenosis) with increased size of gland, ± increased heterogeneous signal on T2WI, ductal ectasia, ± Gd contrast enhancement. *Chronic parotiditis* *MRI:* Chronic disease from nonobstructive causes (autoimmune disorders, granulomatous diseases, radiation treatment), with progressive atrophy, ± increased or decreased signal on T2WI, ± fatty replacement, ± Gd contrast enhancement. *CT:* Chronic disease from nonobstructive causes, with progressive atrophy, ± increased or decreased attenuation, ± fatty replacement.	*Sialadenitis* is defined as a primary infection of a salivary gland. *Acute parotiditis* is usually secondary to bacterial or viral infections, and less commonly fungal and parasitic infections. Can also result from ductal obstruction by sialolith(s). Bacteria commonly associated with parotiditis include *Staphylococcus aureus, Streptococcus pneumoniae,* and *Haemophilus influenzae.* The most common viral infection is due to a paramyxovirus, which can cause acute painful swelling (mumps). Factors associated with parotiditis include the relatively wide anatomic opening of Stensen's duct into the oral cavity, enabling retrograde passage of oral cavity infections, the normal serous type of salivary secretions lacking IgA antibodies, and conditions causing decreased saliva flow. *Chronic sialadenitis* can result from obstruction by sialoliths associated with secondary infection, or from nonobstructive diseases, such as sarcoidosis, autoimmune disorders (Sjögren's syndrome, IgG4 disease, etc.), and radiation treatment. Granulomatous infectious diseases associated with chronic parotiditis include tuberculosis, toxoplasmosis, actinomyosis, and syphilis. Parotiditis/sialadenitis can result in xerostomia.
Sialolithiasis and sialadenitis (**Fig. 4.103**)	*MRI:* Calculi typically have low signal on T1- and T2-weighted imaging (T2WI). Dilatation of ducts with high signal on T2WI may be seen within the parotid gland. Calculi can also be seen as low-signal foci on susceptibility-weighted imaging. The parotid gland may be enlarged, with increased signal on T2WI and increased gadolinium contrast enhancement compared with the contralateral normal gland. MR sialography using heavily weighted T2WI via 3D constructive interference in the steady-state technique or 3D fast/turbo spin-echo techniques can show dilated ducts with high signal and intraluminal defects from stones. *CT:* Calculi typically have high attenuation. *Sialography:* Water-soluble non-ionic iodine contrast is placed via a catheter and shows filling defects for radiopaque or radiolucent stones in salivary ducts on radiographs or CT. *Ultrasound:* Echogenic focus with acoustic shadowing.	Sialolithiasis refers to the formation of calculi within salivary ducts, and it is the most common disorder of major salivary glands. Results from deposition of calcium salts over a core of desquamated epithelial cells, mucus, foreign bodies, or bacteria. Can occur as single or multiple ductal stones per patient. Sialoliths can measure up to 9 mm (mean size ranges from 3 to 4 mm). Sialoliths (calculi) occur more frequently in Wharton's duct (up to 80% of cases) than in Stensen's duct, because of its upward configuration and its saliva, which has relatively high concentrations of phosphates and hydroxyapatites and is more alkaline and viscous than the parotid saliva. Sialoliths also occur in Stensen's duct, which can result in diffuse parotid gland enlargement and susceptibility to superimposed infection. Calculi can also occur within other ducts of the parotid gland. Treatment can be via sialendoscopic extraction or surgery.

(continued on page 398)

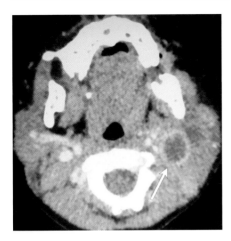

Fig. 4.100 A 2-year-old male with sialadenitis, parotiditis, and intraparotid abscess. Axial CT shows diffuse enlargement of the left parotid gland, which has ill-defined margins and contains an abscess (*arrow*) with a thin rim of contrast enhancement.

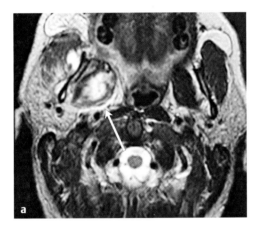

Fig. 4.101 A 39-year-old man with sialadenitis, parotiditis, and abscess. **(a)** Axial T2-weighted imaging shows diffuse enlargement of right parotid gland, which has increased signal and **(b)** shows increased gadolinium contrast enhancement on axial fat-suppressed T1-weighted imaging compared with the left parotid gland. Also seen is an abscess involving the deep portion of the right parotid gland, which has high signal centrally on T2-weighted imaging (*arrow* in **a**) and is surrounded by a rim of gadolinium contrast enhancement on fat-suppressed T1-weighted imaging (*arrow* in **b**).

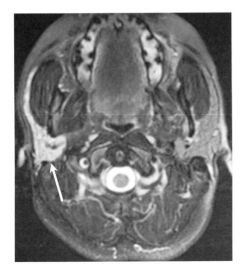

Fig. 4.102 A 43-year-old woman with chronic sialadenitis in the right parotid gland. Axial fat-suppressed T2-weighted imaging shows atrophy and increased signal in the right parotid gland (*arrow*).

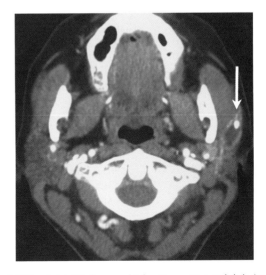

Fig. 4.103 Axial CT shows a high-attenuation sialolith (*arrow*) obstructing the left parotid duct.

Table 4.5 *(cont.)* Lesions of the parotid space

Lesions	Imaging Findings	Comments
Reactive adenopathy (**Fig. 4.104**)	*MRI:* Enlarged intraparotid lymph nodes usually have intermediate signal on T1-weighted imaging and slightly high signal on T2-weighted imaging (T2WI), + gadolinium (Gd) contrast enhancement, ± enlargement of parotid gland, with or without ill-defined margins. Involved glands typically show increased signal on T2WI and fat-suppressed T2WI and increased Gd contrast enhancement compared with the contralateral normal gland. *CT:* Enlarged intraparotid lymph nodes, ± contrast enhancement, ± enlargement of parotid gland, with or without ill-defined margins.	Unlike the other major salivary glands, the parotid normally contains lymph nodes because it becomes encapsulated after development of the lymphatic system. As a result, infections in the parotid gland and adjacent soft tissues can cause abnormally enlarged parotid lymph nodes.
Juvenile recurrent parotiditis (**Fig. 4.105**)	*MRI: Acute inflammation:* Enlarged glands often have low to low-intermediate signal on T1-weighted imaging (T1WI) and intermediate and/or slightly high to high signal on T2-weighted imaging (T2WI), + small foci of high signal on T2WI and constructive interference in steady state (CISS) imaging (MR sialography) from dilated ducts measuring between 1 and 4 mm (sialectasis), + gadolinium (Gd) contrast enhancement. *Chronic changes:* Parotid glands often have low-intermediate signal on T1- and T2WI, ± small foci of high signal on T2WI and CISS from dilated ducts associated with acinar degeneration measuring between 1 and 4 mm (sialectasis). Usually minimal to no Gd contrast enhancement. *CT: Acute inflammation:* Enlarged glands that have intermediate attenuation, + small foci of low attenuation from dilated ducts, ± contrast enhancement. *Chronic changes:* Parotid glands often have intermediate attenuation. *Ultrasound:* Multiple, round, hypoechoic zones are seen that correspond to sites of sialectasis. Color Doppler shows hypervasculization in acute inflammation and hypovascularization during the chronic phases.	Recurrent, nonobstructive, noninfectious, inflammatory disorder resulting in painful unilateral or bilateral episodic parotid swelling with sialectasia. Sialendoscopy shows white ductal layers lacking normal covering blood vessels, mucous plugs, and ductal strictures with less than 50% luminal narrowing. Often associated with fever and malaise. Initial onset is typically in prepubertal children ranging in age from 6 months to 16 years, with most cases found in children 3–6 years old. Usually occurs as one or two episodes or more per year. Episodes can last for days or weeks. Second most common childhood disease of major salivary glands after mumps. Treatment includes supportive care with hydration and warm compresses, as well as sialendoscopy, which includes irrigation of the ductal system, dilating strictures with high-pressure saline or balloon dilatation, and intraductal steroid injection.
Benign lymphoepithelial lesions (HIV, AIDS) (**Fig. 4.106** and **Fig. 4.107**)	*MRI:* Multiple, bilateral, intraparotid, cystic lesions of varying sizes that have low signal on T1-weighted imaging (T1WI) and high signal on T2-weighted imaging (T2WI), as well as solid lesions with intermediate signal on T1WI and slightly high signal on T2WI. Usually lack gadolinium contrast enhancement. Parotid glands are often enlarged. Lesions usually occur in association with cervical lymphadenopathy and lymphoid hyperplasia at Waldeyer's ring and involve the adenoids. *CT:* Multiple, bilateral, intraparotid, cystic lesions of varying sizes that have low attenuation, as well as solid lesions with intermediate attenuation.	Head and neck findings commonly associated with HIV infection include cervical lymphadenopathy, or pharyngitis (herpes, *Candida*) and Kaposi sarcoma. A less common abnormality related to HIV infection is cystic and solid lesions in the parotid glands. Cystic lesions, referred to as cystic lymphoepithelial lesions (CLEL) or benign lymphoepithelial lesions (BLEL), occur in up to 6% of HIV-positive patients and result from lymph node enlargement with interstitial lymphoid infiltrates. Hyperplastic lymphoid tissue compresses salivary acini causing atrophy and cyst formation from ductal obstruction. Cysts are lined by epithelial cells associated with reactive lymphoid stroma. Atrophic acini can be replaced with epithelial and myoepithelial cells, resulting in solid lesions. Lesions are immunoreactive to EMA, CD20, CD3, and the HIV p24 antigen.

(continued on page 400)

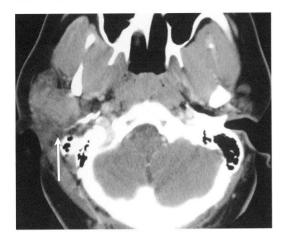

Fig. 4.104 An 18-year-old woman with an abnormally enlarged lymph node with ill-defined margins in the right parotid gland representing reactive adenopathy (*arrow*) on contrast-enhanced axial CT.

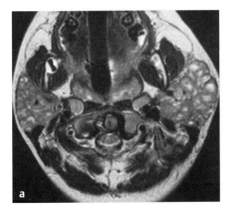

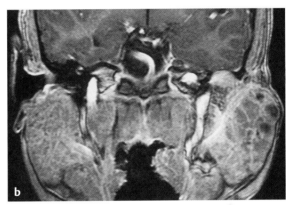

Fig. 4.105 A 9-year-old female with recurrent juvenile parotiditis. **(a)** Axial T2-weighted imaging shows enlargement of both parotid glands, which have heterogeneous intermediate signal and contain small foci of high signal. **(b)** Both parotid glands show heterogeneous gadolinium contrast enhancement on coronal T1-weighted imaging.

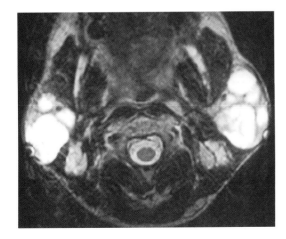

Fig. 4.106 A 36-year-old woman with HIV infection and benign lymphoepithelial lesions in both parotid glands, which have high signal on axial T2-weighted imaging.

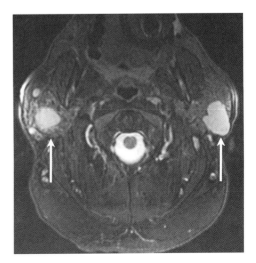

Fig. 4.107 A 51-year-old man with HIV infection and benign lymphoepithelial lesions in both parotid glands, which have high signal on axial fat-suppressed T2-weighted imaging (*arrows*).

Table 4.5 *(cont.)*   Lesions of the parotid space

Lesions	Imaging Findings	Comments
Sjögren's syndrome (**Fig. 4.108** and **Fig. 4.109**)	*MRI:* Parotid glands have heterogeneous low-intermediate signal on T1-weighted imaging (T1WI) and variable mixed low, intermediate, and/or high signal on T2-weighted imaging (T2WI) and fat-suppressed T2WI. Globular zones with high signal on T2WI can occur from saliva within dilated ducts. In the early phases of disease, the involved glands may be enlarged. Over time, the glands decrease in size from apoptosis, with increased fat deposition resulting in progressive increase in signal on T1WI. Zones of low signal on T2WI can also occur in late disease phases from fibrous tissue and lymphocyte aggregates. In the later disease phases, the ADCs of involved glands can become lower than those of normal lacrimal glands. *CT:* Parotid glands can be enlarged in the early phases of disease or atrophic in later phases.	Common autoimmune disease in which a mononuclear lymphocyte infiltration can occur in one or more exocrine glands (lacrimal, parotid, submandibular, and minor salivary glands), resulting in acinar cell destruction and impaired gland function. Usually occurs in adults between 40 and 60 years old, with a female predominance of over 90%. Histopathologic findings include periductal accumulation of lymphocytes and plasma cells associated with acinar destruction, which progresses peripherally to centrally. Aggregates of lymphocytes can result in a localized mass referred to as a benign lymphoepithelial lesion (BLEL) or Godwin tumor. Sjögren's syndrome can be a primary disorder or a secondary form associated with other autoimmune diseases, such as rheumatoid arthritis and systemic lupus erythematosus. Patients present with decreased lacrimal and salivary gland function, xerostomia, and keratoconjunctivitis sicca.
Sarcoidosis	*MRI:* Single or multiple lesions with low to intermediate signal on T1-weighted imaging and slightly high signal on T2-weighted imaging (T2WI) and fat-suppressed T2WI. After gadolinium (Gd) contrast administration, lesions typically show Gd contrast enhancement. *CT:* Single or multiple lesions with soft tissue attenuation with sharply defined margins in 85% and ill-defined margins in the remainder. *Nuclear medicine:* Increased uptake of gallium-67 citrate and F-18 FDG glucose. Symmetric uptake involving the parotid and lacrimal glands is referred to as the *panda sign* and can be seen with sarcoid, with Sjögren's syndrome, and after radiation treatment.	Sarcoidosis is a multisystem, noncaseating, granulomatous disease of uncertain cause that can involve the CNS in 5 to 15% of cases. If untreated, it can be associated with severe neurologic deficits, such as encephalopathy, cranial neuropathies, and myelopathy. Sarcoid involves the parotid glands in up to 30% of cases and presents as painless, nodular or multinodular enlargement of the glands from lesions composed of noncaseating epithelioid granulomas. Sarcoid in the parotid glands in association with uveitis and facial nerve paralysis is defined as the Heerfordt syndrome. Treatment includes oral corticosteroids and surgical debulking.
Kimura disease	*MRI:* Single or multiple lesions with ill-defined margins, mean size of 4 cm, intermediate signal on T1-weighted imaging, slightly high to high signal on T2-weighted imaging, and moderate or mild gadolinium contrast enhancement. *CT:* Ill-defined lesions with intermediate attenuation. Associated lymphadenopathy occurs in up to 80% of cases.	Kimura disease, also referred to eosinophilic lymphogranuloma, is an immune-mediated inflammatory disease with multiple or solitary lesions in the head and neck (parotid gland, buccal space, lacrimal gland, submandibular gland, subcutaneous tissue). Lesions have a folliculoid configuration containing eosinophils, lymphocytes, plasma cells, and mast cells, in association with stromal fibrosis and vascular proliferation. May represent a self-limited autoimmune response with altered T-cell regulation and IgE-mediated type 1 hypersensitivity. Patients typically have > 10% hypereosinophilia and elevated IgE levels (800–35,000 IU/mL). Usually occurs in Asian males (mean age = 32 years). Treatment includes surgery, systemic corticosteroids, cytotoxic medications, and/or cyclosporine.

(continued on page 402)

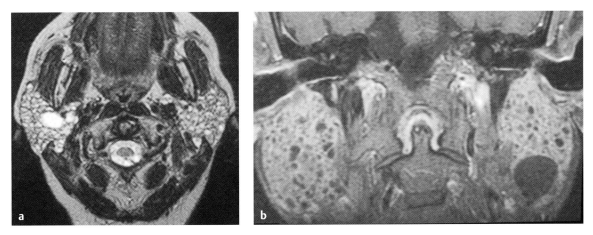

Fig. 4.108 A 66-year-old woman with Sjögren's syndrome. **(a)** Both parotid glands are enlarged and have mixed low, intermediate, and high signal on axial T2-weighted imaging. Globular zones with high signal on T2-weighted imaging are seen from saliva within dilated ducts. **(b)** Both parotid glands show gadolinium contrast enhancement on coronal fat-suppressed T1-weighted imaging except at intraglandular cystic sites.

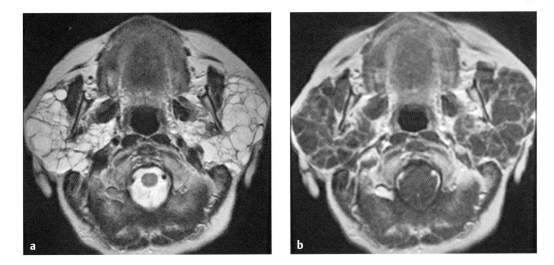

Fig. 4.109 A 65-year-old woman with Sjögren's syndrome. Both parotid glands are enlarged and contain many cystic zones, which have **(a)** high signal on axial T2-weighted imaging and **(b)** low signal on axial T1-weighted imaging from fluid-filled dilated ducts adjacent to atrophied gland parenchyma.

Table 4.5 *(cont.)* Lesions of the parotid space

Lesions	Imaging Findings	Comments
Congenital/Developmental		
First branchial cleft cyst (**Fig. 4.110**)	*MRI:* Circumscribed lesion that often has low-intermediate signal on T1-weighted imaging and high signal on T2-weighted imaging, usually with no gadolinium contrast enhancement unless there is superimposed infection. *CT:* Circumscribed, cystic lesion with low to intermediate attenuation depending on the proportions of protein and water. First branchial cleft cysts can be located adjacent to the external auditory canal (type 1) or adjacent to the superficial portion of the parotid gland, ± extension into the parapharyngeal space, posterior to the submandibular gland, and/or up to the external auditory canal (type 2).	Branchial cleft cysts are developmental anomalies involving the branchial apparatus. The branchial apparatus consists of four major and two rudimentary arches of mesoderm lined by ectoderm externally and endoderm internally within pouches that form at the end of the fourth week of gestation. The mesoderm contains a dominant artery, nerve, cartilage, and muscle. The four major arches are separated by clefts. Each arch develops into a defined neck structure, with eventual obliteration of the branchial clefts. The first arch forms the external auditory canal, eustachian tube, middle ear, and mastoid air cells. First branchial cleft cysts can be located adjacent to the external auditory canal (type 1 first branchial cleft cyst) or superficial portion of the parotid gland, ± extension into the parapharyngeal space, posterior to the submandibular gland, and/or up to the external auditory canal (type 2). Cysts are lined by squamous epithelium (90%), ciliated columnar epithelium (8%), or both types (2%). Sebaceous glands, salivary tissue, lymphoid tissue, and cholesterol crystals in mucoid fluid can also occur. Typically asymptomatic unless complicated by infection.
Hemangioma (**Fig. 4.111**)	*MRI:* Circumscribed or poorly marginated structures in bone marrow or soft tissue with intermediate-high signal on T1-weighted imaging (often isointense to marrow fat) and high signal on T2-weighted imaging (T2WI) and fat-suppressed T2WI, typically with gadolinium contrast enhancement, ± expansion of bone. *CT:* Expansile bone lesions with a radiating pattern of bony trabeculae oriented toward the center. Hemangiomas in soft tissue have mostly intermediate attenuation, ± zones of fat attenuation.	Benign lesions of bone or soft tissue composed of capillary, cavernous, and/or malformed venous vessels. Considered to be a hamartomatous disorder. Occur in patients 1 to 84 years old (median age = 33 years).
Venolymphatic malformation (**Fig. 4.112**)	Can be circumscribed lesions or can occur in an infiltrative pattern with extension into soft tissue and between muscles. *MRI:* Often contain single or multiple cystic zones that can be large (macrocystic type) or small (microcystic type), and that have predominantly low signal on T1-weighted imaging (T1WI) and high signal on T2-weighted imaging (T2WI) and fat-suppressed T2WI. Fluid–fluid levels and zones with high signal on T1WI and variable signal on T2WI may result from cysts containing hemorrhage, high protein concentration, and/or necrotic debris. Septa between the cystic zones can vary in thickness and gadolinium (Gd) contrast enhancement. Nodular zones within the lesions can have variable degrees of Gd contrast enhancement. Microcystic lesions typically show more Gd contrast enhancement than the macrocystic type. *CT:* The macrocystic malformations are usually low-attenuation cystic lesions (10–25 HU) separated by thin walls, ± intermediate or high attenuation, which can result from hemorrhage or infection, ± fluid–fluid levels.	Benign vascular anomalies (also referred to as lymphangioma or cystic hygroma) that primarily result from abnormal lymphangiogenesis. Up to 75% occur in the head and neck. Can be observed in utero with MRI or sonography, at birth (50–65%), or in the first 5 years of life. Approximately 85% are detected by age 2. Lesions are composed of endothelium-lined lymphatic ± venous channels interspersed within connective tissue stroma.

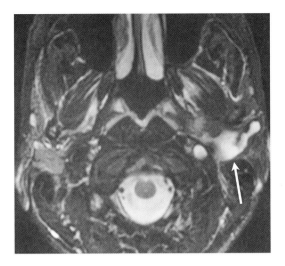

Fig. 4.110 Axial fat-suppressed T2-weighted imaging shows a first branchial cleft cyst (type 2) with high signal located in the superficial portion of the left parotid gland and extending toward the left parapharyngeal space (*arrow*).

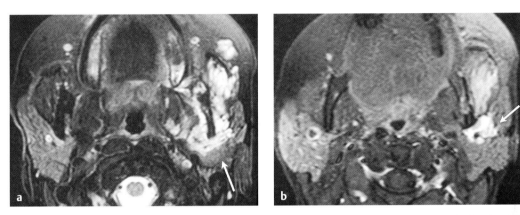

Fig. 4.111 An 18-year-old man with a hemangioma involving the left parotid gland and left masseter muscle that has **(a)** high signal on axial fat-suppressed T2-weighted imaging (*arrow*) and **(b)** gadolinium contrast enhancement on axial fat-suppressed T1-weighted imaging (*arrow*).

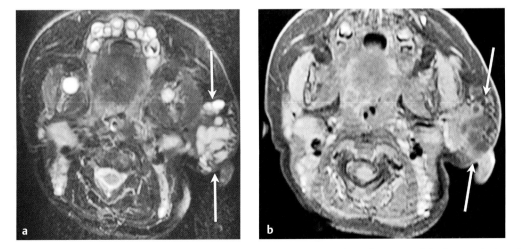

Fig. 4.112 **(a)** A 2-month-old female with a venolymphatic malformation involving the soft tissues of the face, including the left parotid space, which has high signal on axial fat-suppressed T2-weighted imaging (*arrows*). **(b)** Most of the lesion lacks gadolinium contrast enhancement on axial fat-suppressed T1-weighted imaging (*arrows*), except for a small nodular zone at the anterior portion of the lesion.

4.6 Masticator Space and Mandible

The margins of the masticator are the superficial layer of the deep cervical fascia where it splits to surround the muscles of mastication (medial and lateral pterygoid, masseter, and temporalis muscles) and posterior body and ramus of the mandible (**Fig. 4.113**). Also included within the masticator space are the branches of the mandibular (V3) division of the trigeminal nerve, branches of the internal maxillary artery, and inferior alvelolar nerve, artery, and vein. The inner (medial) portion of the fascia extends from inferior margin of the mandible along the inner margin of the medial pterygoid muscle to attach to the skull base at the medial margin of the foramen ovale. This fascial layer separates the masticator space from the prestyloid parapharyngeal space. Neoplasms involving the masticator space can result in perineural tumor spread superiorly along the V3 division of the trigeminal nerve through the foramen ovale, resulting in intracranial tumor extension. The masticator space is located anterolateral to the parapharyngeal space, and lesions in the masticator space displace the parapharyngeal fat posteromedially. The outer superficial layer of the deep cervical fascia extends from the inferior margin of the mandible along the outer surface of the masseter muscle to its attachment at the zygomatic arch, separating the masticator and parotid spaces. Fascia attached at the anterior margin of the mandibular ramus forms the anterior border of the masticator space, separating it from the buccal space.

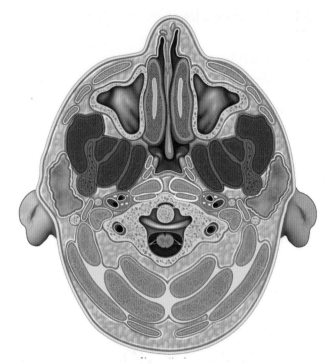

Fig. 4.113 Axial view shows the masticator space in color.

Table 4.6   Lesions involving the masticator space

- Benign Soft Tissue Tumors
  - Schwannoma
  - Neurofibroma
  - Hemangioma
  - Lipoma
  - Venolymphatic malformation
  - Meningioma
  - Juvenile nasopharyngeal angiofibroma
- Nonmalignant Tumors and Tumorlike Lesions of the Mandible
  - Odontogenic radicular (periapical) cyst
  - Odontogenic follicular (dentigerous) cyst
  - Keratocystic odontogenic tumor
  - Primordial cyst
  - Stafne cyst (static bone cavity or cyst)
  - Residual cyst
  - Bone cyst
  - Osteoma
  - Bone island
  - Torus mandibularis
  - Ameloblastoma
  - Ossifying fibroma (cemento-ossifying fibroma)
  - Odontoma
  - Cementoblastoma
  - Calcifying epithelial odontogenic tumor (Pindborg tumor)
  - Odontogenic myxoma
  - Osteochondroma
  - Osteoid osteoma
  - Osteoblastoma
  - Giant cell tumor
  - Giant cell granuloma
- Malignant Soft Tissue Neoplasms
  - Direct extension from squamous cell carcinoma or malignant salivary gland tumor
  - Non-Hodgkin lymphoma (NHL)
  - Rhabdomyosarcoma
- Malignant Neoplasms Involving the Mandible
  - Metastatic malignancies
  - Myeloma
  - Lymphoma
  - Osteosarcoma
  - Chondrosarcoma
  - Ewing's sarcoma
- Tumorlike Osseous Lesions
  - Fibrous dysplasia
  - Florid cemento-osseous dysplasia
  - Paget disease
  - Osteonecrosis
- Inflammatory Lesions
  - Osteomyelitis, periapical abscess
  - Juvenile mandibular chronic osteomyelitis/ chronic recurrent multifocal osteomyelitis
  - Langerhans' cell histiocytosis
- Traumatic Lesions
  - Mandibular fractures
- Developmental Anomalies
  - Pierre Robin syndrome
  - Mandibular hypoplasia
  - Hemifacial microsomia (Goldenhar syndrome, oculoauriculovertebral spectrum)
  - Treacher Collins syndrome
  - Bifid mandibular condyle

Table 4.6 Lesions involving the masticator space

Lesion	Imaging Findings	Comments
Benign Soft Tissue Tumors		
Schwannoma (**Fig. 4.114**)	*MRI:* Circumscribed spheroid or ovoid lesions with low-intermediate signal on T1-weighted imaging, high signal on T2-weighted imaging (T2WI) and fat-suppressed T2WI, and usually prominent gadolinium (Gd) contrast enhancement. High signal on T2WI and Gd contrast enhancement can be heterogeneous in large lesions due to cystic degeneration and/or hemorrhage. *CT:* Circumscribed spheroid or ovoid lesions with intermediate attenuation, + contrast enhancement. Large lesions can have cystic degeneration and/or hemorrhage.	Schwannomas are benign encapsulated tumors that contain differentiated neoplastic Schwann cells. They most commonly occur as solitary, sporadic lesions. Multiple schwannomas are often associated with neurofibromatosis type 2 (NF2), which is an autosomal dominant disease involving a gene mutation at chromosome 22q12. In addition to schwannomas, patients with NF2 can also have multiple meningiomas and ependymomas. The incidence of NF2 is 1/37,000 to 1/50,000 newborns. Age at presentation is 22 to 72 years (mean age = 46 years). Peak incidence is in the fourth to sixth decades. Many patients with NF2 present in the third decade with bilateral vestibular schwannomas.
Neurofibroma	*MRI:* *Solitary neurofibromas* are circumscribed spheroid, ovoid, or lobulated extra-axial lesions with low-intermediate signal on T1-weighted imaging (T1WI), intermediate-high signal on T2-weighted imaging (T2WI), and prominent gadolinium (Gd) contrast enhancement. High signal on T2WI and Gd contrast enhancement can be heterogeneous in large lesions. *Plexiform neurofibromas* appear as curvilinear and multinodular lesions involving multiple nerve branches and have low to intermediate signal on T1WI and intermediate or slightly high to high signal on T2WI and fat-suppressed T2WI, with or without bands or strands of low signal. Lesions usually show Gd contrast enhancement. *CT:* Ovoid or fusiform lesions with low-intermediate attenuation. Lesions can show contrast enhancement. Often erode adjacent bone.	Neurofibromas are benign nerve sheath tumors that contain mixtures of Schwann cells, perineural-like cells, and interlacing fascicles of fibroblasts associated with abundant collagen. Unlike schwannomas, neurofibromas lack Antoni A and B regions and cannot be separated pathologically from the underlying nerve. Neurofibromas most frequently occur as sporadic, localized, solitary lesions, less frequently as diffuse or plexiform lesions. Multiple neurofibromas are typically seen in neurofibromatosis type 1 (NF1), which is an autosomal dominant disorder (1/2,500 births) caused by mutations of the neurofibromin gene on chromosome 17q11.2. NF1 is the most common type of neurocutaneous syndrome and is associated with neoplasms of the central and peripheral nervous systems (optic gliomas, astrocytomas, plexiform and solitary neurofibromas) and skin (café-au-lait spots, axillary and inguinal freckling). Also associated with meningeal and skull dysplasias, as well as hamartomas of the iris (Lisch nodules).
Hemangioma (**Fig. 4.115**)	*MRI:* Circumscribed or poorly marginated structures in bone marrow or soft tissue with intermediate-high signal on T1-weighted imaging (often isointense to marrow fat) and high signal on T2-weighted imaging (T2WI) and fat-suppressed T2WI, typically with gadolinium contrast enhancement, ± expansion of bone. *CT:* Expansile bone lesions with a radiating pattern of bony trabeculae oriented toward the center. Hemangiomas in soft tissue have mostly intermediate attenuation, ± zones of fat attenuation.	Benign lesions of bone or soft tissue composed of capillary, cavernous, and/or malformed venous vessels. Considered to be a hamartomatous disorder. Occur in patients 1 to 84 years old (median age = 33 years).
Lipoma (See **Fig. 4.89**)	*MRI:* Lipomas have MRI signal isointense to subcutaneous fat on T1-weighted imaging (high signal). On T2-weighted imaging, signal suppression occurs with frequency-selective fat saturation techniques or with a short time to inversion recovery (STIR) method. Typically there is no gadolinium contrast enhancement or peripheral edema. *CT:* Lipomas have CT attenuation similar to subcutaneous fat and typically no contrast enhancement or peripheral edema.	Common benign hamartomas composed of mature white adipose tissue without cellular atypia. Most common soft tissue tumor, representing 16% of all soft tissue tumors.

(continued on page 408)

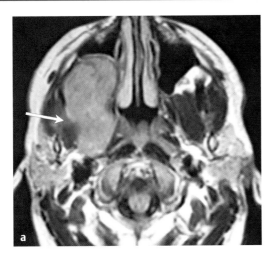
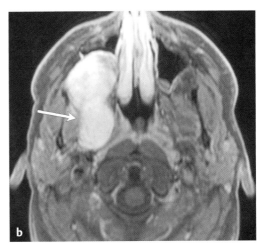

Fig. 4.114 A 30-year-old man with a schwannoma involving the right trigeminal nerve and extending into the right masticator space that has **(a)** heterogeneous high signal on axial T2-weighted imaging (*arrow*) and **(b)** gadolinium contrast enhancement on axial fat-suppressed T1-weighted imaging (*arrow*).

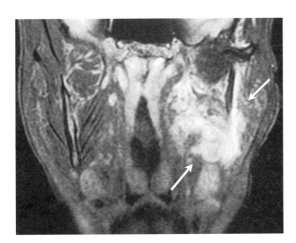

Fig. 4.115 Coronal fat-suppressed T2-weighted imaging of a 33-year-old woman shows a hemangioma (*arrows*) with high signal involving the left masticator space.

Table 4.6 *(cont.)* Lesions involving the masticator space

Lesion	Imaging Findings	Comments
Venolymphatic malformation (See **Fig. 4.112**)	Can be circumscribed lesions or can occur in an infiltrative pattern with extension into soft tissue and between muscles. *MRI:* Often contain single or multiple cystic zones that can be large (macrocystic type) or small (microcystic type), and that have predominantly low signal on T1-weighted imaging (T1WI) and high signal on T2-weighted imaging (T2WI) and fat-suppressed T2WI. Fluid–fluid levels and zones with high signal on T1WI and variable signal on T2WI may result from cysts containing hemorrhage, high protein concentration, and/or necrotic debris. Septa between the cystic zones can vary in thickness and gadolinium (Gd) contrast enhancement. Nodular zones within the lesions can have variable degrees of Gd contrast enhancement. Microcystic lesions typically show more Gd contrast enhancement than the macrocystic type. *CT:* The macrocystic malformations are usually low-attenuation cystic lesions (10–25 HU) separated by thin walls, ± intermediate or high attenuation, which can result from hemorrhage or infection, ± fluid–fluid levels.	Benign vascular anomalies (also referred to as lymphangioma or cystic hygroma) that primarily result from abnormal lymphangiogenesis. Up to 75% occur in the head and neck. Can be observed in utero with MRI or sonography, at birth (50–65%), or within the first 5 years, and ~ 85% are detected by age 2. Lesions are composed of endothelium-lined lymphatic ± venous channels interspersed within connective tissue stroma.
Meningioma (**Fig. 4.116**)	Extra-axial dura-based intracranial or spinal lesions. Some meningiomas can invade bone or occur predominantly within bone. Occasionally, meningiomas can extend inferiorly through the foramen ovale into the masticator space. *MRI:* Tumors often have intermediate signal on T1-weighted imaging, intermediate to slightly high signal on T2-weighted imaging, and typically prominent gadolinium contrast enhancement, ± calcifications, ± hyperostosis and/or invasion of adjacent skull. Some meningiomas have high signal on diffusion-weighted imaging. *CT:* Tumors have intermediate attenuation, usually prominent contrast enhancement, ± calcifications, ± hyperostosis of adjacent bone.	Benign, slow-growing tumors involving cranial and/or spinal dura that are composed of neoplastic meningothelial (arachnoidal or arachnoid cap) cells. Usually solitary and sporadic, but can also occur as multiple lesions in patients with neurofibromatosis type 2 (NF2). Most are benign, although ~ 5% have atypical histologic features. Anaplastic meningiomas are rare and amount to < 3% of meningiomas. Meningiomas account for up to 26% of primary intracranial tumors. Annual incidence is 6 per 100,000. Meningiomas typically occur in adults (> 40 years old) and in women more than in men. Can result in compression of adjacent brain parenchyma, encasement of arteries, and compression of dural venous sinuses. Rarely, invasive/malignant types occur.
Juvenile nasopharyngeal angiofibroma (**Fig. 4.117**; see **Fig. 3.34**)	*MRI:* The origin of juvenile nasopharyngeal angiofibromas is the pterygopalatine fossa. The lesions grow medially into the nasal cavity and nasopharynx via the sphenopalatine foramen, laterally into the pterygomaxillary fissure, and superiorly via the inferior orbital fissure into the orbital apex, ± middle cranial fossa via the superior orbital fissure. Lesions often have intermediate signal on T1-weighted imaging and slightly high to high signal on T2-weighted imaging, ± flow voids, and prominent gadolinium contrast enhancement. *CT:* Lesions often have intermediate attenuation, ± hemorrhage, and erosion and/or remodeling of adjacent bone, such as widening of the pterygopalatine/pterygomaxillary fossae and/or sphenopalatine foramina and vidian canals.	Benign, cellular, and vascularized mesenchymal lesion/malformation that occurs in the posterolateral nasal wall or nasopharynx from testosterone-sensitive cells, associated with high propensity to hemorrhage. Composed of thin-walled slitlike or dilated vessels of varying sizes lined by endothelial cells within fibrous stroma containing spindle, round, or stellate cells and varying amounts of collagen. Immunoreactive to platelet-derived growth factor B, insulin-like growth factor type II, vimentin, and smooth muscle actin. Typically occurs in males (peak incidence in the second decade), 1 in 5,000–60,000. Lesions have locally aggressive growth with erosion and/or remodeling of adjacent bone and can spread through skull base foramina. Treatment can include embolization or hormonal therapy, and, if necessary, surgical resection.

(continued on page 410)

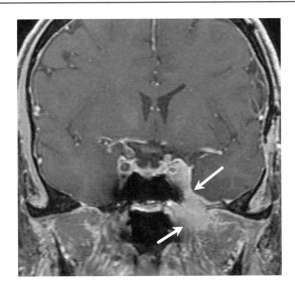

Fig. 4.116 Coronal T1-weighted imaging of a 59-year-old woman shows a gadolinium-enhancing meningioma (*arrows*) in the left trigeminal cistern (Meckel's cave) that extends inferiorly through the left foramen ovale, causing an indentation on the left lateral pterygoid muscle.

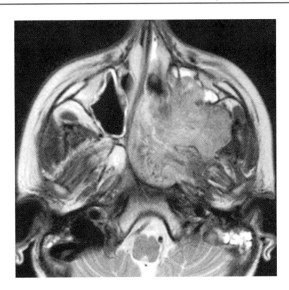

Fig. 4.117 An 11-year-old male with a juvenile nasopharyngeal angiofibroma in the left nasopharynx associated with erosion and remodeling of adjacent bone. The lesion extends into the left nasal cavity and nasopharynx, laterally into the pterygomaxillary fissure, and anteriorly into the left maxillary sinus. The lesion has heterogeneous slightly high to high signal on axial T2-weighted imaging.

Table 4.6 *(cont.)* Lesions involving the masticator space

Lesion	Imaging Findings	Comments
Nonmalignant Tumors and Tumorlike Lesions of the Mandible		
Odontogenic radicular (periapical) cyst (**Fig. 4.118**)	*MRI:* Cyst contents have variable signal on T1-weighted imaging related to protein concentration and usually have slightly high to high signal on T2-weighted imaging. A thin peripheral rim of gadolinium contrast enhancement is often present. *CT:* Circumscribed zone of decreased attenuation at the apex of a tooth and adjacent mandible, ± thin rim of sclerotic bone, ± cortical expansion from the cyst, ± resorption of tooth apex and adjacent teeth, ± displacement of adjacent teeth and mandibular canal.	Most common type of odontogenic cyst. Results from trauma, dental caries, and/or chronic infection of a tooth causing periapical periodontitis, periapical abscess, and/or periapical granuloma. Borders can consist of a thin rim of cortical bone lined by squamous epithelium. Usually occurs in adults between 30 and 50 years old. Treatment includes tooth extraction and periodontal therapy.
Odontogenic follicular (dentigerous) cyst (**Fig. 4.119** and **Fig. 4.120**)	*MRI:* Circumscribed lesions with high signal on T2-weighted imaging (T2WI), ± zones of low signal on T2WI. Thin peripheral gadolinium contrast enhancement is seen along the walls of the lesion. The unerupted tooth has low signal on T1- and T2WI. *CT:* Well-circumscribed radiolucent lesion adjacent to the crown of an unerupted tooth, ± thin sclerotic margin. The roots of the affected tooth are usually outside of the lesion. Can become large adjacent to the roots of other teeth. Cortical bone margins are usually intact, except for in large lesions.	Most common mandibular cyst of odontogenic cell origin and is associated with unerupted teeth, usually the third molar. Fluid collects between the epithelium and tooth enamel. Often presents in patients between 30 and 40 years old. Usually occurs as a solitary lesion, but multiple lesions can be seen with mucopolysaccharidoses and cleidocranial dysplasia. Treatment includes enucleation for small lesions and surgical drainage with marsupialization for large lesions.
Keratocystic odontogenic tumor (**Fig. 4.121** and **Fig. 4.122**)	*MRI:* Circumscribed lesions with intermediate signal on T1-weighted imaging and intermediate to high signal on T2-weighted imaging related to variable protein content. Thin peripheral gadolinium contrast enhancement is seen along the walls of the lesion. *CT:* Well-circumscribed unilocular or multilocular radiolucent lesions in the mandibular body or ramus, ± thin sclerotic margins, ± associated impacted tooth, ± cortical thinning, and expansion of mandibular body.	Benign, locally aggressive tumors derived from the stratified keratinizing squamous epithelium of the dental lamina and overlying alveolar mucosa. Account for up to 17% of jaw cysts. Often present in patients between the second and fourth decades. Can be solitary or multiple in association with the basal cell nevus syndrome (Gorlin-Goltz syndrome). Treatment includes curettage, decompression, and marsupialization.

(continued on page 412)

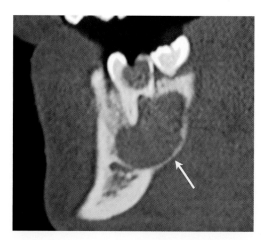

Fig. 4.118 Sagittal CT of a 29-year-old man shows a circumscribed zone of decreased attenuation at the apex of a tooth and adjacent mandible associated with a thin rim of expanded sclerotic bone (*arrow*) representing a radicular cyst. The radicular cyst is associated with a cavity involving the crown of the tooth.

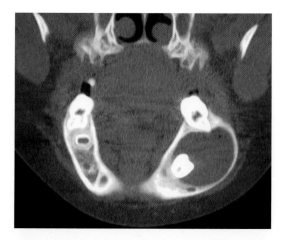

Fig. 4.119 Coronal CT of a 9-year-old male shows a well-circumscribed expansile radiolucent lesion adjacent to the crown of an unerupted tooth representing an odontogenic follicular (dentigerous) cyst.

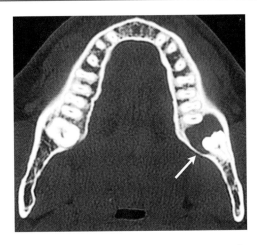

Fig. 4.120 Axial CT of a 41-year-old man shows a well-circumscribed expansile radiolucent lesion adjacent to the crown of an unerupted molar tooth (*arrow*) representing an odontogenic follicular (dentigerous) cyst.

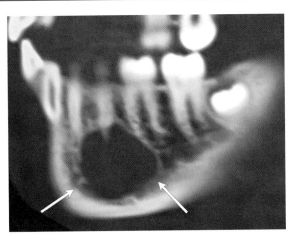

Fig. 4.121 Sagittal CT of a 12-year-old male shows a well-circumscribed unilocular radiolucent lesion in the mandibular body (*arrows*) representing a keratocystic odontogenic tumor (keratocyst).

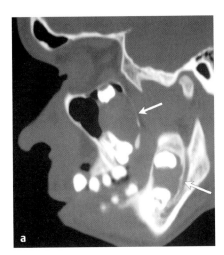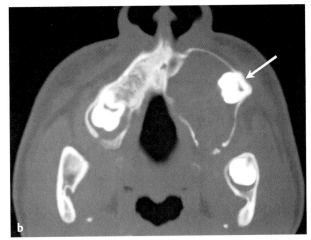

Fig. 4.122 **(a)** Sagittal and **(b)** axial CT images of a 16-year-old male with Gorlin-Goltz syndrome show well-circumscribed radiolucent lesions (*arrows*) in the mandibular body and maxilla with thinned, expanded cortical margins and impacted teeth representing keratocystic odontogenic tumors (keratocysts).

Table 4.6 *(cont.)* Lesions involving the masticator space

Lesion	Imaging Findings	Comments
Primordial cyst	*CT:* Nonexpansile radiolucent lesion in the mandible that has well-defined, thin, sclerotic margins.	Developmental abnormality that results from cystic degeneration of a dental follicle before tooth formation.
Stafne cyst (static bone cavity or cyst) **(Fig. 4.123)**	*CT:* Round or ovoid circumscribed radiolucent zone with a cortical defect at the medial aspect of the mandibular body near the angle, usually occurring below the mandibular canal. Usually measures < 2 cm. Fat is usually present within the osseous defect, ± submandibular salivary gland tissue.	Developmental pseudocystic variant that is typically an incidental finding on CT, with inward bowing of the lingual aspect of the mandibular bony cortex into the medullary space at the angle of the mandible.
Residual cyst	*CT:* Nonexpansile radiolucent lesion in the mandible that has well-defined margins at the site of surgery or dental extraction.	Localized radiolucent changes in the mandible after surgery and/or dental extraction.
Bone cyst **(Fig. 4.124)**	*MRI:* Circumscribed lesions ± a peripheral rim of low signal on T1- and T2-weighted imaging (T2WI) adjacent to normal medullary bone. Usually contain fluid with low to low-intermediate signal on T1-weighted imaging (T1WI) and high signal on T2WI. Fluid–fluid levels may occur. For bone cysts without pathologic fracture, thin peripheral gadolinium (Gd) contrast enhancement can be seen at the margins of lesions. Bone cysts with pathologic fracture can have heterogeneous or homogeneous low-intermediate or slightly high signal on T1WI, and heterogeneous or homogeneous high signal on T2WI and fat-suppressed T2WI. Cysts complicated by fracture can have internal septations and fluid–fluid levels, as well as irregular peripheral Gd contrast enhancement at internal septations. *CT:* Round or ovoid radiolucent zone within the mandibular body, ± circumscribed or slightly irregular margins, ± thin sclerotic margins, and cortical thinning and/or expansion.	Intramedullary nonneoplastic cavities filled with serous or serosanguinous fluid. In the mandible, bone cysts have been proposed to arise from trauma that caused hemorrhage and eventual bone resorption.
Osteoma **(Fig. 4.125)**	*MRI:* Well-circumscribed mandibular lesions with low signal on T1- and T2-weighted imaging and typically no significant gadolinium contrast enhancement. *CT:* Well-circumscribed mandibular lesions with high attenuation.	Benign primary bone tumors composed of dense lamellar, woven, and/or compact cortical bone. Account for less than 1% of primary benign bone tumors. Present in patients 16 to 74 years old, most frequently in the sixth decade.
Bone island **(Fig. 4.126)**	*MRI:* Typically appears as a well-circumscribed zone of dense bone with low signal on T1-weighted imaging, T2-weighted imaging (T2WI), and fat-suppressed T2WI in bone marrow. No associated finding of bone destruction or periosteal reaction. *CT:* Usually appears as a circumscribed, radiodense, ovoid or spheroid focus in medullary bone that may or may not contact the endosteal surface of cortical bone.	Bone islands (enostoses) are nonneoplastic intramedullary zones of mature, compact, lamellar bone that are considered to be developmental anomalies resulting from localized failure of bone resorption during skeletal maturation.

(continued on page 414)

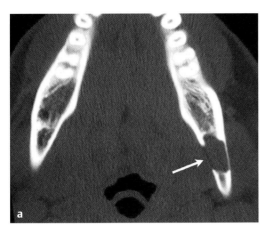
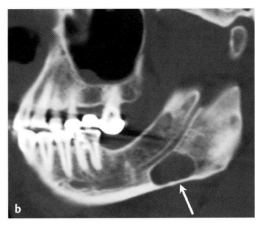

Fig. 4.123 **(a)** Axial and **(b)** sagittal CT images of a 57-year-old man show an ovoid circumscribed radiolucent zone with a cortical defect at the medial aspect of the left mandibular body (*arrows*) near the angle, representing a Stafne cyst (static bone cavity or cyst).

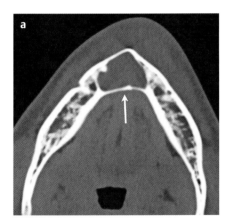
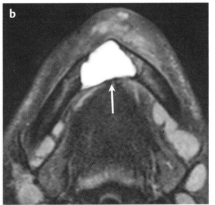
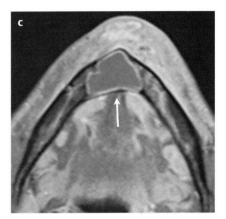

Fig. 4.124 **(a)** Axial CT of a 16-year-old female with a bone cyst shows a radiolucent slightly expansile lesion of the mandible (*arrow*) that has thinned cortical margins and **(b)** high signal on axial T2-weighted imaging (*arrow*), and that **(c)** shows only a minimal peripheral thin rim of gadolinium contrast enhancement on axial fat-suppressed T1-weighted imaging (*arrow*).

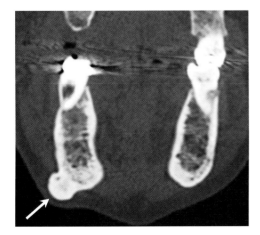
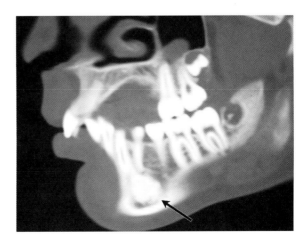

Fig. 4.125 Coronal CT of a 90-year-old woman shows an osteoma (*arrow*) at the outer cortical surface of the lower right mandible that has circumscribed margins and high attenuation.

Fig. 4.126 Sagittal CT of a 12-year-old female who has a circumscribed radiodense ovoid bone island involving the medullary portion of the mandible (*arrow*).

Table 4.6 *(cont.)* Lesions involving the masticator space

Lesion	Imaging Findings	Comments
Torus mandibularis (**Fig. 4.127**)	*MRI:* Well-circumscribed mandibular lesions with low signal on T1- and T2-weighted imaging and no significant gadolinium contrast enhancement. *CT:* Well-circumscribed lesions involving the inner margin of the mandible with high attenuation.	Localized benign outgrowth (exostosis) of bone at the lingual side of the mandible superior to the insertion of the mylohyoid muscle. Composed of compact bone. Can also occur at the hard palate (torus palatinus).
Ameloblastoma (**Fig. 4.128** and **Fig. 4.129**)	*MRI:* Tumors often have circumscribed margins and can have mixed low, intermediate, and/or high signal on T1-weighted imaging, T2-weighted imaging (T2WI), and fat-suppressed T2WI. Cystic portions have high signal on T2WI. Lesions can show heterogeneous irregular gadolinium contrast enhancement. *CT:* Lesions are often radiolucent, with associated bone expansion and cortical thinning, ± hyperostotic margins.	The most common odontogenic tumor, ameloblastomas are slow-growing, benign, locally aggressive, epithelial odontogenic tumors that contain epithelioid cells (basaloid and/or squamous types) associated with regions of spindle cells and fibrous stroma. These odontogenic tumors fail to form calcified tooth enamel or dentin. There are five subtypes: unicystic (5%), solid and multicystic, desmoplastic, peripheral, and malignant. Eighty percent of ameloblastomas occur in the mandible, and they typically lack metastatic potential, except for the malignant subtype.
Ossifying fibroma (cemento-ossifying fibroma) (**Fig. 4.130**)	*MRI:* Expansile, well-circumscribed osseous lesions that often have low-intermediate signal on T1-weighted imaging and mixed low, intermediate, and/or slightly high to high signal on T2-weighted imaging. Usually show heterogeneous gadolinium contrast enhancement. *CT:* Expansile, well-circumscribed lesions involving bone containing varying proportions of low, intermediate, and/or high attenuation based on the composition of fibrous, calcified, and ossified contents, ± thin sclerotic margins. Large lesions tend to cause tooth displacement and root resorption.	Benign, rare, slow-growing fibro-osseous tumor composed of proliferating fibroblasts within fibrous stroma, with varying amounts of woven and lamellar bone and cementumlike material replacing normal bone. Most commonly occur in the mandible, followed by the maxilla and paranasal sinuses. Female/male ratio of 2–9/1, age range 7 to 55 years (most common in second to fourth decades). Two juvenile subtypes (trabecular and psammomatoid) occur in children < 15 years old and have cell-rich fibrous stroma and can show more rapid growth. The psammomatoid type contains small, uniform ossicles, and the trabecular type contains trabeculae and osteoid and woven bone. Treatment is surgical excision or curettage, with recurrence rates of 8 to 28%.

(continued on page 416)

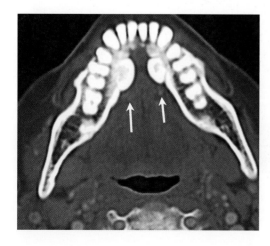

Fig. 4.127 Bilateral tori mandibulari. Axial CT shows well-circumscribed lesions involving the inner margins of the mandible with high attenuation (*arrows*).

Fig. 4.128 Ameloblastoma. **(a)** Axial CT shows a radiolucent lesion with associated bone expansion and cortical thinning involving the left mandible (*arrows*) and that has **(b)** mostly high signal on axial T2-weighted imaging (*arrows*).

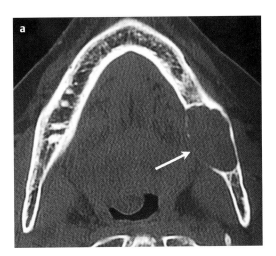

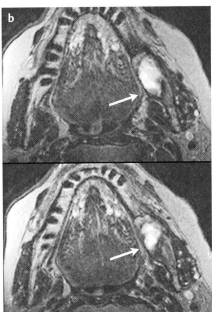

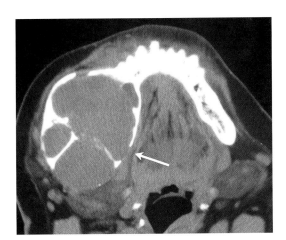

Fig. 4.129 Ameloblastoma. Axial CT of a 57-year-old woman shows a large radiolucent lesion with associated bone expansion and cortical thinning involving the right mandible (*arrow*).

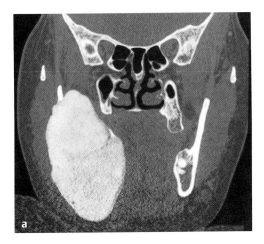

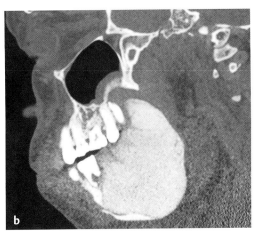

Fig. 4.130 **(a)** Coronal and **(b)** sagittal CT images show a large ossifying fibroma involving the right mandible that has high attenuation and portions with thin sclerotic margins.

Table 4.6 *(cont.)* Lesions involving the masticator space

Lesion	Imaging Findings	Comments
Odontoma **(Fig. 4.131)**	*CT:* Lesions usually have zones with high attenuation between roots of teeth, ± peripheral radiolucent zone, ± impacted, partially formed tooth.	Common odontogenic lesion of the mandible. Usually presents in the second decade and is often asymptomatic. Fifty percent of odontomas are associated with an impacted tooth. Considered a hamartoma rather than a neoplasm. Composed of varying amounts of epithelial and mesenchymal odontogenic tissue (dentin, enamel, etc.), with or without a recognizable tooth. Complex odontomas have mixtures of various tooth elements with amorphous calcifications, whereas compound odontomas also contain a partially formed tooth. Treatment is surgical excision. Lesions typically do not recur after surgery.
Cementoblastoma **(Fig. 4.132)**	*CT:* Rounded lesion with high attenuation immediately adjacent to a tooth root, usually with blurring of the periodontal ligament space.	Rare benign neoplasm of cementoblastic origin that occurs adjacent to the roots of teeth. Usually occurs in patients < 25 years old and can be associated with complaints of pain. Lesions are composed of cementumlike material with basophilic lines, cementoblasts with large nuclei arranged in a linear pattern adjacent to the calcified tissue, cementocytes within lacunae, and osteoclast giant cells. Histologically, cementoblastoma appears similar to osteoid osteoma and osteoblastoma. Treatment is surgical resection.
Calcifying epithelial odontogenic tumor (Pindborg tumor) **(Fig. 4.133)**	*MRI:* Lesions have low-intermediate signal on T1-weighted imaging (T1WI) and slightly high to high signal on T2-weighted imaging (T2WI), as well as zones of low signal on T1- and T2WI related to calcifications. Tumors show heterogeneous gadolinium contrast enhancement. *CT:* Expansile lesions involving bone containing varying proportions of low, intermediate, and/ or high attenuation based on the composition of cellular, fibrous, and calcified contents, ± thin sclerotic margins, ± cortical discontinuities. Large lesions tend to cause tooth displacement and root resorption.	Rare odontogenic tumor that accounts for less than 1% of odontogenic neoplasms. Two-thirds of tumors occur in the mandible, with the remainder in the maxilla. These slow-growing, locally aggressive tumors usually occur in patients between 20 and 60 years old and are composed of polyhedral epithelial cells with mild to moderate nuclear pleomorphism arranged in sheets or strands; mitotic figures are rare. Degenerated epithelial cells with amyloid and calcifications are usually present. Treatment includes resection with tumor-free surgical margins to avoid local recurrence, which occurs in up to 14% of cases.

(continued on page 418)

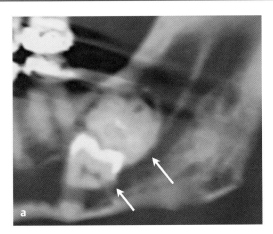

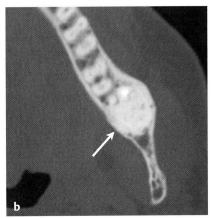

Fig. 4.131 Odontoma. **(a)** Sagittal and **(b)** axial CT images of a 69-year-old woman show an impacted, partially formed molar tooth and an adjacent zone with high attenuation between roots of bordering teeth (*arrows*).

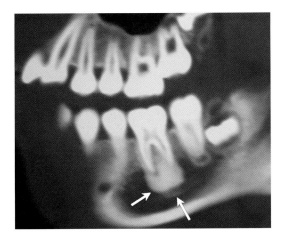

Fig. 4.132 Sagittal CT of a 12-year-old female shows a cementoblastoma with high attenuation immediately adjacent to the first molar tooth root, as well as partial blurring of the periodontal ligament space (*arrows*).

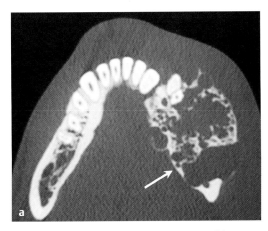

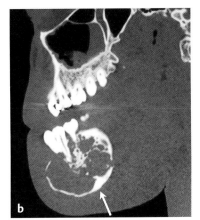

Fig. 4.133 **(a)** Axial and **(b)** sagittal CT images of a 29-year-old man with a calcifying epithelial odontogenic tumor (Pindborg tumor) involving the left mandible that has expanded, thinned, discontinuous bone margins and contains zones of low, intermediate, and/or high attenuation (*arrows*). Also seen are tooth displacement and root resorption.

Table 4.6 *(cont.)*   Lesions involving the masticator space

Lesion	Imaging Findings	Comments
Odontogenic myxoma (**Fig. 4.134**)	*MRI:* Tumors often have circumscribed margins, and can have mixed low and intermediate signal on T1-weighted imaging and heterogensous slightly high and high signal on T2-weighted imaging (T2WI). Myxoid portions have high signal on T2WI. Lesions show heterogeneous irregular gadolinium contrast enhancement. *CT:* Lesions occur as unilocular or multilocular radiolucent zones with associated bone expansion, cortical scalloping and thinning, ± cortical interruption, ± fine bone trabeculae, ± extension into adjacent structures, such as the nasal or oral cavities, paranasal sinuses, or orbits. In the maxilla, lesions often occur in the premolar, molar, and tuberosity areas. In the mandible, lesions often occur in the body and ramus.	Rare, benign, locally invasive, non-encapsulated tumor that arises from the odontogenic ectomesenchyme of a developing tooth or undifferentiated mesenchymal cells in the periodontal ligament. Tumors contain loosely arranged spindle, round, and/or stellate cells within myxoid stroma. Account for 3 to 9% of odontogenic tumors, and typically occur in patients between 10 and 40 years old (mean = 31 years), with a female/male ratio of 2/1. These tumors occur in the maxilla and mandible and only rarely in other bones. Treatment is surgical excision and reconstruction.
Osteochondroma (**Fig. 4.135**)	*MRI:* Circumscribed protruding lesion arising from outer cortex, with a central zone that has intermediate signal on T1- and T2-weighted imaging similar to marrow, surrounded by a peripheral zone of low signal on T1- and T2-weighted imaging. A cartilaginous cap is usually present in children and young adults. Increased malignant potential when cartilaginous cap is > 2 cm thick. *CT:* Circumscribed sessile or protuberant osseous lesion, with a central zone contiguous with the medullary space of bone, with or without a cartilaginous cap.	Benign cartilaginous tumors arising from defect at periphery of growth plate during bone formation, with resultant bone outgrowth covered by a cartilaginous cap. Usually benign lesions unless associated with pain and increasing size of cartilaginous cap. Osteochondromas are common lesions, accounting for 14 to 35% of primary bone tumors. Occur with a median age of 20 years, and up to 75% percent of patients are less than 20 years old.
Osteoid osteoma (**Fig. 4.136**)	*MRI:* A spheroid or ovoid zone (nidus) measuring less than 1.5 cm is seen in bone cortex or medullary bone that has irregular, distinct or indistinct margins. The nidus is usually surrouned by dense fusiform thickening of bone cortex that has low signal on T1-weighted imaging (T1WI), T2-weighted imaging (T2WI), and fat-suppressed (FS) T2WI relative to the adjacent region of cortical thickening. The nidus can have low-intermediate signal on T1WI and proton density-weighted imaging and low-intermediate or high signal on T2WI and FS T2WI. Calcifications in the nidus can be seen as low signal on T2WI. After gadolinium contrast administration, variable degrees of enhancement are seen at the nidus. Poorly defined zones of high signal on T2WI and FS T2WI, and corresponding Gd contrast enhancement, can be seen in the marrow adjacent to the nidus as well as within the extraosseous soft tissues. *CT:* Intraosseous, circumscribed, radiolucent lesion < 1.5 cm in diameter with low-intermediate attenuation that can show contrast enhancement. The nidus is surrounded by a zone of high attenuation (reactive bone sclerosis).	Benign osteoblastic lesion composed of a circumscribed nidus of < 1.5 cm, and usually surrounded by reactive bone formation. These lesions are usually painful and have limited growth potential. Osteoid osteoma accounts for 11 to 13% of primary benign bone tumors. Occurs in patients 6 to 30 years old (median age = 17 years). Approximately 75% occur in patients < 25 years old. Usually occur in long bones, and rarely involve the mandible or maxilla.

(continued on page 420)

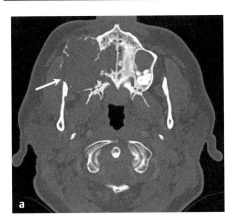
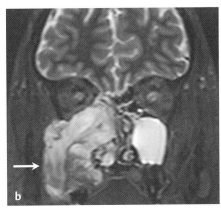
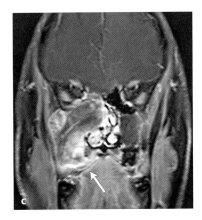

Fig. 4.134 A 32-year-old man with an odontogenic myxoma. **(a)** Axial CT shows a lesion (*arrow*) with soft tissue attenuation in the right maxillary sinus associated with expansion of thinned and interrupted cortical margins. **(b)** The lesion has mixed low, intermediate, slightly high, and high signal on coronal T2-weighted imaging (*arrow*) and **(c)** heterogeneous irregular gadolinium contrast enhancement on coronal fat-suppressed T1-weighted imaging (*arrow*).

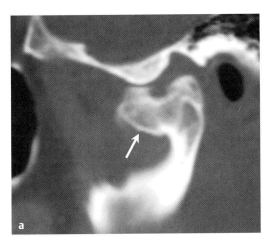
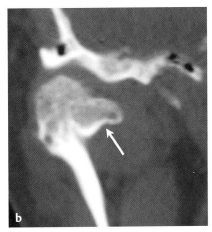

Fig. 4.135 **(a)** Sagittal and **(b)** coronal CT images of a 57-year-old woman show an osteochondroma (*arrows*) involving the anteromedial portion of the mandible.

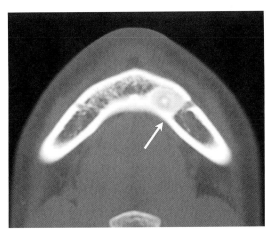

Fig. 4.136 Axial CT of the mandible of a 15-year-old male shows an osteoid osteoma (*arrow*) with the nidus measuring < 1.5 cm and surrounded by a zone of high attenuation (reactive bone sclerosis).

Table 4.6 *(cont.)* Lesions involving the masticator space

Lesion	Imaging Findings	Comments
Osteoblastoma	*MRI:* Spheroid or ovoid zone measuring > 1.5 to 2 cm located within medullary and/or cortical bone. Can have irregular, distinct or indistinct margins. Tumors have low-intermediate signal on T1-weighted imaging and low-intermediate and/or high signal on T2-weighted imaging (T2WI) and fat-suppressed (FS) T2WI. Calcifications or areas of mineralization can be seen as zones of low signal on T2WI. After gadolinium (Gd) contrast administration, osteoblastomas show variable degrees of enhancement. Zones of thickened cortical bone and medullary sclerosis are often seen adjacent to osteoblastomas. Poorly defined zones of high signal on T2WI and FS T2WI, and corresponding Gd contrast enhancement, can be seen in the marrow adjacent to osteoblastomas as well as within the extraosseous soft tissues. ± secondary aneurysmal bone cysts.	Rare, benign, bone-forming tumors that are histologically related to osteoid osteomas. Osteoblastomas are larger than osteoid osteomas and show progressive enlargement. Osteoblastomas typically produce well-vascularized osteoid with woven bone spicules surrounded by osteoblasts. Account for 3–6% of primary benign bone tumors and < 1–2% of all primary bone tumors. Rarely involve the craniofacial bones, mandible more commonly than maxilla. For lesions in the maxilla and mandible, age at presentation ranges from 3 to 61 years (mean age = 26 years). For lesions in long bones, median age of 15 years and mean age of 20 years have been reported.
	CT: Expansile radiolucent lesion > 1.5 cm surrounded by bony sclerosis. Lesions can show contrast enhancement. The radiolucent lesions typically arise in medullary bone and may or may not contain internal calcifications.	
Giant cell tumor	*MRI:* Often well-defined lesions with thin low-signal margins on T1- and T2-weighted imaging (T2WI). Solid portions of giant cell tumors often have low to intermediate signal on T1-weighted imaging, intermediate to high signal on T2WI, and high signal on fat-suppressed T2WI. Signal heterogeneity on T2WI is not uncommon. Zones of low signal on T2WI and T2* imaging may be seen secondary to hemosiderin. Aneurysmal bone cysts can be seen in 14% of giant cell tumors, resulting in cystic zones with variable signal and fluid–fluid levels, ± cortical destruction and extraosseous tumor extension.	Aggressive tumors composed of neoplastic, ovoid, mononuclear cells and scattered multinucleated osteoclast-like giant cells (derived from fusion of marrow mononuclear cells). Giant cell tumor is occasionally associated with Paget disease in older patients. Up to 10% of all giant cell tumors are malignant. Account for ~ 5 to 9.5% of all bone tumors and up to 23% of benign bone tumors. Median at presentation = 30 years, and 80% occur in patients more than 20 years old. Tumors typically occur in long bones, and rarely in the spine, skull, or mandible.
	CT: Radiolucent lesions with relatively narrow zones of transition. Zones of cortical thinning are typical. Expansion and zones of cortical destruction are commonly seen. No matrix mineralization.	
Giant cell granuloma **(Fig. 4.137)**	*MRI:* Lesions have heterogeneous low and/or intermediate signal on T1-weighted imaging and proton density-weighted imaging; and low, intermediate, and/or high signal on T2-weighted imaging, as well as peripheral rimlike and central gadolinium contrast enhancement on fat-suppressed T1WI.	Giant cell granulomas (also known as solid aneurysmal bone cysts) are reactive granulomatous lesions that have histologic features similar to brown tumors. Lesions contain multinucleated giant cells adjacent to sites of hemorrhage, as well as fibroblasts. Osteoid formation adjacent to sites of hemorrhage can be seen. Lesions usually occur in patients less than 30 years old and are most frequently found in the mandible, maxilla, and small bones of the hands and feet. Lesions in long bones have also been referred to as solid variants of aneurysmal bone cysts.
	CT: Typically radiolucent lesions, ± bone expansion with or without intact, thin cortical margins. Extraosseous extension of lesions may occur.	

(continued on page 422)

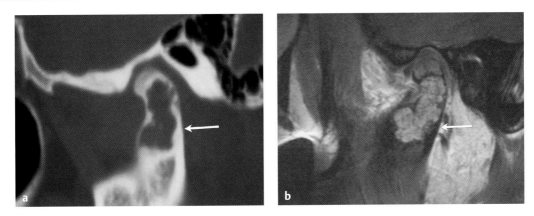

Fig. 4.137   **(a)** Sagittal CT of a 15-year-old female shows a radiolucent giant cell granuloma in the mandible (*arrow*) that has **(b)** heterogeneous gadolinium contrast enhancement on sagittal T1-weighted imaging (*arrow*).

Table 4.6 *(cont.)*   Lesions involving the masticator space

Lesion	Imaging Findings	Comments
Malignant Soft Tissue Neoplasms		
Direct extension from squamous cell carcinoma or malignant salivary gland tumor (**Fig. 4.138** and **Fig. 4.139**)	*MRI:* Malignant lesions from the oral cavity, oropharynx, nasopharynx, and parapharyngeal space can extend into the masticator space to involve muscles and bone. Tumors often have intermediate signal on T1-weighted imaging, intermediate to slightly high signal on T2-weighted imaging, and gadolinium contrast enhancement. Can be large lesions (± necrosis and/or hemorrhage). Contrast-enhancing perineural tumor spread can occur, with potential intracranial extension through the foramen ovale. *CT:* Tumors have intermediate attenuation and mild contrast enhancement and can be large, ± necrosis and/or hemorrhage, as well as bone destruction.	Malignant tumors from the oral cavity, oropharynx, nasopharynx, and parapharyngeal space can invade the masticator space. Common tumors in this category include: squamous cell carcinoma, adenoid cystic carcinoma, adenocarcinoma, and mucoepidermoid carcinoma. Once these tumors have invaded the masticator space, they can result in perineural tumor spread and potentially extend intracranially via the foramen ovale along the third division of CN V.
Non-Hodgkin lymphoma (NHL) (See **Fig. 4.53**)	*MRI:* Lesions have low-intermediate signal on T1-weighted imaging and intermediate to slightly high signal on T2-weighted imaging, + gadolinium contrast enhancement. Can be locally invasive and associated with bone erosion/destruction, intracranial extension with meningeal involvement (up to 5%). B-cell NHL often occurs in the maxillary sinuses, whereas T-cell NHL frequently occurs in the midline, including the septum. *CT:* Lesions have low-intermediate attenuation and may show contrast enhancement, ± bone destruction.	Lymphomas are a group of lymphoid tumors whose neoplastic cells typically arise within lymphoid tissue (lymph nodes and reticuloendothelial organs). Most lymphomas in the nasopharynx, nasal cavity, and paranasal sinuses are NHL (B-cell NHL is more common than T-cell NHL) and more commonly are related to disseminated disease than to primary sinonasal tumors. Sinonasal lymphoma has a poor prognosis, with 5-year survival of less than 65%.
Rhabdomyosarcoma (**Fig. 4.140**)	*MRI:* Tumors can have circumscribed and/or poorly defined margins and typically have low-intermediate signal on T1-weighted imaging and heterogeneous signal (various combinations of intermediate, slightly high, and/or high signal) on T2-weighted imaging (T2WI) and fat-suppressed T2WI. Tumors show variable degrees of gadolinium contrast enhancement, ± bone destruction and invasion. *CT:* Soft tissue lesions that usually can have circumscribed or irregular margins. Calcifications are uncommon. Tumors can have mixed CT attenuation, with solid zones of soft tissue attenuation, cystic appearing and/or necrotic zones, and occasional foci of hemorrhage, ± bone invasion and destruction.	Malignant mesenchymal tumors with rhabdomyoblastic differentiation that occur primarily in soft tissue, and only very rarely in bone. There are three subgroups of rhabdomyosarcoma: embryonal (50 to 70%), alveolar (18 to 45%), and pleomorphic (5 to 10%). Embryonal and alveolar rhabdomyosarcomas occur primarily in children < 10 years old, and pleomorphic rhabdomyosarcomas occur mostly in adults (median age in the sixth decade). Alveolar and pleomorphic rhabdomyosarcomas occur frequently in the extremities. Embryonal rhabdomyosarcomas occur mostly in the head and neck.

(continued on page 424)

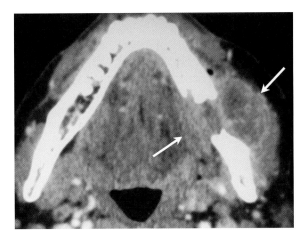

Fig. 4.138 Axial CT of a 64-year-old man shows a squamous cell carcinoma (*arrows*) with heterogeneous contrast enhancement that extends through and destroys the left mandible within the masticator space.

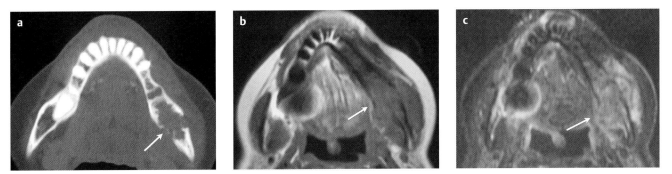

Fig. 4.139 **(a)** Axial CT of a 59-year-old woman who has a squamous cell carcinoma (*arrow*) that extends through and destroys the left mandible. **(b)** The lesion has intermediate signal on axial T1-weighted imaging (*arrow*) and **(c)** mixed slightly high and high signal on axial fat-suppressed T2-weighted imaging (*arrow*).

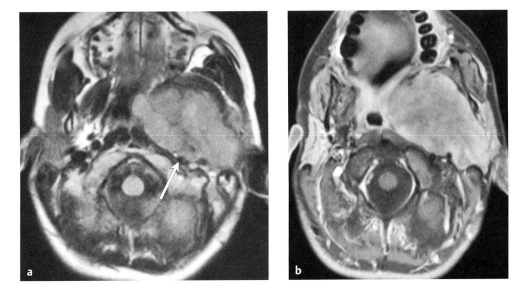

Fig. 4.140 **(a)** A 14-year-old male with a rhabdomyosarcoma in the left parapharyngeal and masticator spaces that has irregular margins and heterogeneous high signal on axial T2-weighted imaging (*arrow*). **(b)** The lesion shows gadolinium contrast enhancement on axial fat-suppressed T1-weighted imaging. The large tumor invades and anteriorly displaces the left medial pterygoid muscle.

Table 4.6 *(cont.)* Lesions involving the masticator space

Lesion	Imaging Findings	Comments
Malignant Neoplasms Involving the Mandible		
Metastatic malignancies	Single or multiple well-circumscribed or poorly defined lesions involving bone. *MRI:* Single or multiple well-circumscribed or poorly defined lesions involving bone, with low-intermediate signal on T1-weighted imaging, intermediate to high signal on T2-weighted imaging, and usually gadolinium contrast enhancement, ± bone destruction, ± compression of neural tissue or vessels. *CT:* Lesions are usually radiolucent and may also be sclerotic, ± extraosseous tumor extension, usually + contrast enhancement, ± compression of neural tissue or vessels.	Metastatic lesions represent proliferating neoplastic cells that are located in sites or organs separated or distant from their origins. Metastatic carcinoma is the most frequent malignant tumor involving bone. In adults, metastatic lesions to bone occur most frequently from carcinomas of the lung, breast, prostate, kidney, and thyroid, as well as from sarcomas. Primary malignancies of the lung, breast, and prostate account for 80% of bone metastases. Metastatic tumor may cause variable destructive or infiltrative changes in single or multiple sites.
Myeloma **(Fig. 4.141)**	Multiple myeloma or single plasmacytoma are well-circumscribed or poorly defined lesions involving bone. *MRI:* Well-circumscribed or poorly defined lesions involving bone, with low-intermediate signal on T1-weighted imaging, intermediate to high signal on T2-weighted imaging, and usually show gadolinium contrast enhancement, + bone destruction. *CT:* Lesions have low-intermediate attenuation, usually with contrast enhancement and bone destruction.	Multiple myeloma are malignant tumors composed of proliferating antibody-secreting plasma cells derived from single clones. Multiple myeloma is primarily located in bone marrow. A solitary myeloma or plasmacytoma is an infrequent variant in which a neoplastic mass of plasma cells occurs at a single site of bone or soft tissues. In the United States, 14,600 new cases occur each year. Multiple myeloma is the most common primary neoplasm of bone in adults. Median age at presentation = 60 years. Most patients are more than 40 years old.
Lymphoma	*MRI:* Lesions have low-intermediate signal on T1-weighted imaging, intermediate to slightly high signal on T2-weighted imaging, and gadolinium contrast enhancement. Can be locally invasive and associated with bone erosion/destruction. *CT:* Lesions have low-intermediate attenuation and may show contrast enhancement, ± bone destruction.	Lymphomas are a group of lymphoid tumors whose neoplastic cells typically arise within lymphoid tissue (lymph nodes and reticuloendothelial organs). Unlike leukemia, lymphomas usually arise as discrete masses. Lymphomas are subdivided into Hodgkin disease (HD) and non-Hodgkin lymphoma (NHL). Distinction between HD and NHL is useful because of differences in clinical and histopathologic features, as well as treatment strategies. HD typically arises in lymph nodes and often spreads along nodal chains, whereas NHL frequently originates at extranodal sites and spreads in an unpredictable pattern. Almost all primary lymphomas of bone are B-cell NHL.

Lesion	Imaging Findings	Comments
Osteosarcoma	*MRI:* Tumors often have poorly defined margins and commonly extend from the marrow through destroyed bone cortex into adjacent soft tissues. Tumors usually have low-intermediate signal on T1-weighted imaging. Zones of low signal often correspond to areas of tumor calcification/mineralization and/or necrosis. Zones of necrosis typically have high signal on T2-weighted imaging (T2WI), whereas mineralized zones usually have low signal on T2WI. Tumors can have variable signal on T2WI and fat-suppressed (FS) T2WI depending upon the relative amounts of calcified/mineralized osteoid, chondroid, fibroid, and hemorrhagic and necrotic components. Tumors may have low, low-intermediate, and intermediate to high signal on T2WI and FS T2WI. After gadolinium contrast administration, osteosarcomas typically show prominent enhancement in nonmineralized/calcified portions of the tumors. *CT:* Tumors have low-intermediate attenuation, usually with matrix mineralization/ossification, and often show contrast enhancement (usually heterogeneous).	Osteosarcomas are malignant tumors composed of proliferating neoplastic spindle cells, which produce osteoid and/or immature tumoral bone. Occur in children as primary tumors; in adults, osteosarcomas are associated with Paget disease, irradiated bone, chronic osteomyelitis, osteoblastoma, giant cell tumor, and fibrous dysplasia.
Chondrosarcoma	*MRI:* Lesions have low-intermediate signal on T1-weighted imaging, high signal on T2-weighted imaging (T2WI) and FS T2WI,, ± matrix mineralization with low signal on T2WI, + gadolinium contrast enhancement (usually heterogeneous). Chondrosarcomas can be locally invasive, associated with bone erosion/destruction, encasement of vessels and nerves. *CT:* Lesions have low-intermediate attenuation associated with localized bone destruction, ± chondroid matrix calcifications, + contrast enhancement.	Chondrosarcomas are malignant tumors containing cartilage formed within sarcomatous stroma, and they can contain areas of calcification/chondroid-matrix mineralization, myxoid material, and/or ossification. Chondrosarcomas rarely arise within synovium. Chondrosarcomas represent 12–21% of malignant bone lesions, 21–26% of primary sarcomas of bone, and 9–14% of all bone tumors.

(continued on page 426)

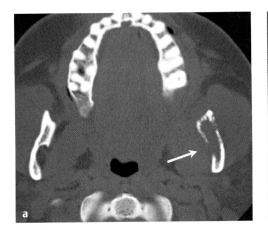 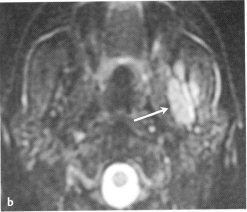

Fig. 4.141 **(a)** Axial CT of a 54-year-old woman with myeloma shows a radiolucent destructive lesion involving the left mandible (*arrow*). **(b)** The lesion has high signal on axial fat-suppressed T2-weighted imaging (*arrow*).

Table 4.6 *(cont.)*   Lesions involving the masticator space

Lesion	Imaging Findings	Comments
Ewing's sarcoma (**Fig. 4.142**)	*MRI:* Destructive lesions involving bone, with low-intermediate signal on T1-weighted imaging and mixed low, intermediate, and high signal on T2-weighted imaging, + gadolinium contrast enhancement (usually heterogeneous). *CT:* Destructive lesions involving bone, with low-intermediate attenuation, can show contrast enhancement (usually heterogeneous).	Malignant primitive tumor of bone composed of undifferentiated small cells with round nuclei. Ewing's sarcomas commonly have translocations involving chromosomes 11 and 22: t(11;22) (q24:q12), which results in fusion of the FL1-1 gene at 11q24 to the EWS gene at 22q12. Accounts for 6 to 11% of primary malignant bone tumors, 5 to 7% of primary bone tumors. Usually occurs between the ages of 5 and 30, in males more than in females, and is locally invasive, with high metastatic potential. Rarely involve the mandible. Tumors are locally invasive, and have high metastatic potential.
Tumorlike Osseous Lesions		
Fibrous dysplasia (**Fig. 4.143**)	*MRI:* Features depend on the proportions of bony spicules, collagen, fibroblastic spindle cells, and hemorrhagic and/or cystic changes. Lesions are usually well circumscribed, and have low or low-intermediate signal on T1-weighted imaging. On T2-weighted imaging, lesions have variable mixtures of low, intermediate, and/or high signal, often surrounded by a low-signal rim of variable thickness. Internal septations and cystic changes are seen in a minority of lesions. Bone expansion is commonly seen. All or portions of the lesions can show gadolinium contrast enhancement in a heterogeneous diffuse or peripheral pattern. *CT:* Lesions involving the mandible are often associated with bone expansion. Lesions have variable density and attenuation on radiographs and CT, respectively, depending on the degree of mineralization and number of the bony spicules in the lesions. Attenuation coefficients can range from 70 to 400 Hounsfield units. Lesions can have a ground-glass radiographic appearance secondary to the mineralized spicules of immature woven bone in fibrous dysplasia. Sclerotic borders of varying thickness can be seen surrounding parts or all of the lesions.	Benign medullary fibro-osseous lesion of bone, most often sporadic involving a single site, referred to as monostotic (80–85%), or in multiple locations (polyostotic fibrous dysplasia). Results from developmental failure in the normal process of remodeling primitive bone to mature lamellar bone, with resultant zone or zones of immature trabeculae within dysplastic fibrous tissue. The lesions do not mineralize normally and can result in cranial neuropathies from neuroforaminal narrowing, facial deformities, sinonasal drainage disorders, and sinusitis. McCune-Albright syndrome accounts for 3% of polyostotic fibrous dysplasia and may include the presence of pigmented cutaneous macules (sometimes referred to as café-au-lait spots) with irregular indented borders that are ipsilateral to bone lesions, precocious puberty, and/or other endocrine disorders, such as acromegaly, hyperthyroidism, hyperparathyroidism, and Cushing's syndrome. *Leontiasis ossea* is a rare form of polyostotic fibrous dyplasia that involves the craniofacial bones, resulting in facial enlargement and deformity. Age at presentation ranges from < 1 year to 76 years, but 75% occur before the age of 30 years. Median age for monostotic fibrous dysplasia = 21 years; mean and median ages for polyostotic fibrous dysplasia are between 8 and 17 years. Most cases are diagnosed in patients between 3 and 20 years old.
Florid cemento-osseous dysplasia (**Fig. 4.144**)	*CT:* Radiolucent zones adjacent to roots of multiple teeth, ± diffuse, lobular, or irregularly shaped sclerotic zones, ± expansion of thinned cortical bone margins.	Reactive nonneoplastic disorder involving the mandible and maxilla in which there are accumulating collections of cementum and bone within a cellular fibrovascular stroma. Usually occurs in middle-aged women (fourth to fifth decades). Patients are usually asymptomatic. The condition can be associated with complications related to oral surgery or from dental or periodontal inflammatory disease.

(continued on page 428)

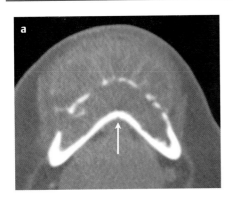
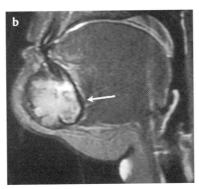
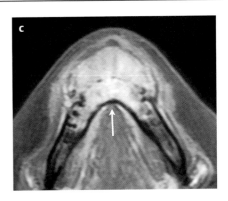

Fig. 4.142 **(a)** Axial CT of a 17-year-old male with Ewing's sarcoma shows a radiolucent destructive lesion involving the anterior portion of the mandible (*arrow*) with extraosseous tumor extension. **(b)** The tumor has mixed low, slightly high, and high signal on sagittal fat-suppressed T2-weighted imaging (*arrow*) and **(c)** shows gadolinium contrast enhancement on axial fat-suppressed T1-weighted imaging (*arrow*).

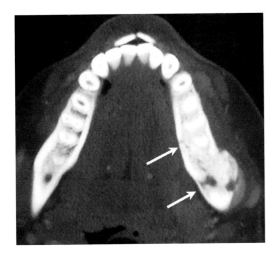

Fig. 4.143 Axial CT of a 16-year-old female shows fibrous dysplasia involving the left mandible, seen as osseous expansion with a "ground glass" appearance (*arrows*).

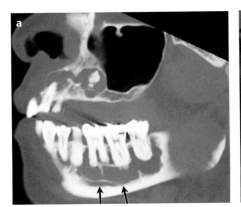
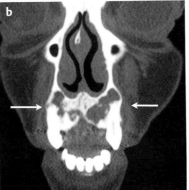
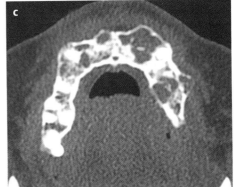

Fig. 4.144 **(a)** Sagittal, **(b)** coronal, and **(c)** axial images of a 43-year-old woman with florid cemento-osseous dysplasia shows radiolucent zones adjacent to roots of multiple teeth, irregularly shaped sclerotic zones, and expansion of thinned cortical bone margins (*arrows*).

Table 4.6 *(cont.)* Lesions involving the masticator space

Lesion	Imaging Findings	Comments
Paget disease (**Fig. 4.145**)	*MRI:* Most cases involving the mandible are in the late or inactive phases. Findings include osseous expansion and cortical thickening with low signal on T1- and T2-weighted imaging. The inner margins of the thickened cortex can be irregular and indistinct. Zones of low signal on T1- and T2-weighted imaging can be seen in the diploic marrow secondary to thickened bone trabeculae. Marrow in late or inactive phases of Paget's disease can have signal similar to normal marrow, contain focal areas of fat signal, have low signal on T1- and T2-weighted imaging secondary to regions of sclerosis, or have areas of high signal on fat-suppressed T2-weighted imaging from edema or persistent fibrovascular tissue. *CT:* Lesions often have mixed intermediate and high attenuation in the marrow, irregular/indistinct borders between marrow and inner margins of cortical bone, and osseous expansion.	Paget disease is a chronic skeletal disease in which there is disordered bone resorption and woven bone formation, resulting in osseous deformity. A paramyxovirus may be an etiologic agent. Paget disease is polyostotic in up to 66% of patients. Paget disease is associated with a risk of less than 1% for developing secondary sarcomatous changes. It occurs in 2.5–5% of Caucasians more than 55 years old, and 10% of those more than 85 years old. Can result in narrowing of neuroforamina, with cranial nerve compression and basilar impression, ± compression of brainstem.
Osteonecrosis (**Fig. 4.146**)	*MRI:* Zones with low-intermediate signal on T1-weighted imaging and high and/or low signal on T2-weighted imaging (T2WI) and fat-suppressed T2WI, as well as variable heterogeneous gadolinium contrast enhancement. *CT:* Zones of abnormal decreased attenuation (bone lysis), ± zones with increased attenuation (sclerosis), + focal sites of medullary and cortical bone destruction, ± periosteal new bone formation, ± late sequestrum, bone deformity.	Osteonecrosis of the mandible can be caused by radiation treatment for malignant tumors, bisphosphonate medications that are used to treat osteoporosis, Paget disease, lytic bone metastases, myeloma, or hypercalcemia (from malignant origin). Lesions can be associated with pain.
Inflammatory Lesions		
Osteomyelitis, periapical abscess (**Fig. 4.147** and **Fig. 4.148**)	*MRI:* Zones with low-intermediate signal on T1-weighted imaging and high signal on T2-weighted imaging (T2WI) and fat-suppressed T2WI, ± high signal on diffusion-weighted imaging and low signal on ADC. Usually shows heterogeneous gadolinium contrast enhancement in marrow and adjacent soft tissues. *CT:* Zones of abnormal decreased attenuation, focal sites of bone destruction, infection/abscess of adjacent soft tissue. Osteomyelitis from infected teeth results in tooth resorption, periapical abscess with lucency, and adjacent osteolysis.	Osteomyelitis (bone infection) can result from surgery, trauma, hematogenous dissemination from another source of infection, or direct extension of infection from adjacent sites, such as the teeth, oral cavity, floor of the mouth, nasopharynx, and parotid space.

(continued on page 430)

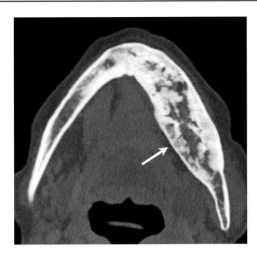

Fig. 4.145 Axial CT of a 90-year-old woman with Paget disease involving the left mandible (*arrow*) with mixed intermediate and high attenuation in the marrow, irregular/indistinct borders between the marrow and inner margins of cortical bone, and osseous expansion.

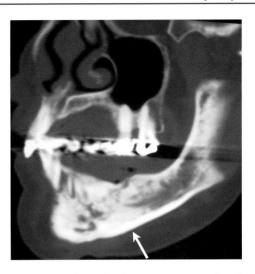

Fig. 4.146 Sagittal CT of radiation treatment-related osteonecrosis of the mandible (*arrow*) shows mixed irregular zones of decreased attenuation (bone lysis) and increased attenuation (sclerosis), as well as focal sites of medullary bone destruction.

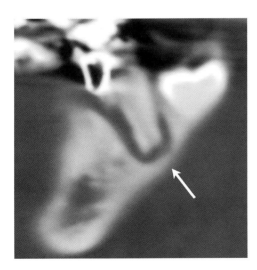

Fig. 4.147 Sagittal CT shows a periapical abscess that is seen as a zone of abnormal decreased attenuation adjacent to the root/apex of a mandibular tooth (*arrow*), representing a focal site of bone destruction from infection.

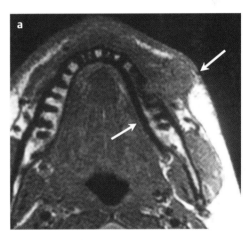

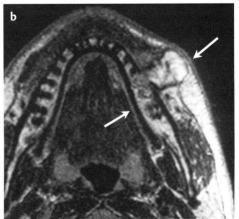

Fig. 4.148 **(a)** A 21-year-old man with osteomyelitis involving the marrow of the left mandible that has abnormal low signal on axial T1-weighted imaging (*arrows*) and **(b)** high signal on axial T2-weighted imaging (*arrows*) and is associated with cortical bone destruction and extraosseous extension of infection.

Table 4.6 *(cont.)* Lesions involving the masticator space

Lesion	Imaging Findings	Comments
Juvenile mandibular chronic osteomyelitis/ chronic recurrent multifocal osteomyelitis (**Fig. 4.149**)	Multifocal lesions that occur in metaphyses of tubular bones (distal femur, proximal and distal tibia and fibula), clavicles, vertebrae, pelvis, and/or mandible. *MRI:* Heterogeneous abnormal high signal on fat-suppressed T2-weighted imaging in marrow and periosteal soft tissues, with gadolinium contrast enhancement. *CT:* Radiolucent ground-glass and/or sclerotic osseous lesions with proliferative lamellated or "onion skin" periosteal bone formation and hyperostosis. Enlargement of the mandibular nerve canal is often seen.	Painful autoinflammatory osseous disorder of unknown cause with histopathology of acute and chronic osteomyelitis. There is no identifiable infectious agent, so it is a diagnosis of exclusion. Usually occurs in children and adolescents (median age = 10 years), in females (85%) more often than in males (15%). Multi-episodic skeletal disorder that can occur over 7 to 25 years. Seventy-five percent of lesions occur in at least one long bone, and approximately 10% of lesions involve the mandible. Symptomatic treatment with NSAIDs. Can be associated with acne or palmoplantar pustulosis (SAPHO syndrome).
Langerhans' cell histiocytosis	Single or multiple circumscribed soft tissue lesions in marrow associated with focal bony destruction/ erosion and with extension extracranially, intracranially, or both. *MRI:* Lesions typically have low-intermediate signal on T1-weighted imaging and heterogeneous slightly high to high signal on T2-weighted imaging (T2WI) and fat-suppressed (FS) T2WI. Poorly defined zones of high signal on T2WI and FS T2WI are usually seen in the marrow and soft tissues peripheral to the lesions secondary to inflammatory changes. Lesions typically show prominent gadolinium contrast enhancement in marrow and extraosseous soft tissue portions. *CT:* Lesions usually have low-intermediate attenuation, + contrast enhancement, ± enhancement of the adjacent dura.	Disorder of reticuloendothelial system in which bone marrow–derived dendritic Langerhans' cells infiltrate various organs as focal lesions or in diffuse patterns. Langerhans' cells have eccentrically located ovoid or convoluted nuclei within pale to eosinophilic cytoplasm. Lesions often consist of Langerhans' cells, macrophages, plasma cells, and eosinophils. Lesions are immunoreactive to S-100, CD1a, CD-207, HLA-DR, and β_2-microglobulin. Prevalence of 2 per 100,000 children less than 15 years old; only a third of lesions occur in adults. Localized lesions (eosinophilic granuloma) can be single or multiple in the skull, usually at the skull base. Single lesions are commonly seen in males more than in females, in patients < 20 years old. Proliferation of histiocytes in medullary bone results in localized destruction of cortical bone with extension into adjacent soft tissues.
Traumatic Lesions		
Mandibular fractures (**Fig. 4.150**)	*CT:* Fractures are classified into those involving the alveolar ridge and teeth and those involving the ramus, with or without involvement of the coronoid or condyle. Condylar fractures are further classified based on fracture location and displacement or dislocation. CT is more accurate and sensitive in detecting condylar fractures than panoramic radiographs.	Mandibular trauma can occur as an isolated injury or in association with other craniofacial fractures. Up to 67% of mandibular fractures occur at more than one site: 36% of mandibular fractures involve the condylar process, 21% the body, 20% the angle, 14% the region of the symphysis, 3% the ramus or alveolar process, and 2% the coronoid. Imaging is important for identifying the fracture findings for surgical planning. Complications include fragment malunion, pseudarthrosis, osteomyelitis, and ischemic necrosis.
Developmental Anomalies		
Pierre Robin syndrome (**Fig. 4.151**)	*CT and MRI:* Micrognathia from congenital mandibular hypoplasia, with mandible/maxilla length ratio of less than 0.75, posterior positioning of the tongue (narrowing the airway), and U-shaped/arched palate, ± cleft palate.	Micrognathia from hypoplasia of the mandible associated with posterior displacement of the tongue (glossoptosis) and arched or cleft palate. Occurs in 1 in 8,500 births. Results from hypoplasia of the mandible during formation before 9 weeks of gestation. Clinical findings include upper airway obstruction, respiratory distress, feeding difficulties, and failure to thrive. Can occur as an isolated finding in an otherwise normal neonate, or in association with hemifacial microsomia (Goldenhar syndrome, oculoauriculovertebral spectrum) and Treacher Collins syndrome. Surgical treatment with mandibular distraction osteogenesis is commonly performed for patients with upper airway obstruction, respiratory distress, and/or difficulty feeding.

(continued on page 432)

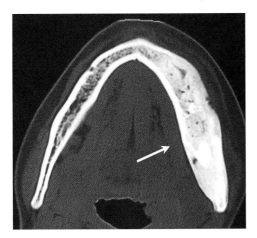

Fig. 4.149 Axial CT shows chronic osteomyelitis in the left mandible with mixed ground-glass appearance and irregular sclerotic hyperostosis (*arrow*).

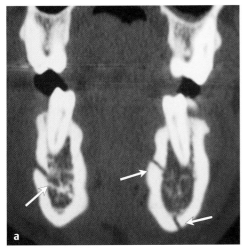
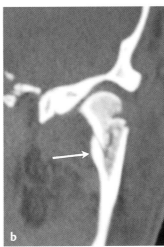

Fig. 4.150 **(a,b)** Coronal CT of examples of mandibular fractures (*arrows*).

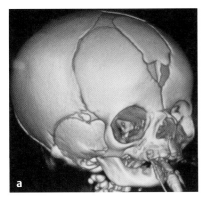
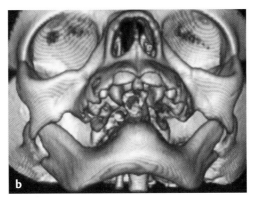
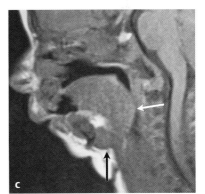
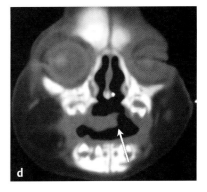

Fig. 4.151 Neonate with Pierre Robin syndrome. **(a,b)** Volume-rendered CT shows mandibular hypoplasia. **(c)** Sagittal T1-weighted imaging shows a U-shaped/arched palate and posterior positioning of the tongue (*arrows*), resulting in narrowing of the airway. **(d)** Coronal CT shows a cleft palate (*arrow*).

Table 4.6 *(cont.)*　Lesions involving the masticator space

Lesion	Imaging Findings	Comments
Mandibular hypoplasia (**Fig. 4.152**)	Symmetric or asymmetric hypoplasia of the posterior portions of the mandible.	Hypoplasia of the mandible that is less severe than that in Pierre Robin syndrome and that can be symmetric or asymmetric. Can be associated with hemifacial microsomia (Goldenhar syndrome, oculoauriculovertebral spectrum) and Treacher Collins syndrome.
Hemifacial microsomia (Goldenhar syndrome, oculoauriculovertebral spectrum) (**Fig. 4.153**; see **Fig. 1.162** and **Fig. 3.23**)	Facial asymmetry from unilateral and/or bilateral hypoplasia of the mandible, maxillae, and zygomatic arches, atresia or stenosis of the external auditory canals, hypoplasia of the middle ear, malformations and/or fusion of the ossicles, oval window atresia, and abnormal position of CN VII.	Asymmetric abnormal development of the first and second branchial arches related to the autosomal dominant mutation of the *TCOF1* gene on chromosome 5q32-q33.1. Results in deafness/hearing loss and airway narrowing.
Treacher Collins syndrome (**Fig. 4.154**; see also **Fig. 3.24**)	Bilateral symmetric hypoplasia of the mandible (± absence of the mandibular rami—retrognathia), maxillae, and zygomatic arches, ± cleft palate, atresia of the external auditory canals, ossicular hypoplasia, deformed pinnae, and colobomas.	Autosomal dominant mutation of *TCOF1* gene on chromosome 5q32 results in impaired function of the gene product treacle protein. Deficiency of treacle protein causes apoptosis of embryonic neural crest cells, leading to bilateral symmetric hypoplasia of first branchial arch structures, such as the maxillae, mandibles, and zygomatic arches.
Bifid mandibular condyle (**Fig. 4.155**)	*CT:* Duplicate mandibular condyles originate from the neck of the condyle. Can be oriented in the mediolateral or anteroposterior planes. Can be unilareral or bilateral. Some cases are associated with ankylosis of the temporomandibular joint.	Rare anomaly of unknown etiology and pathogenesis in which there are two mandibular condyles. Can be asymptomatic or symptomatic.

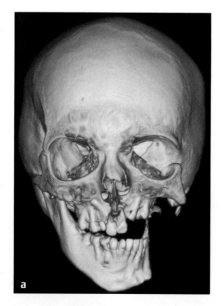 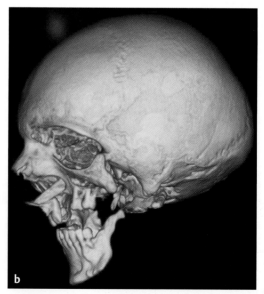

Fig. 4.152　**(a)** Coronal and **(b)** sagittal volume-rendered CT shows asymmetric hypoplasia of the posterior portions of the left mandible.

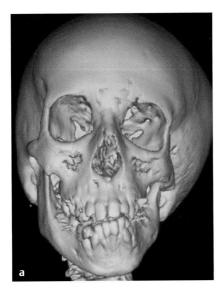
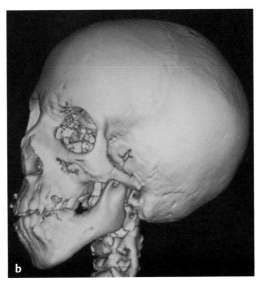

Fig. 4.153 **(a)** Coronal and **(b)** sagittal CT of a patient with hemifacial microsomia (Goldenhar syndrome, oculoauriculovertebral spectrum) shows asymmetric hypoplasia of the left mandible and left maxilla.

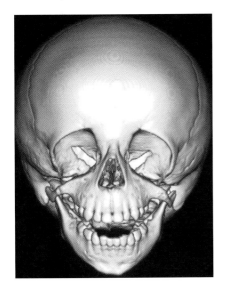

Fig. 4.154 Coronal volume-rendered CT of a 3-year-old male with Treacher Collins syndrome shows bilateral symmetric hypoplasia of the mandible, maxillae, and zygomatic arches.

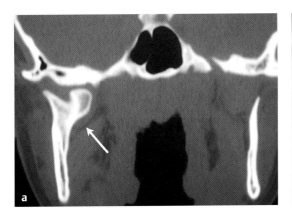
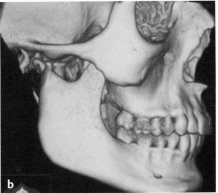

Fig. 4.155 **(a)** Coronal CT (*arrow*) and **(b)** and sagittal volume-rendered CT show a bifid right mandibular condyle.

4.7 Temporomandibular Joint (TMJ)

The maxillae, mandible, muscles of mastication, TMJ, and TMJ discs are derived from the first branchial arch. The TMJ begins to develop during the eighth week of gestation. The TMJ is a diarthrodial hinge joint that enables rotation and forward and backward translation of the mandible in a gliding motion during the process of chewing food (**Fig. 4.156**). In the closed-mouth position, the mandibular condyles are located within the mandibular fossae on each side at the undersurface of the squamosal portions of the temporal bones. With mouth opening, there is counterclockwise rotation of the mandibular condyles and forward translation of the mandible to a more anterior location beneath inferior protuberances of the temporal bones, referred to as the articular eminence on each side. The TMJ contains a biconcave, avascular fibrocartilage disc that separates the synovial joint into superior and inferior compartments. The TMJ disc has a triangular anterior band, a thin central intermediate zone, and a posterior band. The anterior band measures 2 mm in thickness and is continuous with the joint capsule. The thin intermediate zone is normally interposed between the inferior surface of the temporal bone and superior surface of the mandibular condyle in the open-mouth position. The posterior band measures 3 mm in thickness and is contiguous posteriorly with a bilaminar zone consisting of a superior fibroelastic layer and an inferior fibrous layer with intervening tissue containing blood vessels, nerves, and loose elastic fibers. The bilaminar zone is referred to as retrodiscal tissue. The superior layer attaches to the postglenoid process at the posterior and lateral aspects of the articular fossa. The inferior lamina attaches to the condylar neck. The superior layer prevents abnormal slipping of the disc with mouth opening, and the inferior layer limits abnormal movement of the disc over the condyle. The medial and lateral aspects of the disc attach to the medial and lateral poles of the mandibular condyle and do not attach to the joint capsule. The main muscles involved with mastication include the lateral and medial pterygoid, masseter, and temporalis muscles. The superior belly of the lateral pterygoid muscle attaches to the anteromedial margins of the mandibular neck and superomedial joint capsule, which is contiguous with the anterior band of the disc. The inferior belly of the lateral pterygoid muscle attaches to the neck of the condyloid process. The movement of mouth opening occurs from the actions of the lateral pterygoid muscles in association with other muscles, such as stylohyoid, mylohyoid, and geniohyoid muscles. The movement of mouth closing occurs from the actions of the masseter, medial pterygoid, and temporalis muscles. A unique feature of the TMJ is that the articular surfaces of the temporal bone and mandibular condyles are covered by fibrocartilage, unlike other synovial joints, where the articular surfaces are covered by hyaline cartilage.

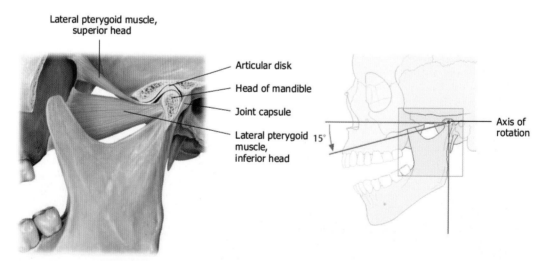

Fig. 4.156 Lateral view of the anatomic relationships at the temporomandibular joint (TMJ). From THIEME Atlas of Anatomy: Head and Neuroanatomy, © Thieme 2007, Illustration by Karl Wesker.

Table 4.7 Temporomandibular joint (TMJ) abnormalities

- TMJ disc: normal appearance (closed mouth/ open mouth)
- TMJ disc displacement: anterior position (closed mouth) with recapture with mouth opening— anterior displacement with reduction
- TMJ disc displacement: anterior displacement without recapture with mouth opening
- TMJ: stuck disc

- TMJ: perforated disc
- TMJ: posterior disc displacement
- Osteoarthritis
- Synovial osteochondromatosis
- Synovial chondroma/chondromatosis
- Rheumatoid arthritis
- Juvenile idiopathic arthritis
- Calcium pyrophosphate deposition (CPPD) disease
- Pigmented villonodular synovitis (PVNS)
- Synovial cyst

Table 4.7 Temporomandibular joint (TMJ) abnormalities

Abnormality/Lesion	Imaging Findings	Comments
TMJ disc: normal appearance (closed mouth/open mouth) **(Fig. 4.157)**	*MRI:* The TMJ disc is a biconcave structure with low signal on T1-weighted imaging, proton density-weighted imaging, and T2-weighted imaging. *In the closed-mouth position*, the posterior band is located above the condylar head in the 12 o'clock position. *In the open-mouth position,* the mandibular condyles rotate and translate anteriorly, with the intermediate zone of the disc interposed between the temporal eminences and the condylar heads.	MRI is the optimal test to evaluate the postion of the disc in closed- and open-mouth positions. The posterior band and bilaminar zone are best seen on the open-mouth view. MRI is typically obtained in coronal and oblique sagittal planes to optimally visualize the position of the discs relative to the mandibular condyles.

(continued on page 436)

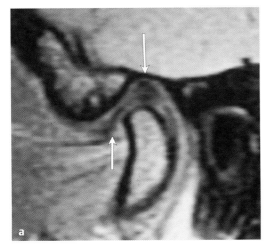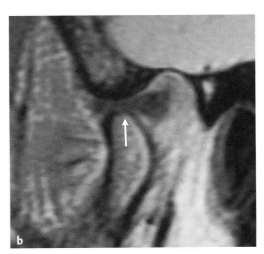

Fig. 4.157 Sagittal proton-density weighted imaging shows normal shape and position of the temporomandibular joint (TMJ) disc (*arrows*) in the **(a)** closed-mouth and **(b)** open-mouth positions.

Table 4.7 *(cont.)* Temporomandibular joint (TMJ) abnormalities

Abnormality/Lesion	Imaging Findings	Comments
TMJ disc displacement: anterior position (closed mouth) with recapture with mouth opening—anterior displacement with reduction (**Fig. 4.158**)	*MRI: In the closed-mouth position,* the disc is anteriorly displaced relative to the condyle. *In the open-mouth position,* the mandibular condyle rotates and translates anteriorly, with the intermediate zone of the disc interposed between the temporal eminence and the condylar head.	Anterior and anterolateral disc displacements account for 80%. Disc displacement is complete if the entire medial-lateral dimension is displaced or is partial if it is not. With partial displacement, the lateral portion is more commonly involved than the medial portion. A reciprocal click is observed with recapture of the disc during mouth opening.
TMJ disc displacement: anterior displacement without recapture with mouth opening (**Fig. 4.159** and **Fig. 4.160**)	*MRI: In the closed-mouth position,* the disc is anteriorly displaced relative to the condyle. *In the open-mouth position,* there is decreased condylar rotation and decreased anterior translation of the mandible, with continued anterior displacement of the disc relative to the condyle. The posterior band is located anterior to the condyle.	With anterior disc displacement without reduction, there is decreased mouth opening, with deviation of the mandible to the affected side (closed lock). Injury can progress to flattened irregular deformity or perforation of the disc. Often the anterior band becomes thin and the posterior band becomes thickened and rounded.
TMJ: stuck disc (**Fig. 4.161**)	*MRI: In the closed-mouth position,* the disc can be in the normal position or anteriorly displaced relative to the condyle. *In the open-mouth position,* there is decreased condylar rotation and anterior translation of the mandible with no change in disc position.	Disorder in which the disc is tethered by adhesions and does not change position with mouth opening. Can be associated with pain and reduced condylar translation.

(continued on page 438)

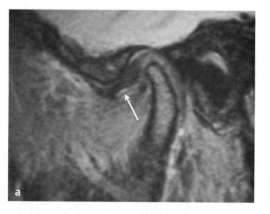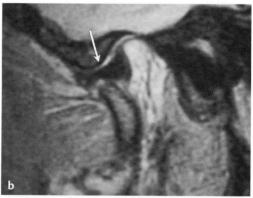

Fig. 4.158 **(a)** Sagittal T2-weighted imaging of a 17-year-old female shows anterior position/displacement of the temporomandibular joint (TMJ) disc (*arrow*) relative to the mandibular condyle in the closed-mouth position. **(b)** In the open-mouth position, there is recapture of the disc (*arrow*), which is referred to as anterior disc displacement with reduction.

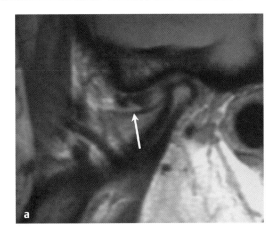
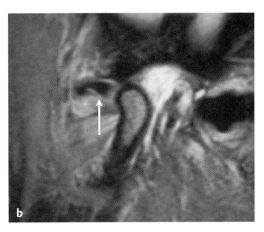

Fig. 4.159 **(a)** Sagittal PDWI of a 41-year-old woman shows anterior position/displacement of the temporomandibular joint (TMJ) disc (*arrow*) relative to the mandibular condyle in the closed-mouth position. **(b)** In the open-mouth position, there is persistent anterior displacement of the disc (*arrow*), which is referred to as anterior disc displacement without recapture.

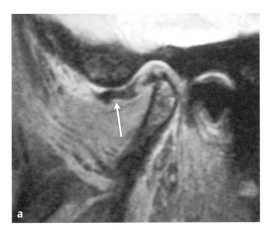
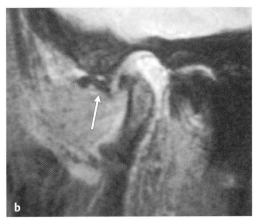

Fig. 4.160 **(a)** Sagittal T2-weighted imaging of a 56-year-old woman shows anterior position/displacement of the temporomandibular joint (TMJ) disc (*arrow*) relative to the mandibular condyle in the closed-mouth position. **(b)** In the open-mouth position, there is persistent anterior displacement of the deformed disc (*arrow*), which is referred to as anterior disc displacement without recapture.

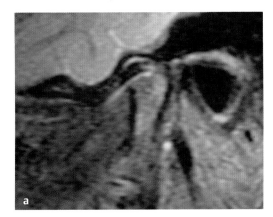
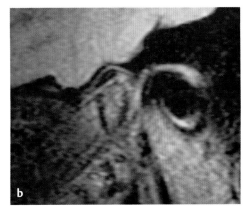

Fig. 4.161 Stuck disc. **(a)** Sagittal T2-weighted imaging shows the temporomandibular joint (TMJ) disc in normal position relative to the mandibular condyle in the closed-mouth position. **(b)** In the open-mouth position, there is decreased rotation and anterior translation of the mandible, with no change in disc position.

Table 4.7 *(cont.)* Temporomandibular joint (TMJ) abnormalities

Abnormality/Lesion	Imaging Findings	Comments
TMJ: perforated disc (**Fig. 4.162**)	*MRI:* Disc deformity, disc displacement, and absence of visualization or stretching of the posterior temporal attachment, ± condylar bone changes, ± joint effusion.	Occurs in up to 15% of TMJ disc displacements, more commonly with anteriorly displaced disc with nonreduction than with discs that reduce in the open-mouth position.
TMJ: posterior disc displacement (**Fig. 4.163**)	*MRI:* Displacement of the posterior band beyond the 1 o'clock position relative to the mandibular condylar head.	Rare disorder, accounts for < 0.01% of disc displacements. Patients often present with acute locking of the jaw upon mouth opening.
Osteoarthritis (**Fig. 4.164** and **Fig. 4.165**)	*MRI:* Deformity and/or osteophyte involving mandibular condyle, ± deformed and/or displaced disc. *CT:* Flattening deformity, sclerosis, and/or erosion of condylar articular surface, ± osteophytes.	Osteoarthritis is a common chronic degenerative disease of articular cartilage within synovial joints associated with sclerosis and remodeling of subchondral bone. In the TMJ, it is associated with pain during chewing motions.
Synovial osteochondromatosis (**Fig. 4.166**)	*MRI:* Features of osteochondromatosis are dependent on the relative proportions of cartilage, calcified cartilage, and mineralized osseous tissue within the lesions. Calcifications result in low signal on T1-weighted imaging (T1WI), proton density-weighted imaging (PDWI), T2-weighted imaging (T2WI), and fat-suppressed (FS) T2WI. Lesions with extensive calcification can have signal voids. Mature ossifications can have peripheral low signal on T1WI and T2WI surrounding a central region with fat signal. Noncalcified portions of the lesions can have low to intermediate signal on T1WI, intermediate signal on PDWI, and slightly high to high signal on T2WI and FS T2WI. Lesions can show irregular, thin, peripheral and/or septal gadolinium contrast enhancement. *CT:* Multiple foci with chondroid-type calcification within the TMJ.	Primary synovial osteochondromatosis is a benign disorder that results from cartilaginous and osseous metaplastic proliferation in synovium of joints. The osteocartilaginous nodules can become detached, forming intra-articular loose bodies. Secondary synovial osteochondromatosis occurs from avulsion of osteochondral fragments into the joint, forming loose bodies, which can enlarge via nutrient supply from synovial fluid.
Synovial chondroma/chondromatosis	*MRI:* Foci with low to intermediate signal on T1-weighted imaging (that is, iso- or hyperintense relative to muscle), intermediate signal on proton density-weighted imaging, and slightly high to high signal on T2-weighted imaging (T2WI) and fat-suppressed T2WI. Low-signal septae on T2WI can be seen within the lesions. Synovial chondromas can show irregular, thin, peripheral and/or septal gadolinium contrast enhancement. *CT:* Synovial chondromas are typically radiolucent.	Primary synovial chondromatosis accounts for < 1% of benign soft tissue tumors and is a benign disorder that results from cartilaginous metaplastic proliferation in synovium of joints. Usually occurs in patients from 25 to 65 years old (mean age = 44 years). The cartilaginous nodules can become detached, forming intra-articular loose bodies. Metaplasia of connective tissue into cartilage can also occur in bursae and in tendon sheaths. Secondary synovial chondromatosis occurs from avulsion of hyaline cartilage into the joint, forming loose bodies, which can enlarge via nutrient supply from synovial fluid.

(continued on page 440)

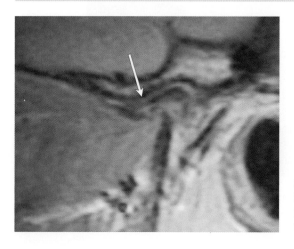

Fig. 4.162 Closed-mouth position sagittal proton density-weighted imaging of a 20-year-old man with juvenile idiopathic arthritis shows an eroded mandibular condyle with a deformed and perforated temporomandibular joint (TMJ) disc (*arrow*).

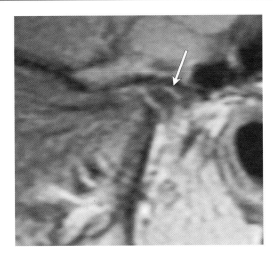

Fig. 4.163 Attempted open-mouth position on sagittal proton density-weighted imaging of a 20-year-old man with juvenile idiopathic arthritis (same patient as in **Fig. 4.162**) shows posterior displacement of the deformed temporomandibular joint (TMJ) disc (*arrow*) relative to the mandibular condyle.

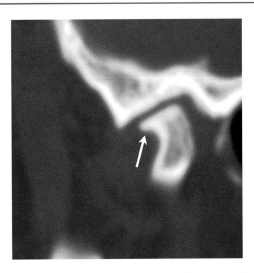

Fig. 4.164 Sagittal CT shows osteoarthritic changes at the temporomandibular joint (TMJ) (*arrow*), with joint space narrowing, flattening of the condylar head, osteophytes, and reactive osteosclerosis.

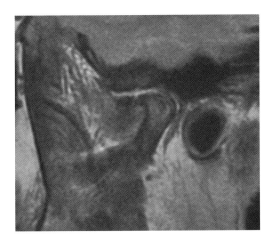

Fig. 4.165 Sagittal T2-weighted imaging shows osteoarthritic changes at the temporomandibular joint (TMJ), with joint space narrowing, flattening of the condylar head, osteophytes, and small joint effusion.

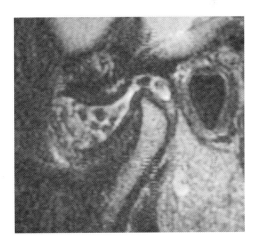

Fig. 4.166 Sagittal T2-weighted imaging of a 33-year-old woman shows a large, high-signal joint effusion in the temporomandibular joint (TMJ). The effusion contains multiple osteochondral bodies with low signal, representing synovial osteochondromatosis.

Table 4.7 *(cont.)*   Temporomandibular joint (TMJ) abnormalities

Abnormality/Lesion	Imaging Findings	Comments
Rheumatoid arthritis (**Fig. 4.167**)	*MRI:* Hypertrophied synovium seen with rheumatoid arthritis can be diffuse, nodular, and/or villous and usually has low to intermediate or intermediate signal on T1-weighted imaging (T1WI), proton density-weighted imaging, and FLAIR. On T2-weighted imaging (T2WI), hypertrophied synovium can have low to intermediate, intermediate, and/or slightly high to high signal, which is typically lower than joint fluid. Signal heterogeneity of hypertrophied synovium on T2WI can result from variable amounts of fibrin, hemosiderin, and fibrosis. Chronic, fibrotic, nonvascular synovium usually has low signal on T1WI and T2WI. Hypertrophied synovium can show prominent homogeneous or variable heterogeneous gadolinium contrast enhancement. Joint effusions can be seen, ± erosion of mandibular condyle, glenoid fossa, and articular eminence. *CT:* Zones of erosion and/or destruction of bone.	Rheumatoid arthritis is a chronic multisystem disease of unknown etiology with persistent inflammatory synovitis involving articular joints and tendon sheaths in a symmetric distribution. Can result in progressive destruction of cartilage and bone, leading to joint dysfunction. Affects ~ 1% of the world population. Eighty percent of adult patients present between the ages of 35 and 50 years.
Juvenile idiopathic arthritis (**Fig. 4.168**)	*MRI:* Joint effusion and synovial thickening > 3 mm. Involved synovium can have low-intermediate signal on T1-weighted imaging and intermediate or mixed intermediate, slightly high to high signal on T2-weighted imaging (T2WI), ± zones of low signal on T2WI from hemosiderin/fibrin, ± bone marrow edema. Gadolinium contrast enhancement of thickened synovium is usually seen. Quantitative assessment of dynamic contrast enhancement can correlate with disease activity and response to treatment. *CT:* Flattening deformity of condylar heads, ± bone erosions and condylar resorption. Micrognathia can occur in advanced disease from abnormal condylar growth and development.	Inflammatory arthritis in children, with a prevalence of 16–150/100,000. Usually begins in children < 16 years old and persists for at least 6 weeks. Rheumatoid factor is positive in only 5–10%. Synovial proliferation occurs, containing inflammatory cells, and is associated with increased secretion of synovial fluid and eventual pannus formation. Can result in articular and bone erosion, leading to joint dysfunction and disability. Often involves the knee and TMJ. Oligoarticular form (50–60%) involves less than five joints in the first 6 months; systemic type (10–20%) involves more than five joints and is associated with fever, myalgias, adenopathy, hepatosplenomegaly, and serositis. TMJ involvement can result in micrognathia, facial dysmorphism, pain, and poor mouth opening. Can be treated with NSAIDs, methotrexate, systemic corticosteroids, and biologic therapy.
Calcium pyrophosphate deposition (CPPD) disease (**Fig. 4.169**)	Radiographs and CT show chondrocalcinosis and synovial thickening, ± erosion of adjacent bone. *MRI:* Hypertrophy of synovium, which can have low-intermediate signal on T1- and T2-weighted imaging. Small zones of low signal correspond to calcifications seen with CT. Involved synovium can have heterogeneous gadolinium contrast enhancement.	CPPD disease is a common disorder, usually in older adults, in which there is deposition of CPPD crystals, resulting in calcifications of hyaline and fibrocartilage. The disease is associated with cartilage degeneration, subchondral cysts, and osteophyte formation. Symptomatic CPPD disease is referred to as pseudogout because of overlapping clinical features. Usually occurs in the knee, hip, shoulder, elbow, and wrist, and rarely at the odontoid-C1 articulation and TMJ.

(continued on page 442)

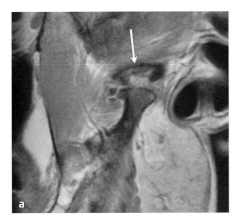
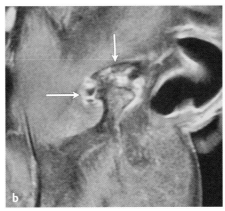

Fig. 4.167 **(a)** A 61-year-old woman with rheumatoid arthritis who has erosive changes involving the cortical bone margins along the temporal fossa and condylar head (*arrow*) on sagittal T1-weighted imaging. **(b)** Postcontrast sagittal fat-suppressed T1-weighted imaging shows gadolinium contrast enhancement of hypertrophied synovium (*arrows*) within the temporomandibular joint (TMJ).

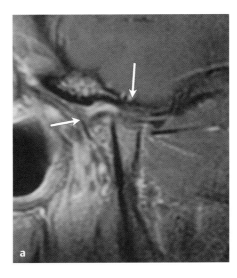
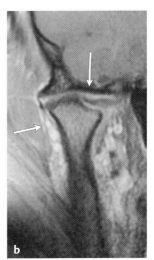

Fig. 4.168 Postcontrast **(a)** sagittal and **(b)** coronal T1-weighted imaging of a 20-year-old man with juvenile idiopathic arthritis shows a joint effusion with gadolinium-enhancing synovium (*arrows*) associated with a flattening deformity of the condylar head.

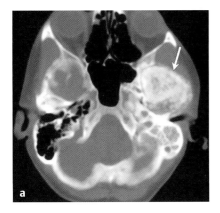
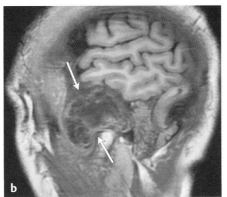
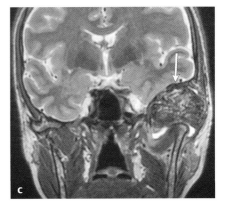
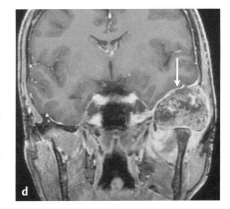

Fig. 4.169 **(a)** A 61-year-old woman with calcium pyrophosphate deposition disease involving the left temporomandibular joint (TMJ), which is seen as a synovial mass with dense chondrocalcinosis (*arrow*) associated with erosion of adjacent bone on axial CT. **(b)** The hypertrophied synovial mass has mixed low and intermediate signal on sagittal T1-weighted imaging (*arrows*); **(c)** mixed low, intermediate, and high signal (*arrow*) on coronal T2-weighted imaging (with a small joint effusion with high signal); and **(d)** heterogeneous gadolinium contrast enhancement on coronal T1-weighted imaging (*arrow*).

Table 4.7 *(cont.)* Temporomandibular joint (TMJ) abnormalities

Abnormality/Lesion	Imaging Findings	Comments
Pigmented villonodular synovitis (PVNS) **(Fig. 4.170)**	*MRI:* Often appears as irregular, multinodular, and/or diffuse thickening of synovium. Occasionally occurs as a single nodular intra-articular lesion. Lesions often have low or low-intermediate signal on T1-weighted imaging, proton density-weighted imaging, FLAIR, and T2-weighted imaging (T2WI). Areas of low signal on T2- and T2*-weighted imaging are secondary to hemosiderin in PVNS. Areas of slightly high to high signal on T2WI and fat-suppressed T2WI can also occur from edema and/or inflammatory reaction. Joint effusions are usually present, rarely with fluid–fluid levels. PVNS can show gadolinium contrast enhancement in irregular heterogeneous and/or homogeneous patterns. *CT:* Synovial thickening ± erosion of adjacent bone.	Benign lesions of proliferative synovium (tendon sheaths, joints, and bursae) containing zones of recent or remote hemorrhage. PVNS has histopathologic features similar to those of giant cell tumors of the tendon sheath/nodular synovitis, although PVNS lesions have frondlike or villous growth patterns and contain large amounts of hemosiderin. PVNS accounts for < 1% of benign and all soft-tissue tumors. Patients range in age from 9 to 74 years, (mean age = 38 years, median age = 32 years).
Synovial cyst **(Fig. 4.171)**	*MRI:* Spheroid or ovoid circumscribed collections that often show a site of communication with the adjacent joint. The contents of the synovial cyst usually have low to intermediate signal on T1-weighted imaging (T1WI), FLAIR, and proton density-weighted imaging, and high signal on T2-weighted imaging (T2WI) and fat-suppressed (FS) T2WI. A thin or slightly thick rim of low signal on T2WI and FS T2WI is typically seen at the periphery of the cysts. Some synovial cysts may have intermediate to high signal on T1WI and/or intermediate or low signal on T2WI secondary to calcifications, and/or hemorrhage. After gadolinium contrast administration, thin marginal enhancement may be seen. *CT:* Circumscribed structure with fluid attenuation in contents.	Synovium-lined fluid collections that frequently occur at or near joints of the extremities and occasionally occur at facet joints of the spine, as well as bursae and tendon sheaths. In adults, synovial cysts are often associated with osteoarthritis, rheumatoid arthritis, and trauma.

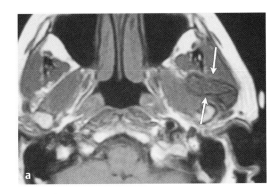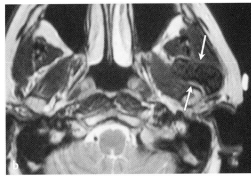

Fig. 4.170 A 58-year-old woman with pigmented villonodular synovitis involving the left temporomandibular joint (TMJ) that is seen as a lesion (*arrows*) anterior to the upper left mandible and that has a peripheral rim of low signal surrounding a central zone with mixed low and intermediate signal on axial **(a)** T1-weighted imaging (*arrows*) and **(b)** T2-weighted imaging (*arrows*).

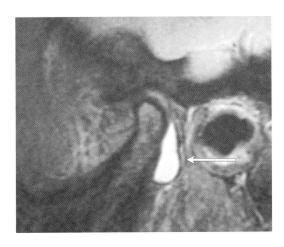

Fig. 4.171 Sagittal T2-weighted imaging shows a synovial cyst (*arrow*) with circumscribed high signal dorsal to the neck of the mandible in a 40-year-old woman.

4.8 Lesions Involving the Oropharynx, Oral Cavity, and Floor of the Mouth

The oral cavity includes the anterior two-thirds of the tongue, the buccal mucosa, the upper and lower alveolar ridges, the hard palate, the retromolar trigone, the floor of the mouth, and the lips (**Fig. 4.172**). Posterior to the oral cavity is the oropharynx. The oral cavity and oropharynx are divided by the anterior tonsillar pillars and the junction between the hard and soft palate. Both the oral cavity and oropharynx are lined by squamous epithelium.

The oropharynx includes the posterior third of the tongue, the lingual and palatine tonsils, the anterior and posterior tonsillar pillars, the posterior and lateral pharyngeal walls, the soft palate superiorly, and the valleculae and epiglottis inferiorly.

The floor of the mouth consists of the mylohyoid muscle sling that attaches to the lower inner surface of the mandible laterally, mandibular symphysis anteriorly, and hyoid bone posteriorly. The mylohyoid muscle sling separates the floor of the mouth from the right and left submandibular spaces inferiorly. The extrinsic muscles of the tongue and geniohyoid muscles are also located at the floor of the mouth.

The bilateral sublingual spaces are located above the mylohyoid sling and lateral to the paired genioglossus muscles, which extend from the anterior portion of the mandible posteriorly into the tongue. Each sublingual space contains fat, the sublingual gland, lingual nerve, lingual artery and vein, hyoglossus muscle, minor salivary glands, Wharton's duct, and the deep portion of the submandibular gland. The hyoglossus muscle separates the medially positioned lingual artery from the lingual vein and Wharton's duct, which are located lateral to the muscle.

The hypopharynx extends from the epiglottis to the upper esophageal sphincter and includes the piriform sinuses lateral to the upper larynx.

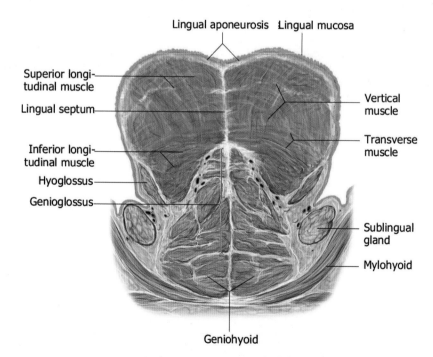

Fig. 4.172 Coronal view of the structures within the oral cavity and floor of the mouth. From THIEME Atlas of Anatomy: Head and Neuroanatomy, © Thieme 2007, Illustration by Karl Wesker.

Table 4.8 Lesions involving the oropharynx, oral cavity, and floor of the mouth

- Developmental/Congenital Abnormalities
  - Epidermal inclusion cyst: epidermoid
  - Epidermal inclusion cyst: dermoid
  - Teratoma
  - Venolymphatic malformation
  - Lingual thyroglossal duct cyst
  - Lingual thyroid
  - Foregut duplication cyst of the tongue
- Benign Neoplasms
  - Pleomorphic adenoma of sublingual gland or minor salivary gland
  - Lipoma
  - Hemangioma
  - Schwannoma
- Tumorlike Lesions
  - Simple ranula
  - Plunging (diving) ranula
- Malignant Tumors
  - Squamous cell carcinoma
  - Adenoid cystic carcinoma
  - Adenocarcinoma and mucoepidermoid carcinoma
  - Non-Hodgkin lymphoma
  - Metastatic malignancies
  - Rhabdomyosarcoma
- Inflammatory Lesions
  - Phlegmon/abscess at the floor of the mouth
  - Ludwig angina
  - Granulomatosis with polyangiitis
  - Submandibular duct stone/sialadenitis

Table 4.8 Lesions involving the oropharynx, oral cavity, and floor of the mouth

Lesion	Imaging Findings	Comments
Developmental/Congenital Abnormalities		
Epidermal inclusion cyst: epidermoid (**Fig. 4.173** and **Fig. 4.174**)	*MRI:* Well-circumscribed spheroid or multilobulated ectodermal-inclusion cystic lesions with low-intermediate signal on T1-weighted imaging, high signal on T2-weighted imaging and diffusion-weighted imaging, mixed low, intermediate, or high signal on FLAIR images, and no gadolinium contrast enhancement. Occur more frequently at the floor of the mouth in the midline than in the submandibular space. *CT:* Well-circumscribed spheroid or multilobulated ectodermal-inclusion cystic lesions with low-intermediate attenuation, ± bone erosion.	Nonneoplastic congenital or acquired lesions filled with desquamated cells and keratinaceous debris surrounded by a wall lined by simple squamous epithelium. Lesions result from congenital inclusion of epidermal elements during embryonic development of the first and second branchial arches, or from trauma. Often occur in patients between 5 and 50 years old (mean age = 30 years).

(continued on page 446)

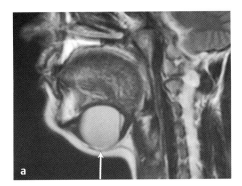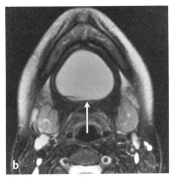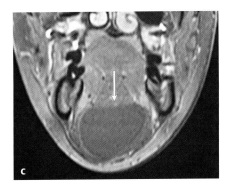

Fig. 4.173 A 17-year-old female with an epidermoid cyst at the floor of the mouth which has high signal on **(a)** sagittal and **(b)** axial T2-weighted imaging (*arrows*), and **(c)** low signal without gadolinium contrast enhancement on coronal fat-suppressed T1-weighted imaging (*arrow*).

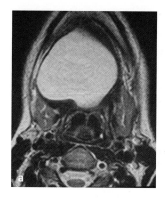
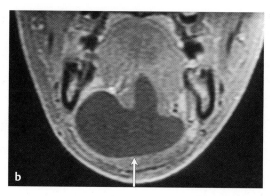
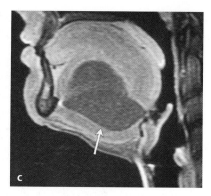

Fig. 4.174 **(a)** A 14-year-old female with an epidermoid cyst (*arrows*) at the floor of the mouth that has high signal on axial T2-weighted imaging. The lesion has low signal without gadolinium contrast enhancement on **(b)** coronal and **(c)** sagittal fat-suppressed T1-weighted imaging (*arrows*).

Table 4.8 *(cont.)*   Lesions involving the oropharynx, oral cavity, and floor of the mouth

Lesion	Imaging Findings	Comments
Epidermal inclusion cyst: dermoid (**Fig. 4.175** and **Fig. 4.176**)	*MRI:* Well-circumscribed spheroid or multilobulated lesions, usually with high signal on T1-weighted images, variable low, intermediate, and/or high signal on T2-weighted imaging, and no gadolinium contrast enhancement. *CT:* Well-circumscribed spheroid or multilobulated lesions, usually with low attenuation, ± fat–fluid or fluid–debris levels.	Nonneoplastic congenital or acquired ectodermal-inclusion cystic lesions filled with lipid material, cholesterol, desquamated cells, and keratinaceous debris surrounded by a wall lined by keratinizing squamous epithelium. Lesions result from congenital inclusion of dermal elements during embryonic development of the first and second branchial arches, or from trauma. Dermoid csysts occur in males slightly more than in females, ± related clinical symptoms. If a dermoid cyst ruptures, it can cause chemical inflammation. Occurs more commonly in the submandibular space than in the floor of the mouth.
Teratoma	*MRI:* Lesions usually have circumscribed margins and can contain various combinations and proportions of zones with low, intermediate, and/or high signal on T1-weighted imaging (T1WI), T2-weighted imaging (T2WI), and fat-suppressed (FS) T2WI. Can contain teeth and zones of bone formation, as well as amorphous, clumplike, and/or curvilinear calcifications with low signal on T1WI, T2WI, and FS T2WI. Fluid–fluid and fat–fluid levels may be seen within teratomas. Gadolinium contrast enhancement is usually seen in solid portions and septa. Invasion of adjacent tissue and bone destruction, as well as metastases, are findings associated with malignant teratomas. *CT:* Can contain zones with low and intermediate attenuation with or without calcifications.	Teratomas are neoplasms that arise from displaced embryonic germ cells (multipotent germinal cells) and contain various combinations of cells and tissues derived from more than one germ layer (endoderm, mesoderm, ectoderm). Teratomas are the second most common type of germ cell tumors, occur in children and in males more than in females. There are benign or malignant types, composed of derivatives of ectoderm, mesoderm, and/or endoderm. Mature teratomas have differentiated cells from ectoderm (brain, skin, and/or choroid plexus), mesoderm (cartilage, bone, muscle, and/or fat), and endoderm (cysts with enteric or respiratory epithelia). Immature teratomas contain partially differentiated ectodermal, mesodermal, or endodermal cells.

(continued on page 448)

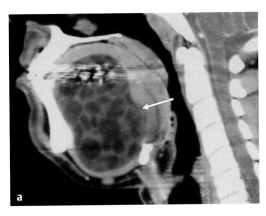
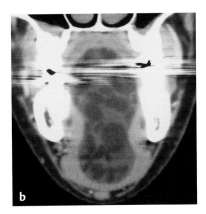

Fig. 4.175 A 30-year-old woman with a large dermoid cyst (*arrow*) at the floor of the mouth that has mixed low and intermediate attenuation on **(a)** sagittal (*arrow*) and **(b)** coronal CT.

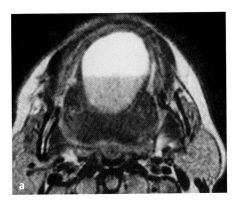
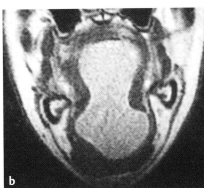
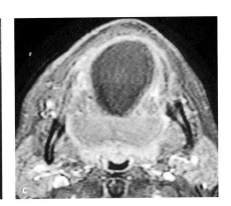

Fig. 4.176 A 75-year-old woman with a dermoid cyst at the floor of the mouth that has high signal on **(a)** axial and **(b)** coronal T2-weighted imaging, and **(c)** low signal without gadolinium contrast enhancement on axial fat-suppressed T1-weighted imaging. A fluid–fluid level is seen on axial T2-weighted imaging **(a)**.

Table 4.8 *(cont.)* Lesions involving the oropharynx, oral cavity, and floor of the mouth

Lesion	Imaging Findings	Comments
Venolymphatic malformation (**Fig. 4.177**)	Can be circumscribed lesions or occur in an infiltrative pattern with extension into soft tissue and between muscles. *MRI:* Often contain single or multiple cystic zones that can be large (macrocystic type) or small (microcystic type), and that have predominantly low signal on T1-weighted imaging (T1WI) and high signal on T2-weighted imaging (T2WI) and fat-suppressed T2WI. Fluid–fluid levels and zones with high signal on T1WI and variable signal on T2WI may result from cysts containing hemorrhage, high protein concentration, and/or necrotic debris. Septa between the cystic zones can vary in thickness and gadolinium (Gd) contrast enhancement. Nodular zones within the lesions can have variable degrees of Gd contrast enhancement. Microcystic lesions typically show more Gd contrast enhancement than the macrocystic type.	Benign vascular anomalies (also referred to as lymphangioma and cystic hygroma) that primarily result from abnormal lymphangiogenesis. Up to 75% occur in the head and neck. Can be observed in utero with MRI or sonography, at birth (50–65%), or within the first 5 years, and ~ 85% are detected by age 2. Lesions are composed of endothelium-lined lymphatic ± venous channels interspersed within connective tissue stroma. Account for less than 1% of benign soft tissue tumors and 5.6% of all benign lesions of infancy and childhood. Can occur in association with Turner syndrome and Proteus syndrome.
Lingual thyroglossal duct cyst (**Fig. 4.178**)	*MRI:* Well-circumscribed spheroid or ovoid lesion at the tongue base that usually has low signal on T1-weighted imaging (T1WI) and diffusion-weighted imaging and high signal on T2-weighted imaging (T2WI). The wall of the thyroglossal duct cyst is typically thin, without gadolinium (Gd) contrast enhancement. Thyroglossal cysts complicated by hemorrhage, current or prior infection can have elevated protein with intermediate to slightly high signal on T1WI and T2WI. The walls of such cysts can be thick and show Gd contrast enhancement. Nodular Gd contrast enhancement involving the wall of a thyroglossal duct cyst can be seen with a potentially malignant lesion. *CT:* Well-circumscribed lesion with low (mucoid) attenuation ranging from 10 to 25 Hounsfield units, surrounded by a thin wall. Occasionally contain thin septations. Thyroglossal duct cysts complicated by infection can have increased attenuation, thick walls, and loss/indistinctness of adjacent tissue planes. *Ultrasound:* Can be well-circumscribed anechoic cysts with through transmission or have a pseudosolid appearance related to elevated protein concentration.	Thyroglossal duct cyst is the most common congenital mass in the neck and is related to altered development of the thyroid gland. The follicular cells of the thyroid gland develop from endodermal cells (median thyroid anlage) located between the first and second pharyngeal arches in the first 3 weeks of gestation. At 24 days of gestation, a small pit (thyroid bud) forms within the thyroid anlage that progressively develops into a bilobed diverticulum that extends inferiorly along the midline adjacent to the aortic primordium. A small channel (thyroglossal duct) temporarily exists between the dorsal portion of the tongue (foramen cecum) and the inferiorly descending thyroid primordium. The thyroglossal duct normally involutes by the tenth week of gestation. The descending thyroid primordium and thyroglossal duct course anterior to the hyoid bone and loop slightly posterior to the inferior margin of the hyoid bone before descending anterior to the thyrohyoid membrane, thyroid cartilage, and trachea. The thyroglossal duct extends between the sternohyoid and sternothyroid strap muscles. The descending thyroid primordium reaches is normal position in the lower neck at 7 weeks of gestation. The parafollicular cells (C cells) of the thyroid develop from endodermal cells (lateral thyroid anlage) at the fourth pharyngeal pouch and migrate to join and merge with the descending thyroid primordium from the median thyroid anlage. Up to two-thirds of thyroglossal duct cysts occur in the infrahyoid neck and can be midline or extend laterally within, or deep to, the strap muscles. Nearly 50% present in patients younger than 20 years, as a progressively enlarging neck lesion.

(continued on page 450)

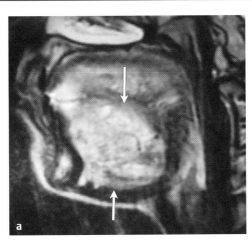 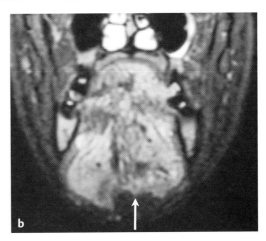

Fig. 4.177 **(a)** A 20-year-old woman with a venolymphatic malformation involving the lower tongue that has heterogeneous, mostly high signal on sagittal T2-weighted imaging (*arrows*) and **(b)** shows gadolinium contrast enhancement on coronal fat-suppressed T1-weighted imaging (*arrow*).

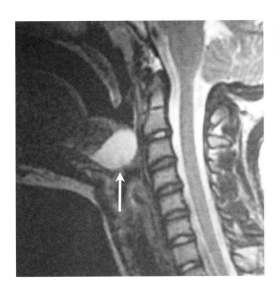

Fig. 4.178 An 11-year-old female with a lingual thyroglossal duct cyst that is seen as a circumscribed lesion at the base of the tongue and foramen cecum (*arrow*) with high signal on sagittal T2-weighted imaging.

Table 4.8 *(cont.)*   Lesions involving the oropharynx, oral cavity, and floor of the mouth

Lesion	Imaging Findings	Comments
Lingual thyroid (**Fig. 4.179** and **Fig. 4.180**)	*MRI:* Circumscribed lesions with low-intermediate signal on T1-weighted imaging and low, intermediate, or slightly high signal on T2-weighted imaging. Variable degrees of gadolinium contrast enhancement. *CT:* Circumscribed ovoid or spheroid lesion at the dorsal portion (base) of the tongue that shows slightly increased attenuation (~ 70 HU), and prominent contrast enhancement, ± low-attenuation thyroid nodules, ± calcifications. *Nuclear medicine:* Iodine-123, iodine-131, or technetium 99m pertechnetate uptake in ectopic thyroid tissue in the tongue and lack of normal uptake in normal orthotopic location of thyroid bed.	The normal thyroid gland is located below the larynx, posterior to the strap muscles, medial to the carotid arteries, and anterolateral to the trachea. Lingual thyroid tissue is a rare developmental anomaly in which ectopic thyroid tissue is located in the posterior portion of the tongue secondary to lack of normal embryologic descent of the primitive thyroid gland along the thyroglossal duct from the foramen cecum at the tongue base down to the lower neck. Represents up to 90% of cases of ectopic thyroid. Can be asymptomatic or can occur in association with dysphagia, dysphonia, and/or stridor.
Foregut duplication cyst of the tongue (**Fig. 4.181**)	*MRI:* Well-circumscribed spheroid or ovoid lesions within the anterior portion of the tongue. Can have low signal on T1-weighted imaging (T1WI) and high signal on T2-weighted imaging (T2WI). Cysts with high protein content or hemorrhage can have intermediate to high signal on T1WI and T2WI, ± fluid–fluid levels. Usually show no gadolinium contrast enhancement. *CT:* Circumscribed lesion in the anterior tongue with low-intermediate attenuation. Usually no contrast enhancement.	During the fourth week of gestation, the primitive endodermal gut tube forms. The cranial portion of the gut tube is the foregut, which gives rise to the pharynx, respiratory tract, esophagus, stomach, and proximal duodenum. A foregut duplications cyst is a malformation considered to be a choristoma, in which there is a mass of histologically normal foregut alimentary tissue in an abnormal location, with attachment to the gastrointestinal tract wall but typically without actual communication with the intestinal lumen. Foregut duplication cysts occur from persistent communication between the ventrally located endoderm and the dorsally located ectoderm secondary to developmental failure of separation of the notochord and foregut. Obliteration of portions of a dorsal enteric sinus can result in cysts lined by stratified ciliated respiratory-type or gastrointestinal epithelial cells. Includes bronchogenic, esophageal, or neurenteric cysts. Lingual duplication cysts account for 0.3% of foregut duplication cysts. Associated with increased risk of airway obstruction. Often present in infancy.

(continued on page 452)

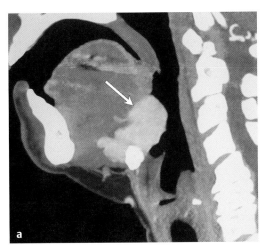
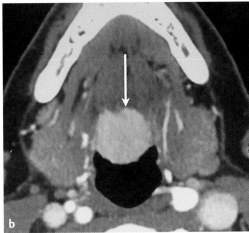

Fig. 4.179 A 52-year-old woman with a lingual thyroid that is seen as a high-attenuation enhancing lesion at the base of the tongue on (a) sagittal and (b) axial CT (*arrows*).

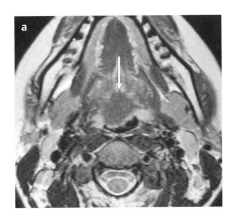
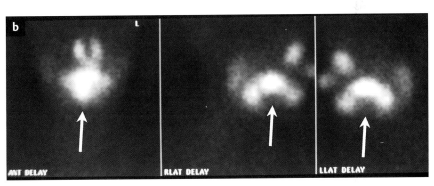

Fig. 4.180 (a) A 22-year-old woman with a lingual thyroid seen at the base of the tongue with low-intermediate signal on axial T2-weighted imaging (*arrow*). (b) Radionuclide exam shows iodine-123 uptake in ectopic thyroid tissue in the tongue (*arrows*) and lack of normal uptake in the normal orthotopic location of the thyroid bed.

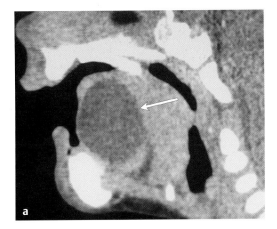
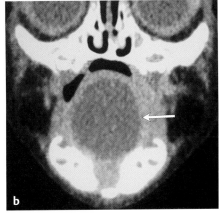

Fig. 4.181 (a) Sagittal and (b) coronal CT of a 2-month-old male show a foregut duplication cyst with fluid attenuation (*arrows*) in the anterior tongue.

Table 4.8 *(cont.)* Lesions involving the oropharynx, oral cavity, and floor of the mouth

Lesion	Imaging Findings	Comments
Benign Neoplasms		
Pleomorphic adenoma of sublingual gland or minor salivary gland (**Fig. 4.182**)	*MRI:* Circumscribed lesions with low-intermediate signal on T1-weighted imaging, slightly high signal on T2-weighted imaging (T2WI) and fat-suppressed T2WI, and usually show gadolinium contrast enhancement. *CT:* Circumscribed or lobulated lesions with intermediate attenuation, + contrast enhancement.	Pleomorphic adenomas arise from sublingual gland or minor salivary gland and rests in the sublingual space. Composed of modified myoepithelial cells associated with sparse stromal elements. Usually occur in patients between 20 and 60 years old. Other, rare types of minor salivary gland adenomas include myoepithelioma and oncocytoma.
Lipoma (**Fig. 4.183**)	*MRI:* Lipomas have MRI signal isointense to subcutaneous fat on T1-weighted imaging (high signal). On T2-weighted imaging, signal suppression occurs with frequency-selective fat saturation techniques or with a short time to inversion recovery (STIR) method. Typically there is no gadolinium contrast enhancement or peripheral edema. *CT:* Lipomas have CT attenuation similar to subcutaneous fat and typically no contrast enhancement or peripheral edema.	Common benign hamartomas composed of mature white adipose tissue without cellular atypia. Most common soft tissue tumor, representing 16% of all soft tissue tumors.
Hemangioma (**Fig. 4.184**)	*MRI:* Circumscribed or poorly marginated structures (< 4 cm in diameter) in bone marrow or soft tissue with intermediate-high signal on T1-weighted imaging (often isointense to marrow fat) and high signal on T2-weighted imaging (T2WI) and fat-suppressed T2WI, typically with gadolinium contrast enhancement, ± expansion of bone. *CT:* Expansile bone lesions with a radiating pattern of bony trabeculae oriented toward the center. Hemangiomas in soft tissue have mostly intermediate attenuation, ± zones of fat attenuation.	Benign lesions of bone or soft tissue composed of capillary, cavernous, and/or malformed venous vessels. Considered to be a hamartomatous disorder. Occur in patients 1 to 84 years old (median age = 33 years).

(continued on page 454)

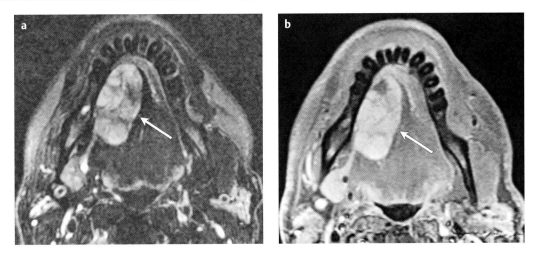

Fig. 4.182 **(a)** A 62-year-old man with a pleomorphic adenoma of the right sublingual gland that has circumscribed margins and mixed low, intermediate, slightly high, and high signal on axial fat-suppressed T2-weighted imaging (*arrow*). **(b)** The adenoma shows heterogeneous gadolinium contrast enhancement on axial fat-suppressed T1-weighted imaging (*arrow*).

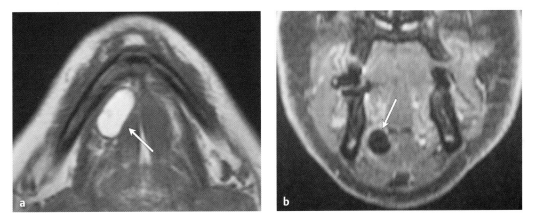

Fig. 4.183 **(a)** Sublingual lipoma on the right that has high signal on axial T1-weighted imaging (*arrow*) and **(b)** nulled signal on postcontrast fat-suppressed T1-weighted imaging (*arrow*).

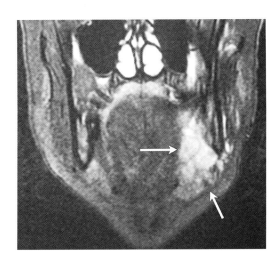

Fig. 4.184 A 33-year-old woman with a hemangioma involving the left lower portion of the tongue and floor of the mouth that has high signal on coronal fat-suppressed T2-weighted imaging (*arrows*).

Table 4.8 *(cont.)*   Lesions involving the oropharynx, oral cavity, and floor of the mouth

Lesion	Imaging Findings	Comments
Schwannoma (**Fig. 4.185**)	*MRI:* Circumscribed ovoid or spheroid lesions with low-intermediate signal on T1-weighted imaging, high signal on T2-weighted imaging (T2WI) and fat-suppressed T2WI, and usually prominent gadolinium (Gd) contrast enhancement. High signal on T2WI and Gd contrast enhancement can be heterogeneous in large lesions due to cystic degeneration and/or hemorrhage. *CT:* Circumscribed spheroid or ovoid lesions with intermediate attenuation, + contrast enhancement. Large lesions can have cystic degeneration and/or hemorrhage.	Schwannomas are benign encapsulated tumors that contain differentiated neoplastic Schwann cells. They most commonly occur as solitary, sporadic lesions. Multiple schwannomas are often associated with neurofibromatosis type 2 (NF2), which is an autosomal dominant disease involving a gene mutation at chromosome 22q12. In addition to schwannomas, patients with NF2 can also have multiple meningiomas and ependymomas. The incidence of NF2 is 1/37,000 to 1/50,000 newborns. Age at presentation is 22 to 72 years (mean age = 46 years). Peak incidence is in the fourth to sixth decades. Many patients with NF2 present in the third decade with bilateral vestibular schwannomas.
Tumorlike Lesions		
Simple ranula (**Fig. 4.186**)	*MRI:* Circumscribed structures in the floor of the mouth with low signal on T1-weighted imaging, FLAIR, and diffusion-weighted imaging, and high signal on T2-weighted imaging. Typically show no gadolinium contrast enhancement unless there is superimposed infection. *CT:* Circumscribed lesions with fluid attenuation in the contents.	Simple ranulas are mucous retention cysts lined by epithelial cells that arise from the sublingual gland or minor salivary gland. Can result from trauma or inflammation of salivary glands. Can occasionally extend into the submandibular space through a defect in the mylohyoid muscle.

(continued on page 456)

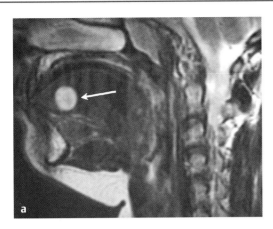
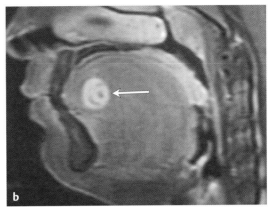

Fig. 4.185 **(a)** A 13-year-old female with a small schwannoma within the tongue that has high signal on sagittal T2-weighted imaging (*arrow*) and **(b)** shows gadolinium contrast enhancement on sagittal fat-suppressed T1-weighted imaging (*arrow*).

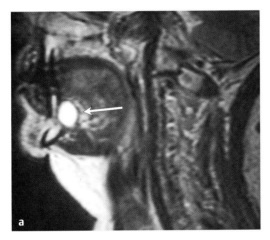
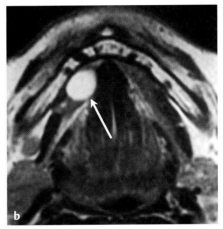

Fig. 4.186 A 60-year-old woman with a simple ranula at the right floor of the mouth that has high signal on **(a)** sagittal and **(b)** axial T2-weighted imaging (*arrows*).

Table 4.8 *(cont.)* Lesions involving the oropharynx, oral cavity, and floor of the mouth

Lesion	Imaging Findings	Comments
Plunging (diving) ranula (**Fig. 4.187**, **Fig. 4.188**, and **Fig. 4.189**)	*MRI:* Circumscribed structures in the floor of the mouth with low signal on T1-weighted imaging, FLAIR, and diffusion-weighted imaging, and high signal on T2-weighted imaging. The ruptured portion of the ranula often has a tubular shape prior to its inferior extension into the submandibular space. Typically shows no gadolinium contrast enhancement unless there is superimposed infection. *CT:* Circumscribed lesions with fluid attenuation.	Plunging or diving ranulas are ranulas that rupture and extend posteriorly beyond the dorsal margin of the mylohyoid muscle, with subsequent inferior extension into the submandibular space. The ruptured portion of the lesion is not enclosed by an epithelial lining and is therefore considered a pseudocyst.
Malignant Tumors		
Squamous cell carcinoma (**Fig. 4.190**)	*MRI:* Lesions in the nasal cavity, paranasal sinuses, nasopharynx and oropharynx, ± perineural spread. Lesions have intermediate signal on T1-weighted imaging, intermediate to slightly high signal on T2-weighted imaging, and mild gadolinium contrast enhancement. Can be large lesions (± necrosis and/or hemorrhage). *CT:* Tumors have intermediate attenuation and mild contrast enhancement and can be large lesions (± necrosis and/or hemorrhage).	Malignant epithelial tumors of both keratinizing and nonkeratinizing types. Account for 80% of malignant oropharyngeal tumors and 3% of malignant tumors of the head and neck. Occur in adults, usually more than 55 years old, and in males more than in females. Associated with occupational or other exposure to tobacco smoke, nickel, chlorophenols, chromium, mustard gas, radium, and material in the manufacture of wood products.

(continued on page 458)

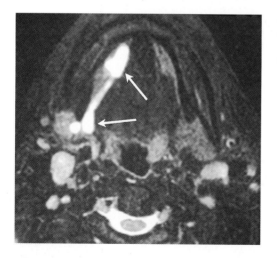

Fig. 4.187 A 38-year-old woman with a plunging (diving) ranula with high signal on axial fat-suppressed T2-weighted imaging (*arrows*) extending from the anterior right floor of the mouth posteriorly to the dorsal margin of the mylohyoid margin on the right.

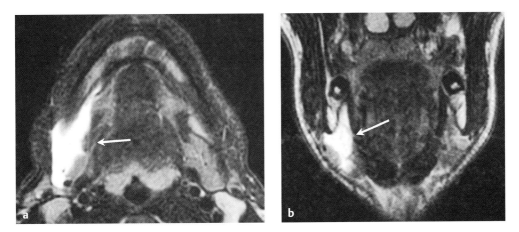

Fig. 4.188   An 18-year-old man with a plunging (diving) ranula with high signal on **(a)** axial fat-suppressed T2-weighted imaging (*arrow*) and **(b)** coronal T2-weighted imaging (*arrow*) extending posteriorly from the right floor of the mouth below the dorsal margin of the mylohyoid muscle.

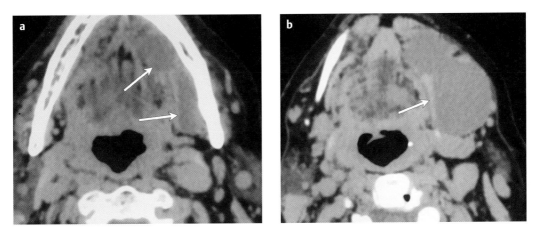

Fig. 4.189   **(a,b)** Axial CT images show a large plunging (diving) ranula on the left that has fluid attenuation (*arrows*).

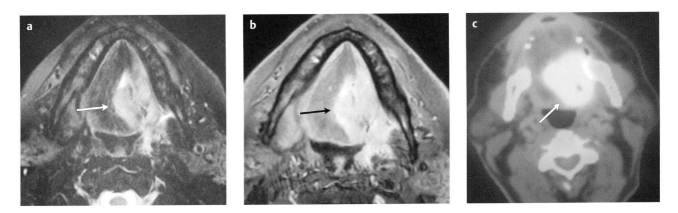

Fig. 4.190   A 64-year-old man with a squamous cell carcinoma involving the left portion of the tongue that extends across the midline and that has **(a)** heterogeneous high signal on axial fat-suppressed T2-weighted imaging (*arrow*), **(b)** gadolinium contrast enhancement on axial fat-suppressed T1-weighted imaging (*arrow*), and **(c)** abnormally high uptake of F-18 FDG on axial PET/CT (*arrow*).

Table 4.8 *(cont.)*   Lesions involving the oropharynx, oral cavity, and floor of the mouth

Lesion	Imaging Findings	Comments
Adenoid cystic carcinoma **(Fig. 4.191)**	*MRI:* Lesions involving major or minor salivary glands in the oral cavity. Lesions have intermediate signal on T1-weighted imaging, intermediate to high signal on T2-weighted imaging, and variable mild, moderate, or prominent gadolinium contrast enhancement. *CT:* Tumors have intermediate attenuation and variable mild, moderate, or prominent contrast enhancement. Destruction of adjacent bone is commonly seen.	Basaloid tumor of salivary gland origin composed of neoplastic epithelial and myoepithelial cells. Morphologic tumor patterns include tubular, cribriform, and solid. Accounts for 10% of epithelial salivary neoplasms. Most commonly involves the parotid, submandibular, and minor salivary glands (palate, tongue, buccal mucosa, floor of the mouth, and other locations, including the prestyloid parapharyngeal space). Perineural tumor spread is common, ± facial nerve paralysis. Usually occurs in adults > 30 years old. Solid type has the worst prognosis. Up to 90% of patients die within 10–15 years of diagnosis.
Adenocarcinoma and mucoepidermoid carcinoma **(Fig. 4.192)**	*MRI:* Malignant lesions in the oral cavity that often have intermediate signal on T1-weighted imaging, intermediate to high signal on T2-weighted imaging, and variable mild, moderate, or prominent gadolinium contrast enhancement. Can be associated with bone destruction and perineural tumor spread. *CT:* Tumors have intermediate attenuation and variable mild, moderate, or prominent contrast enhancement. Destruction of adjacent bone is commonly seen.	Second and third most common malignant tumors derived from salivary glands. Adenocarcinomas contain small to medium-size neoplastic cells with oval nuclei, typically immunoreactive to cytokeratin, vimentin, and S-100 protein. Mucoepidermoid carcinomas often have solid portions with basaloid or cuboidal neoplastic cells and cystic portions containing sialomucin lined by mucous cells with peripheral nuclei within pale cytoplasm. Tumors usually are intermediate to high grade and often are advanced at presentation, ± metastases, ± perineural tumor spread.
Non-Hodgkin lymphoma	*MRI:* Lesions have low-intermediate signal on T1-weighted imaging and intermediate to slightly high signal on T2-weighted imaging, + gadolinium contrast enhancement. Can be locally invasive and associated with bone erosion/destruction. *CT:* Lesions have low-intermediate attenuation and may show contrast enhancement, ± bone destruction.	Lymphomas are a group of tumors whose neoplastic cells typically arise within lymphoid tissue (lymph nodes and reticuloendothelial organs). Most lymphomas in the nasopharynx, nasal and oral cavities, and paranasal sinuses are non-Hodgkin lymphomas (B-cell types are more common than T-cell types) and more commonly are related to disseminated disease than to primary sinonasal tumors. Sinonasal lymphoma has a poor prognosis, with a 5-year survival of less than 65%.
Metastatic malignancies	*MRI:* Circumscribed spheroid lesions that often have low-intermediate signal on T1-weighted imaging, intermediate to high signal on T2-weighted imaging, ± hemorrhage, calcifications, and cysts, and variable gadolinium contrast enhancement. *CT:* Lesions usually have low-intermediate attenuation, ± hemorrhage, calcifications, and cysts, variable contrast enhancement, ± bone destruction, ± compression of neural tissue or vessels.	Primary extracranial tumor source: lung > breast > GI > GU > melanoma. Can occur as single or multiple well-circumscribed or poorly defined lesions. Metastatic tumor may cause variable destructive or infiltrative changes in single or multiple sites.
Rhabdomyosarcoma	*MRI:* Tumors can have circumscribed and/or poorly defined margins and typically have low-intermediate signal on T1-weighted imaging and heterogeneous signal (various combinations of intermediate, slightly high, and/or high signal) on T2-weighted imaging (T2WI) and fat-suppressed T2WI. Tumors show variable degrees of gadolinium contrast enhancement, ± bone destruction and invasion. *CT:* Soft tissue lesions that usually can have circumscribed or irregular margins. Calcifications are uncommon. Tumors can have mixed CT attenuation, with solid zones of soft tissue attenuation, cystic appearing and/or necrotic zones, and occasional foci of hemorrhage, ± bone invasion and destruction.	Malignant mesenchymal tumors with rhabdomyoblastic differentiation that occur primarily in soft tissue, and only very rarely in bone. There are three subgroups of rhabdomyosarcoma: embryonal (50–70%), alveolar (18–45%), and pleomorphic (5–10%). Embryonal and alveolar rhabdomyosarcomas occur primarily in children < 10 years old, and pleomorphic rhabdomyosarcomas occur mostly in adults (median age in the sixth decade). Alveolar and pleomorphic rhabdomyosarcomas occur frequently in the extremities. Embryonal rhabdomyosarcomas occur mostly in the head and neck.

(continued on page 460)

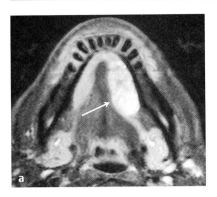
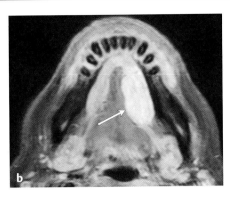
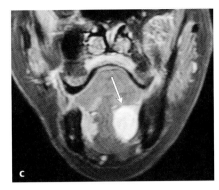

Fig. 4.191 A 51-year-old man with adenoid cystic carcinoma (*arrows*) involving the left sublingual gland that has heterogeneous high signal on **(a)** axial fat-suppressed T2-weighted imaging (*arrow*). The lesion shows gadolinium contrast enhancement on **(b)** axial and **(c)** coronal fat-suppressed T1-weighted imaging (*arrows*).

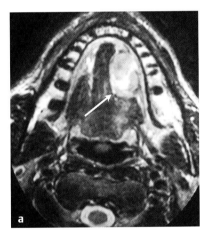
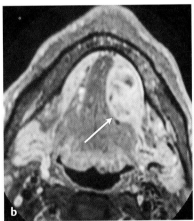
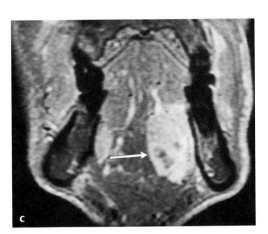

Fig. 4.192 **(a)** A 63-year-old man with adenocarcinoma involving the left sulingual gland that has heterogeneous slightly high and high signal on axial T2-weighted imaging (*arrow*). The lesion shows heterogeneous gadolinium contrast enhancement on **(b)** axial and **(c)** coronal fat-suppressed T1-weighted imaging (*arrows*).

Table 4.8 *(cont.)* Lesions involving the oropharynx, oral cavity, and floor of the mouth

Lesion	Imaging Findings	Comments
Inflammatory Lesions		
Phlegmon/abscess at the floor of the mouth (**Fig. 4.193**)	*MRI:* Phlegmon appears as soft tissue thickening at the floor of the mouth, with poorly defined slightly high to high signal on T2-weighted imaging (T2WI) and fat-suppressed T2WI. Abscesses are collections with high signal on T2WI and diffusion-weighted imaging surrounded by a peripheral rim of gadolinium contrast enhancement. *CT:* Abscesses appear as a fluid collection with rim enhancement and adjacent abnormal soft tissue thickening. Abnormal soft tissue thickening without a rim-enhancing collection is seen with a phlegmon.	Infections involving the floor of the mouth can result from spread of dental/mandibular infections, trauma, bacteremia/sepsis, and/or calculi obstructing the submandibular duct.
Ludwig angina (**Fig. 4.194**)	*CT:* Extensive abnormal soft tissue thickening with ill-defined margins and containing low-attenuation fluid zones involving the floor of the mouth and that often extend into the submandibular, pharyngeal, and/or parapharyngeal spaces, ± narrowing or obstruction of the airway.	Severe cellulitis at the floor of the mouth that can progress and extend inferiorly into the mediastinum, causing chest pain. Commonly results from infection of teeth and mandible, with involvement of adjacent soft tissues, or as a complication of dental surgery. Considered a life-threatening condition, it has a mortality rate of up to 10%. Often requires surgical management.
Granulomatosis with polyangiitis	*MRI:* Poorly defined zones of mucosal soft tissue thickening, with low-intermediate signal on T1-weighted imaging, slightly high to high signal on T2-weighted imaging, and gadolinium contrast enhancement within the nasal cavity, paranasal sinuses, nasopharynx, oropharynx, orbits, infratemporal fossa, and external auditory canal, ± invasion and destruction of bone and cartilage, ± extension into the skull base with involvement of the dura, leptomeninges, brain, or venous sinuses. *CT:* Zones with soft tissue attenuation, ± bone destruction.	Multisystem autoimmune disease with necrotizing granulomas in the respiratory tract, focal necrotizing angiitis of small arteries and veins of various tissues, and glomerulonephritis. Can involve the oral cavity, paranasal sinuses, orbits, skull base, dura, leptomeninges, and the temporal bone. Typically, positive immunoreactivity to cytoplasmic antineutrophil cytoplasmic antibody (c-ANCA). Treatment includes corticosteroids, cyclophosphamide, and anti-TNF agents.
Submandibular duct stone/ sialadenitis (**Fig. 4.195**)	*MRI:* Calculi typically have low signal on T1-weighted imaging and T2-weighted imaging (T2WI). Dilatation of ducts with high signal on T2WI may be seen within the submandibular gland. Calculi can also be seen low-signal foci on susceptibility-weighted imaging. The submandibular gland may be enlarged, with increased signal on T2WI and increased gadolinium contrast enhancement compared with the contralateral normal gland. MR sialography using heavily weighted T2WI via 3D constructive interference in the steady state technique or 3D fast/turbo spin echo techniques can show dilated ducts with high signal and intraluminal defects from stones. *CT:* Calculi typically have high attenuation. Dilated ducts can be seen proximal to the obstructing stone as well as within the submandibular gland. The submandibular gland can be enlarged and show increased contrast enhancement.	Sialolithiasis is the formation of calculi within salivary ducts and is the most common disorder of major salivary glands. Results from deposition of calcium salts over a core of desquamated epithelial cells, mucus, foreign bodies, or bacteria. Can occur as single or multiple ductal stones per patient. Sialoliths can measure up to 9 mm (mean size ranges from 3 to 4 mm). Sialoliths (calculi) occur more frequently in Wharton's duct of the submandibular gland (up to 80% of cases) than Stensen's duct of the parotid gland because of its upward configuration and its saliva, relatively high concentrations of phosphates and hydroxyapatites, and is more alkaline and viscous than the parotid saliva. Sialoliths can result in diffuse submandibular gland enlargement and susceptibility to superimposed infection. Treatment can be via sialendoscopic extraction or surgery.

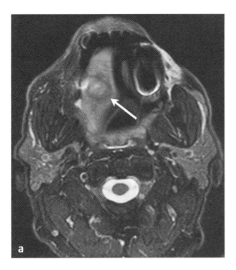
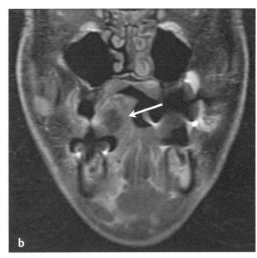

Fig. 4.193 **(a)** A 64-year-old man with a phlegmon with early abscess formation in the right side of the oral cavity on axial fat-suppressed T2-weighted imaging (*arrow*). **(b)** There is corresponding abnormal gadolinium contrast enhancement on coronal fat-suppressed T1-weighted imaging (*arrow*).

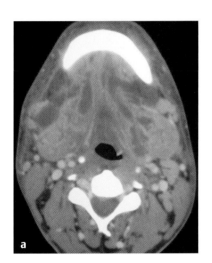
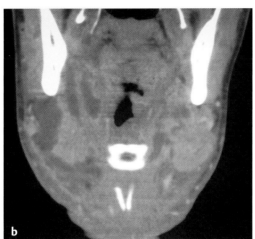

Fig. 4.194 Ludwig angina. **(a)** Axial and **(b)** coronal CT images of a 52-year-old man show extensive, abnormal, irregular soft tissue thickening containing low-attenuation fluid zones in the floor of the mouth and extending into the submandibular spaces bilaterally.

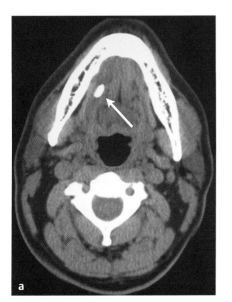
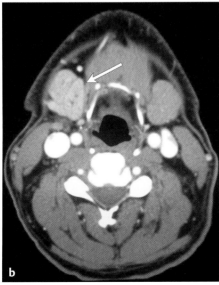

Fig. 4.195 **(a)** Axial CT of a 36-year-old man shows a stone (*arrow*) in the right submandibular (Wharton's) duct. **(b)** Axial postcontrast CT shows asymmetric enlargement and increased contrast enhancement of the right submandibular gland (*arrow*) compared to the normal left submandibular gland, representing inflammation related to the ductal obstruction.

4.9 Submandibular Space Lesions

The submandibular space is the most inferior anatomic space of the suprahyoid neck and is located below the mylohyoid muscle and above the hyoid bone. The superficial layer of the deep cervical fascia splits and encloses the submandibular space. The inner fascial layer is adjacent to the lower border of the mylohyoid muscle, and the outer fascial layer is adjacent to the inner margin of the platysma muscle. There is continuity between both sides of the submandibular space because of lack of an intervening fascial layer. The submandibular space is contiguous posteriorly with the sublingual space and inferior portion of the prestyloid parapharyngeal space, and inferiorly with the anterior cervical space. Contained within the submandibular space are the superficial portions of the submandibular glands, anterior bellies of the jugulodigastric muscles, facial veins and arteries, hypoglossal nerve, fat, and lymph nodes. The marginal branch of the facial nerve is located between the outer margin of the submandibular gland and the platysma muscle. The submandibular glands are the second largest salivary glands and are located in the submandibular triangles between the anterior and posterior bellies of the jugulodigastric muscles and the lower border of the mandible. Lymphatic drainage into the submental (Level 1A) and submandibular (Level 1B) nodes occurs from tumors involving the anterior two-thirds of the tongue, floor of the mouth, and sublingual and submandibular glands. Lymphatic drainage from submandibular gland tumors also involves the deep cervical and jugular nodes (usually Level II nodes).

Table 4.9   Submandibular space lesions

- Developmental/Congenital Abnormalities
  - Epidermoid
  - Dermoid
  - Teratoma
  - Venolymphatic malformation
  - Thyroglossal duct cyst
  - Branchial cleft cyst
- Benign Neoplasms
  - Pleomorphic adenoma of submandibular gland
  - Lipoma
  - Hemangioma
  - Schwannoma
  - Paraganglioma
- Tumorlike Lesions
  - Plunging (diving) ranula
  - Castleman's disease
- Malignant Tumors
  - Adenocarcinoma and mucoepidermoid carcinoma
  - Adenoid cystic carcinoma
  - Acinic cell carcinoma
  - Squamous cell carcinoma
  - Non-Hodgkin lymphoma (NHL)
  - Leukemia
  - Metastatic malignancies
- Inflammatory Lesions
  - Lymphadenitis (reactive adenopathy; presuppurative and suppurative adenopathy)
  - Phlegmon/abscess
  - Ludwig angina
  - Viral lymphadenopathy
  - Submandibular duct stone/sialadenitis
  - Sjögren's syndrome
  - Sarcoidosis

Table 4.9 Submandibular space lesions

Lesion	Imaging Findings	Comments
Developmental/Congenital Abnormalities		
Epidermoid (See **Fig. 4.173** and **Fig. 4.174**)	*MRI:* Well-circumscribed spheroid or multilobulated ectodermal-inclusion cystic lesions with low-intermediate signal on T1-weighted imaging, high signal on T2- and diffusion-weighted imaging, mixed low, intermediate, or high signal on FLAIR images, and no gadolinium contrast enhancement. Epidermoids occur more frequently at the floor of the mouth in the midline than in the submandibular space. *CT:* Well-circumscribed spheroid or multilobulated extra-axial ectodermal-inclusion cystic lesions with low-intermediate attenuation.	Nonneoplastic congenital or acquired lesions filled with desquamated cells and keratinaceous debris surrounded by a wall lined by simple squamous epithelium. Lesions result from congenital inclusion of epidermal elements during embryonic development of the first and second branchial arches, or from trauma. Often occur in patients between 5 and 50 years old (mean age = 30 years).
Dermoid (**Fig. 4.196**; see **Fig. 4.175**)	*MRI:* Well-circumscribed spheroid or multilobulated lesions, usually with high signal on T1-weighted imaging, variable low, intermediate, and/or high signal on T2-weighted imaging, and no gadolinium contrast enhancement. *CT:* Well-circumscribed spheroid or multilobulated lesions, usually with low attenuation, ± fat–fluid or fluid–debris levels.	Nonneoplastic congenital or acquired ectodermal-inclusion cystic lesions filled with lipid material, cholesterol, desquamated cells, and keratinaceous debris surrounded by a wall lined by keratinizing squamous epithelium. Lesions result from congenital inclusion of dermal elements during embryonic development of the first and second branchial arches, or from trauma. Occur in males slightly more than in females, ± related clinical symptoms. If a dermoid cyst ruptures, it can cause chemical inflammation. Occurs more commonly in the submandibular space than in the floor of the mouth.
Teratoma	*MRI:* Lesions usually have circumscribed margins and can contain various combinations and proportions of zones with low, intermediate, and/or high signal on T1-weighted imaging (T1WI), T2-weighted imaging (T2WI), and fat-suppressed (FS) T2WI. May contain teeth and zones of bone formation, as well as amorphous, clumplike, and/or curvilinear calcifications with low signal on T1WI, T2WI, and FS T2WI. Fluid–fluid and fat–fluid levels may be seen within teratomas. Gadolinium contrast enhancement is usually seen in solid portions and septa. Invasion of adjacent tissue and bone destruction, as well as metastases, are findings associated with malignant teratomas. *CT:* Can contain zones with low and intermediate attenuation with or without calcifications.	Teratomas are neoplasms that arise from displaced embryonic germ cells (multipotent germinal cells) and contain various combinations of cells and tissues derived from more than one germ layer (endoderm, mesoderm, ectoderm). They are the second most common type of germ cell tumors, occur in children, are found in males more than in females, have benign and malignant types, and are composed of derivatives of ectoderm, mesoderm, and/or endoderm. Mature teratomas have differentiated cells from ectoderm (brain, skin), mesoderm (cartilage, bone, muscle, and/or fat), and endoderm (cysts with enteric or respiratory epithelia). Immature teratomas contain partially differentiated ectodermal, mesodermal, or endodermal cells.

(continued on page 464)

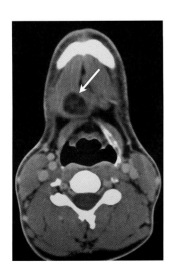

Fig. 4.196 Axial CT shows a dermoid cyst (*arrow*) with low attenuation in the submandibular space.

Table 4.9 *(cont.)*   Submandibular space lesions

Lesion	Imaging Findings	Comments
Venolymphatic malformation (See **Fig. 4.177**)	Can be circumscribed lesions or occur in an infiltrative pattern with extension into soft tissue and between muscles. *MRI:* Often contain single or multiple cystic zones that can be large (macrocystic type) or small (microcystic type), and that have predominantly low signal on T1-weighted imaging (T1WI) and high signal on T2-weighted imaging (T2WI) and fat-suppressed T2WI. Fluid–fluid levels and zones with high signal on T1WI and variable signal on T2WI may result from cysts containing hemorrhage, high protein concentration, and/or necrotic debris. Septa between the cystic zones can vary in thickness and gadolinium (Gd) contrast enhancement. Nodular zones within the lesions can have variable degrees of Gd contrast enhancement. Microcystic lesions typically show more Gd contrast enhancement than the macrocystic type.	Benign vascular anomalies (also referred to as lymphangioma or cystic hygroma) that primarily result from abnormal lymphangiogenesis. Up to 75% occur in the head and neck. Can be observed in utero with MRI or sonography, at birth (50–65%), or within the first 5 years, and ~ 85% are detected by age 2. Lesions are composed of endothelium-lined lymphatic ± venous channels interspersed within connective tissue stroma. Account for less than 1% of benign soft tissue tumors and 5.6% of all benign lesions of infancy and childhood. Can occur in association with Turner syndrome and Proteus syndrome.
Thyroglossal duct cyst (**Fig. 4.197**; see **Fig. 4.178**)	*MRI:* Well-circumscribed spheroid or ovoid lesion at the tongue base that usually has low signal on T1-weighted imaging (T1WI) and diffusion-weighted imaging and high signal on T2-weighted imaging (T2WI). The wall of the thyroglossal duct cyst is typically thin, without gadolinium (Gd) contrast enhancement. Thyroglossal duct cysts complicated by hemorrhage, current or prior infection can have elevated protein, with intermediate to slightly high signal on T1WI and T2WI. The walls of such cysts can be thick and show Gd contrast enhancement. Nodular Gd contrast enhancement involving the wall of a thyroglossal duct cyst can be seen with a potentially malignant lesion. *CT:* Well-circumscribed lesion with low (mucoid) attenuation ranging from 10 to 25 Hounsfield units, surrounded by a thin wall. Occasionally contain thin septations. Thyroglossal duct cysts complicated by infection can have increased attenuation, thick walls, and loss/indistinctness of adjacent tissue planes. *Ultrasound:* Can be well-circumscribed anechoic cysts with through transmission or have a pseudosolid appearance related to elevated protein concentration.	Thyroglossal duct cyst is the most common congenital mass in the neck and is related to altered development of the thyroid gland. The follicular cells of the thyroid gland develop from endodermal cells (median thyroid anlage) located between the first and second pharyngeal arches in the first 3 weeks of gestation. At 24 days of gestation, a small pit (thyroid bud) forms within the thyroid anlage that progressively develops into a bilobed diverticulum that extends inferiorly along the midline adjacent to the aortic primordium. A small channel (thyroglossal duct) temporarily exists between the dorsal portion of the tongue (foramen cecum) and the inferiorly descending thyroid primordium. The thyroglossal duct normally involutes by the tenth week of gestation. The descending thyroid primordium and thyroglossal duct course anterior to the hyoid bone and loop slightly posterior to the inferior margin of the hyoid bone before descending anterior to the thyrohyoid membrane, thyroid cartilage, and trachea. The thyroglossal duct extends between the sternohyoid and sternothyroid strap muscles. The descending thyroid primordium reaches it normal position in the lower neck at 7 weeks of gestation. The parafollicular cells (C cells) of the thyroid develop from endodermal cells (lateral thyroid anlage) at the fourth pharyngeal pouch and migrate to join and merge with the descending thyroid primordium from the median thyroid anlage. Up to two-thirds of thyroglossal duct cysts occur in the infrahyoid neck and can be midline or extend laterally within, or deep to, the strap muscles. Nearly 50% present in patients less than 20 years old as a progressively enlarging neck lesion.

Lesion	Imaging Findings	Comments
Branchial cleft cyst (**Fig. 4.198**)	*MRI:* Circumscribed lesion that often has low-intermediate signal on T1-weighted imaging and high signal on T2-weighted imaging. Usually there is no gadolinium contrast enhancement unless there is superimposed infection. *CT:* Circumscribed, cystic lesion with low to intermediate attenuation depending on the proportions of protein and water. *First branchial cleft cysts* can be located adjacent to the external auditory canal (type 1 first branchial cleft cyst) or superficial portion of the parotid gland, ± extension into the parapharyngeal space, posterior to the submandibular gland, and/or up to the external auditory canal (type 2). *Second branchial cleft cysts* can be anterior to the sternocleidomastoid muscle (SCM) and medial to the carotid arteries (type 1), anteromedial to the SCM with or without extension posterior to the carotid sheath (type 2), or extend into the parapharyngeal space and between the internal and external carotid arteries (type 3). *Third branchial cleft cysts* are located at the lower anterior margin of the SCM at the level of the upper thyroid lobe, ± extension into the sinus tract posterior to the carotid artery and glossopharyngeal nerve, passing through the thyroid membrane above the level of the internal branch of the superior laryngeal nerve into base of the piriform sinus. *Fourth branchial cleft cysts* occur in the lower third of the neck laterally and anterior to the lower SCM and level of the aortic arch, ± visible connecting sinus tract on the right below the subclavian artery or on the left below the aortic arch that extends superiorly and dorsal to the carotid artery up to the level of the hypoglossal nerve and then downward along the SCM to the piriform sinus.	Branchial cleft cysts are developmental anomalies involving the branchial apparatus. The branchial apparatus consists of four major and two rudimentary arches of mesoderm lined by ectoderm externally and endoderm internally within pouches that form at the end of the fourth week of gestation. The mesoderm contains a dominant artery, nerve, cartilage, and muscle. The four major arches are separated by clefts. Each arch develops into a defined neck structure, with eventual obliteration of the branchial clefts. The first arch forms the external auditory canal, eustachian tube, middle ear, and mastoid air cells. The second arch develops into the hyoid bone and tonsillar and supratonsillar fossae. The third and fourth arches develop into the pharynx below the hyoid bone. Branchial anomalies include cysts, sinuses, and fistulae. Second branchial cleft cysts account for up to 90% of all branchial cleft malformations. Cysts are lined by squamous epithelium (90%), ciliated columnar epithelium (8%), or both types (2%). Sebaceous glands, salivary tissue, lymphoid tissue, and cholesterol crystals in mucoid fluid can also occur. There are four types of second branchial cleft cysts. Type 1 is located anterior to the SCM and deep to the platysma muscle. Type 2 (the most common type) is located at the anteromedial surface of the SCM, lateral to the carotid space and posterior to the submandibular gland. Type 3 is located lateral to the pharyngeal wall and medial to the carotid arteries, ± extension between the external and internal carotid arteries (*beak sign*). Type 4 is located between the medial aspect of the carotid sheath and pharynx at the level of the tonsillar fossa and can extend superiorly to the skull base. Typically asymptomatic unless complicated by infection.

(continued on page 466)

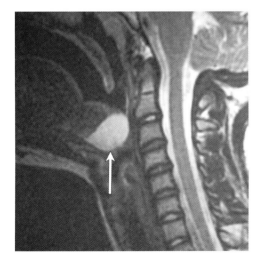

Fig. 4.197 An 11-year-old female with a lingual thyroglossal duct cyst, which is seen as a circumscribed lesion at the base of the tongue and foramen cecum (*arrow*), with high signal on sagittal T2-weighted imaging.

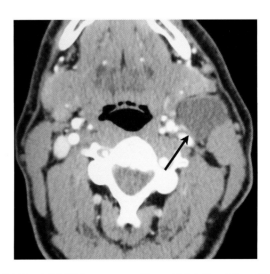

Fig. 4.198 Axial CT shows a second branchial cleft cyst (type 2) posterior to the left submandibular gland, anteromedial to the left SCM, and lateral to the carotid sheath (*arrow*).

Table 4.9 *(cont.)* Submandibular space lesions

Lesion	Imaging Findings	Comments
Benign Neoplasms		
Pleomorphic adenoma of submandibular gland (**Fig. 4.199**)	*MRI:* Circumscribed lesions with low-intermediate signal on T1-weighted imaging, slightly high signal on T2-weighted imaging (T2WI) and fat-suppressed T2WI, and usually gadolinium contrast enhancement. *CT:* Circumscribed or lobulated lesions with intermediate attenuation, + contrast enhancement.	Pleomorphic adenomas arise from the submandibular gland or salivary gland and rests in the submandibular space. Composed of modified myoepithelial cells associated with sparse stromal elements. Usually occur in patients between 20 and 60 years old. Other, rare types of minor salivary gland adenomas include myoepithelioma and oncocytoma.
Lipoma (See **Fig. 4.183**)	*MRI:* Lipomas have MRI signal isointense to subcutaneous fat on T1-weighted imaging (high signal). On T2-weighted imaging, signal suppression occurs with frequency-selective fat saturation techniques or with a short time to inversion recovery (STIR) method. Typically there is no gadolinium contrast enhancement or peripheral edema. *CT:* Lipomas have CT attenuation similar to subcutaneous fat and typically no contrast enhancement or peripheral edema.	Common benign hamartomas composed of mature white adipose tissue without cellular atypia. Most common soft tissue tumor, representing 16% of all soft tissue tumors.
Hemangioma (**Fig. 4.200**)	*MRI:* Circumscribed or poorly marginated structures (< 4 cm in diameter) in bone marrow or soft tissue with intermediate-high signal on T1-weighted imaging (often isointense to marrow fat) and high signal on T2-weighted imaging (T2WI) and fat-suppressed T2WI, typically with gadolinium contrast enhancement, ± expansion of bone. *CT:* Expansile bone lesions with a radiating pattern of bony trabeculae oriented toward the center. Hemangiomas in soft tissue have mostly intermediate attenuation, ± zones of fat attenuation.	Benign lesions of bone or soft tissue composed of capillary, cavernous, and/or malformed venous vessels. Considered to be a hamartomatous disorder. Occur in patients 1 to 84 years old (median age = 33 years).
Schwannoma (**Fig. 4.201**)	*MRI:* Circumscribed spheroid or ovoid lesions with low-intermediate signal on T1-weighted imaging, high signal on T2-weighted imaging (T2WI) and fat-suppressed T2WI, and usually prominent gadolinium (Gd) contrast enhancement. High signal on T2WI and Gd contrast enhancement can be heterogeneous in large lesions due to cystic degeneration and/or hemorrhage. *CT:* Circumscribed spheroid or ovoid lesions with intermediate attenuation, + contrast enhancement. Large lesions can have cystic degeneration and/or hemorrhage.	Schwannomas are benign encapsulated tumors that contain differentiated neoplastic Schwann cells. They most commonly occur as solitary, sporadic lesions. Multiple schwannomas are often associated with neurofibromatosis type 2 (NF2), which is an autosomal dominant disease involving a gene mutation at chromosome 22q12. In addition to schwannomas, patients with NF2 can also have multiple meningiomas and ependymomas. The incidence of NF2 is 1/37,000 to 1/50,000 newborns. Age at presentation is 22 to 72 years (mean age = 46 years). Peak incidence is in the fourth to sixth decades. Many patients with NF2 present in the third decade with bilateral vestibular schwannomas.

(continued on page 468)

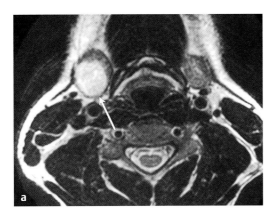

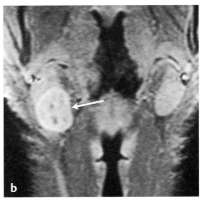

Fig. 4.199 **(a)** A 21-year-old man with a pleomorphic adenoma in the right submandibular gland that has high signal on axial T2-weighted imaging (*arrow*). **(b)** The adenoma shows gadolinium contrast enhancement on coronal fat-suppressed T1-weighted imaging (*arrow*).

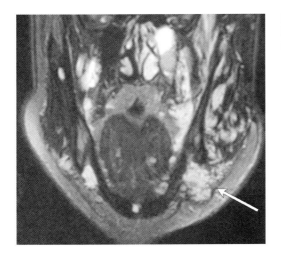

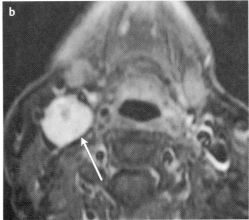

Fig. 4.200 A 2-year-old male with a hemangioma (*arrow*) with high signal on fat-suppressed T2-weighted imaging involving the soft tissues of the left submandibular and masticator spaces as well as the left side of the tongue.

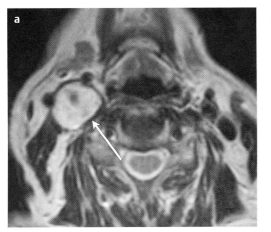

Fig. 4.201 **(a)** Axial T2-weighted imaging shows a schwannoma posterior to the right submandibular gland that has high signal (*arrow*). **(b)** The tumor shows gadolinium contrast enhancement on axial fat-suppressed T1-weighted imaging (*arrow*) and displaces the right carotid artery and jugular vein anteriorly.

Table 4.9 *(cont.)*   Submandibular space lesions

Lesion	Imaging Findings	Comments
Paraganglioma (**Fig. 4.202**)	*MRI:* Circumscribed lesion with intermediate signal on T1-weighted imaging and often heterogeneous intermediate to slightly high signal on T2-weighted imaging, ± small flow voids, + gadolinium contrast enhancement. Can have associated erosive bone changes. *CT:* Spheroid or ovoid lesions with low-intermediate attenuation. Lesions can show contrast enhancement. Often erode adjacent bone.	Benign encapsulated neuroendocrine tumors that arise from neural crest cells associated with autonomic ganglia (paraganglia) throughout the body. Paraganglia cells are chemoreceptors involved in the detection of oxygen, carbon dioxide, and pH. Lesions are also referred to as chemodectomas and are named according to location (carotid body tumor at the carotid artery bifurcation in the neck, glomus typanicum in the middle ear, glomus jugulare in the jugular foramen, etc.). Paragangliomas are the most common tumor of the middle ear. Tumors are typically not immunoreactive to cytokeratins 5/7 and 7, p63, SMA, and S-100 protein.
Tumorlike Lesions		
Plunging (diving) ranula (**Fig. 4.203**; see **Fig. 4.187, Fig. 4.188,** and **Fig. 4.189**)	*MRI:* Circumscribed structures in the floor of the mouth with low signal on T1-weighted imaging, FLAIR, and diffusion-weighted imaging and high signal on T2-weighted imaging. The ruptured portion of the ranula often has a tubular shape prior to its inferior extension into the submandibular space. Typically show no gadolinium contrast enhancement unless there is superimposed infection. *CT:* Circumscribed lesions with fluid attenuation.	Ranulas are mucous retention cysts lined by epithelial cells that arise from the sublingual gland or minor salivary gland. Can result from trauma or inflammation of salivary glands. Plunging or diving ranulas are ranulas that rupture and extend posteriorly beyond the dorsal margin of the mylohyoid muscle, with subsequent inferior extension into the submandibular space. The ruptured portion of the lesion is not enclosed by an epithelial lining and is therefore considered a pseudocyst.
Castleman's disease (See **Fig. 6.16**)	*CT and MRI:* *Multicentric:* Multiple enlarged lymph nodes in the thorax, abdomen, and/or neck, + contrast enhancement, ± calcifications. Lymph node uptake of gallium-67 on radionuclear examinations, and F-18 FDG on PET/CT, are seen with active disease. *Unicentric:* Solitary mass lesion, intermediate attenuation on CT, + contrast enhancement. Intermediate signal on T1-weighted imaging and intermediate to slightly high signal on T2-weighted imaging, + gadolinium contrast enhancement.	Also known as angiofollicular lymph node hyperplasia or giant lymph node hyperplasia. Adenopathy occurs in the thorax (70%), abdomen and pelvis (10 to 15%), and neck (10 to 15%). Can be a unicentric or multicentric disorder. Multicentric Castleman's disease consists of multiple enlarged lymph nodes with extensive accumulation of polyclonal plasma cells in the interfollicular regions. Patients with this type can also have hepatosplenomegaly and usually have a worse prognosis than those with the unicentric type. One variant of the multicentric type occurs in immunocompromised or HIV patients related to infection by the HHV-8 virus. Treatment includes chemotherapy and rituximab. The lymph nodes in unicentric Castleman's disease contain hyalinized vascular follicles with interfollicular capillary proliferations. This type can be treated with surgery and/or radiation and usually has a favorable prognosis.

(continued on page 470)

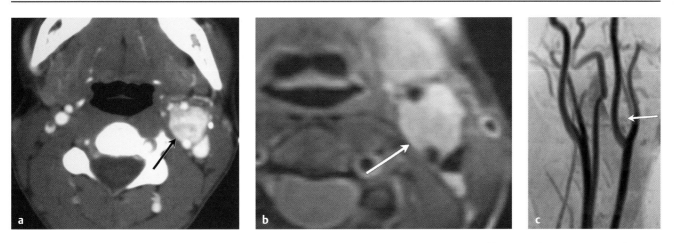

Fig. 4.202   **(a)** Postcontrast axial CT and **(b)** axial fat-suppressed T1-weighted imaging of a 30-year-old woman show a contrast-enhancing paraganglioma (*arrows*) splaying apart the left internal and external carotid arteries, as also seen on **(c)** oblique coronal MRA (*arrow*).

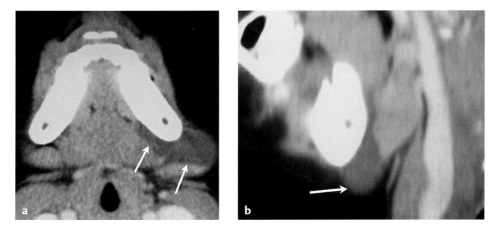

Fig. 4.203   **(a)** Axial and **(b)** sagittal contrast-enhanced CT images of a 4-year-old male show a plunging (diving) ranula (*arrows*) that has fluid attenuation and extends from the floor of the mouth posteriorly and inferiorly below the mylohyoid muscle.

Table 4.9 *(cont.)* Submandibular space lesions

Lesion	Imaging Findings	Comments
Malignant Tumors		
Adenocarcinoma and mucoepidermoid carcinoma (See **Fig. 4.192**)	*MRI:* Malignant lesions in the submandibular gland that often have intermediate signal on T1-weighted imaging, intermediate to high signal on T2-weighted imaging, and variable mild, moderate, or prominent gadolinium contrast enhancement. Can be associated with bone destruction and perineural tumor spread. *CT:* Tumors have intermediate attenuation and variable mild, moderate, or prominent contrast enhancement. Destruction of adjacent bone can be seen.	Mucoepidermoid carcinomas are the most common malignant tumors derived from the submandibular glands. Mucoepidermoid carcinomas account for up to 15% of salivary gland tumors, and 50% occur in the major salivary glands (> 80% occur in the parotid glands, 13% involve the submandibular glands, 4% involve the sublingual glands). Adenocarcinomas contain small to medium-size neoplastic cells with oval nuclei, typically immunoreactive to cytokeratin, vimentin, and S-100 protein. Mucoepidermoid carcinomas often have solid portions with basaloid or cuboidal neoplastic cells and cystic portions containing sialomucin lined by mucous cells with peripheral nuclei within pale cytoplasm. Most commonly occur in the maxillary sinus and nasal cavity. Tumors usually are intermediate to high grade and often are advanced at presentation, ± metastases, ± perineural tumor spread.
Adenoid cystic carcinoma (**Fig. 4.204**; see **Fig. 4.191**)	*MRI:* Lesions involving the submandibular gland. Lesions have intermediate signal on T1-weighted imaging, intermediate to high signal on T2-weighted imaging, and variable mild, moderate, or prominent gadolinium contrast enhancement. *CT:* Tumors have intermediate attenuation and variable mild, moderate, or prominent contrast enhancement. Destruction of adjacent bone is commonly seen.	Basaloid tumor of salivary gland origin composed of neoplastic epithelial and myoepithelial cells. Morphologic tumor patterns include tubular, cribriform, and solid. Accounts for 10% of epithelial salivary neoplasms. Most commonly involves the parotid, submandibular, and minor salivary glands (palate, tongue, buccal mucosa, floor of the mouth, and other locations. Perineural tumor spread is common, ± facial nerve paralysis. Usually occurs in adults > 30 years old. Solid type has the worst prognosis. Up to 90% of patients die within 10–15 years of diagnosis.
Acinic cell carcinoma (See **Fig. 4.94** and **Fig. 4.95**)	*MRI:* Lesions can be solid or solid and cystic. Tumors range in size from 1 to 5 cm (mean = 3 cm). Tumors have low or intermediate signal on T1-weighted imaging and intermediate to high signal on T2-weighted imaging, ± cystic and/or hemorrhagic zones. Tumors show variable mild or moderate heterogeneous gadolinium contrast enhancement. *CT:* Tumors have intermediate attenuation and variable mild, moderate, or prominent contrast enhancement. Destruction of adjacent bone is commonly seen.	Malignant epithelial tumor involving salivary glands composed of tumor cells showing differentiation toward serous acinar cells. The large neoplastic acinar cells have polygonal shapes, round eccentric nuclei within basophilic granular cytoplasm containing PAS-positive zymogen-like granules. Immunoreactive to cytokeratin, transferrin, lactoferrin, a_1-antitrypsin, IgA, and amylase. Occurs in children and in adults more than 20 years old, usually between 38 and 46 years. Accounts for 3% of all salivary gland tumors: 80% occur in the parotid gland, 17% involve the minor salivary glands, 4% occur in the submandibular gland, and 1% involve the sublingual gland. Can be bilateral. Local recurrence rate of 35%. Prognosis is poor for Ki-67 indices of > 10%.
Squamous cell carcinoma (See **Fig. 4.190**)	*MRI:* Lesions in the nasal and oral cavities, floor of the mouth, paranasal sinuses, and nasopharynx, ± intracranial extension via bone destruction or perineural spread. Lesions have intermediate signal on T1-weighted imaging, intermediate to slightly high signal on T2-weighted imaging, and mild gadolinium contrast enhancement. Can be large lesions (± necrosis and/or hemorrhage). *CT:* Tumors have intermediate attenuation and mild contrast enhancement and can be large lesions (± necrosis and/or hemorrhage).	Malignant epithelial tumors that have both keratinizing and nonkeratinizing types. Account for 80% of malignant oropharyngeal tumors and 3% of malignant tumors of the head and neck. Can arise in major salivary glands from metaplasia secondary to chronic inflammation or from metastatic disease. Occur in adults, usually > 55 years old, in males more than in females. Associated with occupational or other exposure to tobacco smoke, nickel, chlorophenols, chromium, mustard gas, radium, and material in the manufacture of wood products.

(continued on page 472)

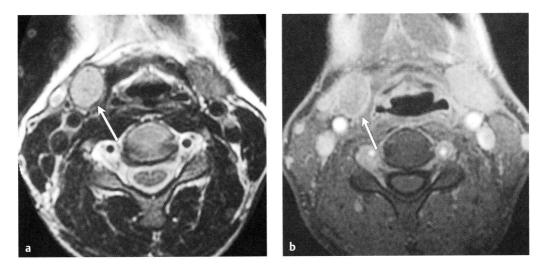

Fig. 4.204 **(a)** Axial T2-weighted imaging of a 32-year-old woman shows an adenoid cystic carcinoma in the right submandibular gland that has slightly high signal (*arrow*). **(b)** The lesion shows mild gadolinium contrast enhancement on axial fat-suppressed T1-weighted imaging (*arrow*).

Table 4.9 *(cont.)* Submandibular space lesions

Lesion	Imaging Findings	Comments
Non-Hodgkin lymphoma (NHL) (**Fig. 4.205**)	*MRI:* Lesions have low-intermediate signal on T1-weighted imaging and intermediate to slightly high signal on T2-weighted imaging, + gadolinium contrast enhancement. Can be locally invasive and associated with bone erosion/destruction. *CT:* Lesions in the submandibular gland have low-intermediate attenuation and may show contrast enhancement, ± bone destruction. Lymphoma also presents in the submandibular space as multiple abnormally enlarged lymph nodes measuring > 15 mm in the short axis.	Lymphomas are a group of tumors whose neoplastic cells typically arise within lymphoid tissue (lymph nodes and reticuloendothelial organs). Primary lymphomas rarely occur in the submandibular gland and are usually NHL (B-cell NHL is more common than T-cell NHL). More commonly occurs as secondary neoplasm from disseminated disease than as primary tumors. Poor prognosis, with 5-year survival of less than 65%.
Leukemia (**Fig. 4.206**)	*MRI:* Acute lymphoblastic leukemia (ALL), chronic lymphocytic leukemia (CLL), acute myelogenous leukemia (AML), and chronic myelogenous leukemia (CML) infiltrate marrow and can appear as diffuse or poorly defined zones of low-intermediate signal on T1-weighted imaging (T1WI) and proton density-weighted imaging and as intermediate-slightly high to high signal on fat-suppressed (FS) T2-weighted imaging. Focal or geographic regions with similar signal alteration can also be seen. After gadolinium (Gd) contrast administration, ALL, CLL, AML, and CML may show Gd contrast enhancement on T1WI and FS T1WI. *CT:* CLL patients with Richter's transformation commonly have cervical lymphadenopathy.	Lymphoid neoplasms that have widespread involvement of the bone marrow as well as tumor cells in peripheral blood. ALL occurs the most frequently in children and adolescents and can be associated with lymphadenopathy. CLL is the most common type of leukemia in the Western world and usually occurs in adults over 50 years old. CLL is the most indolent type of leukemia. CLL usually presents as an asymptomatic lymphocytosis and follows a protracted clinical course. Four percent of CLL patients develop an aggressive B-cell lymphoma (*Richter's transformation*). Myelogenous leukemias represent neoplasms derived from abnormal myeloid progenitor cells that, if normal, would form erythrocytes, monocytes, granulocytes, and platelets. AML usually occurs in adolescents and young adults and accounts for ~ 20% of childhood leukemias. CML occurs in adults more than 25 years old.
Metastatic malignancies (**Fig. 4.207** and **Fig. 4.208**)	*MRI:* Circumscribed spheroid lesions that often have low-intermediate signal on T1-weighted imaging, intermediate to high signal on T2-weighted imaging, ± hemorrhage, calcifications, and cysts, and variable gadolinium contrast enhancement. *CT:* Lesions usually have low-intermediate attenuation, ± hemorrhage, calcifications, and cysts, and variable contrast enhancement, ± bone destruction, ± compression of neural tissue or vessels.	Primary extracranial tumor source: lung > breast > GI > GU > melanoma. Can occur as single or multiple well-circumscribed or poorly defined lesions. Metastatic tumor may cause variable destructive or infiltrative changes in single or multiple sites.

(continued on page 474)

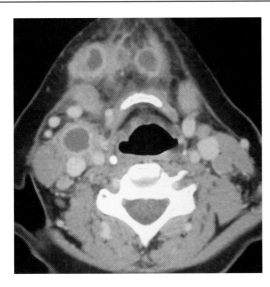

Fig. 4.205 Axial contrast-enhanced CT of a non-Hodgkin lymphoma shows abnormally enlarged lymph nodes that have low attenuation centrally surrounded by peripheral rims of enhancement.

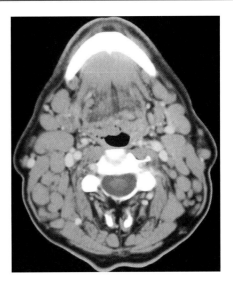

Fig. 4.206 Axial CT of multiple enlarged cervical lymph nodes in a patient with history of chronic lymphocytic leukemia (CLL) and development of aggressive B-cell lymphoma (Richter's transformation).

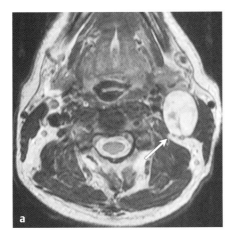 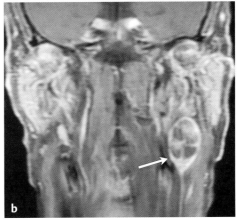

Fig. 4.207 **(a)** Axial T2-weighted imaging shows an abnormally enlarged lymph node (*arrow*) due to metastatic squamous cell carcinoma associated with human papilloma virus that has heterogeneous high signal. **(b)** The lesion shows heterogeneous gadolinium contrast enhancement on coronal fat-suppressed T1-weighted imaging (*arrow*).

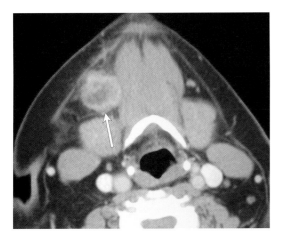

Fig. 4.208 Axial CT of a 60-year-old woman with an abnormally enlarged lymph node (*arrow*) due to metastatic squamous cell carcinoma. The lymph node has an irregular central zone with decreased attenuation and has ill-defined peripheral margins related to extracapsular tumor extension.

Table 4.9 *(cont.)* Submandibular space lesions

Lesion	Imaging Findings	Comments
Inflammatory Lesions		
Lymphadenitis (reactive adenopathy; presuppurative and suppurative adenopathy) (**Fig. 4.209**; see **Fig. 4.71** and **Fig. 4.72**)	*MRI:* Enlarged *presuppurative* nodes have intermediate signal on T1-weighted imaging (T1WI), slightly high signal on T2-weighted imaging (T2WI), and gadolinium (Gd) contrast enhancement. *Suppurative* nodes have low-intermediate signal on T1WI, slightly high to high signal on T2WI, and rim Gd contrast enhancement. Irregular increased signal on T2WI and Gd contrast enhancement are typically seen in the adjacent soft tissue. *CT:* *Reactive adenopathy:* Enlarged lymph nodes measure less than 12 mm, with preservation of nodal architecture, ± prominent single hilar vessel or branching vascular pattern. *Presuppurative* enlarged lymph nodes are associated with loss of the fatty hilum, slightly decreased attenuation, increased contrast enhancement, and reticulation of adjacent fat. *Suppurative* lymph nodes are typically enlarged and have low attenuation centrally surrounded by a rim of contrast enhancement.	Enlarged lymph nodes of the submandibular region (1A = submental and 1B = submandibular nodes) that typically measure less than 12 mm, with preservation of nodal architecture, can result from infections of the anterior oral cavity, lip, and sinonasal structures, which is referred to as *reactive adenopathy* or *presuppurative adenitis*. In children, lymphadenitis can result from upper respiratory viral infections as well as bacteria, such as *Staphylococcus aureus* and *Streptococcus pyogenes*. Infection by the gram-negative bacillus *Bartonella henselae* can result in self-limited regional granulomatous adenitis. This infection usually occurs in patients less than 30 years old and is often related to contact with cats (cat-scratch disease). Other infectious granulomatous diseases causing lymphadenopathy result from bacteria like *Mycobacterium tuberculosis, M. avium intracellulare, M. bovis,* and *M. kansasii*. Enlarged lymph nodes can undergo liquefactive necrosis (suppurative adenitis)—resulting in purulent lymph nodes, which measure up to 4.5 cm. Treatment with IV antibiotics is usually effective when the suppurative low-attenuation nodes measure < 2 cm. Larger suppurative lymph nodes usually require surgical drainage, especially with airway compromise. In adults, suppurative adenitis often results from trauma and procedural or surgical complications. Gram-positive cocci are common pathogens for suppurative adenitis in adults.
Phlegmon/abscess (**Fig. 4.210**; see **Fig. 4.193**)	*MRI:* Phlegmon appears as soft tissue thickening at the floor of the mouth with poorly defined slightly high to high signal on T2-weighted imaging (T2WI) and FS T2WI. Abscesses appear as collections with high signal on T2WI and diffusion-weighted imaging surrounded by a peripheral rim of gadolinium contrast enhancement. *CT:* Abscesses appear as a fluid collection with rim enhancement and adjacent abnormal soft tissue thickening. Abnormal soft tissue thickening without a rim-enhancing collection is seen with a phlegmon.	Infections involving the floor of the mouth and submandibular space can result from spread of dental/mandibular infections, trauma, bacteremia/sepsis, and/or calculi obstructing the submandibular duct.
Ludwig angina (**Fig. 4.211**)	*CT:* Extensive abnormal soft tissue thickening with ill-defined margins containing small low-attenuation fluid zones. The abnormality extends into the submandibular, pharyngeal, and/or parapharyngeal spaces, ± narrowing or obstruction of the airway.	Severe cellulitis at the floor of the mouth that can progress and extend inferiorly into the submandibular space and mediastinum, causing chest pain. Commonly results from infection of the mandible and adjacent soft tissues or as a complication of dental surgery. Considered a life-threatening condition, with a mortality rate of up to 10%.

(continued on page 476)

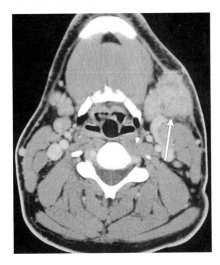

Fig. 4.209 Axial CT shows an abnormally enlarged lymph node with ill-defined margins (*arrow*) representing presuppurative lymphadenitis secondary to infection by the gram-negative bacillus *Bartonella henselae* (cat-scratch disease).

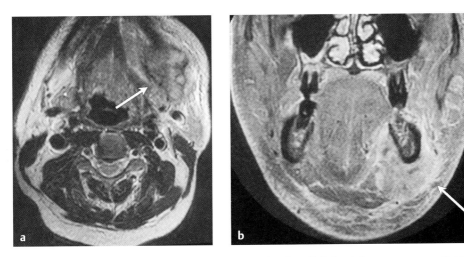

Fig. 4.210 **(a)** A 55-year-old man with a phlegmon in the left neck that has ill-defined, heterogeneous, slightly high signal on axial T2-weighted imaging (*arrow*) and **(b)** irregular, poorly defined gadolinium contrast enhancement on coronal fat-suppressed T1-weighted imaging (*arrow*).

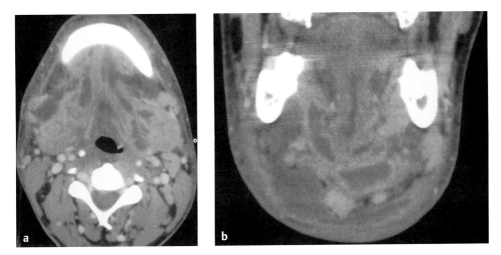

Fig. 4.211 Ludwig angina. **(a)** Axial and **(b)** coronal CT images of a 52-year-old man show extensive, abnormal, irregular soft tissue thickening containing low-attenuation fluid zones in the floor of the mouth extending into the submandibular spaces bilaterally.

Table 4.9 *(cont.)*   Submandibular space lesions

Lesion	Imaging Findings	Comments
Viral lymphadenopathy **(Fig. 4.212)**	*CT and MRI:* Multiple enlarged lymph nodes in the neck, + contrast enhancement. Often associated with enlargement of adenoids and palatine tonsils, ± enlargement of parotid and submandibular glands.	In young adults, generalized lymphadenopathy can result from Epstein-Barr virus infection (mononucleosis). Mononucleosis is a self-limited disease that is often associated with fever, malaise, pharyngotonsillitis, lymphadenopathy, and/or hepatosplenomegaly. Can involve major salivary glands. Other causes of viral lymphadenopathy include infection by cytomegalovirus, Mumps paramyxovirus, and by human T-cell lymphotropic virus type III (HIV), which can result in AIDS.
Submandibular duct stone/ sialadenitis **(Fig. 4.213, Fig. 4.214,** and **Fig. 4.215)**	*MRI:* Calculi typically have low signal on T1-weighted imaging and T2-weighted imaging (T2WI). Dilatation of ducts with high signal on T2WI may be seen in the submandibular gland. Calculi can also be seen as low-signal foci on susceptibility-weighted imaging. The submandibular gland may be enlarged from inflammation, with increased signal on T2WI and increased gadolinium contrast enhancement compared with the contralateral normal gland. MR sialography using heavily weighted T2WI via 3D constructive interference in the steady state technique or 3D fast/ turbo spin echo techniques can show dilated ducts with high signal and intraluminal defects from stones. *CT:* Calculi typically have high attenuation. Dilated ducts can be seen proximal to the obstructing stone as well as within the submandibular gland. The submandibular gland can be enlarged and can show increased contrast enhancement.	Sialolithiasis is the formation of calculi within salivary ducts, and it is the most common disorder of major salivary glands. It results from deposition of calcium salts over a core of desquamated epithelial cells, mucus, foreign bodies, or bacteria. Can occur as single or multiple ductal stones per patient. Sialoliths can measure up to 9 mm (mean size ranges from 3 to 4 mm). Sialoliths (calculi) occur more frequently in Wharton's duct of the submandibular gland (up to 80% of cases) than in Stensen's duct of the parotid gland because of its upward configuration and its saliva, which has relatively high concentrations of phosphates and hydroxyapatites, and is more alkaline and viscous than the parotid saliva. Sialoliths can result in diffuse submandibular gland enlargement and susceptibility to superimposed infection. Treatment can be via sialendoscopic extraction or surgery.

(continued on page 478)

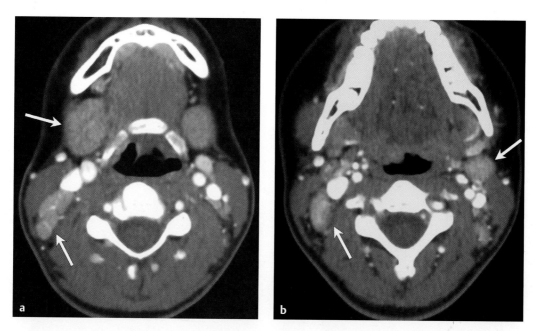

Fig. 4.212   **(a,b)** Axial CT of a 22-year-old woman with Epstein-Barr virus infection (mononucleosis) shows asymmetric enlargement of the right submandibular gland (*upper arrow* in **a**) and multiple enlarged contrast-enhancing cervical lymph nodes (*arrows* in **b**, *lower arrow* in **a**).

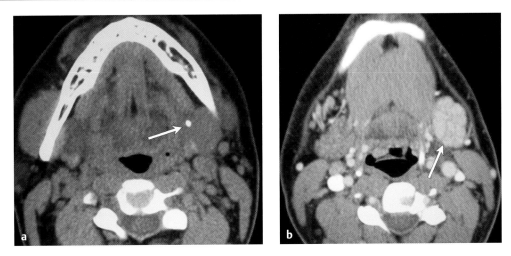

Fig. 4.213 **(a)** Axial non-enhanced CT shows a stone (*arrow*) in the left submandibular duct that on postcontrast axial CT **(b)** is associated with enlargement and asymmetric increased contrast enhancement of the left submandibular gland (*arrow*) due to inflammation.

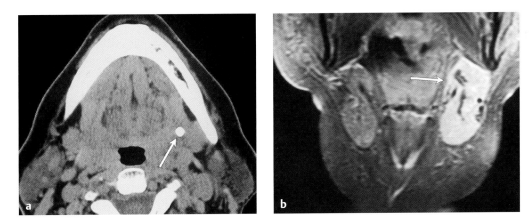

Fig. 4.214 **(a)** Axial non-enhanced CT shows a stone (*arrow*) in the left submandibular duct that on coronal fat-suppressed T1-weighted imaging **(b)** is associated with enlargement and asymmetric increased gadolinium contrast enhancement of the left submandibular gland (*arrow*) due to inflammation related to ductal obstruction.

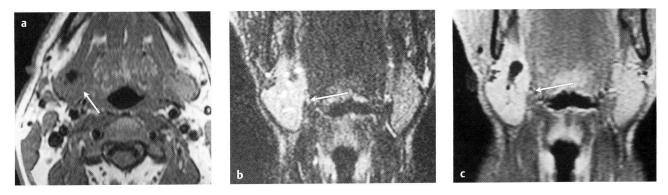

Fig. 4.215 **(a)** Axial T1-weighted imaging shows a stone with low signal in the right submandibular gland duct (*arrow*) that on **(b)** coronal fat-suppressed T2-weighted imaging shows enlargement and asymmetric increased signal involving the right submandibular gland (*arrow*). **(c)** There is corresponding increased gadolinium contrast enhancement involving the right submandibular gland (*arrow*) on postcontrast coronal fat-suppressed T1-weighted imaging due to inflammation related to ductal obstruction.

Table 4.9 *(cont.)*   Submandibular space lesions

Lesion	Imaging Findings	Comments
Sjögren's syndrome (See **Fig. 4.108** and **Fig. 4.109**)	*MRI:* Parotid glands have heterogeneous low-intermediate signal on T1-weighted imaging (T1WI), and variable mixed low, intermediate, and/or high signal on T2-weighted imaging (T2WI) and FS T2WI. Globular zones with high signal on T2WI can occur from saliva within dilated ducts. In the early phases of disease, the involved glands may be enlarged. Over time, the glands decrease in size from apoptosis, with increased fat deposition resulting in progressive increase in signal on T1WI. Zones of low signal on T2WI can also occur in late disease phases from fibrous tissue and lymphocyte aggregates. In the later disease phases, the ADCs of involved glands can become lower than normal lacrimal glands. *CT:* Parotid glands can be enlarged in the early phases of disease, or atrophic in later phases.	Common autoimmune disease in which a mononuclear lymphocyte infiltration can occur in one or more exocrine glands (lacrimal, parotid, submandibular, and minor salivary glands), resulting in acinar cell destruction and impaired gland function. Usually occurs in adults between 40 and 60 years old, with a female predominance of over 90%. Histopathologic findings include periductal accumulation of lymphocytes and plasma cells associated with acinar destruction, which progresses peripherally to centrally. Aggregates of lymphocytes can result in a localized mass referred to as a benign lymphoepithelial lesion (BLEL) or Godwin tumor. Sjögren's syndrome can be a primary disorder or secondary, associated with other autoimmune diseases, such as rheumatoid arthritis and systemic lupus erythematosus. Patients present with decreased lacrimal and salivary gland function, xerostomia, and keratoconjunctivitis sicca.
Sarcoidosis	*MRI:* Single or multiple lesions with low to intermediate signal on T1-weighted imaging and slightly high signal on T2-weighted imaging (T2WI) and FS T2WI. After gadolinium (Gd) contrast administration, lesions typically show Gd contrast enhancement. *CT:* Single or multiple lesions with soft tissue attenuation and sharply defined margins (in 85%; ill-defined margins in the remainder). *Nuclear medicine:* Increased uptake of gallium-67 citrate and F-18 FDG glucose.	Sarcoidosis is a multisystem noncaseating granulomatous disease of uncertain cause that can involve the CNS in 5 to 15% of cases. If untreated, it can be associated with severe neurologic deficits, such as encephalopathy, cranial neuropathies, and myelopathy. Sarcoid can involve the major salivary glands in up to 30% of cases, and it presents as painless nodular or multinodular enlargement of the glands from lesions composed of noncaseating epithelioid granulomas. Treatment includes oral corticosteroids and surgical debulking.

4.10 Buccal Space Lesions

The buccal space includes the soft tissues of the cheek. The buccal space is located lateral to the buccinator muscle (which originates above the maxillary alveolar ridge and inserts on the pterygomandibular raphe adjacent to the superior pharyngeal constrictor); posterior to the muscles of facial expression (greater and lesser zygomatic muscles and risorius muscle), which are enclosed by the superficial layer of the deep cervical fascia; anterior to the masticator space (which includes the masseter muscle, lateral and medial pterygoid muscles, and mandible); and anterior to the parotid space. Superiorly, the buccal fat is contiguous with the fat of the infratemporal fossa. The inferior portion of the buccal space is continuous with the submandibular space. The lack of fascial separation of the buccal space from the parotid and submandibular spaces and the infratemporal fossa allows a pathway for infections and tumors. The predominant component of the buccal space is adipose tissue (buccal fat pad). Other structures within the buccal space include the facial and buccal artery, facial vein, lymphatic channels, branches of CN V and CN VII, parotid duct, accessory parotid lobules, and minor salivary glands. The parotid duct courses around the masseter muscle and extends medially into the buccal mucosa at the level of the second maxillary molar tooth.

Table 4.10 Buccal space lesions

- Developmental Variants
  - Accessory parotid lobule
  - Accessory parotid tissue
  - Epidermoid
  - Dermoid
- Benign Tumors
  - Lipoma
  - Hemangioma
  - Juvenile angiofibroma
  - Venolymphatic malformation
  - Schwannoma
  - Neurofibroma
  - Pleomorphic adenoma of accessory parotid tissue or minor salivary gland
  - Myxoma

- Tumorlike Lesions
  - Hematoma
  - Foreign body
- Malignant Neoplasms
  - Adenoid cystic carcinoma
  - Adenocarcinoma and mucoepidermoid carcinoma
  - Squamous cell carcinoma
  - Rhabdomyosarcoma
  - Metastatic malignancies
  - Non-Hodgkin lymphoma (NHL)
- Inflammatory Disease
  - Cellulitis
  - Abscess

Table 4.10 Buccal space lesions

Lesion	Imaging Findings	Comments
Developmental Variants		
Accessory parotid lobule (**Fig. 4.216**)	*CT and MRI:* Accessory parotid lobule extends along the course of the parotid duct, which is continuous with the parotid gland. Tissue has intermediate attenuation on CT and MRI signal isointense relative to the parotid gland.	Developmental variant in which the parotid gland extends anteriorly along the course of the parotid duct within the buccal space.
Accessory parotid tissue (**Fig. 4.217**)	*CT and MRI:* Accessory parotid tissue along the parotid duct, which is separate from the parotid gland. Tissue has intermediate attenuation on CT and MRI signal isointense relative to the parotid gland.	Developmental variant with localized parotid tissue adjacent to the parotid duct, anterior to and separate from the parotid gland. Occurs in up to 21% of patients. Rarely, tumors occur in accessory parotid tissue (70% benign, 30% malignant).

(continued on page 480)

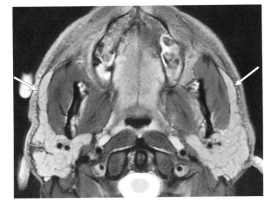

Fig. 4.216 Axial fat-suppressed T2-weighted imaging shows bilateral accessory parotid lobules (*arrows*).

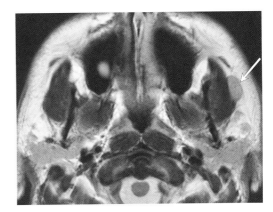

Fig. 4.217 Axial T2-weighted imaging shows accessory parotid tissue (*arrow*) with signal similar to the parotid gland.

Table 4.10 *(cont.)* Buccal space lesions

Lesion	Imaging Findings	Comments
Epidermoid	*MRI:* Well-circumscribed spheroid or multilobulated ectodermal-inclusion cystic lesions with low-intermediate signal on T1-weighted imaging, high signal on T2- and diffusion-weighted imaging, mixed low, intermediate, or high signal on FLAIR images, and no gadolinium contrast enhancement. Occur more frequently at the floor of the mouth in the midline than in the submandibular space. *CT:* Well-circumscribed spheroid or multilobulated extra-axial ectodermal-inclusion cystic lesions with low-intermediate attenuation, ± bone erosion.	Nonneoplastic congenital or acquired lesions filled with desquamated cells and keratinaceous debris surrounded by a wall lined by simple squamous epithelium. Lesions result from congenital inclusion of epidermal elements during embryonic development of the first and second branchial arches or from trauma. Often occur in patients between 5 and 50 years old (mean = 30 years).
Dermoid	*MRI:* Well-circumscribed spheroid or multilobulated lesions, usually with high signal on T1-weighted imaging, variable low, intermediate, and/or high signal on T2-weighted imaging, and no gadolinium contrast enhancement. *CT:* Well-circumscribed spheroid or multilobulated lesions, usually with low attenuation, ± fat–fluid or fluid–debris levels.	Nonneoplastic congenital or acquired ectodermal-inclusion cystic lesions filled with lipid material, cholesterol, desquamated cells, and keratinaceous debris surrounded by a wall lined by keratinizing squamous epithelium. Lesions result from congenital inclusion of dermal elements during embryonic development of the first and second branchial arches or from trauma. Occur in males slightly more than in females, ± related symptoms.
Benign Tumors		
Lipoma	*MRI:* Lipomas have MRI signal isointense to subcutaneous fat on T1-weighted imaging (high signal). On T2-weighted imaging, signal suppression occurs with frequency-selective fat saturation techniques or with a short time to inversion recovery (STIR) method. Typically there is no gadolinium contrast enhancement or peripheral edema. *CT:* Lipomas have CT attenuation similar to subcutaneous fat and typically show no contrast enhancement or peripheral edema.	Common benign hamartomas composed of mature white adipose tissue without cellular atypia. Most common soft tissue tumor, representing 16% of all soft tissue tumors.
Hemangioma **(Fig. 4.218)**	*MRI:* Circumscribed or poorly marginated structures (< 4 cm in diameter) in bone marrow or soft tissue with intermediate-high signal on T1-weighted imaging (often isointense to marrow fat) and high signal on T2-weighted imaging (T2WI) and fat-suppressed T2WI, typically with gadolinium contrast enhancement, ± expansion of bone. *CT:* Expansile bone lesions with a radiating pattern of bony trabeculae oriented toward the center. Hemangiomas in soft tissue have mostly intermediate attenuation, ± zones of fat attenuation.	Benign lesions of bone or soft tissue composed of capillary, cavernous, and/or malformed venous vessels. Considered to be a hamartomatous disorder. Occur in patients 1 to 84 years old (median age = 33 years).
Juvenile angiofibroma **(Fig. 4.219)**	*MRI:* Origin of lesion is the pterygopalatine fossa. The lesions grow medially into the nasal cavity and nasopharynx via the sphenopalatine foramen, laterally into the pterygomaxillary fissure, superiorly via the inferior orbital fissure into the orbital apex, ± anteriorly into the maxillary sinus, ± middle cranial fossa via the superior orbital fissure. Lesions often have intermediate signal on T1-weighted imaging, slightly high to high signal on T2-weighted imaging, ± flow voids, and prominent gadolinium contrast enhancement. *CT:* Lesions often have intermediate attenuation, ± hemorrhage, as well as erosion and/or remodeling of adjacent bone, such as widening of the pterygopalatine/pterygomaxillary fossae and/or sphenopalatine foramina and vidian canals.	Benign, cellular, and vascularized mesenchymal lesion/malformation that occurs in the posterolateral nasal wall or nasopharynx from testosterone-sensitive cells, associated with high propensity to hemorrhage. Composed of thin-walled slitlike or dilated vessels of varying sizes lined by endothelial cells within fibrous stroma containing spindle, round, or stellate cells and varying amounts of collagen. Immunoreactive to platelet-derived growth factor B, insulin-like growth factor type II, vimentin, and smooth muscle actin. Typically occurs in males, with peak incidence in the second decade, and total incidence of 1 in 5,000–60,000. Lesions have locally aggressive growth, with erosion and/or remodeling of adjacent bone, and can spread through skull-base foramina. Treatment can include embolization or hormonal therapy, and, if necessary, surgical resection.

Lesion	Imaging Findings	Comments
Venolymphatic malformation	Can be circumscribed lesions or occur in an infiltrative pattern with extension into soft tissue and between muscles. *MRI:* Often contain single or multiple cystic zones that can be large (macrocystic type) or small (microcystic type), and that have predominantly low signal on T1-weighted imaging (T1WI) and high signal on T2-weighted imaging (T2WI) and fat-suppressed (FS) T2WI. Fluid–fluid levels and zones with high signal on T1WI and variable signal on T2WI may result from cysts containing hemorrhage, high protein concentration, and/or necrotic debris. Septa between the cystic zones vary in thickness and gadolinium (Gd) contrast enhancement. Nodular zones within the lesions can have variable degrees of Gd contrast enhancement. Microcystic lesions typically show more Gd contrast enhancement than the macrocystic type.	Benign vascular anomalies (also referred to as lymphangioma and cystic hygroma) that primarily result from abnormal lymphangiogenesis. Up to 75% occur in the head and neck. Can be observed in utero with MRI or sonography, at birth (50–65%) or within the first 5 years, and ~ 85% are detected by age 2. Lesions are composed of endothelium-lined lymphatic ± venous channels interspersed within connective tissue stroma. Account for less than 1% of benign soft tissue tumors and 5.6% of all benign lesions of infancy and childhood. Can occur in association with Turner syndrome and Proteus syndrome.
Schwannoma	*MRI:* Circumscribed spheroid or ovoid lesions with low-intermediate signal on T1-weighted imaging, high signal on T2-weighted imaging (T2WI) and fat-suppressed T2WI, and usually prominent gadolinium (Gd) contrast enhancement. High signal on T2WI and Gd contrast enhancement can be heterogeneous in large lesions due to cystic degeneration and/or hemorrhage. *CT:* Circumscribed spheroid or ovoid lesions with intermediate attenuation, + contrast enhancement. Large lesions can have cystic degeneration and/or hemorrhage.	Schwannomas are benign encapsulated tumors that contain differentiated neoplastic Schwann cells. They most commonly occur as solitary, sporadic lesions. Multiple schwannomas are often associated with neurofibromatosis type 2 (NF2), which is an autosomal dominant disease involving a gene mutation at chromosome 22q12. In addition to schwannomas, patients with NF2 can also have multiple meningiomas and ependymomas. The incidence of NF2 is 1/37,000 to 1/50,000 newborns. Age at presentation is 22 to 72 years (mean age = 46 years). Peak incidence is in the fourth to sixth decades. Many patients with NF2 present in the third decade with bilateral vestibular schwannomas.

(continued on page 482)

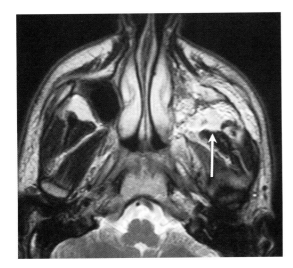

Fig. 4.218 A 9-year-old male with a hemangioma involving the soft tissues of the left face, left maxilla, left maxillary sinus, and left masticator and buccal spaces. The infiltrative lesion has high signal on axial T2-weighted imaging (*arrow*).

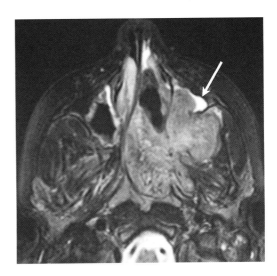

Fig. 4.219 An 11-year-old male with a juvenile nasopharyngeal angiofibroma. Axial fat-suppressed T2-weighted imaging shows a large lesion (*arrow*) in the left nasopharynx associated with erosion and remodeling of adjacent bone. The lesion extends into the left nasal cavity, laterally into the pterygomaxillary fissure, and anteriorly into the left maxillary sinus. The lesion has heterogeneous slightly high to high signal.

Table 4.10 *(cont.)* Buccal space lesions

Lesion	Imaging Findings	Comments
Neurofibroma (**Fig. 4.220**)	*MRI:* *Solitary neurofibromas* are circumscribed spheroid, ovoid, or lobulated extra-axial lesions with low-intermediate signal on T1-weighted imaging (T1WI), intermediate-high signal on T2-weighted imaging (T2WI), and prominent gadolinium (Gd) contrast enhancement. High signal on T2WI and Gd contrast enhancement can be heterogeneous in large lesions. *Plexiform neurofibromas* appear as curvilinear and multinodular lesions involving multiple nerve branches and have low to intermediate signal on T1WI and intermediate or slightly high to high signal on T2WI and fat-suppressed T2WI, with or without bands or strands of low signal. Lesions usually show Gd contrast enhancement. *CT:* Ovoid or fusiform lesions with low-intermediate attenuation. Lesions can show contrast enhancement. Often erode adjacent bone.	Neurofibromas are benign nerve sheath tumors that contain mixtures of Schwann cells, perineural-like cells, and interlacing fascicles of fibroblasts associated with abundant collagen. Unlike schwannomas, neurofibromas lack Antoni A and B regions and cannot be separated pathologically from the underlying nerve. Neurofibromas most frequently occur as sporadic, localized, solitary lesions, less frequently as diffuse or plexiform lesions. Multiple neurofibromas are typically seen in neurofibromatosis type 1 (NF1), which is an autosomal dominant disorder (1/2,500 births) caused by mutations of the neurofibromin gene on chromosome 17q11.2. NF1 is the most common type of neurocutaneous syndrome and is associated with neoplasms of the central and peripheral nervous systems (optic gliomas, astrocytomas, plexiform and solitary neurofibromas) and skin (café-au-lait spots, axillary and inguinal freckling). Also associated with meningeal and skull dysplasias, as well as hamartomas of the iris (Lisch nodules).
Pleomorphic adenoma of accessory parotid tissue or minor salivary gland (**Fig. 4.221**)	*MRI:* Circumscribed lesions with low-intermediate signal on T1-weighted imaging, slightly high signal on T2-weighted imaging (T2WI) and fat-suppressed T2WI, and usually gadolinium contrast enhancement. *CT:* Circumscribed or lobulated lesions with intermediate attenuation, + contrast enhancement.	Pleomorphic adenoma is the most common type of benign salivary gland tumor, composed of modified myoepithelial cells associated with sparse stromal elements. Most arise from the submucosa of the nasal septum or lateral sinus wall. Usually occur in patients between 20 and 60 years old. Other, rare types of adenomas include myoepithelioma and oncocytoma.
Myxoma (**Fig. 4.222**)	*MRI:* Lesions usually have low or low-intermediate signal on T1-weighted imaging and proton density-weighted imaging and high signal on T2-weighted imaging (T2WI) and FS T2WI. Myxomas can have heterogeneous mild or moderate degrees of gadolinium contrast enhancement in noncystic portions. Can occur in muscle or subcutaneous fat. *CT:* Spheroid or ovoid lesions with low-intermediate attenuation.	Myxomas are benign lesions that contain fibroblasts (spindle cells) and abundant mucoid material (glycosaminoglycans, other mucopolysaccharides). Account for 3% of benign soft tissue tumors/lesions and 2% of all soft tissue tumors/lesions. Occur in adults 24 to 74 years old (average age = 52 years).

(continued on page 484)

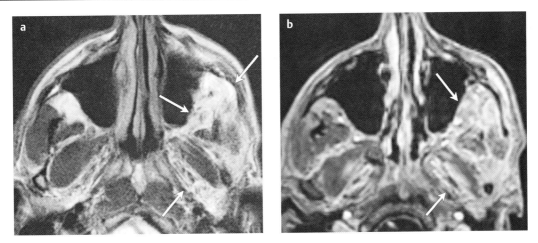

Fig. 4.220 A 38-year-old man with a plexiform neurofibroma with ill-defined margins involving the left maxilla and left masticator and buccal spaces that has **(a)** heterogeneous high signal on axial T2-weighted imaging (*arrows*) and **(b)** irregular gadolinium contrast enhancement on axial T1-weighted imaging (*arrows*).

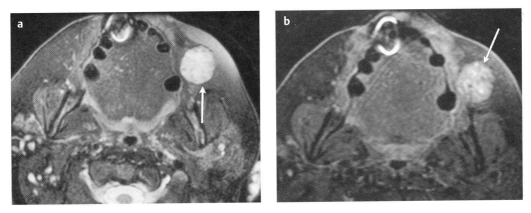

Fig. 4.221 **(a)** Axial fat-suppressed T2-weighted imaging shows a pleomorphic adenoma of accessory left parotid tissue (*arrow*). **(b)** The adenoma shows gadolinium contrast enhancement on axial fat-suppressed T1-weighted imaging (*arrow*).

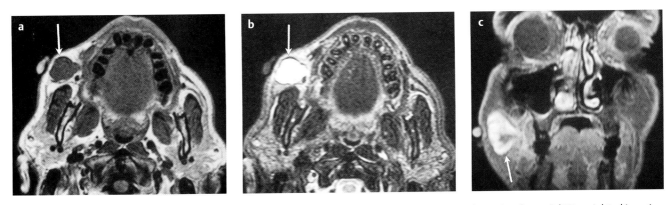

Fig. 4.222 A 52-year-old man with a myxoma in the right buccal space that has **(a)** low-intermediate signal on axial T1-weighted imaging (*arrow*), **(b)** high signal on axial T2-weighted imaging (*arrow*), and **(c)** heterogeneous gadolinium contrast enhancement on coronal fat-suppressed T1-weighted imaging (*arrow*).

Table 4.10 *(cont.)* Buccal space lesions

Lesion	Imaging Findings	Comments
Tumorlike Lesions		
Hematoma	*MRI: Acute hematomas* (< 3–7 days) have mostly intermediate signal similar to muscle on T1-weighted imaging (T1WI) and mixed low-intermediate and/or high signal relative to muscle on proton density-weighted imaging (PDWI), T2-weighted imaging (T2WI), and fat-suppressed (FS) T2WI. Poorly defined zones of high signal on PDWI, T2WI, and FS T2WI may also be seen peripheral to the hematoma, representing adjacent edema. *Subacute hematomas* (1 week to 3 months) have high and/or intermediate signal on T1WI, and high signal on FS T1WI, PDWI, T2WI, and FS T2WI. Peripheral and central zones of low signal on PDWI, T2WI, and FS T2WI can be seen in mid to late subacute hematomas secondary to the presence of hemosiderin from breakdown of blood cells and oxidation/metabolism of hemoglobin. Mild peripheral gadolinium contrast may be seen. *Chronic hematomas* (> 3 months) usually have high signal on T1WI, PDWI, T2WI, and FS T2WI. A thick peripheral rim of low signal on T2WI from hemosiderin is often seen with chronic hematomas. Chronic hematomas often evolve eventually into zones with low-intermediate signal on T1WI and T2WI secondary to fibrosis and residual hemosiderin.	Hematomas are extravascular collections of red and white blood cells that can result from trauma, surgery, or coagulopathy (hemophilia, thrombocytopenia, medications/coumadin/heparin, and sepsis). An acute hematoma is defined as one less than a few days old. A subacute hematoma is of 1 week to 3 months duration, and chronic hematomas are older than 3 months. Hemophilic pseudotumors are chronic, slow-growing, encapsulated cystic lesions in bone or soft tissues secondary to recurrent hemorrhage that occur in 1–2% of patients with hemophilia.
Foreign body **(Fig. 4.223)**	*MRI:* Gadolinium contrast enhancement surrounding nonmetallic foreign bodies can be seen. *CT:* CT is the optimal test to safely evaluate for metallic foreign bodies and can detect metal fragments of < 1 mm. Metal fragments have high attenuation and can show streak artifacts. Glass fragments > 1.5 mm can be detected in more than 96% of cases, whereas smaller glass fragments < 0.5 mm are detected in ~ 50%. Wood foreign bodies have low attenuation that can be similar to air, although they have geometric shapes with peripheral inflammation that may suggest the diagnosis.	Penetrating traumatic injuries involving the face can be associated with foreign bodies in the subcutaneous tissue. If metallic foreign bodies are suspected, CT should be done prior to MRI because of potential safety issues. Retained foreign bodies can result in cellulitis and abscess formation.
Malignant Neoplasms		
Adenoid cystic carcinoma	*MRI:* Lesions involving major or minor salivary glands in the oral cavity. Lesions have intermediate signal on T1-weighted imaging, intermediate to high signal on T2-weighted imaging, and variable mild, moderate, or prominent gadolinium contrast enhancement. *CT:* Tumors have intermediate attenuation and variable mild, moderate, or prominent contrast enhancement. Destruction of adjacent bone is commonly seen.	Basaloid tumor of salivary gland origin composed of neoplastic epithelial and myoepithelial cells. Morphologic tumor patterns include tubular, cribriform, and solid. Accounts for 10% of epithelial salivary neoplasms. Most commonly involves the parotid, submandibular, and minor salivary glands (palate, tongue, buccal mucosa, floor of the mouth, and other locations). Perineural tumor spread is common, ± facial nerve paralysis. Usually occurs in adults > 30 years old. Solid type has the worst prognosis. Up to 90% of patients die within 10–15 years of diagnosis.

Lesion	Imaging Findings	Comments
Adenocarcinoma and mucoepidermoid carcinoma (**Fig. 4.224**)	*MRI:* Malignant lesions in the oral cavity that often have intermediate signal on T1-weighted imaging, intermediate to high signal on T2-weighted imaging, and variable mild, moderate, or prominent gadolinium contrast enhancement. Can be associated with bone destruction and perineural tumor spread. *CT:* Tumors have intermediate attenuation and variable mild, moderate, or prominent contrast enhancement. Destruction of adjacent bone can be seen.	Second and third most common malignant sinonasal tumors derived from salivary glands. Adenocarcinomas contain small to medium-size neoplastic cells with oval nuclei, typically immunoreactive to cytokeratin, vimentin, and S-100 protein. Mucoepidermoid carcinomas often have solid portions with basaloid or cuboidal neoplastic cells and cystic portions containing sialomucin lined by mucous cells with peripheral nuclei within pale cytoplasm. Most commonly occur in the maxillary sinus and nasal cavity. Tumors usually are intermediate to high grade and often are advanced at presentation, ± metastases, ± perineural tumor spread.

(continued on page 486)

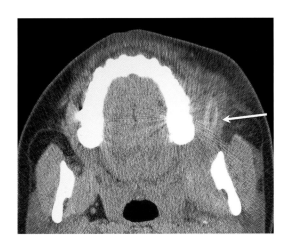

Fig. 4.223 Axial CT of a 35-year-old woman shows a wood foreign body (*arrow*) in the left buccal space with adjacent inflammatory reaction.

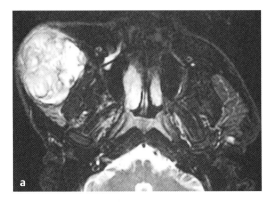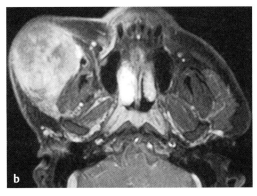

Fig. 4.224 **(a)** A 44-year-old man with an adenocarcinoma in the right buccal space that has heterogeneous high signal on axial fat-suppressed T2-weighted imaging. **(b)** The lesion shows heterogeneous gadolinium contrast enhancement on axial fat-suppressed T1-weighted imaging.

Table 4.10 *(cont.)* Buccal space lesions

Lesion	Imaging Findings	Comments
Squamous cell carcinoma (**Fig. 4.225**)	*MRI:* Lesions in the nasal and oral cavities, floor of the mouth, paranasal sinuses, oropharynx and nasopharynx, ± intracranial extension via bone destruction or perineural spread. Lesions have intermediate signal on T1-weighted imaging, intermediate to slightly high signal on T2-weighted imaging, and mild gadolinium contrast enhancement. Can be large lesions (± necrosis and/or hemorrhage). *CT:* Tumors have intermediate attenuation and mild contrast enhancement and can be large (± necrosis and/or hemorrhage).	Malignant epithelial tumors that include both keratinizing and nonkeratinizing types. Account for 80% of malignant oropharyngeal tumors and 3% of malignant tumors of the head and neck. Occur in adults (usually > 55 years old) and in males more than in females. Associated with occupational or other exposure to tobacco smoke, nickel, chlorophenols, chromium, mustard gas, radium, and material in the manufacture of wood products.
Rhabdomyosarcoma	*MRI:* Tumors can have circumscribed and/or poorly defined margins and typically have low-intermediate signal on T1-weighted imaging and heterogeneous signal (various combinations of intermediate, slightly high, and/or high signal) on T2-weighted imaging (T2WI) and fat-suppressed T2WI. Tumors show variable degrees of gadolinium contrast enhancement, ± bone destruction and invasion. *CT:* Soft tissue lesions that usually can have circumscribed or irregular margins. Calcifications are uncommon. Tumors can have mixed CT attenuation, with solid zones of soft tissue attenuation, cystic appearing and/or necrotic zones, and occasional foci of hemorrhage, ± bone invasion and destruction.	Malignant mesenchymal tumors with rhabdomyoblastic differentiation that occur primarily in soft tissue and only very rarely in bone. There are three subgroups of rhabdomyosarcoma: embryonal (50–70%), alveolar (18–45%), and pleomorphic (5–10%). Embryonal and alveolar rhabdomyosarcomas occur primarily in children < 10 years old, and pleomorphic rhabdomyosarcomas occur mostly in adults (median age in the sixth decade). Alveolar and pleomorphic rhabdomyosarcomas occur frequently in the extremities. Embryonal rhabdomyosarcomas occur mostly in the head and neck.
Metastatic malignancies (**Fig. 4.226**)	*MRI:* Circumscribed spheroid lesions that often have low-intermediate signal on T1-weighted imaging and intermediate to high signal on T2-weighted imaging, ± hemorrhage, calcifications, and cysts. Variable gadolinium contrast enhancement. *CT:* Lesions usually have low-intermediate attenuation, ± hemorrhage, calcifications, and cysts. Variable contrast enhancement, ± bone destruction, ± compression of neural tissue or vessels.	Primary extracranial tumor source: lung > breast > GI > GU > melanoma. Can occur as single or multiple well-circumscribed or poorly defined lesions Metastatic tumor may cause variable destructive or infiltrative changes in single or multiple sites.
Non-Hodgkin lymphoma (NHL)	*MRI:* Lesions have low-intermediate signal on T1-weighted imaging and intermediate to slightly high signal on T2-weighted imaging, + gadolinium contrast enhancement. Can be locally invasive and associated with bone erosion/destruction. *CT:* Lesions have low-intermediate attenuation and may show contrast enhancement, ± bone destruction.	Lymphomas are a group of tumors whose neoplastic cells typically arise within lymphoid tissue (lymph nodes and reticuloendothelial organs). Most lymphomas in the nasopharynx, nasal and oral cavities, and paranasal sinuses are NHL (B-cell NHL is more common than T-cell NHL) and more commonly are related to disseminated disease than to primary sinonasal tumors. Sinonasal lymphoma has a poor prognosis, with a 5-year survival rate of less than 65%.

(continued on page 488)

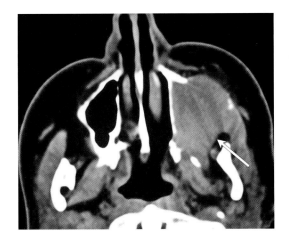

Fig. 4.225 Axial CT of a 56-year-old woman with a squamous cell carcinoma in the left maxillary sinus that is associated with bone destruction and extension anteriorly into the left buccal space and posteriorly into the left pterygomaxillary fissure (*arrow*).

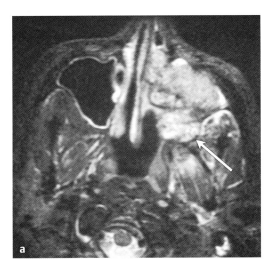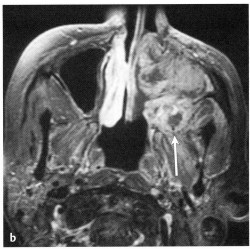

Fig. 4.226 **(a)** A 70-year-old woman with metastatic renal cell carcinoma involving the left maxillary sinus that has heterogeneous high signal on axial fat-suppressed T2-weighted imaging (*arrow*). **(b)** The lesion shows heterogeneous gadolinium contrast enhancement on axial fat-suppressed T1-weighted imaging (*arrow*). The tumor is associated with bone destruction and extension anteriorly into the left buccal space and posteriorly into the left pterygomaxillary fissure and left masticator space.

Table 4.10 *(cont.)* Buccal space lesions

Lesion	Imaging Findings	Comments
Inflammatory Disease		
Cellulitis (**Fig. 4.227**)	*MRI:* Soft tissue thickening involving the buccal space, with poorly defined, slightly high to high signal on T2-weighted imaging (T2WI) and fat-suppressed T2WI, as well as gadolinium (Gd) contrast enhancement. Abscesses appear as collections with high signal on T2WI and diffusion-weighted imaging, surrounded by a peripheral rim of Gd contrast enhancement. *CT:* Abnormal soft tissue thickening with contrast enhancement.	Infections involving the buccal space can result from spread of dental/maxillary infections, sinusitis trauma, bacteremia/sepsis, and/or calculi obstructing the parotid duct.
Abscess	*MRI:* Poorly defined zone with slightly high to high signal on T2-weighted imaging (T2WI) and fat-suppressed T2WI surrounding a collection with high signal on T2WI and diffusion-weighted imaging, with a peripheral rim of gadolinium contrast enhancement. *CT:* Fluid collection with rim enhancement and adjacent abnormal soft tissue thickening.	Cellulitis from infections involving the buccal space can progress to abscess formation. Infections can result from spread of dental/maxillary disease, sinusitis, trauma, bacteremia/sepsis, and/or calculi obstructing the parotid duct.

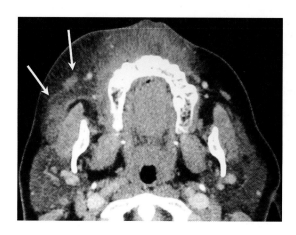

Fig. 4.227 Axial CT shows poorly defined zones of soft tissue attenuation in the right buccal space (*arrows*) representing cellulitis from a right maxillary dental infection.

References

Ansa Cervicalis

1. Banneheka S. Anatomy of the ansa cervicalis: nerve fiber analysis. Anat Sci Int 2008;83(2):61–67
2. Khaki AA, Shokouhi G, Shoja MM, et al. Ansa cervicalis as a variant of spinal accessory nerve plexus: a case report. Clin Anat 2006;19(6):540–543

Benign Lymphoepithelial Parotid Lesions (HIV)

3. Ihrler S, Steger W, Riederer A, Zietz C, Vogl I, Löhrs U. [HIV-associated cysts of the parotid glands. An histomorphologic and magnetic resonance tomography study of formal pathogenesis]. Laryngorhinootologie 1996;75(11):671–676
4. Kothari KS, Madiwale CV, Deshpande AA. Cystic lymphoepithelial lesion of the parotid as an early indicator of HIV infection. J Postgrad Med 2009;55(2):135–136
5. Shah GV. MR imaging of salivary glands. Neuroimag Clin N Am 2004;777–808

Branchial Cleft Cyst

6. Acierno SP, Waldhausen JHT. Congenital cervical cysts, sinuses and fistulae. Otolaryngol Clin North Am 2007;40(1):161–176, vii–viii
7. Ahn JY, Kang SY, Lee CH, Yoon PH, Lee KS. Parapharyngeal branchial cleft cyst extending to the skull base: a lateral transzygomatic-transtemporal approach to the parapharyngeal space. Neurosurg Rev 2005;28(1):73–76
8. Dallan I, Seccia V, Bruschini L, Ciancia E, Franceschini SS. Parapharyngeal cyst: considerations on embryology, clinical evaluation, and surgical management. J Craniofac Surg 2008;19(6):1487–1490
9. Gaddikeri S, Vattoth S, Gaddikeri RS, et al. Congenital cystic neck masses: embryology and imaging appearances, with clinicopathological correlation. Curr Probl Diagn Radiol 2014;43(2):55–67
10. Gupta M, Gupta M. A rare parapharyngeal space branchial cleft cyst. BMJ Case Reports April 29, 2013;pii: bcr2013008952. doi: 10.1136/bcr-2013-008952
11. Joshi MJ, Provenzano MJ, Smith RJH, Sato Y, Smoker WRK. The rare third branchial cleft cyst. AJNR Am J Neuroradiol 2009;30(9):1804–1806
12. Shin JH, Lee HK, Kim SY, et al. Parapharyngeal second branchial cyst manifesting as cranial nerve palsies: MR findings. AJNR Am J Neuroradiol 2001;22(3):510–512

Buccal Space Lesions

13. Falavigna A, Righesso O, Volquind D, Teles AR. Intramuscular myxoma of the cervical paraspinal muscle. Eur Spine J 2009;18(Suppl 2):245–249
14. Frison L, Goudot P, Yachouh J. [Soft tissue myxoma of the face]. Rev Stomatol Chir Maxillofac 2010;111(1):21–24
15. Kalsi JS, Pring M, Hughes C, Fasanmade A. Presentation of intramuscular myxoma as an unusual neck lump. J Oral Maxillofac Surg 2013;71(5):e210–e214
16. Kim HC, Han MH, Moon MH, Kim JH, Kim IO, Chang KH. CT and MR imaging of the buccal space: normal anatomy and abnormalities. Korean J Radiol 2005;6(1):22–30
17. Kurabayashi T, Ida M, Tetsumura A, Ohbayashi N, Yasumoto M, Sasaki T. MR imaging of benign and malignant lesions in the buccal space. Dentomaxillofac Radiol 2002;31(6):344–349
18. Newberry TR, Kaufmann CR, Miller FR. Review of accessory parotid gland tumors: pathologic incidence and surgical management. Am J Otolaryngol 2014;35(1):48–52
19. Tart RP, Kotzur IM, Mancuso AA, Glantz MS, Mukherji SK. CT and MR imaging of the buccal space and buccal space masses. Radiographics 1995;15(3):531–550
20. Tu AS, Geyer CA, Mancall AC, Baker RA. The buccal space: a doorway for percutaneous CT-guided biopsy of the parapharyngeal region. AJNR Am J Neuroradiol 1998;19(4):728–731

Calcifying Epithelial Odontogenic Tumor

21. Ching AS, Pak MW, Kew J, Metreweli C. CT and MR imaging appearances of an extraosseous calcifying epithelial odontogenic tumor (Pindborg tumor). AJNR Am J Neuroradiol 2000;21(2):343–345

22. Deboni MCZ, Naclério-Homem MdaG, Pinto Junior DS, Traina AA, Cavalcanti MGP. Clinical, radiological and histological features of calcifying epithelial odontogenic tumor: case report. Braz Dent J 2006;17(2):171–174
23. Hada MS, Sable M, Kane SV, Pai PS, Juvekar SL. Calcifying epithelial odontogenic tumor: a clinico-radio-pathological dilemma. J Cancer Res Ther 2014;10(1):194–196
24. Misra SR, Lenka S, Sahoo SR, Mishra S. Giant Pindborg tumor (calcifying epithelial odontogenic tumor): an unusual case report with radiologic-pathologic correlation. J Clin Imaging Sci 2013;3(Suppl 1):11
25. Singh N, Sahai S, Singh S, Singh S. Calcifying epithelial odontogenic tumor (Pindborg tumor). Natl J Maxillofac Surg 2011;2(2):225–227
26. Venkateswarlu M, Geetha P, Lakshmi Kavitha N. CT imaging findings of a calcifying epithelial odontogenic tumour. Br J Radiol 2012;85(1009):e14–e16

Carotid Space Anatomy

27. Kuwada C, Mannion K, Aulino JM, Kanekar SG. Imaging of the carotid space. Otolaryngol Clin North Am 2012;45(6):1273–1292
28. Warshafsky D, Goldenberg D, Kanekar SG. Imaging anatomy of deep neck spaces. Otolaryngol Clin North Am 2012;45(6):1203–1221

Castleman's Disease

29. Cronin DMP, Warnke RA. Castleman disease: an update on classification and the spectrum of associated lesions. Adv Anat Pathol 2009;16(4):236–246
30. Enomoto K, Nakamichi I, Hamada K, et al. Unicentric and multicentric Castleman's disease. Br J Radiol 2007;80(949):e24–e26
31. Hillier JC, Shaw P, Miller RF, et al. Imaging features of multicentric Castleman's disease in HIV infection. Clin Radiol 2004;59(7):596–601
32. Koşucu P, Ahmetoğlu A, Imamoğlu M, Cay A, Cobanoğlu U, Gümele HR. Multicentric Castleman's disease in a child with subpectoral involvement. Pediatr Radiol 2003;33(8):570–573
33. Roca B. Castleman's disease. A review. AIDS Rev 2009;11(1):3–7
34. Wen L, Zhang D, Zhang ZG. CT characteristics of cervical Castleman's disease. Clin Imaging 2005;29(2):141–143

Cat-Scratch Disease

35. Dong PR, Seeger LL, Yao L, Panosian CB, Johnson BL Jr, Eckardt JJ. Uncomplicated cat-scratch disease: findings at CT, MR imaging, and radiography. Radiology 1995;195(3):837–839
36. Gielen J, Wang XL, Vanhoenacker F, et al. Lymphadenopathy at the medial epitrochlear region in cat-scratch disease. Eur Radiol 2003;13(6):1363–1369
37. Mele FM, Friedman M, Reznik AM. MR imaging of the knee: findings in cat-scratch disease. AJR Am J Roentgenol 1996;166(5):1232–1233
38. Wang CW, Chang WC, Chao TK, Liu CC, Huang GS. Computed tomography and magnetic resonance imaging of cat-scratch disease: a report of two cases. Clin Imaging 2009;33(4):318–321

Cervical Lymph Nodes

39. Hoang JK, Vanka J, Ludwig BJ, Glastonbury CM. Evaluation of cervical lymph nodes in head and neck cancer with CT and MRI: tips, traps, and a systematic approach. AJR Am J Roentgenol 2013;200(1):W17-25
40. Restrepo R, Oneto J, Lopez K, Kukreja K. Head and neck lymph nodes in children: the spectrum from normal to abnormal. Pediatr Radiol 2009;39(8):836–846

Dermoid in Floor of Mouth

41. Boko E, Amaglo K, Kpemissi E. A bulky dermoid cyst of the floor of the mouth. Eur Ann Otorhinolaryngol Head Neck Dis 2014;131(2):131–134
42. Gordon PE, Faquin WC, Lahey E, Kaban LB. Floor-of-mouth dermoid cysts: report of 3 variants and a suggested change in terminology. J Oral Maxillofac Surg 2013;71(6):1034–1041

Developmental Anomalies of Mandible

43. Balaji SM. Bifid mandibular condyle with temporomandibular joint ankylosis—a pooled data analysis. Dent Traumatol 2010;26(4):332–337
44. Baxter DJG, Shroff MM. Developmental maxillofacial anomalies. Semin Ultrasound CT MR 2011;32(6):555–568
45. Gitton Y, Heude E, Vieux-Rochas M, et al. Evolving maps in craniofacial development. Semin Cell Dev Biol 2010;21(3):301–308

46. Heude E, Rivals I, Couly G, Levi G. Masticatory muscle defects in hemifacial microsomia: a new embryological concept. Am J Med Genet A 2011;155A(8):1991–1995

47. López-López J, Ayuso-Montero R, Salas EJ, Roselló-Llabrés X. Bifid condyle: review of the literature of the last 10 years and report of two cases. Cranio 2010;28(2):136–140

48. MacArthur CJ. Prenatal diagnosis of fetal cervicofacial anomalies. Curr Opin Otolaryngol Head Neck Surg 2012;20(6):482–490

49. Pirttiniemi P, Peltomäki T, Müller L, Luder HU. Abnormal mandibular growth and the condylar cartilage. Eur J Orthod 2009;31(1):1–11

50. Scott AR, Tibesar RJ, Sidman JD. Pierre Robin sequence: evaluation, management, indications for surgery, and pitfalls. Otolaryngol Clin North Am 2012;45(3):695–710, ix

51. Suri M. Craniofacial syndromes. Semin Fetal Neonatal Med 2005; 10(3):243–257

52. Tan TY, Kilpatrick N, Farlie PG. Developmental and genetic perspectives on Pierre Robin sequence. Am J Med Genet C Semin Med Genet 2013;163C(4):295–305

Epidermoid in Floor of Mouth

53. Yilmaz I, Yilmazer C, Yavuz H, Bal N, Ozluoglu LN. Giant sublingual epidermoid cyst: a report of two cases. J Laryngol Otol 2006;120(3):E19

Floor of the Mouth Anatomy

54. Becker M. Oral cavity, oropharynx, and hypopharynx. Semin Roentgenol 2000;35(1):21–30

55. Warshafsky D, Goldenberg D, Kanekar SG. Imaging anatomy of deep neck spaces. Otolaryngol Clin North Am 2012;45(6):1203–1221

Florid Cemento-Osseous Dysplasia

56. Kim JH, Song BC, Kim SH, Park YS. Clinical, radiographic, and histological findings of florid cemento-osseous dysplasia: a case report. Imaging Sci Dent 2011;41(3):139–142

57. Köse TE, Köse OD, Karabas HC, Erdem TL, Ozcan I. Findings of florid cemento-osseous dysplasia: a report of three cases. J Oral Maxillofac Res 2013;4(4):e4

58. Sciubba JJ, Fantasia JE, Kahn LB. Fibro-osseous lesions. In: Atlas of Tumor Pathology, Tumors and Cysts of the Jaw. Washington DC: Armed Forces Institute of Pathology; 2001:141–160

Foregut Duplication Cyst

59. Hammoud A, Hourani M, Akoum M, Rajab M. Foregut duplication cyst: an unusual presentation during childhood. N Am J Med Sci 2012;4(6):287–289

60. Houshmand G, Hosseinzadeh K, Ozolek J. Prenatal magnetic resonance imaging (MRI) findings of a foregut duplication cyst of the tongue: value of real-time MRI evaluation of the fetal swallowing mechanism. J Ultrasound Med 2011;30(6):843–850

61. McMaster WG Jr, Mukherjee K, Parikh AA. Surgical management of a symptomatic foregut duplication cyst. Am Surg 2012; 78(6):E306–E307

Fracture of Mandible

62. Romeo A, Pinto A, Cappabianca S, Scaglione M, Brunese L. Role of multidetector row computed tomography in the management of mandible traumatic lesions. Semin Ultrasound CT MR 2009;30(3):174–180

Inflammatory Diseases of the Salivary Glands

63. Abdullah A, Rivas FFR, Srinivasan A. Imaging of the salivary glands. Semin Roentgenol 2012;48(1):65–74

64. Bonfils P, Moya-Plana A, Badoual C, Nadéri S, Malinvaud D, Laccourreye O. Intraparotid Kimura disease. Eur Ann Otorhinolaryngol Head Neck Dis 2013;130(2):87–89

65. Boyd ZT, Goud AR, Lowe LH, Shao L. Pediatric salivary gland imaging. Pediatr Radiol 2009;39(7):710–722

66. Burke CJ, Thomas RH, Howlett D. Imaging the major salivary glands. Br J Oral Maxillofac Surg 2011;49(4):261–269

67. Capaccio P, Sigismund PE, Luca N, Marchisio P, Pignataro L. Modern management of juvenile recurrent parotitis. J Laryngol Otol 2012;126(12):1254–1260

68. Gadodia A, Seith A, Sharma R, Thakar A. MRI and MR sialography of juvenile recurrent parotitis. Pediatr Radiol 2010;40(8):1405–1410

69. Horikoshi T, Motoori K, Ueda T, et al. Head and neck MRI of Kimura disease. Br J Radiol 2011;84(1005):800–804

70. Howlett DC, Kesse KW, Hughes DV, Sallomi DF. The role of imaging in the evaluation of parotid disease. Clin Radiol 2002;57(8):692–701

71. Kanekar SG, Mannion K, Zacharia T, Showalter M. Parotid space: anatomic imaging. Otolaryngol Clin North Am 2012;45(6):1253–1272

72. Oksüz MO, Werner MK, Aschoff P, Pfannenberg C. 18F-FDG PET/CT for the diagnosis of sarcoidosis in a patient with bilateral inflammatory involvement of the parotid and lacrimal glands (panda sign) and bilateral hilar and mediastinal lymphadenopathy (lambda sign). Eur J Nucl Med Mol Imaging 2011;38(3):603

73. Park SW, Kim HJ, Sung KJ, Lee JH, Park IS. Kimura disease: CT and MR imaging findings. AJNR Am J Neuroradiol 2012;33(4):784–788

74. Wilson KF, Meier JD, Ward PD. Salivary gland disorders. Am Fam Physician 2014;89(11):882–888

Juvenile Mandibular Chronic Osteomyelitis

75. Agarwal A, Kumar N, Tyagi A, De N. Primary chronic osteomyelitis in the mandible: a conservative approach. BMJ Case Reports, published on-line 2014. doi:10.1136/bcr-2013-202448

76. Falip C, Alison M, Boutry N, et al. Chronic recurrent multifocal osteomyelitis (CRMO): a longitudinal case series review. Pediatr Radiol 2013;43(3):355–375

77. Kadom N, Egloff A, Obeid G, Bandarkar A, Vezina G. Juvenile mandibular chronic osteomyelitis: multimodality imaging findings. Oral Surg Oral Med Oral Pathol Oral Radiol Endod 2011;111(3):e38–e43

78. Kuijpers SCC, de Jong E, Hamdy NAT, van Merkesteyn JPR. Initial results of the treatment of diffuse sclerosing osteomyelitis of the mandible with bisphosphonates. J Craniomaxillofac Surg 2011;39(1):65–68

79. Mehra H, Gupta S, Gupta H, Sinha V, Singh J. Chronic suppurative osteomyelitis of mandible: a case report. Craniomaxillofac Trauma Reconstr 2013;6(3):197–200

80. Urade M, Noguchi K, Takaoka K, Moridera K, Kishimoto H. Diffuse sclerosing osteomyelitis of the mandible successfully treated with pamidronate: a long-term follow-up report. Oral Surg Oral Med Oral Pathol Oral Radiol 2012;114(4):e9–e12

Juvenile Nasopharyngeal Angiofibroma

81. Boghani Z, Husain Q, Kanumuri VV, et al. Juvenile nasopharyngeal angiofibroma: a systematic review and comparison of endoscopic, endoscopic-assisted, and open resection in 1047 cases. Laryngoscope 2013;123(4):859–869

82. Griauzde J, Srinivasan A. Imaging of vascular lesions of the head and neck. Radiol Clin North Am 2015;53(1):197–213

83. Khoueir N, Nicolas N, Rohayem Z, Haddad A, Abou Hamad W. Exclusive endoscopic resection of juvenile nasopharyngeal angiofibroma: a systematic review of the literature. Otolaryngol Head Neck Surg 2014;150(3):350–358

84. Szymańska A, Szymański M, Czekajska-Chehab E, Szczerbo-Trojanowska M. Invasive growth patterns of juvenile nasopharyngeal angiofibroma: radiological imaging and clinical implications. Acta Radiol 2014;55(6):725–731

Lemierre Syndrome

85. Hile LM, Gibbons MD, Hile DC. Lemierre syndrome complicating otitis externa: case report and literature review. J Emerg Med 2012;42(4):e77–e80

86. Ridgway JM, Parikh DA, Wright R, et al. Lemierre syndrome: a pediatric case series and review of literature. Am J Otolaryngol 2010;31(1):38–45

87. Righini CA, Karkas A, Tourniaire R, et al. Lemierre syndrome: study of 11 cases and literature review. Head Neck 2014;36(7):1044–1051

88. Syed MI, Baring D, Addidle M, Murray C, Adams C. Lemierre syndrome: two cases and a review. Laryngoscope 2007;117(9):1605–1610

Lesions of the Mandible

89. Dunfee BL, Sakai O, Pistey R, Gohel A. Radiologic and pathologic characteristics of benign and malignant lesions of the mandible. Radiographics 2006;26(6):1751–1768

90. Devenney-Cakir B, Subramaniam RM, Reddy SM, Imsande H, Gohel A, Sakai O. Cystic and cystic-appearing lesions of the mandible: review. AJR Am J Roentgenol 2011;196(6, Suppl):WS66–WS77

91. Shimizu M, Osa N, Okamura K, Yoshiura K. CT analysis of the Stafne's bone defects of the mandible. Dentomaxillofac Radiol 2006; 35(2):95–102

92. Sciubba JJ, Fantasia JE, Kahn LB. Tumors and cysts of the jaw. In: Atlas of Tumor Pathology. Washington DC: Armed Forces Institute of Pathology; 2001

Lesions of the Retropharyngeal and Danger Spaces

93. Bakir S, Tanriverdi MH, Gün R, et al. Deep neck space infections: a retrospective review of 173 cases. Am J Otolaryngol 2012;33(1):56–63
94. Bosemani T, Izbudak I. Head and neck emergencies. Semin Roentgenol 2013;48(1):4–13
95. Debnam JM, Guha-Thakurta N. Retropharyngeal and prevertebral spaces: anatomic imaging and diagnosis. Otolaryngol Clin North Am 2012;45(6):1293–1310
96. Hoang JK, Eastwood JD, Branstetter BF, et al. Masses in the retropharyngeal space: key concepts on multiplanar CT and MR imaging. Neurographics 2011;1:49–55
97. Hoffmann C, Pierrot S, Contencin P, Morisseau-Durand MP, Manach Y, Couloigner V. Retropharyngeal infections in children. Treatment strategies and outcomes. Int J Pediatr Otorhinolaryngol 2011; 75(9):1099–1103
98. Jaworsky D, Reynolds S, Chow AW. Extracranial head and neck infections. Crit Care Clin 2013;29(3):443–463
99. Kato H, Kanematsu M, Kato Z, et al. Necrotic cervical nodes: usefulness of diffusion-weighted MR imaging in the differentiation of suppurative lymphadenitis from malignancy. Eur J Radiol 2013;82(1):e28–e35
100. Maroldi R, Farina D, Ravanelli M, Lombardi D, Nicolai P. Emergency imaging assessment of deep neck space infections. Semin Ultrasound CT MR 2012;33(5):432–442
101. Novis SJ, Pritchett CV, Thorne MC, Sun GH. Pediatric deep space neck infections in U.S. children, 2000–2009. Int J Pediatr Otorhinolaryngol 2014;78(5):832–836
102. Ozlugedik S, Ibrahim Acar H, Apaydin N, et al. Retropharyngeal space and lymph nodes: an anatomical guide for surgical dissection. Acta Otolaryngol 2005;125(10):1111–1115
103. Sauer MW, Sharma S, Hirsh DA, Simon HK, Agha BS, Sturm JJ. Acute neck infections in children: who is likely to undergo surgical drainage? Am J Emerg Med 2013;31(6):906–909
104. Schuler PJ, Cohnen M, Greve J, et al. Surgical management of retropharyngeal abscesses. Acta Otolaryngol 2009;129(11):1274–1279
105. Shefelbine SE, Mancuso AA, Gajewski BJ, Ojiri H, Stringer S, Sedwick JD. Pediatric retropharyngeal lymphadenitis: differentiation from retropharyngeal abscess and treatment implications. Otolaryngol Head Neck Surg 2007;136(2):182–188
106. Warshafsky D, Goldenberg D, Kanekar SG. Imaging anatomy of deep neck spaces. Otolaryngol Clin North Am 2012;45(6):1203–1221
107. Williams DW III. An imager's guide to normal neck anatomy. Semin Ultrasound CT MR 1997;18(3):157–181

Lingual Thyroid

108. Toso A, Colombani F, Averono G, Aluffi P, Pia F. Lingual thyroid causing dysphagia and dyspnoea. Case reports and review of the literature. Acta Otorhinolaryngol Ital 2009;29(4):213–217
109. Zander DA, Smoker WRK. Imaging of ectopic thyroid tissue and thyroglossal duct cysts. Radiographics 2014;34(1):37–50

Lymphoid Hyperplasia

110. Bhatia KSS, King AD, Vlantis AC, Ahuja AT, Tse GM. Nasopharyngeal mucosa and adenoids: appearance at MR imaging. Radiology 2012;263(2):437–443

Mandibular Osteonecrosis

111. García-Ferrer L, Bagán JV, Martínez-Sanjuan V, et al. MRI of mandibular osteonecrosis secondary to bisphosphonates. AJR Am J Roentgenol 2008;190(4):949–955
112. Popovic KS, Kocar M. Imaging findings in bisphosphonate-induced osteonecrosis of the jaws. Radiol Oncol 2010;44(4):215–219

Masticator Space

113. Connor SEJ, Davitt SM. Masticator space masses and pseudomasses. Clin Radiol 2004;59(3):237–245
114. Fernandes T, Lobo JC, Castro R, Oliveira MI, Som PM. Anatomy and pathology of the masticator space. Insights Imaging 2013;4(5):605–616
115. Meltzer DE, Shatzkes DR. Masticator space: imaging anatomy for diagnosis. Otolaryngol Clin North Am 2012;45(6):1233–1251

116. Wei Y, Xiao J, Zou L. Masticator space: CT and MRI of secondary tumor spread. AJR Am J Roentgenol 2007;189(2):488–497

Nasopharyngeal Carcinoma

117. King AD, Vlantis AC, Bhatia KSS, et al. Primary nasopharyngeal carcinoma: diagnostic accuracy of MR imaging versus that of endoscopy and endoscopic biopsy. Radiology 2011;258(2):531–537
118. King AD, Vlantis AC, Tsang RKY, et al. Magnetic resonance imaging for the detection of nasopharyngeal carcinoma. AJNR Am J Neuroradiol 2006;27(6):1288–1291

Neck Development

119. Grevellec A, Tucker AS. The pharyngeal pouches and clefts: Development, evolution, structure and derivatives. Semin Cell Dev Biol 2010;21(3):325–332
120. Prosser JD, Myer CM III. Branchial cleft anomalies and thymic cysts. Otolaryngol Clin North Am 2015;48(1):1–14
121. Som PM, Smoker WRK, Reidenberg JS, et al. Embryology and anatomy of the neck. In: Head and Neck Imaging. 5th ed. St. Louis, MO: Elsevier Mosby; 2011:2117–2180

Neuroglial Heterotopia

122. Hagiwara A, Nagai N, Ogawa Y, Suzuki M. A case of nasal glial heterotopia in an adult. Case Rep Otolaryngol 2014;2014:354672
123. Husein OF, Collins M, Kang DR. Neuroglial heterotopia causing neonatal airway obstruction: presentation, management, and literature review. Eur J Pediatr 2008;167(12):1351–1355

Odontogenic Myxoma

124. Gupta S, Grover N, Kadam A, Gupta S, Sah K, Sunitha JD. Odontogenic myxoma. Natl J Maxillofac Surg 2013;4(1):81–83
125. Kheir E, Stephen L, Nortje C, van Rensburg LJ, Titinchi F. The imaging characteristics of odontogenic myxoma and a comparison of three different imaging modalities. Oral Surg Oral Med Oral Pathol Oral Radiol 2013;116(4):492–502
126. Kleiber GM, Skapek SX, Lingen M, Reid RR. Odontogenic myxoma of the face: mimicry of cherubism. J Oral Maxillofac Surg 2014;72(11):2186–2191
127. Sumi Y, Miyaishi O, Ito K, Ueda M. Magnetic resonance imaging of myxoma in the mandible: a case report. Oral Surg Oral Med Oral Pathol Oral Radiol Endod 2000;90(5):671–676

Osteoblastoma of the Mandible and Maxilla

128. Jones AC, Prihoda TJ, Kacher JE, Odingo NA, Freedman PD. Osteoblastoma of the maxilla and mandible: a report of 24 cases, review of the literature, and discussion of its relationship to osteoid osteoma of the jaws. Oral Surg Oral Med Oral Pathol Oral Radiol Endod 2006;102(5):639–650

Osteoid Osteoma of Mandible

129. An SY, Shin HI, Choi KS, et al. Unusual osteoid osteoma of the mandible: report of case and review of the literature. Oral Surg Oral Med Oral Pathol Oral Radiol 2013;116(2):e134–e140
130. Rahsepar B, Nikgoo A, Fatemitabar SA. Osteoid osteoma of subcondylar region: case report and review of the literature. J Oral Maxillofac Surg 2009;67(4):888–893

Parapharyngeal Space

131. Gupta A, Chazen JL, Phillips CD. Imaging evaluation of the parapharyngeal space. Otolaryngol Clin North Am 2012;45(6):1223–1232

Parapharyngeal Space Tumors

132. Cassoni A, Terenzi V, Della Monaca M, et al. Parapharyngeal space benign tumours: our experience. J Craniomaxillofac Surg 2014;42(2):101–105
133. Dimitrijevic MV, Jesic SD, Mikic AA, Arsovic NA, Tomanovic NR. Parapharyngeal space tumors: 61 case reviews. Int J Oral Maxillofac Surg 2010;39(10):983–989
134. El Fiky L, Shoukry T, Hamid O. Pediatric parapharyngeal lesions: criteria for malignancy. Int J Pediatr Otorhinolaryngol 2013;77(12):1955–1959
135. Shin JH, Lee HK, Kim SY, Choi CG, Suh DC. Imaging of parapharyngeal space lesions: focus on the prestyloid compartment. AJR Am J Roentgenol 2001;177(6):1465–1470

136. Shirakura S, Tsunoda A, Akita K, et al. Parapharyngeal space tumors: anatomical and image analysis findings. Auris Nasus Larynx 2010;37(5):621–625

137. Som PM, Sacher M, Stollman AL, Biller HF, Lawson W. Common tumors of the parapharyngeal space: refined imaging diagnosis. Radiology 1988;169(1):81–85

Retrostyloid Parapharyngeal Space Neoplasms

138. Varoquaux A, Fakhry N, Gabriel S, et al. Retrostyloid parapharyngeal space tumors: a clinician and imaging perspective. Eur J Radiol 2013;82(5):773–782

Richter's Transformation

139. Bruzzi JF, Macapinlac H, Tsimberidou AM, et al. Detection of Richter's transformation of chronic lymphocytic leukemia by PET/CT. J Nucl Med 2006;47(8):1267–1273

Salivary Gland Tumors

140. Ban X, Wu J, Mo Y, et al. Lymphoepithelial carcinoma of the salivary gland: morphologic patterns and imaging features on CT and MRI. AJNR Am J Neuroradiol 2014;35(9):1813–1819

141. Christe A, Waldherr C, Hallett R, Zbaeren P, Thoeny H. MR imaging of parotid tumors: typical lesion characteristics in MR imaging improve discrimination between benign and malignant disease. AJNR Am J Neuroradiol 2011;32(7):1202–1207

142. Ellis G, Simpson RHW. Acinic cell carcinoma. In: Barnes L, Eveson JW, Reichart P, Sidransky D, eds. World Health Organization Classification of Tumours. Pathology and Genetics of Head and Neck Tumors. Lyon: IARC Press; 2005:216–218

143. El-Naggar AK, Huvos AG. Adenoid cystic carcinoma. In: Barnes L, Eveson JW, Reichart P, Sidransky D, eds. World Health Organization Classification of Tumours. Pathology and Genetics of Head and Neck Tumors. Lyon: IARC Press; 2005:221–222

144. Eveson JW, Kusafuka K, Stenman G, Nagao T. Pleomorphic adenoma. In: Barnes L, Eveson JW, Reichart P, Sidransky D, eds. World Health Organization Classification of Tumours. Pathology and Genetics of Head and Neck Tumors. Lyon: IARC Press; 2005:254–258

145. Gnepp DR, Brandwein-Gensier MS, El-Naggar AK, Nagao T. Carcinoma ex-pleomorphic adenoma. In: Barnes L, Eveson JW, Reichart P, Sidransky D, eds. World Health Organization Classification of Tumours. Pathology and Genetics of Head and Neck Tumors. Lyon: IARC Press; 2005:242–243

146. Goode RK, El-Naggar AK. Mucoepidermoid carcinoma. In Barnes L, Eveson JW, Reichart P, Sidransky D, eds. World Health Organization Classification of Tumours. Pathology and Genetics of Head and Neck Tumors. Lyon: IARC Press; 2005:219–220

147. Hamilton BE, Salzman KL, Wiggins RH III, Harnsberger HR. Earring lesions of the parotid tail. AJNR Am J Neuroradiol 2003;24(9):1757–1764

148. Kakimoto N, Gamoh S, Tamaki J, Kishino M, Murakami S, Furukawa S. CT and MR images of pleomorphic adenoma in major and minor salivary glands. Eur J Radiol 2009;69(3):464–472

149. Kinoshita T, Ishii K, Naganuma H, Okitsu T. MR imaging findings of parotid tumors with pathologic diagnostic clues: a pictorial essay. Clin Imaging 2004;28(2):93–101

150. Lee YYP, Wong KT, King AD, Ahuja AT. Imaging of salivary gland tumours. Eur J Radiol 2008;66(3):419–436

151. Li J, Gong X, Xiong P, et al. Ultrasound and computed tomography features of primary acinic cell carcinoma in the parotid gland: a retrospective study. Eur J Radiol 2014;83(7):1152–1156

152. Roach MC, Turkington TG, Higgins KA, Hawk TC, Hoang JK, Brizel DM. FDG-PET assessment of the effect of head and neck radiotherapy on parotid gland glucose metabolism. Int J Radiat Oncol Biol Phys 2012;82(1):321–326

153. Simpson RHW, Eveson JW. Warthin tumour. In: Barnes L, Eveson JW, Reichart P, Sidransky D, eds. World Health Organization Classification of Tumours. Pathology and Genetics of Head and Neck Tumors. Lyon: IARC Press; 2005:263–265

154. Suh SI, Seol HY, Kim TK, et al. Acinic cell carcinoma of the head and neck: radiologic-pathologic correlation. J Comput Assist Tomogr 2005;29(1):121–126

Sialolithiasis Involving the Submandibular Gland and Duct

155. Fatemi-Ardekani A, Boylan C, Noseworthy MD. Magnetic resonance imaging sialolithography: direct visualization of calculi in the submandibular gland using susceptibility-weighted imaging (SWI) at 3 Tesla. J Comput Assist Tomogr 2011;35(1):46–49

156. Kiringoda R, Eisele DW, Chang JL. A comparison of parotid imaging characteristics and sialendoscopic findings in obstructive salivary disorders. Laryngoscope 2014;124(12):2696–2701

157. Rzymska-Grala I, Stopa Z, Grala B, et al. Salivary gland calculi—contemporary methods of imaging. Pol J Radiol 2010;75(3):25–37

Stafne Bone Defect

158. Shimizu M, Osa N, Okamura K, Yoshiura K. CT analysis of the Stafne's bone defects of the mandible. Dentomaxillofac Radiol 2006; 35(2):95–102

Temporomandibular Joint

159. Bag AK, Gaddikeri S, Singhal A, et al. Imaging of the temporomandibular joint: An update. World J Radiol 2014;6(8):567–582

160. Peng LW, Yan DM, Wang YG, Li YD. Synovial chondromatosis of the temporomandibular joint: a case report with bilateral occurrence. J Oral Maxillofac Surg 2009;67(4):893–895

161. Petscavage-Thomas JM, Walker EA. Unlocking the jaw: advanced imaging of the temporomandibular joint. AJR Am J Roentgenol 2014;203(5):1047–1058

162. Tomas X, Pomes J, Berenguer J, et al. MR imaging of temporomandibular joint dysfunction: a pictorial review. Radiographics 2006;26(3):765–781

163. Vaid YN, Dunnavant FD, Royal SA, Beukelman T, Stoll ML, Cron RQ. Imaging of the temporomandibular joint in juvenile idiopathic arthritis. Arthritis Care Res (Hoboken) 2014;66(1):47–54

Tonsillar/Peritonsillar Infection

164. Bosemani T, Izbudak I. Head and neck emergencies. Semin Roentgenol 2013;48(1):4–13

165. Brook I. Microbiology and management of peritonsillar, retropharyngeal, and parapharyngeal abscesses. J Oral Maxillofac Surg 2004; 62(12):1545–1550

166. Ormond A, Chao S, Shapiro D, Walner D. Peritonsillar abscess with rapid progression to complete airway obstruction in a toddler. Laryngoscope 2014;124(10):2418–2421

167. Wang AS, Stater BJ, Kacker A. Intratonsillar abscess: 3 case reports and a review of the literature. Int J Pediatr Otorhinolaryngol 2013;77(4):605–607

Tornwaldt Cyst

168. Sekiya K, Watanabe M, Nadgir RN, et al. Nasopharyngeal cystic lesions: Tornwaldt and mucous retention cysts of the nasopharynx: findings on MR imaging. J Comput Assist Tomogr 2014;38(1):9–13

Thrombosis of the Internal Jugular Vein

169. Gallanos M, Hafner JW. Posttraumatic internal jugular vein thrombosis presenting as a painful neck mass in a child. Pediatr Emerg Care 2008;24(8):542–545

170. Ohba K, Matsushita A, Yamashita M, et al. The importance of imaging procedures in evaluating painful neck masses: two patients with a painful internal jugular vein thrombosis. Thyroid 2012;22(5):556–557

Thyroglossal Duct Cyst

171. Ahuja AT, Wong KT, King AD, Yuen EHY. Imaging for thyroglossal duct cyst: the bare essentials. Clin Radiol 2005;60(2):141–148

172. Gaddikeri S, Vattoth S, Gaddikeri RS, et al. Congenital cystic neck masses: embryology and imaging appearances, with clinicopathological correlation. Curr Probl Diagn Radiol 2014;43(2):55–67

173. Sameer KSM, Mohanty S, Correa MMA, Das K. Lingual thyroglossal duct cysts—a review. Int J Pediatr Otorhinolaryngol 2012;76(2):165–168

Tongue Abscess

174. Kim HJ, Lee BJ, Kim SJ, Shim WY, Baik SK, Sunwoo M. Tongue abscess mimicking neoplasia. AJNR Am J Neuroradiol 2006;27(10):2202–2203

175. Ozturk M, Mavili E, Erdogan N, Cagli S, Guney E. Tongue abscesses: MR imaging findings. AJNR Am J Neuroradiol 2006;27(6):1300–1303

Tongue Metastasis

176. Mavili E, Oztürk M, Yücel T, Yüce I, Cağli S. Tongue metastasis mimicking an abscess. Diagn Interv Radiol 2010;16(1):27–29

Tongue Schwannoma

177. Bhola N, Jadhav A, Borle R, Khemka G, Bhutekar U, Kumar S. Schwannoma of the tongue in a paediatric patient: a case report and 20-year review. Case Rep Dent 2014;780762

178. Manna F, Barbi E, Murru F, Bussani R. Lingual schwannoma in pediatric patients. J Craniofac Surg 2012;23(5):e454–e456

Tumors Involving the Oral Cavity and Floor of the Mouth

179. Beil CM, Keberle M. Oral and oropharyngeal tumors. Eur J Radiol 2008;66(3):448–459

180. Edwards RM, Chapman T, Horn DL, Paladin AM, Iyer RS. Imaging of pediatric floor of mouth lesions. Pediatr Radiol 2013;43(5):523–535

181. La'porte SJ, Juttla JK, Lingam RK. Imaging the floor of the mouth and the sublingual space. Radiographics 2011;31(5):1215–1230

182. Lenz M, Greess H, Baum U, Dobritz M, Kersting-Sommerhoff B. Oropharynx, oral cavity, floor of the mouth: CT and MRI. Eur J Radiol 2000;33(3):203–215

183. Stambuk HE, Karimi S, Lee N, Patel SG. Oral cavity and oropharynx tumors. Radiol Clin North Am 2007;45(1):1–20

Chapter 5

Infrahyoid Neck

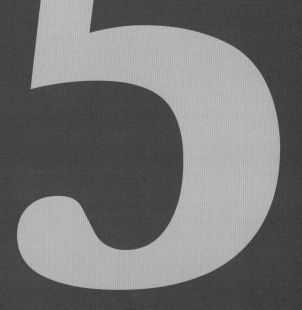

5 Infrahyoid Neck

Table 5.1	Congenital and developmental abnormalities of the infrahyoid neck
Table 5.2	Lesions of the hypopharynx and larynx
Table 5.3	Visceral space: lesions of the thyroid and parathyroid glands
Table 5.4	Visceral space: lesions of the pharynx, esophagus, and trachea
Table 5.5	Lesions of the infrahyoid carotid space
Table 5.6	Abnormalities of the anterior cervical space
Table 5.7	Abnormalities of the posterior cervical space

Introduction

The infrahyoid neck contains fascia-enclosed spaces that can provide relative barriers to the spread of neoplasms and infections, and can be useful in limiting and refining the list of differential diagnoses of various lesions (**Fig. 5.1**).

The superficial fascia includes the subcutaneous tissue, platysma muscle, blood vessels, superficial lymph nodes, and cutaneous nerves. Below the superficial fascia is the deep cervical fascia (DCF). The DCF is composed of three layers: the superficial layer (investing layer), the middle layer (visceral layer), and the deep layer (prevertebral layer).

The superficial layer of the DCF encircles the neck deep to the superficial fascia and extends from the skull base down to the thoracic inlet. The superficial layer of the DCF splits and encloses the sternocleidomastoid and trapezius muscles and has attachments to the hyoid bone, clavicle, scapula, and sternum.

The middle layer of the DCF (visceral fascia) extends from the hyoid bone down to the thoracic inlet anteriorly, and posteriorly from the skull base down into the mediastinum, forming the anterior wall of the retropharyngeal space. The middle layer of the DCF is contiguous superiorly with the buccopharyngeal fascia in the suprahyoid neck. The muscular portion of the middle layer of the DCF encircles the strap muscles, and the visceral portion of the middle layer of the DCF forms the outer border of the visceral space, which contains the hypopharynx, larynx, recurrent laryngeal nerves, trachea, thyroid gland, parathyroid glands, esophagus, and paraesophageal lymph nodes.

The deep layer of the DCF has two portions. The posterior major portion (also referred to as the prevertebral fascial layer) encloses the prevertebral and perivertebral muscles and the vertebral column; it extends from the skull base down to the coccyx. This layer fuses with the anterior longitudinal ligament at the T3 level, resulting in restriction of neoplasm or infection below the T3 level. The alar fascia is a layer of DCF that is located anterior to the prevertebral fascial layer of the DCF, and it extends inferiorly from the skull base to where it fuses with the visceral fascia (middle layer of the deep cervical fascia and inferior extension of the buccopharyngeal fascia), most often at the C7–T1 level. In the suprahyoid neck, the alar fascial layer forms the posterior border of the retropharyngeal space. The inferior border of the retropharyngeal space is usually at the C7–T1 level. Fusion of the visceral fascia with the alar fascia can, however, vary from the C6 to T4 levels. Between the alar fascia and the prevertebral fascia of the DCF is the potential danger space, which consists of loose areolar tissue. The danger space continues inferiorly to the level of the diaphragm between the prevertebral fascia posteriorly and fused alar fascia and visceral fascia anteriorly. Infections or neoplasms that extend into the danger space can spread between the skull base and mediastinum. The prevertebral fascia extends from the skull base to the coccyx, although it fuses with the anterior longitudinal ligament at the T3 level, resulting in restriction of neoplasm or infection below the T3 level.

5.1 Congenital and Developmental Abnormalities of the Infrahyoid Neck

The visceral space is enclosed by the middle layer of the DCF and contains the hypopharynx, larynx, recurrent laryngeal nerves, trachea, thyroid gland, parathyroid glands, esophagus, and paraesophageal lymph nodes. The visceral space is located anterior to the retropharyngeal and danger spaces, anteromedial to the infrahyoid carotid spaces, and medial to the anterior cervical space.

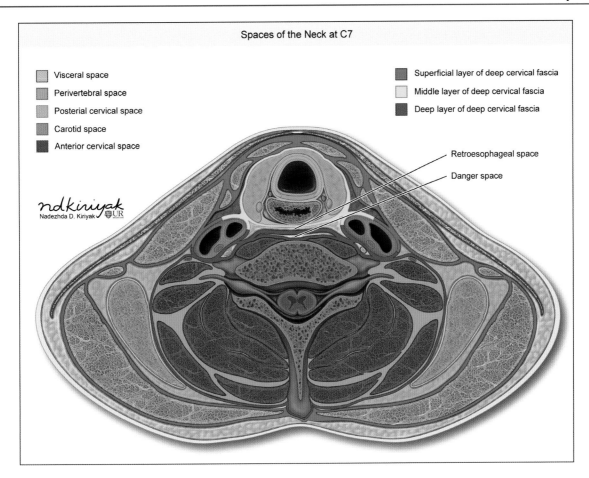

Fig. 5.1   Axial view diagram shows the layers of the deep cervical fascia and the spaces of the infrahyoid neck.

Table 5.1   Congenital and developmental abnormalities of the infrahyoid neck

- Thyroglossal duct cyst
- Ectopic thyroid tissue
- Branchial cleft cyst
- Venolymphatic malformation (lymphangioma)
- Klippel-Trenaunay syndrome
- Hemangioma
- Hemangioendothelioma
- Epidermoid
- Dermoid
- Teratoma
- Esophageal atresia (EA) without or with tracheoesophageal fistula (TEF)
- Neurenteric cysts
- Cervical thymic cyst
- Fibromatosis colli

Table 5.1 Congenital and developmental abnormalities of the infrahyoid neck

Abnormality	Imaging Findings	Comments
Thyroglossal duct cyst (**Fig. 5.2** and **Fig. 5.3**)	*MRI:* Well-circumscribed spheroid or ovoid lesion along the pathway of the thyroglossal duct extending from the tongue base inferiorly in the anterior neck in the midline or laterally within, or deep to, the strap muscles. Thyroglossal duct cysts usually have low signal on T1-weighted imaging (T1WI) and diffusion-weighted imaging and high signal on T2-weighted imaging (T2WI). The wall of a thyroglossal duct cyst is typically thin, without gadolinium (Gd) contrast enhancement. Thyroglossal cysts complicated by hemorrhage or current or prior infection can have elevated protein with intermediate to slightly high signal on T1WI and T2WI. The walls of such cysts can be thick and show Gd contrast enhancement. Nodular Gd contrast enhancement involving the wall of a thyroglossal cyst can be seen with a potentially malignant lesion. *CT:* Well-circumscribed lesion with low (mucoid) attenuation ranging from 10 to 25 HU, surrounded by a thin wall. Occasionally contains thin septations. Thyroglossal cysts complicated by infection can have increased attenuation, thick walls, and loss/indistinctness of adjacent tissue planes. *US:* Can be well-circumscribed, anechoic cysts with through transmission, or may have a pseudosolid appearance related to elevated protein concentration.	Thyroglossal duct cyst is the most common congenital mass in the neck and is related to altered development of the thyroid gland. The follicular cells of the thyroid gland develop from endodermal cells (median thyroid anlage) located between the first and second pharyngeal arches in the first 3 weeks of gestation. At 24 days of gestation, a small pit (thyroid bud) forms within the thyroid anlage that progressively forms a bilobed diverticulum that extends inferiorly along the midline adjacent to the aortic primordium. A small channel (thyroglossal duct) temporarily exists between the dorsal portion of the tongue (foramen cecum) and the inferiorly descending thyroid primordium. The thyroglossal duct normally involutes by the tenth week of gestation. The descending thyroid primordium and thyroglossal duct course anterior to the hyoid bone and loop slightly posterior to the inferior margin of the hyoid bone before descending anterior to the thyrohyoid membrane, thyroid cartilage, and trachea. The thyroglossal duct extends between the sternohyoid and sternothyroid strap muscles. The descending thyroid primordium reaches its normal position in the lower neck at 7 weeks of gestation. The parafollicular cells (C cells) of the thyroid develop from endodermal cells (lateral thyroid anlage) at the fourth pharyngeal pouch and migrate to join and merge with the descending thyroid primordium from the median thyroid anlage. Up to two-thirds of thyroglossal duct cysts occur in the infrahyoid neck and can be midline or extend laterally within, or deep to, the strap muscles. Nearly 50% present in patients < 20 years old as a progressively enlarging neck lesion.

(continued on page 500)

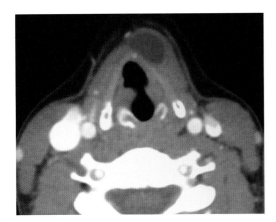

Fig. 5.2 Axial CT of a 45-year-old woman shows a thyroglossal duct cyst located anterior to the left thyroid cartilage that has low (mucoid) attenuation surrounded by a thin wall.

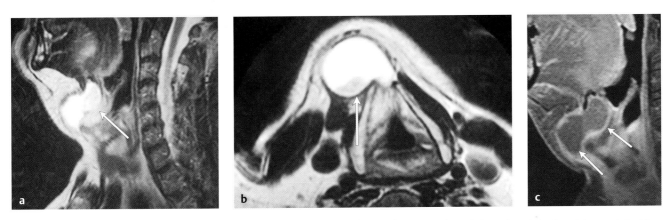

Fig. 5.3 **(a)** Sagittal and **(b)** axial T2-weighted imaging of a 73-year-old man shows an infected thyroglossal duct cyst (*arrows*) that has mostly high signal as well as a dependent component with slightly high signal. **(c)** Postcontrast sagittal fat-suppressed T1-weighted imaging shows irregular peripheral contrast enhancement of the cyst wall (*arrows*) surrounding contents with a fluid–fluid level.

Table 5.1 *(cont.)*   Congenital and developmental abnormalities of the infrahyoid neck

Abnormality	Imaging Findings	Comments
Ectopic thyroid tissue (**Fig. 5.4, Fig. 5.5**, and **Fig. 5.6**)	*CT:* Circumscribed ovoid or spheroid lesion at the dorsal portion (base) of the tongue that shows slightly increased attenuation (~ 70 HU), + contrast enhancement, ± low-attenuation thyroid nodules, ± calcifications. *MRI:* Circumscribed lesions with low-intermediate signal on T1-weighted imaging and low, intermediate, or slightly high signal on T2-weighted imaging. Variable degrees of gadolinium contrast enhancement. *Nuclear medicine:* Iodine-123, iodine-131, or technetium-99m pertechnetate uptake in ectopic thyroid tissue in the tongue and lack of normal uptake in normal orthotopic location of thyroid bed.	The normal thyroid gland is located below the larynx, posterior to the strap muscles, medial to the carotid arteries, and anterolateral to the trachea. Ectopic thyroid tissue results from lack of normal embryologic descent of the primitive thyroid gland along the thyroglossal duct from the foramen cecum at the tongue base down to the lower neck. Lingual thyroid represents up to 90% of cases of ectopic thyroid. Other locations include: adjacent to the hyoid bone, midline infrahyoid neck, and lateral neck. Can be asymptomatic, or may occur in association with dysphagia, dysphonia, and/or stridor.

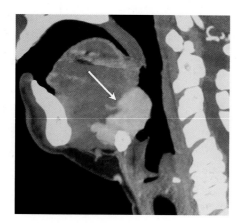

Fig. 5.4 Postcontrast sagittal CT shows enhancing ectopic thyroid tissue at the tongue base (*arrow*).

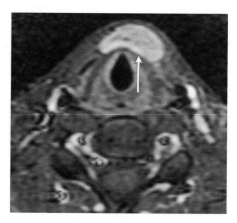

Fig. 5.5 Postcontrast axial fat-suppressed T1-weighted imaging shows enhancing ectopic thyroid tissue (*arrow*).

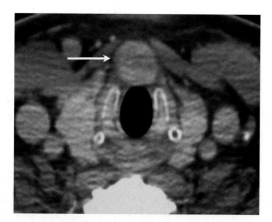

Fig. 5.6 Axial CT shows ectopic thyroid tissue (*arrow*) that has slightly high attenuation that is similar to normally located thyroid tissue in the field of view.

Abnormality	Imaging Findings	Comments
Branchial cleft cyst (**Fig. 5.7**, **Fig. 5.8**, **Fig. 5.9**, and **Fig. 5.10**)	*CT:* Circumscribed, cystic lesion with low to intermediate attenuation depending on the proportions of protein and water. *First branchial cleft cysts* can be located adjacent to the external auditory canal (type 1 first branchial cyst) or superficial portion of the parotid gland ± extension into the parapharyngeal space, posterior to the submandibular gland, and/or up to the external auditory canal (type 2). *Second branchial cleft cysts* can be superficial to the anterior margin of the sternocleidomastoid muscle (SCM) and deep to the platysma muscle (type 1), anteromedial to the upper third of the SCM near the level of the hyoid bone with or without extension posterior to the carotid sheath (type 2), or extend into the parapharyngeal space, and between the internal and external carotid arteries (type 3). Type 4 is located between the medial aspect of the carotid sheath and pharynx at the level of the tonsillar fossa. *Third branchial cleft cysts* are located at the lower anterior margin of the SCM at the level of the upper thyroid lobe, ± extension of sinus tract posterior to the carotid artery and glossopharyngeal nerve, passing through the thyroid membrane above the level of the internal branch of the superior laryngeal nerve into the base of the piriform sinus. *Fourth branchial cleft cysts* occur in the lower third of the neck laterally, and anterior to the lower SCM and level of the aortic arch, ± visible connecting sinus tract on the right below the subclavian artery or on the left below the aortic arch that extends superiorly and dorsal to the carotid artery up to the level of the hypoglossal nerve and then downward along the SCM to the piriform sinus. Can follow the course of the recurrent laryngeal nerve. *MRI:* Circumscribed lesion that often has low-intermediate signal on T1-weighted imaging and high signal on T2-weighted imaging. Usually there is no gadolinium contrast enhancement unless there is superimposed infection.	Branchial cleft cysts are developmental anomalies involving the branchial apparatus. The branchial apparatus consists of four major and two rudimentary arches of mesoderm lined by ectoderm externally and endoderm internally within pouches that form at the end of the fourth week of gestation. The mesoderm contains a dominant artery, nerve, cartilage, and muscle. The four major arches are separated by clefts. Each arch develops into a defined neck structure with eventual obliteration of the branchial clefts. The first arch forms the external auditory canal, eustachian tube, middle ear, and mastoid air cells. The second arch develops into the hyoid bone and tonsillar and supratonsillar fossae. The third and fourth arches develop into the pharynx below the hyoid bone. Branchial anomalies include cysts, sinuses, and fistulae. Second branchial cleft cysts account for up to 90% of all branchial cleft malformations. Cysts are lined by squamous epithelium (90%), ciliated columnar epithelium (8%), or both types (2%). Sebaceous glands, salivary tissue, lymphoid tissue, and cholesterol crystals in mucoid fluid can also occur. There are four types of second branchial cleft cysts. Type 1 is located anterior to the SCM and deep to the platysma muscle; type 2 (the most common type) is located at the anteromedial surface of the SCM, lateral to the carotid space and posterior to the submandibular gland; type 3 is located lateral to the pharyngeal wall and medial to the carotid arteries ± extension between the external and internal carotid arteries ("beak sign"); type 4 is located between the medial aspect of the carotid sheath and pharynx at the level of the tonsillar fossa, and can extend superiorly to the skull base. Typically, branchial cleft cysts are asymptomatic unless complicated by infection.

(continued on page 503)

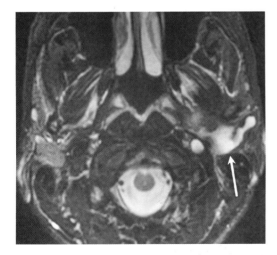

Fig. 5.7 Axial fat-suppressed T2-weighted imaging shows a first branchial cleft cyst (type 2) with high signal located in the superficial portion of the left parotid gland and extending toward the left parapharyngeal space (*arrow*).

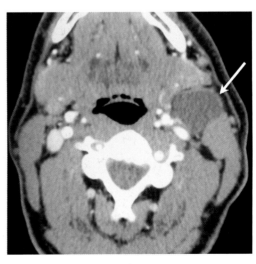

Fig. 5.8 Axial CT shows a second branchial cleft cyst (type 2) anteromedial to the left sternocleidomastoid muscle and lateral to the carotid sheath (*arrow*).

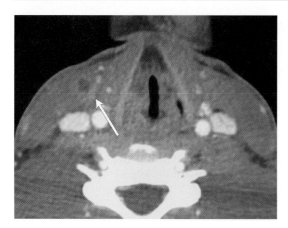

Fig. 5.9 Axial postcontrast CT shows an infected third branchial cleft cyst at the lower anterior margin of the right sternocleidomastoid muscle that has low attenuation centrally surrounded by a thick rim of irregular soft tissue attenuation (*arrow*), with adjacent peripheral ill-defined soft tissue attenuation.

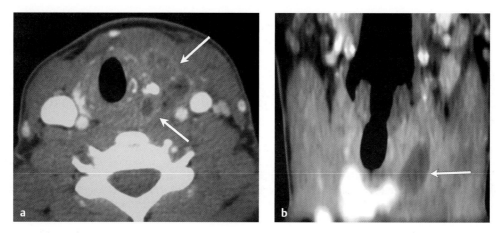

Fig. 5.10 **(a)** Axial and **(b)** coronal CT images show an infected fourth branchial cleft cyst containing zones of low attenuation with irregular peripheral contrast enhancement (*arrows*) located anterior to the lower left sternocleidomastoid muscle, with extension medial to the carotid space to involve the upper left thyroid lobe.

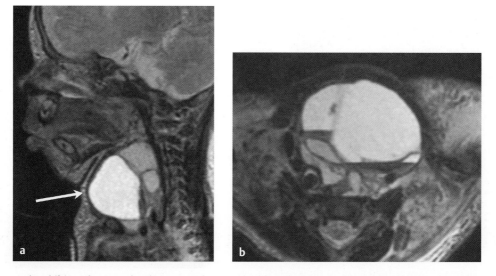

Fig. 5.11 **(a)** Sagittal and **(b)** axial T2-weighted imaging of a 4-week-old male with a venolymphatic malformation (lymphangioma) shows a complex lesion compressing the airway that has multiple fluid–fluid levels with high, intermediate, and low signal (*arrow* in **a**).

Table 5.1 *(cont.)* Congenital and developmental abnormalities of the infrahyoid neck

Abnormality	Imaging Findings	Comments
Venolymphatic malformation (lymphangioma) (**Fig. 5.11**)	Can be circumscribed lesions or occur in an infiltrative pattern, with extension into soft tissue and between muscles. *MRI:* The malformation often contains single or multiple cystic zones, which can be large (macrocystic type) or small (microcystic type), and which have predominantly low signal on T1-weighted imaging (T1WI) and high signal on T2-weighted imaging (T2WI) and fat-suppressed T2WI. Fluid–fluid levels and zones with high signal on T1WI and variable signal on T2WI may result from cysts containing hemorrhage, high protein concentration, and/or necrotic debris. Septa between the cystic zones can vary in thickness and gadolinium (Gd) contrast enhancement. Nodular zones within the lesions can have variable degrees of Gd contrast enhancement. Microcystic malformations typically show more Gd contrast enhancement than the macrocystic type. *CT:* The macrocystic malformations are usually low-attenuation cystic lesions (10–25 HU) separated by thin walls, ± intermediate or high attenuation resulting from hemorrhage or infection, ± fluid–fluid levels.	Benign vascular anomalies (also referred to as lymphangioma or cystic hygroma) that primarily result from abnormal lymphangiogenesis. Up to 75% occur in the head and neck. Can be observed in utero with MRI or sonography, at birth (50–65%), or within the first 5 years. Approximately 85% are detected by age 2. Lesions are composed of endothelium-lined lymphatic ± venous channels interspersed within connective tissue stroma. Account for less than 1% of benign soft tissue tumors and 5.6% of all benign lesions of infancy and childhood. Can occur in association with Turner syndrome and Proteus syndrome.
Klippel-Trenaunay syndrome (**Fig. 5.12**)	*MRI:* Single or multiple cystic-appearing zones that can be large. The cystic-appearing zones can have low signal on T1-weighted imaging (T1WI) and high signal on T2-weighted imaging (T2WI) and fat-suppressed T2WI. Fluid–fluid levels and zones with high signal on T1WI and variable signal on T2WI may result from cysts containing hemorrhage, high protein concentration, and/or necrotic debris. Septa between the cystic zones can vary in thickness and gadolinium contrast enhancement.	Rare congenital disorder involving blood and lymph vessels, consisting of capillary or cavernous hemangiomas and venous varicosities with soft tissue and/or hypertrophy. Can be associated with a consumptive coagulopathy with thrombocytopenia (Kasabach-Merritt syndrome), as well as Parkes-Weber and Proteus syndromes. Lesions in the neck can result in narrowing of the airway, causing respiratory distress.

(continued on page 504)

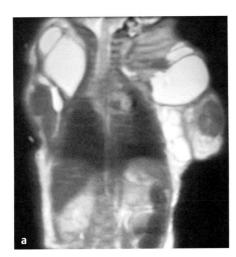 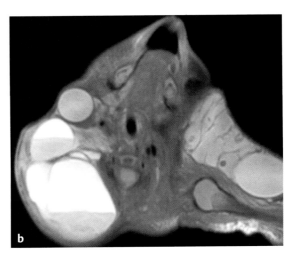

Fig. 5.12 **(a)** Coronal and **(b)** axial T2-weighted images of a 1-day-old neonate (37 weeks' gestation) with Klippel-Trenaunay syndrome show multiple cystic-appearing zones with high signal and fluid–fluid levels with variable signal from hemorrhage, high protein concentration, and/necrotic debris.

Table 5.1 *(cont.)*   Congenital and developmental abnormalities of the infrahyoid neck

Abnormality	Imaging Findings	Comments
Hemangioma (**Fig. 5.13**)	*MRI:* Circumscribed or poorly marginated structures (< 4 cm in diameter) in bone marrow or soft tissue with intermediate-high signal on T1-weighted imaging (often isointense to marrow fat), high signal on T2-weighted imaging (T2WI) and fat-suppressed T2WI, and typically show gadolinium contrast enhancement, ± expansion of bone. *CT:* Expansile bone lesions with a radiating pattern of bony trabeculae oriented toward the center. Hemangiomas in soft tissue have mostly intermediate attenuation, ± zones of fat attenuation.	Benign lesions of bone or soft tissue composed of capillary, cavernous, and/or venous malformations. Considered to be a hamartomatous disorder. Occurs in patients 1 to 84 years old (median age = 33 years).
Hemangioendothelioma (**Fig. 5.14**)	*MRI:* Tumors have lobulated, well-defined or irregular margins and have intermediate signal on T1-weighted imaging and heterogeneous, predominantly high signal on T2-weighted imaging, with or without internal low-signal septations. Flow voids may be seen with the lesions. Tumors show heterogeneous gadolinium contrast enhancement.	Locally aggressive tumors with vascular differentiation and associated Kaposi sarcoma-like fascicular patterns of atypical spindle cells. The tumors rarely metastasize. Frequently occur in patients from 2 weeks to 20 years old (mean age = 3.75 years), but also occur in adults as much as 64 years old. Large lesions can be associated with anemia and consumptive coagulopathy (Kasabach-Meritt syndrome or phenomenon) due to clot activation within the neoplastic vasculature. The prognosis is poorer for large intra-abdominal lesions associated with Kasabach-Merritt syndrome than for those located in the superficial soft tissues with easier surgical access. Tumors can occasionally spread to regional perinodal tissue, but typically do not metastasize to distant sites.
Epidermoid	*MRI:* Well-circumscribed spheroid or multilobulated ectodermal-inclusion cystic lesions with low-intermediate signal on T1-weighted imaging, high signal on T2-weighted imaging and diffusion-weighted imaging, and mixed low, intermediate, or high signal on FLAIR images. There is no gadolinium contrast enhancement. *CT:* Well-circumscribed spheroid or multilobulated extra-axial ectodermal-inclusion cystic lesions with low-intermediate attenuation.	Nonneoplastic congenital or acquired lesions filled with desquamated cells and keratinaceous debris surrounded by a wall lined by simple squamous epithelium. Lesions result from congenital inclusion of epidermal elements during embryonic development of the first and second branchial arches, or from trauma. Often occur in patients between 5 and 50 years old (mean age = 30 years).
Dermoid	*MRI:* Well-circumscribed spheroid or multilobulated lesions, usually with high signal on T1-weighted imaging, variable low, intermediate, and/or high signal on T2-weighted imaging, and no gadolinium contrast enhancement. *CT:* Well-circumscribed spheroid or multilobulated lesions, usually with low attenuation, ± fat–fluid or fluid–debris levels.	Nonneoplastic congenital or acquired ectodermal-inclusion cystic lesions filled with lipid material, cholesterol, desquamated cells, and keratinaceous debris surrounded by a wall lined by keratinizing squamous epithelium. Lesions result from congenital inclusion of dermal elements during embryonic development or from trauma. Occur in males slightly more than in females, ± related clinical symptoms. Can cause chemical inflammation if dermoid cyst ruptures.

(continued on page 506)

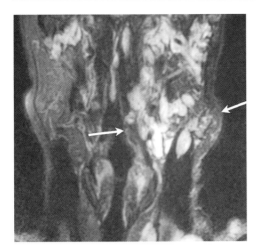

Fig. 5.13 Coronal T2-weighted imaging of a 22-year-old man with hemangiomatosis seen as high signal involving the soft tissues of the left neck and face (*arrows*).

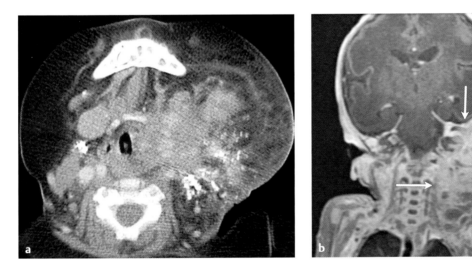

Fig. 5.14 **(a)** Axial CT of a 1-day-old neonate with Kasabach-Merritt syndrome shows a kaposiform hemangioendothelioma in the left lower face and neck with ill-defined margins and mostly soft tissue attenuation, including dystrophic calcifications. **(b)** The lesion shows gadolinium contrast enhancement on coronal T1-weighted imaging (*arrows*).

Table 5.1 (cont.)   Congenital and developmental abnormalities of the infrahyoid neck

Abnormality	Imaging Findings	Comments
Teratoma	*MRI:* Lesions usually have circumscribed margins and can contain various combinations and proportions of zones with low, intermediate, and/or high signal on T1-weighted imaging (T1WI), T2-weighted imaging (T2WI), and fat-suppressed (FS) T2WI. Can contain teeth and zones of bone formation, as well as amorphous, clumplike, and/or curvilinear calcifications with low signal on T1WI, T2WI, and FS T2WI. Fluid–fluid and fat–fluid levels may be seen within teratomas. Gadolinium contrast enhancement is usually seen in solid portions and septa. Invasion of adjacent tissue and bone destruction, as well as metastases, are findings associated with malignant teratomas. *CT:* Can contain zones with low and intermediate attenuation with or without calcifications.	Teratomas are neoplasms that arise from displaced embryonic germ cells (multipotential germinal cells) and contain various combinations of cells and tissues derived from more than one germ layer (endoderm, mesoderm, ectoderm). Second most common type of germ cell tumor. Occurs in children, and in males more than in females. Can be benign or malignant. Mature teratomas have differentiated cells from ectoderm (skin), mesoderm (cartilage, bone, muscle, and/or fat); and endoderm (cysts with enteric or respiratory epithelia). Immature teratomas contain partially differentiated ectodermal, mesodermal, or endodermal cells.
Esophageal atresia (EA) without or with tracheoesophageal fistula (TEF) (**Fig. 5.15**)	*Prenatal ultrasound:* Findings in the third trimester include polyhydramnios, small or absent stomach bubble, and fluid-filled loops of bowel. These findings have a positive predictive value of 56%. *Radiographs and CT:* Findings for *EA without TEF* include a proximal air-filled pouch with gasless abdomen (type A). For *EA with proximal TEF* (type B) or *distal TEF* (type C), findings include a distended air-filled abdomen. Similar findings occur for *EA with TEF* to both esophageal segments (type D). *TEF without EA* is a type H fistula, and can be evaluated with non-ionic water-soluble contrast. Three-dimensional CT with shaded-surface display can also be used to evaluate EA with or without TEF.	Esophageal atresia (EA) without or with tracheoesophageal fistula (TEF) represents a group of congenital malformations involving the foregut, which results from deficient formation of the tracheoesophageal septum that normally separates the developing respiratory and digestive tracts after 22 weeks of gestation. Occurs in 1 per 3,000–5,000 live births. Neonates present with excessive salivation, coughing, regurgitation, inability to swallow food, and respiratory distress from aspiration. Associated with anomalies involving the cardiovascular, neurologic, musculoskeletal, and/or renal systems. Also included in the VACTERL (vertebral defects, anal atresia, tracheoesophageal fistula with esophageal atresia, cardiac anomalies, renal anomalies and limb anomalies) association.
Neurenteric cysts (See **Fig. 1.104**)	*MRI:* Well-circumscribed, spheroid, intradural, extra-axial lesions, with low, intermediate, or high signal on T1- and T2-weighted imaging, and usually no gadolinium contrast enhancement. *CT:* Circumscribed, intradural, extra-axial structures with low-intermediate attenuation. Usually no contrast enhancement.	Neurenteric cysts are malformations in which there is a persistent communication between the ventrally located endoderm and the dorsally located ectoderm secondary to developmental failure of separation of the notochord and foregut. Obliteration of portions of a dorsal enteric sinus can result in cysts lined by endothelium, fibrous cords, or sinuses. Observed in patients < 40 years old. Locations: thoracic > cervical > posterior cranial fossa > craniovertebral junction > lumbar. Usually midline in position and often ventral to the spinal cord or brainstem. Associated with anomalies of the adjacent vertebrae and clivus. Lesions can extend from the spinal canal to the visceral space of the neck.
Cervical thymic cyst (**Fig. 5.16**)	*CT:* Circumscribed, thin-walled lesion usually with fluid attenuation, located in the lateral portion of the visceral space at the level of the thyroid gland, ± nodular zones of wall thickening. Typically shows no contrast enhancement unless there is superimposed infection or hemorrhage. *MRI:* Circumscribed thin-walled lesion, usually with low signal on T1-weighted imaging and high signal on T2-weighted imaging, ± nodular zones of wall thickening. Typically no gadolinium contrast enhancement within the lesion unless there is superimposed infection or hemorrhage. Approximately 50% are contiguous with the mediastinal thymus. Cysts may extend into the carotid sheath between the carotid artery and jugular vein in the suprahyoid neck.	Developmental abnormality of the third branchial pouch involving the thymopharyngeal duct. The thymopharyngeal duct is the embryologic pathway of primordial thymus cells that begin to migrate from the pharynx down to the mediastinum at 8 weeks of gestation. This duct normally involutes after the inferior migration of thymic cells. Cysts can occur along the tract of this duct from the piriform sinus down to the mediastinum. Cyst walls typically contain Hassall's corpuscles. Usually present in the first 2 decades. Often asymptomatic. Can, however, be associated with enlarging neck mass, dysphagia, vocal cord paresis or paralysis, or respiratory distress.

Abnormality	Imaging Findings	Comments
Fibromatosis colli (**Fig. 5.17**)	*MRI:* Lesions appear as fusiform enlargement of the lower sternocleidomastoid muscle (SCM). No discrete focal lesions are usually seen in the enlarged lower SCM. The involved muscle can have low-intermediate signal on T1- and T2-weighted imaging (T2WI), and low, intermediate, and/or slightly high signal on FS T2WI. *CT:* Fusiform swelling of the lower SCM is usually seen.	Fibromatosis colli is a benign form of infantile fibromatosis involving the distal SCM that can occur after abnormal intrauterine positioning or difficult deliveries. The lesions are rare and occur in 0.4% of live births. Most cases are diagnosed in infants < 6 months old. The affected muscle is thickened and shortened, resulting in cervicofacial asymmetry. Lesions contain groups of plump spindle cells within myxoid and/or collagenous ground substance. Torticollis is seen in up to 20% of infants with fibromatosis colli. Can be seen in association with other developmental abnormalities, such as forefoot anomalies (metatarsus adductus, talipes equinovarus) and hip dysplasia with congenital hip dislocation.

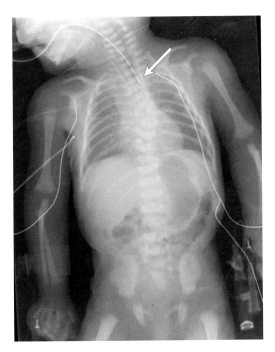

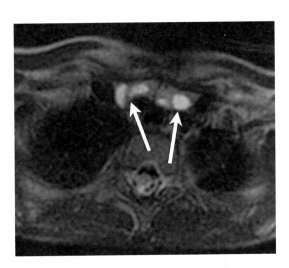

Fig. 5.16 Axial T2-weighted imaging shows small thymic cysts with high signal (*arrows*).

Fig. 5.15 Frontal radiograph of a neonate with esophageal atresia with tracheoesophageal fistula shows a tube terminating in the proximal pouch (*arrow*) and air-filled stomach and bowel.

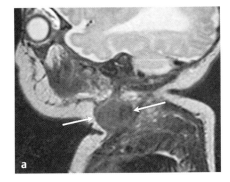

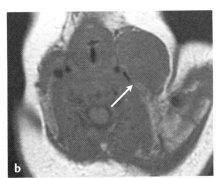

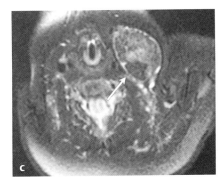

Fig. 5.17 A 5-week-old male infant with fibromatosis colli involving the left sternoclavicular muscle. There is fusiform thickening of the left sternoclavicular muscle that has (**a**) low-intermediate signal on sagittal T2-weighted imaging (*arrows*), (**b**) intermediate signal on axial T1-weighted imaging (*arrow*), and (**c**) mixed low, intermediate, and slightly high signal on axial fat-suppressed T2-weighted imaging (*arrow*).

5.2 Visceral Space of the Infrahyoid Neck

Lesions of the Hypopharynx and Larynx

The hyoid bone is a movable bone that is supported by suprahyoid and infrahyoid muscles, and it separates the supra- and infrahyoid portions of the neck (**Fig. 5.18**). The hyoid bone supports the larynx and hypopharynx. The hypopharynx is the lowermost portion of the pharynx and extends inferiorly and posteriorly from the hyoid bone and valleculae dorsal to the larynx down to the level of the cricoid cartilage (**Fig. 5.19**). The hypopharynx includes the piriform sinuses, the postcricoid zone containing the inferior pharyngeal constrictor muscles and pharyngoesophageal junction, and the posterior hypopharyngeal wall. The posterior pharyngeal wall is the inferior continuation of the posterior oropharyngeal wall and extends from the level of the valleculae down to the level of the inferior margin of the cricoid cartilage and cricopharyngeus muscle.

The piriform sinuses are separated from the upper larynx by the aryepiglottic folds.

The larynx has a cartilaginous framework consisting of the epiglottis, arytenoid, thyroid, and cricoid cartilages as well as the true vocal cords (**Fig. 5.20**). The laryngeal cartilage is composed of hyaline cartilage. The arytenoid, thyroid, and cricoid cartilage often undergo endochondral ossification beginning in the second decade. The hyaline cartilage of the epiglottis, vocal processes at the lower anterior margins of the arytenoids, and corniculate and cuneiform processes do not typically ossify. The epiglottis is a flexible leaf-shaped thin structure composed of elastic cartilage that tapers anteroinferiorly to a point (petiole), where it attaches to the thyroid cartilage above the anterior commissure. The epiglottis prevents swallowed fluid or food from entering the larynx. The upper anterior margin of the thyroid cartilage is connected to the hyoid bone via the thyrohyoid membrane. The lower anterior margin of the thyroid cartilage is connected to the cricoid bone via the cricothyroid membrane. Muscles contributing to the support of the larynx include the thyroarytenoid muscle, which comprises most of the vocal cord, as well as the cricoarytenoid, interarytenoid, and cricothyroid muscles.

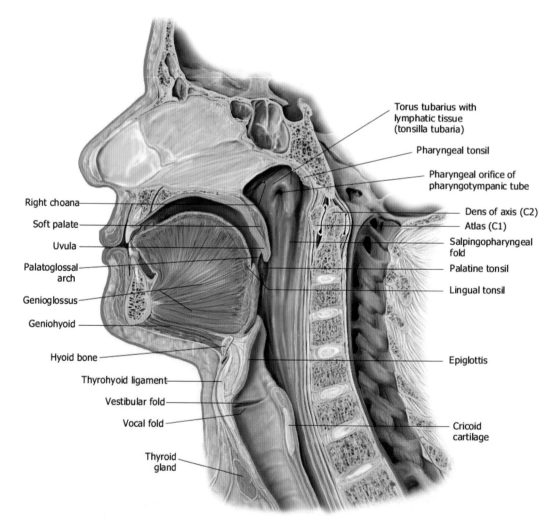

Fig. 5.18 Sagittal view of the hypopharynx and larynx related to adjacent anatomic structures. From THIEME Atlas of Anatomy: Head and Neuroanatomy, © Thieme 2007, Illustration by Karl Wesker.

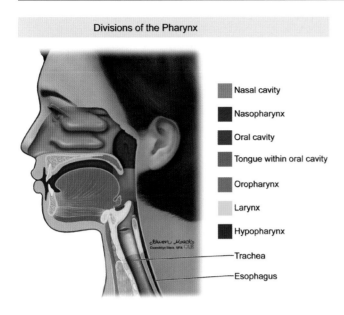

Divisions of the Pharynx

Nasal cavity

Nasopharynx

Oral cavity

Tongue within oral cavity

Oropharynx

Larynx

Hypopharynx

Trachea

Esophagus

Fig. 5.19 Sagittal view of the boundaries of the spaces of the pharynx, hypopharynx, and larynx.

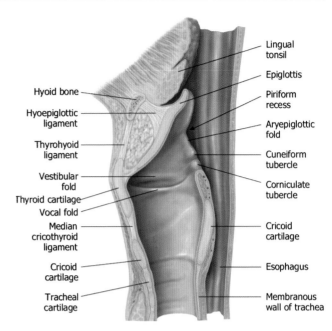

Lingual tonsil

Epiglottis

Hyoid bone

Hyoepiglottic ligament

Thyrohyoid ligament

Vestibular fold

Thyroid cartilage

Vocal fold

Median cricothyroid ligament

Cricoid cartilage

Tracheal cartilage

Piriform recess

Aryepiglottic fold

Cuneiform tubercle

Corniculate tubercle

Cricoid cartilage

Esophagus

Membranous wall of trachea

Fig. 5.20 Sagittal view of the epiglottis and larynx. From THIEME Atlas of Anatomy: Head and Neuroanatomy, © Thieme 2007, Illustration by Karl Wesker.

The larynx can be demarcated into three spaces. The glottic space is at the level of the true vocal cords (**Fig. 5.21**). The ventricle is the thin space between the true and false vocal cords. The upper border of the glottic space is at the inferior margin of the ventricle, and the lower border is 1 cm below the ventricle. The supraglottic portion of the larynx is located superior to the ventricle and below the upper portion of the epiglottis and aryepiglottic folds. The false cords are at the lower portion of the supraglottic larynx. The subglottic region is located between the glottis and inferior margin of the cricoid cartilage.

The preepiglottic space is located between the thyrohyoid membrane anteriorly and infrahyoid portion of the epiglottis posteriorly. The paraglottic (paralaryngeal) space is a paired symmetric space that is located between the laryngeal mucosa and laryngeal cartilage. At its upper border, the paraglottic space is contiguous with the pre-epiglottic space and aryepiglottic folds. In the supraglottic region, the paraglottic space is primarily composed of adipose tissue, which extends down to the level of the false cords. At the level of the glottis, the paraglottic space is located between the thyroarytenoid muscles and vocal cords medially, and thyroid and cricoid cartilages laterally. Because of their anatomic relationships, the preepiglottic and paraglottic spaces are routes of spread of neoplasms above and below the glottis as well as beyond the laryngeal borders, affecting staging and treatment options.

Most malignant tumors involving the hypopharynx and larynx are squamous cell carcinomas (SCC). The current widely accepted staging method for these tumors is

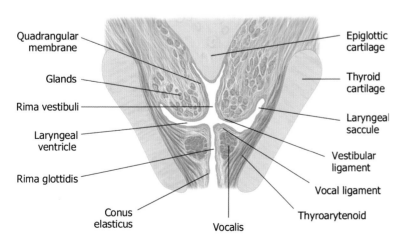

Quadrangular membrane

Glands

Rima vestibuli

Laryngeal ventricle

Rima glottidis

Conus elasticus

Vocalis

Epiglottic cartilage

Thyroid cartilage

Laryngeal saccule

Vestibular ligament

Vocal ligament

Thyroarytenoid

Fig. 5.21 Coronal view illustration shows anatomy of the larynx at the level of the vocal cords. From THIEME Atlas of Anatomy: Head and Neuroanatomy, © Thieme 2007, Illustration by Karl Wesker.

the American Joint Committee on Cancer (AJCC) seventh edition, developed in 2010. Staging of SCC is important for prognosis and treatment planning. The AJCC evaluates tumor size (T), presence of nodes (N), and metastases (M). The TNM classification system (**Box 5.1** and **Box 5.2**) for laryngeal tumors evaluates SCC according to where the neoplasms are located (supraglottis, glottis, subglottis). Supraglottic and glottic carcinomas that have invaded the preepiglottic or paraglottic space are staged as T3 lesions, and are commonly associated with nodal metastases and poor outcomes. Tumor invasion into the preepiglottic space alters surgical planning. Small amounts of tumor invasion into the preepiglottic space are a contraindication for supracricoid laryngectomies with cricohyoidepiglottopexy. A large amount of tumor invasion into the preepiglottic space contraindicates supracricoid laryngectomies with cricohyoidopexy. Tumor involvement of the anterior or posterior commissures limits effectiveness for cure with transoral resection or laser techniques. Standard supraglottic laryngectomies are contraindicated for supraglottic or glottic tumors that extend into the subglottis. Other contraindications for supraglottic laryngectomies include: invasion of cricoid or thyroid cartilage, arytenoid fixation, and extension into the piriform sinus or tongue base (> 1 cm). Tumors extending into the prevertebral space or carotid space with encasement of the carotid artery are typically T4b lesions and are considered unresectable. The presence of malignant nodes reduces survival by 50%. Supraglottic tumors have higher rates of nodal tumor than glottic and subglottic tumors because of the greater lymphovascular network within the paraglottic space. Supraglottic tumors typically metastasize to jugular chain nodes at levels II, III, and IV. Glottic tumors limited to the endolarynx rarely have nodal disease, whereas subglottic tumors spread to level IV, visceral node level VI, and mediastinal nodes.

Box 5.1 TNM System for Hypopharyngeal Squamous Cell Carcinoma

Primary Tumor (T)

- **TX:** *Primary tumor cannot be assessed.*
- **T0:** *No evidence of primary tumor.*
- **T1:** *Tumor < 2 cm and limited to one subsite.*
- **T2:** *Tumor 2–4 cm or more than one site in hypopharynx.*
- **T3:** *Tumor > 4 cm or vocal cord fixation.*
- **T4a:** *Tumor invades any of the following: hyoid bone, thyroid or cricoid cartilage, thyroid gland, esophagus, prelaryngeal strap muscles, or subcutaneous fat.*
- **T4b:** *Tumor invades prevertebral fascia, carotid space, or mediastinum.*

Regional Lymph Nodes (N)

- **NX:** *Regional lymph nodes cannot be assessed.*
- **N0:** *No regional lymph node metastases.*
- **N1:** *Single ipsilateral metastatic lymph node measuring < 3 cm.*
- **N2a:** *Single ipsilateral metastatic lymph node measuring > 3 cm and < 6 cm.*
- **N2b:** *Multiple ipsilateral nodes measuring < 6 cm.*
- **N2c:** *Bilateral or contralateral lymph nodes, none > 6 cm.*
- **N3:** *Metastatic lymph node > 6 cm.*

Distant Metatases (M)

- **MX:** *Distant metastasis cannot be assessed.*
- **M0:** *No distant metastases.*
- **M1:** *Distant metastases*

Box 5.2   TNM System for Laryngeal Squamous Cell Carcinoma

Primary Tumor (T)

Supraglottis

- **T1:** *Tumor limited to one side of supraglottis with normal vocal cord mobility.*
- **T2:** *Tumor invades mucosa of more than one adjacent site of supraglottis, glottis, or outside supraglottis without fixation of larynx.*
- **T3:** *Tumor limited to larynx with vocal cord fixation and/or invades paraglottic space, preepiglottic space, inner margin of laryngeal cartilage.*
- **T4a:** *Moderately advanced local disease. (Tumor invades and extends through the cartilage, and/or invades adjacent extralaryngeal soft tissues.)*
- **T4b:** *Very advanced local disease. (Tumor invades and extends through the cartilage, and invades adjacent extralaryngeal soft tissues that can include the prevertebral and carotid spaces, and mediastinum.)*

Glottis

- **T1:** *Tumor limited to one vocal cord, may involve anterior or posterior commissure, normal cord mobility.*
- **T1a:** *Tumor limited to one vocal cord.*
- **T1b:** *Tumor involves both vocal cords.*
- **T2:** *Tumor extends to supaglottis and/or subglottis, and/or impaired vocal cord mobility.*
- **T3**: *Tumor limited to larynx with vocal cord fixation and/or invades paraglottic space, preepiglottic space, inner margin of thyroid cartilage.*
- **T4a:** *Moderately advanced local disease. (Tumor invades and extends through the outer margin of thyroid cartilage, and/or invades adjacent extralaryngeal soft tissues.)*
- **T4b:** *Very advanced local disease. (Tumor invades and extends through the cartilage, and invades adjacent extralaryngeal soft tissues that can include the prevertebral and carotid spaces and mediastinum.)*

Subglottis

- **Tis:** *Carcinoma in situ.*
- **T1:** *Tumor limited to one side of subglottis.*
- **T2:** *Tumor extends upward to vocal cords without or with impaired cord mobility.*

- **T3:** *Tumor limited to larynx with vocal cord fixation.*
- **T4a:** *Moderately advanced local disease. (Tumor invades and extends through the cricoid or thyroid cartilage, and/or invades adjacent extralaryngeal soft tissues.)*
- **T4b:** *Very advanced local disease. (Tumor invades and extends through the cartilage, and invades adjacent extralaryngeal soft tissues that can include the prevertebral and carotid spaces and mediastinum.)*

Regional Lymph Nodes (N)

- **NX**: *Regional lymph nodes cannot be assessed.*
- **N0**: *No regional lymph node metastases.*
- **N1:** *Single ipsilateral metastatic lymph node measuring < 3 cm.*
- **N2a:** *Single ipsilateral metastatic lymph node measuring > 3 cm and < 6 cm.*
- **N2b:** *Multiple ipsilateral nodes measuring < 6 cm.*
- **N3:** *Metastatic lymph node > 6 cm.*

Distant Metatases (M)

- **M0:** *No distant metastases.*
- **M1:** *Distant metastases.*

Anatomic Stages/Prognostic Groups

- **Stage 0:** *Tis, N0*
- **Stage I:** *T1, N0*
- **Stage II:** *T2, N0*
- **Stage III:** *T3, N0*
  - *T1, N1, M0*
  - *T2, N1, M0*
  - *T3, N1, M0*
- **Stage IVa:** *T4a, N0, M0*
  - *T4a, N1, M0*
  - *T1, N2, M0*
  - *T2, N2, M0*
  - *T3, N2, M0*
  - *T4a, N2, M0*
- **Stage IVb**: *T4b, Any N, M0*
  - *Any T, N3, M0*
- **Stage IVc**: *Any T, Any N, M1*

Table 5.2 Lesions of the hypopharynx and larynx

- Hypopharyngeal Lesions
  - Squamous cell carcinoma (SCC) of the hypopharynx and epiglottis
  - Epiglottitis
- Malignant Laryngeal Lesions
  - Squamous cell carcinoma (SCC)
  - Supraglottic carcinoma
  - Glottic **c**arcinoma
  - Transglottic **c**arcinoma
  - Primary subglottic carcinoma
  - Minor salivary gland tumor
  - Chondrosarcoma
  - Osteosarcoma
  - Lymphoma
  - Metastatic neoplasm
  - Myeloma
  - Vocal cord paralysis/paresis
- Benign Laryngeal Neoplasms
  - Hemangioma
  - Lipoma
  - Schwannoma
  - Paraganglioma
  - Chondroma
- Tumorlike Lesions
  - Laryngocele
  - Thyroglossal duct cyst
  - Fourth branchial cleft cyst
  - Amyloidomas
- Inflammatory Lesions
  - Pyogenic infection
  - Necrotizing fasciitis
  - Laryngeal tuberculosis
  - Relapsing polychondritis
  - Rheumatoid arthritis
- Traumatic Laryngeal Lesions
  - Blunt trauma/laryngeal fracture
  - Hematoma
  - Penetrating trauma
- Other Lesions
  - Postradiation treatment changes
  - Laryngeal chondronecrosis
  - Reinke's edema

Table 5.2 Lesions of the hypopharynx and larynx

Lesions	Imaging Findings	Comments
Hypopharyngeal Lesions		
Squamous cell carcinoma (SCC) of the hypopharynx and epiglottis (**Fig. 5.22, Fig. 5.23**, and **Fig. 5.24**)	*CT and MRI:* Soft tissue tumor with intermediate attenuation on CT and intermediate signal on T1-weighted imaging and intermediate to slightly high signal on T2-weighted imaging, + contrast enhancement, ± paraglottic extension, laryngeal cartilage invasion. SCC of the posterior pharyngeal wall can be seen as asymmetric thickening of the posterior pharyngeal wall, ± invasion of prevertebral space structures. *PET/CT:* Abnormal increased accumulation of F-18 FDG.	SCC in the hypopharynx arises in the piriform sinus (65%), postcricoid region (20%), or posterior pharyngeal wall (15%). Tumors at the medial wall of the piriform sinus can invade the larynx via extension into the epiglottis or paraglottic space, ± laryngeal cartilage invasion. Tumors at the lateral margin of the piriform sinus commonly invade the adjacent soft tissues of the neck. Postcricoid SCC usually spreads submucosally, and is associated with Plummer-Vinson syndrome. SCC of the posterior pharyngeal wall often involves the oropharynx and hypopharynx. At initial diagnosis of SCC of the hypopharynx, 75% of patients have metastases to cervical lymph nodes.

(continued on page 514)

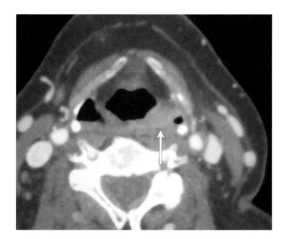

Fig. 5.22   Axial CT of a 50-year-old man shows a squamous cell carcinoma of the hypopharynx involving the left aryepiglottic fold (*arrow*).

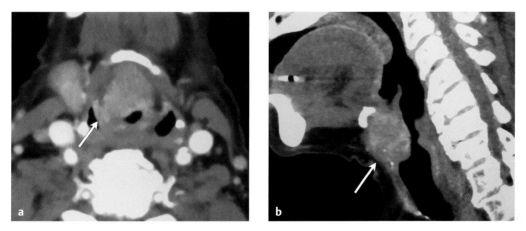

Fig. 5.23   (a) Axial and (b) sagittal CT images of a 69-year-old man show a squamous cell carcinoma of the hypopharynx involving the right aryepiglottic fold (*arrow* in **a**) and that extends inferiorly to the preepiglottic space (*arrow* in **b**).

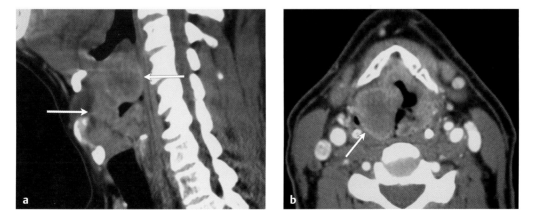

Fig. 5.24   (a) Sagittal and (b) axial CT images of a 51-year-old man show a squamous cell carcinoma enlarging the epiglottis (*arrows* in **a**), with extension inferiorly along the right aryepiglottic fold (*arrow* in **b**).

Table 5.2 *(cont.)*   Lesions of the hypopharynx and larynx

Lesions	Imaging Findings	Comments
Epiglottitis (**Fig. 5.25** and **Fig. 5.26**)	*CT:* Enlarged edematous epiglottis with mucosal contrast enhancement, ± edematous changes involving the tongue, tonsils, hypopharynx, and aryepiglottic folds, ± abscess in neck.	In children, life-threatening infection of the epiglottis that can require emergent intubation. Occurs less frequently in adults. Patients present with fever and abrupt onset of stridor and dysphagia. Infection by *Haemophilus influenzae* was a common etiology before the advent of the related vaccine. Epiglottitis from *H. influenzae* in children often involves the entire supraglottic larynx, tongue base, and/or tonsils and can progress rapidly, causing severe respiratory distress that requires intubation. Other microorganisms resulting in epiglottitis, such as *Streptococcus* and viruses, occur in older children and adults and usually have a more indolent course. In Africa and Asia, granulomatous diseases, such as tuberculosis, syphilis, and leprosy, cause infections of the pharynx, epiglottis, and larynx.
Malignant Laryngeal Lesions		
Squamous cell carcinoma (SCC)		SCC accounts for over 90% of the malignant tumors of the larynx. SCC arises in the supraglottic region (30%), glottic region (65%), and subglottic region (5%). In the United States, 11,000 new cases of laryngeal SCC occur each year. Tumors have squamous differentiation with keratinization and invasive growth. Tumors are graded into well-differentiated, moderately differentiated, and poorly differentiated types. Well-differentiated SCC has features that resemble squamous epithelium, whereas poorly differentiated SCC has immature cells with nuclear pleomorphism and high atypical mitotic activity. Moderately differentiated SCC has features intermediate between well- and poorly differentiated SCC. Tumor classification uses the TNM system.
Supraglottic carcinoma (**Fig. 5.27**)	*CT and MRI:* Soft tissue tumor involving the epiglottis and/or preepiglottic space, aryepiglottic fold, false cord, or ventricle. Tumors often have intermediate attenuation on CT and intermediate signal on T1-weighted imaging and intermediate to slightly high signal on T2-weighted imaging, and loss of normal fat signal in the preepiglottic space, aryepiglottic folds, and false cords. On diffusion-weighted imaging, ADC values can be low/decreased in proportion to the degree of SCC cellularity, stromal content, and nuclear-cytoplasmic ratio. SCC typically shows contrast enhancement. Tumors commonly spread through the paraglottic space. *PET/CT:* Abnormal increased accumulation of F-18 FDG.	SCC that commonly arises in the epiglottis and often invades the preepiglottic space. Can further extend into the lower preepiglottic space, anterior commissure, paraglottic space, glottis, and subglottis (transglottic SCC). Other primary sites of supraglottic SCC include: aryepiglottic folds, false cords, and/or ventricle. Supraglottic SCC spreads to the superior jugular lymph nodes. Lymph node metastases are common and are often bilateral. Tumors extending into the preepiglottic or paraglottic spaces are T3 neoplasms, and treatment by supracricoid laryngectomy with cricohyoidoepiglottopexy is contraindicated. Other treatment includes radiation therapy or combined chemoradiotherapy.

(continued on page 516)

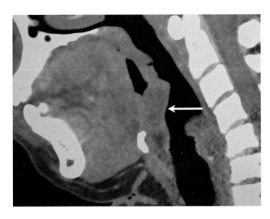

Fig. 5.25 Sagittal CT of a 30-year-old woman shows abnormal thickening of the epiglottis from infection (*arrow*).

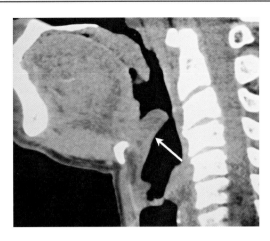

Fig. 5.26 Sagittal CT of a 49-year-old man shows abnormal thickening of the epiglottis from infection (*arrow*).

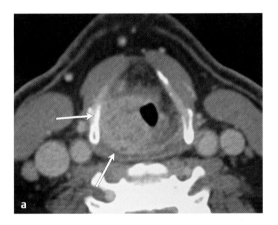

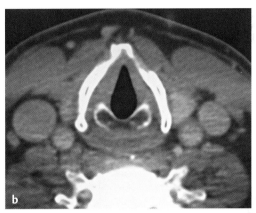

Fig. 5.27 **(a)** Axial CT of a 68-year-old man shows a supraglottic squamous cell carcinoma (*arrows*) involving the right false cord. **(b)** Axial CT more inferiorly shows normal appearance of the true cords with no evidence of tumor extension.

Table 5.2 *(cont.)* Lesions of the hypopharynx and larynx

Lesions	Imaging Findings	Comments
Glottic carcinoma (**Fig. 5.28**, **Fig. 5.29**, and **Fig. 5.30**)	*CT and MRI:* Soft tissue tumor with intermediate attenuation on CT and intermediate signal on T1-weighted imaging and intermediate to slightly high signal on T2-weighted imaging. On diffusion-weighted imaging, ADC values can be low/decreased in proportion to the degree of SCC cellularity, stromal content, and nuclear-cytoplasmic ratio. SCC typically shows contrast enhancement. Involvement of the anterior and/or posterior commissures is seen as a > 2 mm zone of soft tissue thickening, ± invasion of thyroarytenoid muscle and laryngeal cartilage, ± paraglottic or extralaryngeal tumor extension. Subglottic and supraglottic extension is seen as irregular soft tissue thickening of the cricothyroid membrane. *PET/CT:* Abnormal increased accumulation of F-18 FDG.	SCC that usually arises from the anterior half of the vocal cord. Often extends into the anterior commissure without or with associated tumor spread into the thyroarytenoid muscle, contralateral vocal cord, paraglottic space, supraglottis, or subglottis. Often associated with vocal cord paresis or paralysis. Subglottic extension is common. Lymphatic metastases from glottic SCC are uncommon unless tumor has extended into the extralaryngeal soft tissues. Tumors extending into the preepiglottic or paraglottic spaces are T3 neoplasms, and treatment by supracricoid laryngectomy with cricohyoidoepiglottopexy is contraindicated. Other treatment includes radiation therapy or combined chemoradiotherapy.
Transglottic carcinoma (**Fig. 5.31**)	*CT and MRI:* Soft tissue tumor with intermediate attenuation on CT and intermediate signal on T1-weighted imaging and intermediate to slightly high signal on T2-weighted imaging. On diffusion-weighted imaging, ADC values can be low/decreased in proportion to the degree of SCC cellularity, stromal content, and nuclear-cytoplasmic ratio. SCC typically shows contrast enhancement, ± invasion of laryngeal cartilage, ± paraglottic, cricothyroid membrane, and extralaryngeal tumor extension. *PET/CT:* Abnormal increased accumulation of F-18 FDG.	SCC that crosses the ventricle, involving both the glottis and supraglottis at diagnosis. Lymph node metastases occur commonly with transglottic SCC. Treatment by standard horizontal supraglottic laryngectomy is contraindicated. Other treatment includes radiation therapy or combined chemoradiotherapy.
Primary subglottic carcinoma	*CT and MRI:* Soft tissue tumor with intermediate attenuation on CT and intermediate signal on T1-weighted imaging and intermediate to slightly high signal on T2-weighted imaging. On diffusion-weighted imaging, ADC values can be low/decreased in proportion to the degree of SCC cellularity, stromal content, and nuclear-cytoplasmic ratio. SCC typically shows contrast enhancement. *PET/CT:* Abnormal increased accumulation of F-18 FDG.	Uncommon primary location of SCC that often invades the cricoid cartilage and trachea, ± thyroid gland, esophagus. Treatment includes radiation therapy or combined chemoradiotherapy.

(continued on page 518)

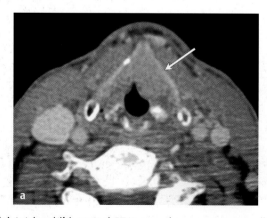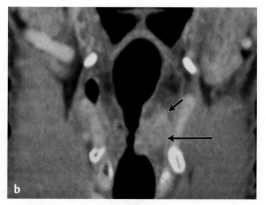

Fig. 5.28 **(a)** Axial and **(b)** coronal CT images show a squamous cell carcinoma involving the left true and false cords (*arrows*).

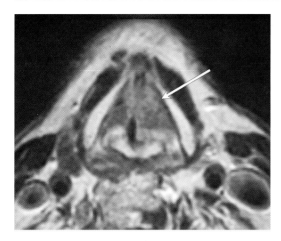

Fig. 5.29 Axial T2-weighted imaging of an 86-year-old man with a squamous cell carcinoma involving the left true cord (*arrow*) that has intermediate signal.

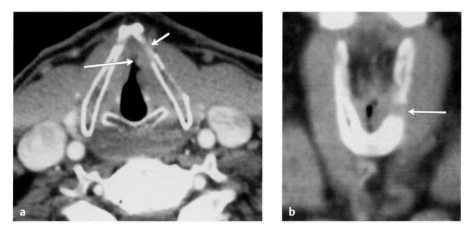

Fig. 5.30 **(a)** Axial and **(b)** coronal CT images of a 70-year-old man show nodular irregularity at the left vocal cord (*arrows* in **a**) from squamous cell carcinoma, which is associated with localized invasion and destruction of the adjacent thyroid cartilage (*arrow* in **b**).

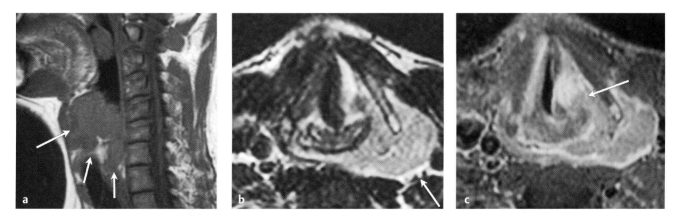

Fig. 5.31 **(a)** A large transglottic squamous cell carcinoma is seen that has intermediate signal on sagittal T1-weighted imaging (*arrows*), **(b)** slightly high signal on axial T2-weighted imaging (*arrow*), and **(c)** gadolinium contrast enhancement on axial fat-suppressed T1-weighted imaging (*arrow*). The tumor involves the left true cord and extends into the paraglottic soft tissues, with invasion and extension through the left thyroid cartilage.

Table 5.2 *(cont.)* Lesions of the hypopharynx and larynx

Lesions	Imaging Findings	Comments
Minor salivary gland tumor	*MRI:* Lesions have intermediate signal on T1-weighted imaging, intermediate-high signal on T2-weighted imaging, variable mild, moderate, or prominent gadolinium contrast enhancement, ± cartilage or bone destruction, perineural tumor spread. *CT:* Tumors have intermediate attenuation, and variable mild, moderate, or prominent contrast enhancement. Destruction of adjacent cartilage and bone is commonly seen.	Minor salivary glands occur throughout the respiratory tract as well as within the larynx. Tumors of the minor salivary glands account for < 1% of laryngeal neoplasms. Most of these neoplasms are malignant and include adenoid cystic carcinomas, mucoepidermoid carcinoma, adenocarcinoma, acinic cell carcinoma, and myoepithelial carcinoma. Usually occur in adults, and are not associated with tobacco smoking. Adenoid cystic carcinomas usually occur in the subglottis, whereas mucoepidermoid carcinomas and adenocarcinomas often occur in the supraglottic larynx.
Chondrosarcoma	*CT:* Lesions have low-intermediate attenuation associated with localized laryngeal cartilage destruction, ± chondroid matrix calcifications, + contrast enhancement. *MRI:* Lesions have low-intermediate signal on T1-weighted imaging, high signal on T2-weighted imaging (T2WI), ± matrix mineralization with low signal on T2WI, + gadolinium contrast enhancement (usually heterogeneous). Locally invasive and associated with laryngeal cartilage erosion/destruction. *PET/CT:* Increased uptake of F-18 FDG with SUVs greater than 2.0.	Chondrosarcomas are malignant tumors containing cartilage formed within sarcomatous stroma. Chondrosarcomas can contain areas of calcification/mineralization, myxoid material, and/or ossification. Chondrosarcomas represent 12–21% of malignant bone lesions, 21–26% of primary sarcomas of bone, and 9–14% of all bone tumors. Most common nonepithelial laryngeal tumor. Accounts for < 1% of laryngeal tumors. Possible increased incidence secondary to radiation treatment or Teflon injection for treatment of vocal cord paralysis.
Osteosarcoma	*CT:* Tumors have low-intermediate attenuation, usually + matrix mineralization/ossification, and often show contrast enhancement (usually heterogeneous). *MRI:* Tumors often have poorly defined margins and commonly extend from the destroyed portions of the laryngeal cartilage into adjacent soft tissues. Tumors usually have low-intermediate signal on T1-weighted imaging. Zones of low signal often correspond to areas of tumor calcification/mineralization and/or necrosis. Zones of necrosis typically have high signal on T2-weighted imaging (T2WI), whereas mineralized zones usually have low signal on T2WI. Tumors can have variable MRI signal on T2WI and fat-suppressed (FS) T2WI depending upon the relative amounts of calcified/mineralized osteoid, chondroid, fibroid, hemorrhagic, and necrotic components. Tumors may have low, low-intermediate, intermediate to high signal on T2WI and FS T2WI. After gadolinium contrast administration, osteosarcomas typically show prominent enhancement in nonmineralized/noncalcified portions of the tumors.	Osteosarcomas are malignant tumors composed of proliferating neoplastic spindle cells, which produce osteoid and/or immature tumoral bone. Occur in children as primary tumors and in adults are associated with Paget disease, irradiated bone, chronic osteomyelitis, osteoblastoma, giant cell tumor, and fibrous dysplasia. Account for < 1% of laryngeal tumors.

Lesions	Imaging Findings	Comments
Lymphoma (**Fig. 5.32**)	*CT:* Lesions have low-intermediate attenuation, may show moderate contrast enhancement, + laryngeal cartilage destruction. *MRI:* Lesions have low-intermediate signal on T1-weighted imaging, intermediate to slightly high signal on T2-weighted imaging, + moderate gadolinium contrast enhancement. Locally invasive and are associated with cartilage and bone erosion/destruction. *PET/CT:* Abnormal increased accumulation of F-18 FDG.	Lymphomas are a group of lymphoid tumors whose neoplastic cells typically arise within lymphoid tissue (lymph nodes, reticuloendothelial organs, and mucosa-associated lymphatic tissue). Unlike leukemia, lymphomas usually arise as discrete masses. Lymphomas are subdivided into Hodgkin disease (HD) and non-Hodgkin lymphoma (NHL). Primary lymphoma of the larynx is rare, and it is often B-cell NHL. Common laryngeal sites of primary lymphoma include: false cords > aryepiglottic folds > true cords > epiglottis. Cervical lymphadenopathy from lymphoma can also secondarily involve the larynx.
Metastatic neoplasm (**Fig. 5.33**)	Single or multiple well-circumscribed or poorly defined lesions involving laryngeal cartilage. *CT:* Lesions usually have soft tissue attenuation, ± sclerosis, ± extralaryngeal tumor extension, usually + contrast enhancement, ± compression of neural tissue or vessels. *MRI:* Single or multiple well-circumscribed or poorly defined lesions involving laryngeal cartilage, with low-intermediate signal on T1-weighted imaging, intermediate-high signal on T2-weighted imaging, and usually gadolinium contrast enhancement, ± cartilage and/or bone destruction, ± compression of neural tissue or vessels. *PET/CT:* Abnormal increased accumulation of F-18 FDG.	Metastatic lesions represent proliferating neoplastic cells that are located in sites or organs separated or distant from their origins. Metastatic carcinoma is the most frequent type of metastatic tumor involving laryngeal cartilage. In adults, metastatic lesions occur most frequently from carcinomas of the lung, breast, prostate, kidney, and thyroid, as well as from sarcomas. Metastatic tumor may cause variable destructive or infiltrative changes in single or multiple sites.

(continued on page 520)

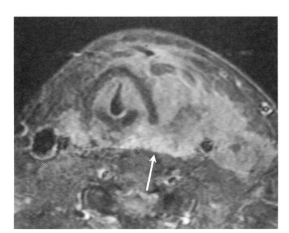

Fig. 5.32 Axial postcontrast fat-suppressed T1-weighted imaging shows a large contrast-enhancing lesion in the left neck from B-cell non-Hodgkin lymphoma (*arrow*) that extends into the left anterior cervical, carotid, and visceral spaces, as well as extending to involve the left paraglottic space and left vocal cord.

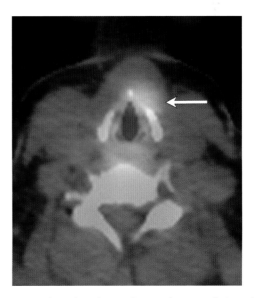

Fig. 5.33 Axial PET/CT shows abnormal accumulation of F-18 FDG in the left thyroid cartilage from metastatic lung carcinoma (*arrow*).

Table 5.2 *(cont.)* Lesions of the hypopharynx and larynx

Lesions	Imaging Findings	Comments
Myeloma (**Fig. 5.34**)	Multiple (myeloma) or single (plasmacytoma) well-circumscribed or poorly defined lesions involving laryngeal cartilage. *CT:* Lesions have low-intermediate attenuation, usually + contrast enhancement, + cartilage and/or bone destruction. *MRI:* Well-circumscribed or poorly defined lesions involving laryngeal cartilage, with low-intermediate signal on T1-weighted imaging, intermediate-high signal on T2-weighted imaging, and usually gadolinium contrast enhancement, + bone destruction. *PET/CT:* Abnormal increased accumulation of F-18 FDG.	Multiple myeloma is a malignancy composed of proliferating antibody-secreting plasma cells derived from single clones. Multiple myeloma primarily is located in bone marrow, but can also occur within laryngeal cartilage. A solitary myeloma or plasmacytoma is an infrequent variant in which a neoplastic mass of plasma cells occurs at a single site of bone or soft tissues. In the United States, 14,600 new cases occur each year. Multiple myeloma is the most common primary neoplasm of bone in adults. Median age at presentation = 60 years. Most patients are > 40 years old.
Vocal cord paralysis/paresis (**Fig. 5.35**)	*CT:* Findings of vocal cord paralysis include: medial position of the vocal cord, dilatation of ipsilateral piriform sinus, thickening and slight medial positioning of the ipsilateral aryepiglottic fold, anteromedial rotation of the ipsilateral arytenoid cartilage, dilatation of ipsilateral valleculae and laryngeal ventricle, and ipsilateral ventricular fullness. Imaging is routinely performed to look for causative lesions along the courses of the recurrent laryngeal nerves. Imaging of the lower neck and upper mediastinum is necessary because the right recurrent laryngeal nerve loops under the right subclavian artery, and the left recurrent laryngeal nerve loops under the aortic arch.	Paralysis of the vocal cord refers to complete cord immobility, whereas paresis refers to partial loss of cord mobility. Usually results from injury, compression, or tumor invasion involving the recurrent laryngeal nerve or proximal vagus nerve, versus less commonly from a lesion involving the central nervous system. The recurrent laryngeal nerve innervates the intrinsic muscles of the larynx, including the thyroarytenoid and posterior cricoarytenoid muscles. The recurrent laryngeal nerve arises as a branch of the vagus nerve in the upper thorax. The right recurrent laryngeal nerve loops under the right subclavian artery before it extends superiorly along the right tracheoesophageal groove as far as its entry into the cricothyroid joint after penetrating the inferior pharyngeal constrictor muscle. The left recurrent laryngeal nerve loops under the aorta before it extends superiorly along the left tracheoesophageal groove as far as its entry into the cricothyroid joint after penetrating the inferior pharyngeal constrictor. Paralysis/paresis can be a complication of surgery, such as thyroidectomy. A causative lesion may not be found on imaging in up to 85% of cases.
Benign Laryngeal Neoplasms		
Hemangioma	*MRI:* Circumscribed or poorly marginated structures (< 4 cm in diameter) in the larynx with intermediate-high signal on T1-weighted imaging (often with portions isointense to marrow fat), high signal on T2-weighted imaging (T2WI) and fat-suppressed T2WI, typically with gadolinium contrast enhancement. *CT:* Usually have mostly intermediate attenuation, ± zones of fat attenuation.	Benign lesions of soft tissue composed of capillary, cavernous, and/or venous malformation. Considered to be a hamartomatous disorder. Classified into infantile and adult types. Adult type (median age = 33 years) usually occurs in the supraglottis or glottis. Infantile type usually presents in the first 3 months, usually occurs in the subglottic region, and is associated with respiratory distress from progressive enlargement. Infantile subglottic hemangiomas are associated with cutaneous hemangiomas in up to 50% of cases.
Lipoma	*MRI:* Lipomas have MRI signal isointense to subcutaneous fat on T1-weighted imaging (high signal), and on T2-weighted imaging, signal suppression occurs with frequency-selective fat saturation techniques or with a short time to inversion recovery (STIR) method. Typically there is no gadolinium contrast enhancement or peripheral edema. *CT:* Lipomas have attenuation similar to subcutaneous fat, and typically there is no contrast enhancement or peripheral edema.	Common benign hamartomas composed of mature white adipose tissue without cellular atypia. Most common soft tissue tumor, representing 16% of all soft tissue tumors. Most common location in the larynx is the aryepiglottic fold.

(continued on page 522)

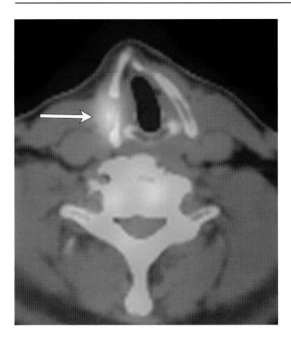

Fig. 5.34 Axial PET/CT shows abnormal accumulation of F-18 FDG in the right thyroid cartilage from myeloma (*arrow*); there is also localized cartilage destruction.

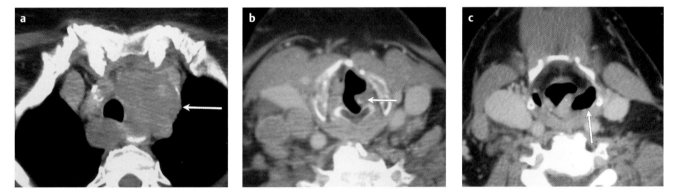

Fig. 5.35 (a) Axial CT of 69-year-old man with lung carcinoma shows the tumor involving the mediastinum, including the aortopulmonary window (*arrow*), which results in compression and invasion of the left recurrent laryngeal nerve. (b) Axial CT shows left vocal cord paralysis with medial rotation of the left arytenoid cartilage (*arrow*). (c) Axial CT shows enlargement of the ipsilateral left piriform sinus (*arrow*).

Table 5.2 *(cont.)* Lesions of the hypopharynx and larynx

Lesions	Imaging Findings	Comments
Schwannoma (**Fig. 5.36**)	*MRI:* Circumscribed ovoid or spheroid lesions, with low-intermediate signal on T1-weighted imaging, high signal on T2-weighted imaging (T2WI) and fat-suppressed T2WI, and usually prominent gadolinium (Gd) contrast enhancement. High signal on T2WI and Gd contrast enhancement can be heterogeneous in large lesions due to cystic degeneration and/or hemorrhage. *CT:* Circumscribed ovoid or spheroid lesions, with intermediate attenuation, + contrast enhancement. Large lesions can have cystic degeneration and/or hemorrhage.	Schwannomas are benign encapsulated tumors that contain differentiated neoplastic Schwann cells. Most commonly occur as solitary, sporadic lesions. Schwannomas rarely occur in the larynx and account for less than 1.5% of benign laryngeal tumors. Most occur in the submucosal space and up to 80% involve the aryepiglottic fold. Multiple schwannomas are often associated with neurofibromatosis type 2 (NF2), which is an autosomal dominant disease involving a gene mutation at chromosome 22q12. In addition to schwannomas, patients with NF2 can also have multiple meningiomas and ependymomas. The incidence of NF2 is 1/37,000 to 1/50,000 newborns. Age at presentation = 22 to 72 years (mean age = 46 years). Peak incidence is in the fourth to sixth decades. Many patients with NF2 present in the third decade with bilateral vestibular schwannomas.
Paraganglioma	*CT:* Well-circumscribed lesions with intermediate attenuation, + contrast enhancement, often with associated erosive bone changes. *MRI:* Well-circumscribed lesions with intermediate signal on T1-weighted imaging and often heterogeneous intermediate to slightly high signal on T2-weighted imaging, ± intratumoral flow voids, + gadolinium contrast enhancement, often with associated erosive bone changes.	Lesions, also referred to as chemodectomas, arise from paraganglia in multiple sites in the body, and are named accordingly (glomus jugulare, tympanicum, vagale, etc.). Paragangliomas are typically well-differentiated neoplasms composed of biphasic collections of chief cells (type 1) arranged in nests or lobules (*zellballen*) surrounded by single layers of sustentacular cells (type 2). Present in patients from 24 to 70 years old (mean age = 47 years). Rarely involve the larynx.
Chondroma (**Fig. 5.37**)	*CT:* Expansile lesion within laryngeal cartilage containing chondroid mineralization. *MRI:* Expansile lesion in laryngeal cartilage with intermediate signal on T1-weighted imaging, often heterogeneous intermediate to slightly high signal on T2-weighted imaging, + intratumoral zones of low signal from chondroid mineralization, + gadolinium contrast enhancement.	Benign cartilaginous laryngeal tumor, accounts for < 1% of laryngeal tumors. Occurs most frequently in the cricoid cartilage (75%), followed by the thyroid cartilage (20%) and other sites for the remainder. Usually occurs in adults in the sixth decade. May be difficult to distinguish from low-grade chondrosarcoma.

(continued on page 524)

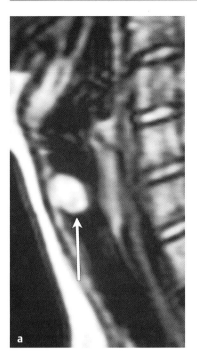
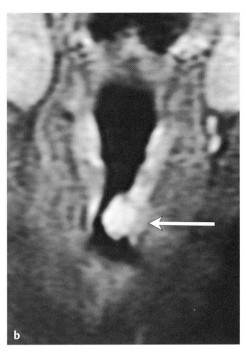

Fig. 5.36 **(a)** A 12-year-old female with a schwannoma at the lower border of the larynx that has high signal on sagittal T2-weighted imaging (*arrow*) and **(b)** shows gadolinium contrast enhancement on coronal fat-suppressed T1-weighted imaging (*arrow*).

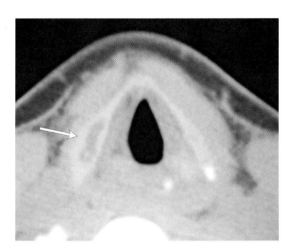

Fig. 5.37 Axial CT shows an expansile chondroma in the right thyroid cartilage (*arrow*) that has low-intermediate attenuation centrally with peripheral slightly high attenuation.

Table 5.2 *(cont.)* Lesions of the hypopharynx and larynx

Lesions	Imaging Findings	Comments
Tumorlike Lesions		
Laryngocele (**Fig. 5.38**, **Fig. 5.39**, **Fig. 5.40**, and **Fig. 5.41**)	*CT:* Well-circumscribed air-filled lesion or cystic structure with low (mucoid) attenuation ranging from 10 to 25 HU or soft tissue attenuation, surrounded by a thin wall. No central contrast enhancement, ± thin peripheral enhancement of wall. Laryngoceles complicated by infection can have increased attenuation, thick walls, and loss/indistinctness of adjacent tissue planes. *MRI:* Air-filled laryngoceles have low signal on all pulse sequences. Fluid-filled laryngoceles are spheroid or ovoid lesions that often have low signal on T1-weighted imaging (T1WI) and diffusion-weighted imaging and high signal on T2-weighted imaging (T2WI). The walls of these cysts are typically thin, without gadolinium (Gd) contrast enhancement. Laryngoceles complicated by hemorrhage or current or prior infection can have elevated protein with intermediate to slightly high signal on T1WI and T2WI. The walls of such cysts can be thick and show Gd contrast enhancement. Nodular Gd contrast enhancement involving the cyst wall can be seen with a potentially malignant lesion. *Ultrasound:* Can be well-circumscribed anechoic cysts with through transmission or may have a pseudosolid appearance related to elevated protein concentration.	At the upper anterior portion of the laryngeal ventricle, there is a pouch (laryngeal saccule, appendix ventriculi laryngis) that extends superiorly between the false vocal cord and inner surface of the thyroid cartilage. A laryngocele is an abnormal enlargement of the laryngeal saccule that extends superiorly within the false vocal cord, where it enters into the laryngeal lumen. Occurs with 7:1 male:female ratio, usually in fifth to sixth decades. Laryngoceles can be air-filled, with or without communication with the ventricle, or filled with fluid or mucus (saccular cysts, or laryngeal mucocele). Laryngoceles are subclassified as internal laryngoceles when limited in location to the paraglottic space of the false cords, and medial to the thyrohyoid membrane. External laryngoceles have a portion that can protrude through the thyrohyoid membrane. Mixed or combined laryngoceles are the most common type and have portions in both locations. Can be symptomatic and can be visible on laryngoscopy as a submucosal bulge of the false cord, particularly when there is extension above the superior margin of the thyroid cartilage. Up to 17% may be associated with a neoplasm. Treatment includes endoscopic laser treatment for small laryngoceles and conventional surgery for large lesions.

(continued on page 526)

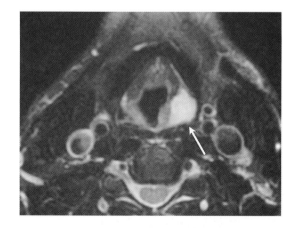

Fig. 5.38 Axial T2-weighted imaging shows a fluid-filled internal laryngocele with high signal (*arrow*) in the left false cord.

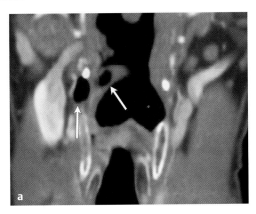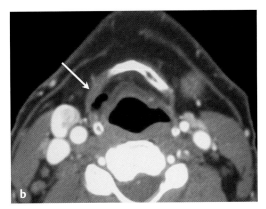

Fig. 5.39   **(a)** Coronal and **(b)** axial CT images show an air-filled laryngocele (*arrows*) in the right false cord extending into the right ary-epiglottic fold.

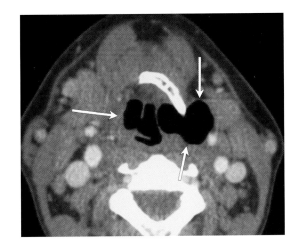

Fig. 5.40   Axial CT shows a mixed air-filled laryngocele on left extending through the thyrohyoid membrane (*left and lower arrows*). Also, an internal air-filled laryngocele is seen on the right (*upper arrow*).

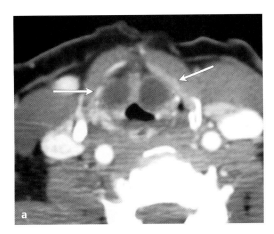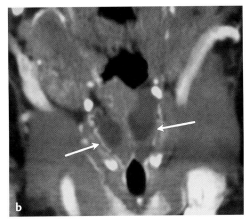

Fig. 5.41   **(a)** Axial and **(b)** coronal images show bilateral fluid-filled laryngoceles (*arrows*).

Table 5.2 *(cont.)* Lesions of the hypopharynx and larynx

Lesions	Imaging Findings	Comments
Thyroglossal duct cyst (**Fig. 5.42**)	*MRI:* Well-circumscribed spheroid or ovoid lesion at the tongue base or along the course of the thyroglossal duct that usually has low signal on T1-weighted imaging (T1WI) and diffusion-weighted imaging and high signal on T2-weighted imaging (T2WI). The wall of the thyroglossal duct cyst is typically thin, without gadolinium (Gd) contrast enhancement. Thyroglossal duct cysts complicated by hemorrhage or current or prior infection can have elevated protein with intermediate to slightly high signal on T1WI and T2WI. The walls of such cysts can be thick and show Gd contrast enhancement. Nodular Gd contrast enhancement involving the wall of a thyroglossal duct cyst can be seen with a potentially malignant lesion. *CT:* Well-circumscribed lesion with low (mucoid) attenuation ranging from 10 to 25 HU, surrounded by a thin wall. Occasionally contain thin septations. Thyroglossal duct cysts complicated by infection can have increased attenuation, thick walls, and loss/indistinctness of adjacent tissue planes. *Ultrasound:* Can be well-circumscribed anechoic cysts with through transmission or may have a pseudosolid appearance related to elevated protein concentration.	Most common congenital mass in the neck and is related to altered development of the thyroid gland with persistence of the embryologic thyroglossal duct between the dorsal portion of the tongue (foramen cecum) and the normal position of the thyroid gland. The thyroglossal duct normally involutes by the tenth week of gestation. The thyroglossal duct courses anterior to the hyoid bone, and loops slightly posterior to the inferior margin of the hyoid bone before descending anterior to the thyrohyoid membrane, thyroid cartilage, and trachea. The thyroglossal duct extends between the sternohyoid and sternothyroid strap muscles. Up to two-thirds of thyroglossal duct cysts occur in the infrahyoid neck and can be midline or extend laterally within or deep to the strap muscles. Nearly 50% present in patients < 20 years old as a progressively enlarging neck lesion.
Third branchial cleft cyst (**Fig. 5.43**)	*CT:* Circumscribed, cystic lesion with low to intermediate attenuation depending on the proportions of protein and water. Can have intermediate attenuation and thickened wall if superimposed infection. *First branchial cleft cysts* can be located adjacent to the external auditory canal (type 1 first branchial cleft cyst) or superficial portion of the parotid gland ± extension into the parapharyngeal space, posterior to the submandibular gland, and/or up to the external auditory canal (type 2). *Second branchial cleft cysts* are often posterolateral to the submandibular gland, anterior or anteromedial to the sternocleidomastoid muscle (SCM) and medial to the carotid arteries, ± extension to the parapharyngeal space, and between the internal and external carotid arteries. Typically, at least 50% of the cyst is located anterior to the ventral margin of the SCM. *Third branchial cleft cysts* are located at the lower anterior margin of the SCM at the level of the upper thyroid lobe or in the posterior cervical space of the upper neck, ± extension of sinus tract posterior to the carotid artery and glossopharyngeal nerve, passing through the thyroid membrane above the level of the internal branch of the superior laryngeal nerve into the base of the piriform sinus. *Fourth branchial cleft cysts* occur in the lower third of the neck laterally, and anterior to the lower SCM and level of the aortic arch, ± visible connecting sinus tract on the right below the subclavian artery or on the left below the aortic arch that extends superiorly and dorsal to the carotid artery up to the level of the hypoglossal nerve and then downward along the SCM to the piriform sinus. *MRI:* Circumscribed lesion that often has low-intermediate signal on T1-weighted imaging and high signal on T2-weighted imaging. Usually there is no gadolinium contrast enhancement unless there is superimposed infection.	Branchial cleft cysts are developmental anomalies involving the branchial apparatus. The branchial apparatus consists of four major and two rudimentary arches of mesoderm lined by ectoderm externally and endoderm internally within pouches that form at the end of the fourth week of gestation. The mesoderm contains a dominant artery, nerve, cartilage, and muscle. The four major arches are separated by clefts. Each arch develops into a defined neck structure, with eventual obliteration of the branchial clefts. The first arch forms the external auditory canal, eustachian tube, middle ear, and mastoid air cells. The second arch develops into the hyoid bone and tonsillar and supratonsillar fossae. The third and fourth arches develop into the pharynx below the hyoid bone. Branchial anomalies include cysts, sinuses, and fistulae. Second branchial cleft cysts account for up to 90% of all branchial cleft malformations. Cysts are lined by squamous epithelium (90%), ciliated columnar epithelium (8%), or both types (2%). Sebaceous glands, salivary tissue, lymphoid tissue, and cholesterol crystals in mucoid fluid can also occur. There are four types of second branchial cleft cysts. Type 1 is located anterior to the sternocleidomastoid muscle (SCM) and deep to the platysma muscle; type 2 (the most common type) is located at the anteromedial surface of the SCM, lateral to the carotid space and posterior to the submandibular gland; type 3 is located lateral to pharyngeal wall and medial to the carotid arteries ± extension between the external and internal carotid arteries ("beak sign"); type 4 is located between the medial aspect of the carotid sheath and pharynx at the level of the tonsillar fossa, and can extend superiorly to the skull base. Branchial cleft cysts are typically asymptomatic unless complicated by infection.

(continued on page 528)

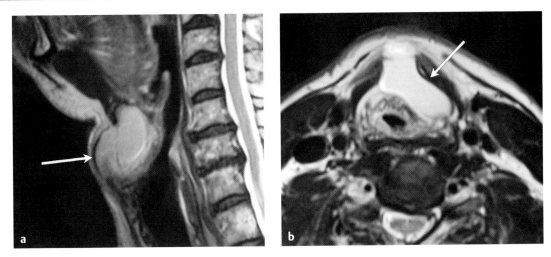

Fig. 5.42 **(a)** Sagittal and **(b)** axial T2-weighted images show a thyroglossal duct cyst (*arrows*) with high signal that extends posteriorly through the superior notch of the thyroid cartilage.

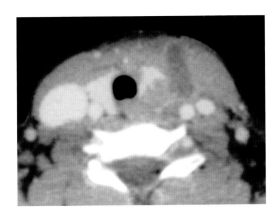

Fig. 5.43 Axial CT shows an infected third branchial cleft cyst containing zones of low attenuation with irregular peripheral contrast enhancement located anterior and medial to the lower left sternocleidomastoid muscle, with extension medial to the carotid space to involve the upper left thyroid lobe.

Table 5.2 *(cont.)*   Lesions of the hypopharynx and larynx

Lesions	Imaging Findings	Comments
Amyloidomas	Amyloidomas can occur as solitary or multifocal lesions with ill-defined margins. *MRI:* Lesions can have low-intermediate or slightly high signal on T1-weighted imaging and variable heterogeneous slightly high to high signal with or without low signal zones on T2-weighted imaging. Variable degrees of gadolinium contrast enhancement can be seen. *CT:* Lesions can have low, intermediate, and/or high attenuation, as well as contrast enhancement.	Amyloidosis is a disease complex that results from the extracellular deposition of insoluble eosinophilic fibrillar protein with a β-pleated configuration. Deposits of amyloid protein can occur in a systemic distribution or as localized lesions. The systemic form often results from plasma cell dyscrasias and hereditary diseases, or due to chronic diseases. Amyloidoma accounts for < 1% of laryngeal lesions. Submucosal lesions occur in the vestibular folds > aryepiglottic folds, subglottis > vocal folds.
Inflammatory Lesions		
Pyogenic infection (**Fig. 5.44** and **Fig. 5.45**)	*CT:* Irregular soft tissue thickening with ill-defined margins (phlegmon) ± rim-enhancing fluid collection (abscess). *MRI:* Irregular soft tissue thickening with poorly defined slightly high signal on T2-weighted imaging (T2WI) and fat-suppressed T2WI (phlegmon). Abscesses are collections with high signal on T2WI surrounded by peripheral rims of gadolinium contrast enhancement. Soft tissue thickening with slightly high to high signal on T2WI is typically seen adjacent to the abscess.	In children, peritonsillar abscess is the most common infection involving the head and neck. Occurs in young children and adults often during times with highest incidence of streptococcal pharyngitis and exudative tonsillitis. The infection can extend into the adjacent parapharyngeal, retropharyngeal, danger, masticator, and/or submandibular spaces, with potential involvement of the hypopharynx, larynx, and mid and lower neck. Other etiologies for retropharyngeal space (RPS) infection include: complications from intubation, nasogastric tubes, surgery, foreign bodies, and necrotizing otitis externa. Infection involving the RPS and danger space can extend into the larynx and/or mediastinum, causing mediastinitis. Infection and abscess formation in the neck can result from inferior extension of dental infections with osteomyelitis. Infections in the neck can also result from extension of pyogenic or tuberculous vertebral osteomyelitis through the prevertebral fascia. Patients with infection in the RPS and danger space often present with odynophagia, dysphagia, stiff neck, head tilted backward, and dyspnea.
Necrotizing fasciitis	*CT:* Extensive abnormal soft tissue thickening with ill-defined margins containing small low-attenuation fluid zones, ± foci of gas from gas-forming bacteria. The abnormality usually involves multiple neck spaces, with thickening and/or contrast enhancement of fascia and muscles.	Acute, rapidly progressive polymicrobial destructive infection that results in liquefaction of connective tissues and fascia. Occurs in diabetic and immunocompromised or immunosuppressed patients. Often involves multiple neck spaces and results in sepsis and descending mediastinitis. Associated with increased mortality of 25–40%. Prompt treatment with broad-spectrum antibiotics, surgical debridement, and hyperbaric oxygen is routinely used for this aggressive disease.
Laryngeal tuberculosis	*MRI:* Bilateral, diffuse, soft tissue lesions in the larynx with low-intermediate signal on T1-weighted imaging and intermediate to high signal on T2-weighted imaging, + solid or rim gadolinium contrast enhancement and restricted or increased diffusion. *CT:* Diffuse, soft tissue attenuation lesions in the larynx, ± calcifications. Destruction of laryngeal cartilage can occur late in the disease process. Usually occurs in association with pulmonary tuberculosis.	Occurs in immunocompromised patients and in immunocompetent patients in developing countries. Caseating granulomas occur in multiple tissues, including the larynx.

(continued on page 530)

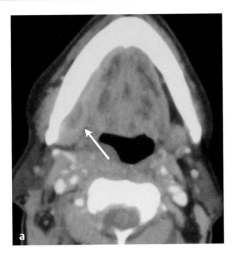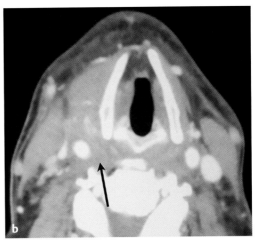

Fig. 5.44   (a) Axial postcontrast CT of a 74-year-old man with a pyogenic abscess (*arrow*) adjacent to the medial margin of the right mandible secondary to a dental infection. **(b)** Axial CT shows inferior extension of the infection along the outer margin of the right thyroid cartilage, with involvement of the right carotid space (*arrow*).

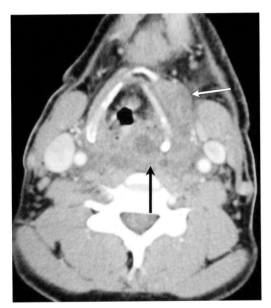

Fig. 5.45   Axial postcontrast CT of a 50-year-old man shows a retropharyngeal abscess extending into the posterior portion of the larynx at the level of the left false cord (*black arrow*), as well as involving the left strap muscle (*white arrow*).

Table 5.2 *(cont.)* Lesions of the hypopharynx and larynx

Lesions	Imaging Findings	Comments
Relapsing polychondritis	*CT:* Findings include subglottic stenosis, tracheobronchial narrowing, densely calcified tracheal and laryngeal cartilage, and "train-track" calcifications of the cricoid cartilage posteriorly. Other findings include nasal cartilage collapse, bronchiectasis, and peripheral bronchial narrowing. *PET/CT:* Abnormal increased uptake of F-18 FDG is seen at sites of active inflammation.	Rare and potentially fatal autoimmune disease in which there are widespread destructive inflammatory lesions of cartilage. Involves hyaline cartilage and fibrocartilage of appendicular joints, as well as cartilage in the ears, nose, larynx, trachea, and bronchi. Patients with laryngeal involvement present with hoarseness, chronic cough, and dyspnea on exertion. The inflammation can also involve the media of arteries, conjunctiva, ocular sclera, and heart valves. Involvement of the larynx, trachea, and/or bronchi occurs in up to 50% of patients, and can be associated with progressive respiratory distress. Peak age at presentation is the fifth decade, with an annual incidence of 3.5 per million, and 3:1 female:male ratio. The combination of auricular chondritis and polyarthritis occurs in 80%. Treatment includes corticosteroids, methotrexate, or cyclophosphamide.
Rheumatoid arthritis	*CT:* Findings include narrowing of the cricothyroid joint (up to 80%), ankylosis at the cricothyroid joint (9%), increase in cartilage density (45%), and edema of the vocal folds (27%). Rarely involves the cricoarytenoid joints.	Chronic multisystem disease of unknown etiology with persistent inflammatory synovitis involving diarthrodial joints in a symmetric distribution. Can result in progressive destruction of cartilage and bone, leading to joint dysfunction. Affects ~ 1% of the world's population. Eighty percent of adult patients present between the ages of 35 and 50 years. Laryngeal involvement is common but often subclinical. Involves the cricothyroid and cricoarytenoid joints, which are synovial joints. Patients can present with hoarsenss, vocal fatigue, and dyspnea.
Traumatic Laryngeal Lesions		
Blunt trauma/ laryngeal fracture (**Fig. 5.46** and **Fig. 5.47**)	*CT:* Axial and/or reformatted sagittal and coronal images can show and characterize fractures of the thyroid and cricoid cartilage, as well as the hyoid bone. Soft tissue emphysema can be seen adjacent to the fracture site. Malrotated arytenoid cartilage can be seen with dislocations involving the cricoarytenoid joint.	Laryngeal fractures commonly result from motor vehicle collisions or sports-related injuries. Paramedian or median vertical fractures of the thyroid cartilage are the most common type of laryngeal fracture, followed by cricoid ring fractures. Cricoarytenoid dislocations are the most common type of cartilage dislocation, followed by dislocations of the cricothyroid joints.
Hematoma (**Fig. 5.48**)	*CT:* Nodular lesion with intermediate to slightly high attenuation and irregular margins, ± osseous or cartilage fracture.	Extravasated blood from trauma can be an isolated finding or can be associated with laryngeal injuries including fractures.
Penetrating trauma	*CT:* ± laryngeal cartilage fractures, hematomas, foreign bodies, and/or subcutaneous emphysema.	Penetrating trauma can result in direct injuries to the larynx, nerves, and/or blood vessels. Can result in respiratory distress and/or vocal cord paresis or paralysis from laryngeal fractures, cartilage dislocations, or nerve injuries.

(continued on page 532)

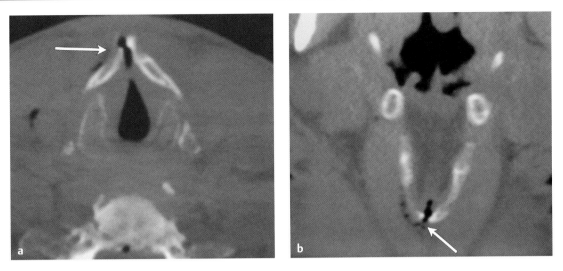

Fig. 5.46 **(a)** Axial and **(b)** coronal CT images show a traumatic fracture (*arrows*) through the anteroinferior portion of the thyroid cartilage.

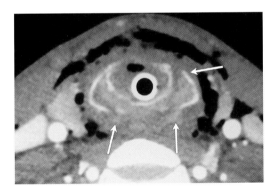

Fig. 5.47 Axial CT of an intubated patient shows traumatic fractures (*arrows*) involving the cricoid cartilage, with extensive subcutaneous emphysema.

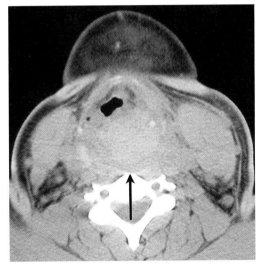

Fig. 5.48 Axial CT of a patient with a history of blunt neck trauma shows a hematoma in the posterior larynx (*arrow*) that has slightly high attenuation.

Table 5.2 *(cont.)*   Lesions of the hypopharynx and larynx

Lesions	Imaging Findings	Comments
Other Lesions		
Postradiation treatment changes (**Fig. 5.49**)	*CT:* Radiation-induced mucositis and submucosal edema are associated with laryngeal findings of thickening of the epiglottis, aryepiglottic folds, and/or false vocal cords, as well as stranding within the preepiglottic and paraglottic fat. Prominent contrast enhancement of the mucosa is often seen. These findings can persist for months to years in up to 50% of patients. Other findings include: thickening of the epidermis and platysma muscle and stranding within the subcutaneous fat. *MRI:* Thickening of the epiglottis, aryepiglottic folds, and/or false vocal cords, which have slightly high to high signal on T2-weighted imaging, as well as prominent contrast enhancement of the mucosa.	Treatment with radiation or chemoradiation for malignant tumors in the neck typically causes an acute inflammation in connective tissue, with increased leukocytes and histiocytes as well as hemorrhage and necrosis (mucositis). Injury to the endothelium of small arteries and veins results in edema from increased vessel permeability. Between 1 and 8 months after treatment, there is progressive deposition of collagen, resulting in sclerosis and fibrosis of connective tissue, as well as occlusion of small blood vessels.
Laryngeal chondronecrosis (**Fig. 5.50**)	*CT:* Sclerosis of laryngeal cartilage, ± cartilage fragmentation, ± cartilage collapse, ± gas bubbles.	Delayed complication of radiation treatment that often occurs more than 1 year after completion of therapy. More common with treatment for T3 and T4 lesions than with treatment for T1 or T2 tumors. Symptoms can be nonspecific and include hoarseness, dysphagia, odynophagia, and pain. Progressive problems that can be associated with chondronecrosis include fistula formation, respiratory distress, and airway obstruction. Chondronecrosis can also occur as a complication of endotracheal intubation.
Reinke's edema (**Fig. 5.51**)	*CT and MRI:* Diffuse swelling of vocal cords without evidence of a focal lesion.	Edematous membranous swelling of the vocal folds resulting in narrowing of the laryngeal airway. Edema involves the superficial lamina propria of the vocal cords (Reinke's space). Associated with activation of CD34+ fibroblasts in stroma of vocal folds. Can result from gastroesophageal or laryngopharyngeal reflux, exposure to tobacco smoke, vocal abuse, or hypothyroidism. Histologic changes include increased exudative fluid in the extracellular matrix and disarrangement of collagenous and elastic fibers. Treatment of cause typically results in resolution.

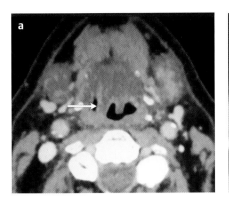

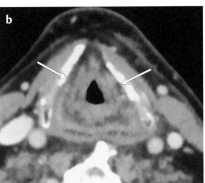

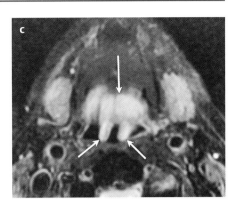

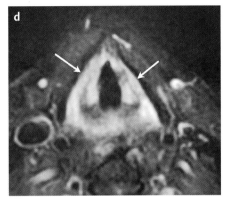

Fig. 5.49 **(a,b)** Axial CT images of a 60-year-old man obtained 2 years after radiation treatment show thickening of the aryepiglottic folds and false vocal cords, as well as stranding within the preepiglottic and paraglottic fat (*arrows*). **(c,d)** Axial fat-suppressed T2-weighted imaging shows abnormal high signal in the aryepiglottic folds, paraglottic soft tissue, and vocal cords (*arrows*).

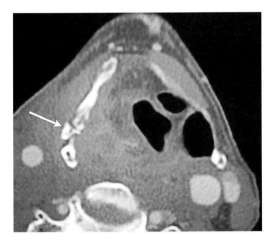

Fig. 5.50 Axial CT of a 56-year-old man shows chondronecrosis with fragmentation of the right thyroid cartilage (*arrow*) from the late effects of prior radiation treatment for Hodgkin disease.

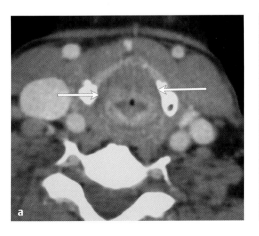

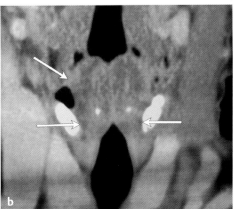

Fig. 5.51 **(a)** Axial and **(b)** coronal CT images of a patient with Reinke's edema show diffuse swelling of the vocal cords (*arrows*) and narrowing of the airway without evidence of a focal lesion.

5.3 Visceral Space: Lesions of the Thyroid and Parathyroid Glands

Thyroid Gland

The paired thyroid and parathyroid glands are located in the visceral space (**Fig. 5.52**) and are endocrine glands, which lack ducts and secrete hormones directly into the bloodstream. The thyroid gland produces triiodothyronine (T_3) and thyroxine (T_4), which are involved in regulation of body metabolism and fetal brain development. Release of T_3 and T_4 from the thyroid gland occurs via feedback regulation involving the hypothalamus, which secretes thyrotropin-releasing hormone (TRH), which stimulates the pituitary gland to secrete thyrotropin-stimulating hormone (TSH). TSH stimulates the production of thyroglobulin in the thyroid gland. Thyroglobulin is a key protein involved in production of T_3 and T_4, which occurs after uptake and concentration of serum iodine in thyroid follicular cells, oxidization of iodine via the enzyme thyroid peroxidase, and iodination of tyrosine within thyroglobulin to form monoiodotyrosine (MIT) and diiodotyrosine (DIT). T_3 is formed by coupling of MIT and DIT, and T_4 is formed by coupling of two molecules of DIT. T_3 and T_4 are subsequently released into the bloodstream after separa-tion from thyroglobulin. T_3 can also be metabolized from T_4 after release from the thyroid gland.

The thyroid gland also produces and secretes calcitonin, which is involved in calcium homeostasis. The parathyroid glands produce and secrete parathyroid hormone, which regulates calcium metabolism through its interaction with receptors in the kidneys, skeletal muscles, and intestines.

The thyroid gland is composed of follicular cells and parafollicular cells. The follicular cells of the thyroid gland develop from endodermal cells (median thyroid anlage), located between the first and second pharyngeal arches, in the first 3 weeks of gestation. At 24 days of gestation, a small pit (thyroid bud) forms within the thyroid anlage that progressively forms a bilobed diverticulum that extends inferiorly along the midline adjacent to the aortic primordium. A small channel (thyroglossal duct) temporarily exists between the dorsal portion of the tongue (foramen cecum) and the inferiorly descending thyroid primordium (**Fig. 5.53**). The thyroglossal duct normally involutes by the tenth week of gestation. The descending thyroid primordium and thyroglossal duct course anterior to the hyoid bone and loop slightly posterior to the inferior margin of the hyoid bone before descending anterior to the thyrohyoid membrane, thyroid cartilage, and trachea. The thyroglossal duct extends between the sternohyoid and sternothyroid strap muscles. The descending thyroid primordium reaches it normal position in the lower neck

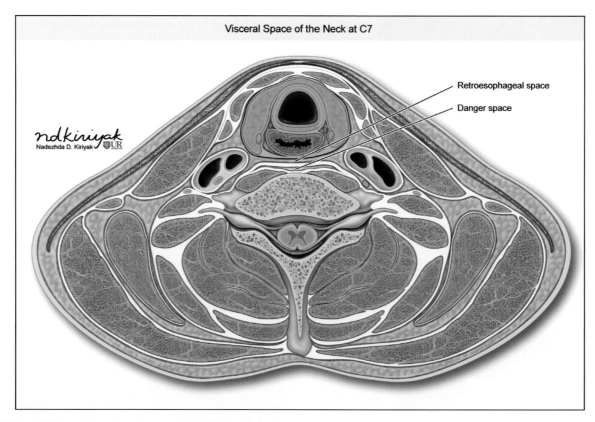

Fig. 5.52 Axial view of the visceral space of the infrahyoid neck in color.

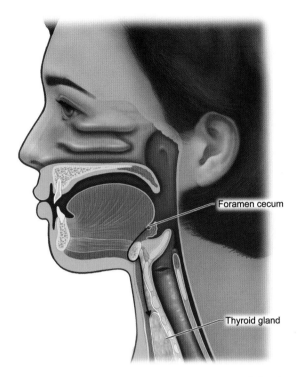

Fig. 5.53 Sagittal illustration shows the pathway of the thryoglossal duct.

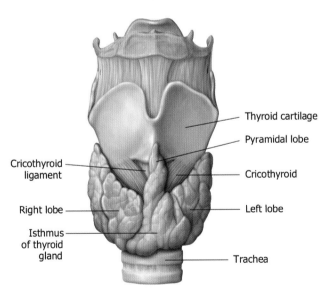

Fig. 5.54 Frontal view of the thyroid gland and adjacent structures. From THIEME Atlas of Anatomy: Head and Neuroanatomy, © Thieme 2007, Illustration by Karl Wesker.

at 7 weeks of gestation. The parafollicular cells (C cells) of the thyroid develop from endodermal cells (lateral thyroid anlage) at the fourth pharyngeal pouch and migrate to join and merge with the descending thyroid primordium from the median thyroid anlage.

The thyroid gland is usually located in the visceral space of the lower neck, anterior and anterolateral to the lower larynx and upper trachea, and posterior to the infrahyoid strap muscles (sternohyoid and sternothyroid muscles). The thyroid gland has left and right lobes, which are usually connected by a midline isthmus (**Fig. 5.54**). Thyroid tissue in the residual lower portion of the embryologic thyroglossal duct results in an elongated pyramidal lobe that attaches inferiorly to either the right or left thyroid lobes. The thyroid gland usually weighs ~ 30 g.

Blood supply to the thyroid gland is from the inferior thyroid artery, derived from the thyrocervical trunk, and the superior thyroid artery, which is the first branch of the external carotid artery (**Fig. 5.55**). Venous drainage is into the internal jugular veins and brachiocephalic veins. Sympathetic innervation of the thyroid gland is via the middle and inferior cervical ganglia, and parasympathetic innervation is from the vagus nerve.

On ultrasonography, the normal thyroid gland shows homogeneous echogenicity. With CT performed without intravenous contrast, the thyroid gland has intermediate to slightly high attenuation, ranging from 80 to 100 HU, related to its intrinsic iodine content. After administration of iodinated contrast, the thyroid gland shows prominent homogeneous contrast enhancement. With MRI, the thyroid gland typically has intermediate signal on T1-weighted imaging that is slightly hyperintense relative to muscle, and intermediate signal on T2-weighted imaging that is slightly hyperintense to muscle. The thyroid gland normally shows prominent gadolinium contrast enhancement. On radionuclide scintigraphy, the normal gland shows uniform uptake of iodine 123 or technetium 99m pertechnetate.

Parathyroid Gland

The parathyroid gland is derived from the third and fourth pharyngeal pouches. The most common configuration is two sets of paired glands located dorsal to the thyroid gland (**Fig. 5.56**). The superior glands arise from the fourth branchial pouch and are usually located posterior to the thyroid gland at the level of the inferior margin of the cricoid cartilage. The inferior glands arise from the third branchial pouch and are located posterior to the inferior portion of the thyroid gland (50%), 1 cm below the thyroid gland (15%), or anywhere from between the angle of the mandible and mediastinum. Ectopic superior glands can occur within the thyroid gland because parafollicular cells of the thyroid also develop from the fourth branchial pouch. Ectopic inferior glands can occur within the thymus or thyrothymic ligament because the thymus is also derived from the third branchial pouch. Parathyroid glands range in size from 5 to 10 mm in craniocaudal dimension, 2 to 4 mm in transverse dimension, and 2 mm in thickness,

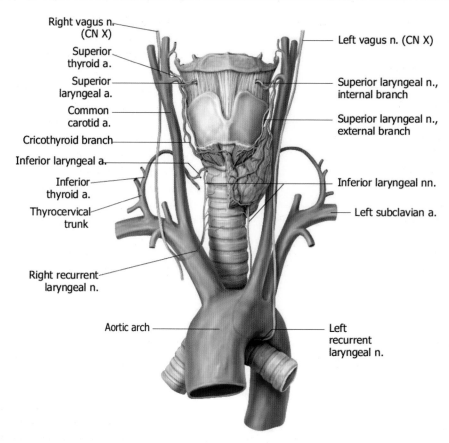

Fig. 5.55 Illustration shows the arterial supply to, and innervation of, the thyroid glands. From THIEME Atlas of Anatomy: Head and Neuroanatomy, © Thieme 2007, Illustration by Karl Wesker.

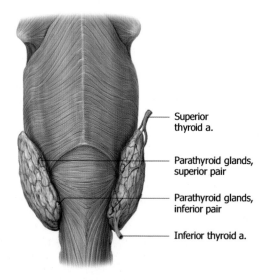

Fig. 5.56 Posterior view of the parathyroid glands and adjacent structures. From THIEME Atlas of Anatomy: Head and Neuroanatomy, © Thieme 2007, Illustration by Karl Wesker.

and weigh up to 40 mg. Parathyroid glands that weigh more than 60 mg are considered abnormal. Most parathyroid adenomas weigh over 100 mg.

The superior and inferior thyroid arteries supply the superior and inferior parathyroid glands, respectively. Venous drainage occurs to the thyroid veins. The parathyroid glands secrete parathyroid hormone proportional to the concentration of calcium in blood, which normally ranges from 8.8 to 10.2 mg/dL. Hypercalcemia results in decreased parathyroid hormone production. Primary hyperparathyroidism refers to excessive autonomous production of parathyroid hormone from sporadic parathyroid adenomas (85%), parathyroid hyperplasia (10%) multiple adenomas (4%), and carcinomas (1%). The incidence of primary hyperparathyroidism is 10 to 300 per million. Primary hyperparathyroidism is 2–3 times more common in women than men, and the average age at presentation is 55 years. Treatment is typically surgery. Secondary hyperparathyroidism consists of elevated parathyroid hormone that results from renal failure, hyperphosphatemia, calcitriol deficiency, and/or vitamin D deficiency. Secondary hyperparathyroidism related to renal failure/end-stage kidney disease is more common than primary hyperparathyroidism. Medical treatment is usually the initial therapy for secondary hyperparathyroidism, although surgery is often done when medical management fails.

Table 5.3 Visceral space: lesions of the thyroid and parathyroid glands

- Developmental Anomalies
  - Thyroglossal duct cyst
  - Ectopic thyroid tissue
- Benign Thyroid Tumors
  - Thyroid adenoma
  - Multinodular goiter
- Tumorlike Thyroid Lesions
  - Thyroid nodule
- Malignant Thyroid Neoplasms
  - Papillary (differentiated) thyroid carcinoma
  - Follicular thyroid carcinoma
  - Medullary carcinoma
  - Poorly differentiated thyroid carcinoma (PDTC)
  - Anaplastic (undifferentiated) thyroid carcinoma (ATC)
- Thyroid lymphoma
- Metastatic tumor
- Infections involving the Thyroid
  - Acute suppurative thyroiditis
  - Subacute (de Quervain) thyroiditis
  - Tuberculous thyroiditis
- Autoimmune Thyroid Diseases
  - Graves disease
  - Hashimoto thyroiditis
  - Riedel's thyroiditis
  - Granulomatous thyroiditis
- Benign Parathyroid Tumors
  - Parathyroid adenoma
  - Parathyroid hyperplasia
  - Multiple parathyroid adenomas
- Malignant Parathyroid Tumors
  - Parathyroid carcinoma

Table 5.3 Visceral space: lesions of the thyroid and parathyroid glands

Lesions	Imaging Findings	Comments
Developmental Anomalies		
Thyroglossal duct cyst (See **Fig. 5.2** and **Fig. 5.3**)	*MRI:* Well-circumscribed spheroid or ovoid lesion at the tongue base or along the pathway of the thyroglossal duct, which usually has low signal on T1-weighted imaging (T1WI) and diffusion-weighted imaging and high signal on T2-weighted imaging (T2WI). The wall of the thyroglossal duct cyst is typically thin without gadolinium (Gd) contrast enhancement. Thyroglossal duct cysts complicated by hemorrhage or current or prior infection can have elevated protein with intermediate to slightly high signal on T1WI and T2WI. The walls of such cysts can be thick and show Gd contrast enhancement. Nodular Gd contrast enhancement involving the wall of a thyroglossal duct cyst can be seen with a potentially malignant lesion. *CT:* Well-circumscribed lesion with low (mucoid) attenuation ranging from 10 to 25 HU, surrounded by a thin wall. Occasionally contains thin septations. Thyroglossal duct cysts complicated by infection can have increased attenuation, thick walls, and loss/indistinctness of adjacent tissue planes. *Ultrasound:* Can be well-circumscribed anechoic cysts with through transmission or can have a pseudosolid appearance related to elevated protein concentration.	Thyroglossal duct cyst is the most common congenital mass in the neck and is related to altered development of the thyroid gland. The follicular cells of the thyroid gland develop from endodermal cells (median thyroid anlage) located between the first and second pharyngeal arches in the first 3 weeks of gestation. At 24 days of gestation, a small pit (thyroid bud) forms within the thyroid anlage, which progressively forms a bilobed diverticulum that extends inferiorly along the midline adjacent to the aortic primordium. A small channel (thyroglossal duct) temporarily exists between the dorsal portion of the tongue (foramen cecum) and the inferiorly descending thyroid primordium. The thyroglossal duct normally involutes by the tenth week of gestation. The descending thyroid primordium and thyroglossal duct course anterior to the hyoid bone and loop slightly posterior to the inferior margin of the hyoid bone before descending anterior to the thyrohyoid membrane, thyroid cartilage, and trachea. The thyroglossal duct extends between the sternohyoid and sternothyroid strap muscles. The descending thyroid primordium reaches its normal position in the lower neck at 7 weeks of gestation. The parafollicular cells (C cells) of the thyroid develop from endodermal cells (lateral thyroid anlage) at the fourth pharyngeal pouch and migrate to join and merge with the descending thyroid primordium from the median thyroid anlage. Up to two-thirds of thyroglossal duct cysts occur in the infrahyoid neck and can be midline or extend laterally within, or deep to, the strap muscles. Nearly 50% present in patients < 20 years old as a progressively enlarging neck lesion.

(continued on page 538)

Table 5.3 *(cont.)* Visceral space: Lesions of the thyroid and parathyroid glands

Lesions	Imaging Findings	Comments
Ectopic thyroid tissue (See **Fig. 5.4**, **Fig. 5.5**, and **Fig. 5.6**)	*CT:* Circumscribed ovoid or spheroid lesion at the dorsal portion (base) of the tongue or along the pathway of the thyroglossal duct that shows slightly increased attenuation (~ 70 HU), prominent contrast enhancement, ± low-attenuation thyroid nodules, ± calcifications. *MRI:* Circumscribed lesions with low-intermediate signal on T1-weighted imaging and low, intermediate, or slightly high signal on T2-weighted imaging. Variable degrees of gadolinium contrast enhancement. *Nuclear medicine:* Iodine 123, iodine 131, or technetium 99m pertechnetate uptake in ectopic thyroid tissue in the tongue or along the course of the thyroglossal duct, and lack of normal uptake in normal orthotopic location of thyroid bed.	The normal thyroid gland is located below the larynx, posterior to the strap muscles, medial to the carotid arteries, and anterolateral to the trachea. Ectopic thyroid tissue results from lack of normal embryologic descent of the primitive thyroid gland along the thyroglossal duct from the foramen cecum at the tongue base down to the lower neck. Lingual thyroid represents up to 90% of cases of ectopic thyroid. Other locations include: adjacent to the hyoid bone, midline infrahyoid neck, and lateral neck. Can be asymptomatic, or can occur in association with dysphagia, dysphonia, and/or stridor.
Benign Thyroid Tumors		
Thyroid adenoma (**Fig. 5.57** and **Fig. 5.58**)	*CT:* Circumscribed ovoid or spheroid lesion often with decreased attenuation relative to the normal gland. Variable contrast enhancement, ± cysts, calcifications, and/or hemorrhage. *MRI:* Circumscribed lesions with low-intermediate signal on T1-weighted imaging (T1WI) and intermediate to high signal on T2-weighted imaging, ± cysts without or with proteinaceous or hemorrhagic content resulting in high signal on T1WI. Lesions show varying degrees of gadolinium contrast enhancement.	Follicular adenomas are benign neoplastic proliferations of follicles enclosed by a fibrous capsule. Usually occur as a solitary lesion within a normal gland. Most often measure less than 4 cm unless there is superimposed hemorrhage or cystic degeneration. Usually adenomas are nonfunctioning lesions, although they can be autogenously functioning. Large lesions may be associated with hyperthyroidism. Occur in adults 20 to 60 years old. Follicular thyroid lesions diagnosed by fine-needle aspiration biopsy are benign adenomas in 85% of cases, but because there is also a 15% chance of malignancy, surgical hemithyroidectomy is usually performed. Hürthle cell adenomas are variants of follicular adenoma that contain numerous granular follicular cells with pink-staining cytoplasm (oncocytic features).
Multinodular goiter (**Fig. 5.59** and **Fig. 5.60**)	*CT: Simple goiters* appear as diffuse enlargement of the thyroid gland. *Multinodular goiters* have multiple nodules that often have low attenuation, ± cystic zones and calcifications. Margins are usually well circumscribed. Can displace and/or compress the trachea and/or esophagus, ± extension inferiorly into the mediastinum. *Ultrasound: Simple goiters* are associated with diffuse enlargement of the thyroid gland that has uniform or heterogeneous echogenicity. *Multinodular goiters* can have heterogeneous echogenicity with multiple hypoechoic nodules, ± cystic or necrotic zones, ± calcifications, ± hemorrhage. Toxic nodules chow increased systolic velocities on color Doppler sonography. *MRI: Simple goiters* show diffuse enlargement of the thyroid gland. *Multinodular goiters* have circumscribed margins and contain multiple nodules. Nodules can have low, intermediate, or high signal on T1-weighted imaging (T1WI) and T2-weighted imaging (T2WI). High signal on T1WI can be secondary to cysts with colloid or hemorrhage. Low signal foci on T1WI and T2WI can occur from calcifications. Can displace and/or compress the trachea and/or esophagus, ± extend inferiorly into the mediastinum. *Nuclear scintigraphy:* Iodine 123, iodine 131, or technetium 99m pertechnetate uptake often occurs in multiple nodules.	Goiter is an enlargement of the thyroid gland without or with multiple nodules (multinodular goiter). Simple diffuse goiters result from inadequate output of thyroid hormone, which causes compensatory hypertrophy of follicular thyroid epithelium. The simple, diffuse, nontoxic goiters usually have an initial phase of follicular cell growth with hyperemia. Patients with simple diffuse goiters are usually euthyroid. Endemic goiters occur in areas when dietary iodine is insufficient. Another type is the simple sporadic goiter, which usually occurs in females with onset around puberty. Eventually, there is often colloid involution that progresses to nodule formation within the goiter (multinodular goiter). Toxic multinodular goiters are associated with hyperthyroidism and have one or more autofunctioning nodules (Plummer's disease). Most toxic goiters occur in patients who initially had nontoxic goiters. Patients present with a neck mass and neck discomfort. Goiters can extend into the mediastinum without or with displacement and compression of the trachea and esophagus, resulting in shortness of breath and dysphagia. Multinodular goiters contain various-sized nodules that contain follicles distended by colloid, papillary hyperplasia, cystic and/or hemorrhagic zones, cholesterol clefts, dystrophic calcifications, ossifications, and necrosis.

(continued on page 540)

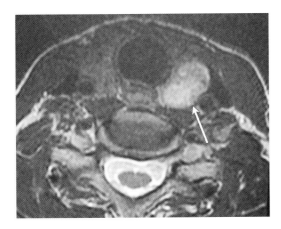

Fig. 5.57 Axial T2-weighted imaging of a 45-year-old woman shows a thyroid adenoma (*arrow*) in the left thyroid lobe. The adenoma has heterogeneous slightly high signal.

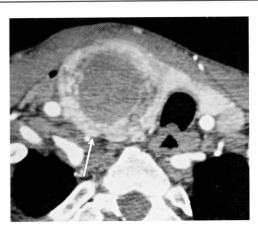

Fig. 5.58 Axial postcontrast CT of a 52-year-old man shows a large adenoma (*arrow*) in the right thyroid lobe that has mixed low-intermediate and slightly high attenuation.

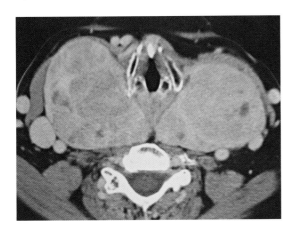

Fig. 5.59 Axial postcontrast CT shows a multinodular goiter with diffuse abnormal enlargement of both thyroid lobes and well-defined margins containing zones with low, intermediate, and slightly high attenuation.

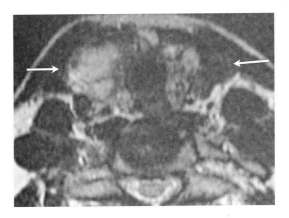

Fig. 5.60 Axial T2-weighted imaging of a 49-year-old woman shows a multinodular goiter with zones of low, intermediate, and slightly high signal in both thyroid lobes (*arrows*).

Table 5.3 *(cont.)*   Visceral space: Lesions of the thyroid and parathyroid glands

Lesions	Imaging Findings	Comments
Tumorlike Thyroid Lesions		
Thyroid nodule (**Fig. 5.61** and **Fig. 5.62**)	*Ultrasound:* Findings associated with *benign nodules* include: solid hypoechoic and predominantly cystic lesion, presence of a sonolucent halo, avascularity, well-defined margins, and an enlarged thyroid with multiple nodules. Colloid cysts are typically hypoechoic with internal linear echogenic bands and "comet tail" reflections from colloid calcifications. Findings associated with increased risk for a *malignant nodule* include: microcalcifications, central hypervascularity, irregular margins, and cervical lymphadenopathy. *CT:* Circumscribed ovoid or spheroid lesion, often with decreased attenuation relative to the normal gland. Variable contrast enhancement, ± cysts, calcifications, and/or hemorrhage. Large size, ill-defined margins, and lymphadenopathy are associated with malignant lesions. *MRI:* Circumscribed lesions with low-intermediate signal on T1-weighted imaging (T1WI) and intermediate to high signal on T2-weighted imaging (T2WI), ± cysts without or with proteinaceous or hemorrhagic content resulting in high signal on T1WI. Colloid cysts can have low, intermediate, or high signal on T1WI and usually have high signal on T2WI. Ill-defined margins and lymphadenopathy are associated with malignant lesions. With *diffusion-weighted imaging*, malignant nodules can have mean apparent diffusion coefficient (ADC) values that are significantly lower than benign nodules, with the cutoff at 0.98×10^{-3} mm^2/sec. Lesions show varying degrees of gadolinium (Gd) contrast enhancement. With dynamic Gd contrast enhancement techniques, conflicting results have been reported. Some studies of benign lesions have shown a rapid inflow and washout pattern of Gd, whereas malignant lesions may or may not show a delayed inflow pattern, with decreased slopes of the time-intensity curves and longer time to peak enhancement. *Nuclear medicine:* Iodine 123, iodine 131, or technetium 99m pertechnetate uptake can be decreased ("cold nodules") or increased ("hot nodules"). The risk for malignancy is higher with cold nodules (20%) than with hot nodules (< 5%). *F-18 FDG PET:* Standardized uptake values > 5 in nodules are associated with an increased risk for malignancy.	Thyroid nodules occur in up to 50% of adults. CT and MRI show incidental thyroid nodules in 15% of examinations. Palpable thyroid nodules, however, occur in only 7% of patients. Most of these lesions are unencapsulated benign follicular nodules that result from cycles of hyperplasia and colloid involution within adenomatous goiters. Benign follicular nodules are composed of varying proportions of benign follicular cells, colloid, and fibrous tissue. Follicular nodules can occur in multinodular goiters, or as adenomatoid or hyperplastic nodules, nodules in Graves disease, or colloid cysts (composed mostly of colloid, with only a minimal amount of follicular cells). Fine-needle aspiration biopsies cannot distinguish between the different types of benign nodules. Most palpable thyroid nodules are benign, although 5 to 7% are malignant tumors. Factors associated with increased likelihood of malignant nodules include: age < 20 years or > 80 years, history of thyroid cancer in one or more first-degree relatives, history of prior external beam radiation treatment, multiple endocrine neoplasia (MEN), familial medullary thyroid cancer (FMTC), MEN2/FMTC-associated *RET* proto-oncogene mutation, and calcitonin > 100 pg/mL.

(continued on page 542)

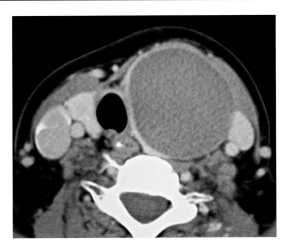

Fig. 5.61 Axial CT of a 59-year-old woman shows a large colloid cyst in the left thyroid lobe; the cyst has well-defined margins.

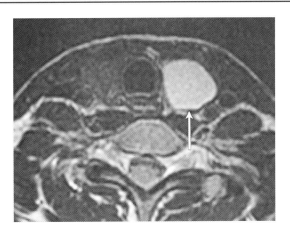

Fig. 5.62 Axial T2-weighted imaging of a 16-year-old female shows a colloid cyst (*arrow*) in the left thyroid lobe that has high signal and well-defined margins.

Table 5.3 *(cont.)* Visceral space: Lesions of the thyroid and parathyroid glands

Lesions	Imaging Findings	Comments
Malignant Thyroid Neoplasms		
Papillary (differentiated) thyroid carcinoma (**Fig. 5.63** and **Fig. 5.64**)	*CT:* Lesion with soft tissue attenuation, often with microcalcifications (< 1 mm), ± macrocalcifications, ± irregular borders, + contrast enhancement. Metastases to regional lymph nodes occur in up to 20%. Features associated with metastatic lymph nodes include calcifications and cystic and/or hemorrhagic changes (up to 70%). *Ultrasound:* Tumors can have irregular shapes and borders, internal echoes, hypervascularity, and/or microcalcifications. *MRI:* Tumors have low-intermediate signal on T1-weighted imaging, intermediate to slightly high signal on T2-weighted imaging, ± cystic and/or hemorrhagic changes. Tumors often show heterogeneous gadolinium contrast enhancement. MRI is useful in the evaluation of tumor spread beyond the thyroid capsule. *Radionuclide scintigraphy:* Postoperative evaluation with iodine 131 is used to assess for recurrent or metastatic tumor. *PET/CT:* Tumors often show increased uptake of F-18 FDG; standardized uptake value (SUV) can be up to 7.	Most common malignant primary tumor of the thyroid gland (accounts for up to 80% of primary malignant tumors). Commonly occurs in young adults. The tumors are often low grade and contain malignant follicular cells arranged in a papillary pattern. Mixed papillary and follicular histologic patterns also occur and are treated like pure papillary types. The tumors can be multifocal within the thyroid gland. Treatment is total thyroidectomy because of the potential for multifocal tumor. Additional subsequent radioactive iodine ablation is often performed. Prognosis is usually favorable, with a 10-year survival of 90%. Factors associated with poor outcome include advanced tumor stage and patient age over 45 years. CT and MRI have a role in staging tumors in patients who have hoarseness, vocal cord paralysis, dysphagia, and stridor.
Follicular thyroid carcinoma (**Fig. 5.65**)	*CT:* Solitary lesion with soft tissue attenuation, often has microcalcifications (< 1 mm), ± macrocalcifications, ± irregular borders, + contrast enhancement. *Ultrasound:* Tumors can have irregular shapes and borders, internal echoes, hypervascularity, and/or microcalcifications. *MRI:* Tumors have low-intermediate signal on T1-weighted imaging, intermediate to slightly high signal on T2-weighted imaging, ± cystic and/or hemorrhagic changes. Tumors often show heterogeneous gadolinium contrast enhancement. MRI is useful in the evaluation of tumor spread beyond the thyroid capsule. *Radionuclide scintigraphy:* Postoperative evaluation with iodine 131 is used to assess for recurrent or metastatic tumor. *PET/CT:* Tumors often show increased uptake of F-18 FDG; standardized uptake value (SUV) can be up to 7.	Low-grade, malignant, solitary tumors composed of neoplastic follicular cells that account for 10% of primary thyroid cancers. A variant of follicular carcinomas is the Hürthle cell carcinoma, which contains oncocytic neoplastic cells. Hürthle cell carcinomas account for 3% of primary thyroid malignant tumors. Both types often have capsular invasion, ± associated vascular invasion. More common in males than in females. Treatment is total thyroidectomy, ± radioactive thyroid ablation. Ten-year survival rate for follicular carcinomas is 85%, and 76% for Hürthle carcinoma. Poor prognosis is associated with patients > 45 years old at diagnosis and with advanced tumor stage. Metastatic tumor usually occurs in the lungs and bone, and less commonly involves lymph nodes.

(continued on page 544)

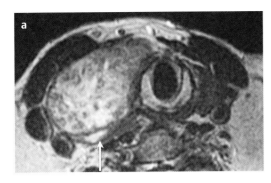 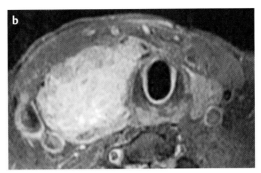

Fig. 5.63   **(a)** Axial T2-weighted imaging of a 76-year-old man shows a papillary thyroid carcinoma (*arrow*) in the right thyroid lobe that has ill-defined margins and contains heterogeneous signal with zones of high, slightly high, intermediate, and low signal. **(b)** The tumor shows heterogeneous gadolinium contrast enhancement on axial fat-suppressed T1-weighted imaging.

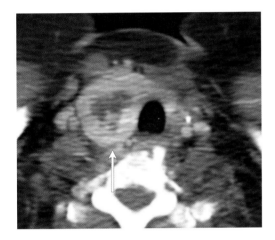

Fig. 5.64   Axial CT of a 43-year-old woman shows a papillary thyroid carcinoma (*arrow*) in the right thyroid lobe that has intermediate attenuation peripherally surrounding an irregular central zone of low attenuation. Several small calcifications are also present in the lesion.

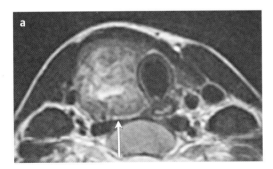 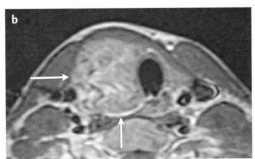

Fig. 5.65   **(a)** Axial T2-weighted imaging shows a follicular thyroid carcinoma (*arrow*) in the right thyroid lobe that has ill-defined margins and heterogeneous signal with zones of intermediate, slightly high, and high signal. **(b)** The neoplasm (*arrows*) has heterogeneous gadolinium contrast enhancement on axial T1-weighted imaging.

Table 5.3 *(cont.)*   Visceral space: Lesions of the thyroid and parathyroid glands

Lesions	Imaging Findings	Comments
Medullary carcinoma (**Fig. 5.66** and **Fig. 5.67**)	*CT:* Solitary lesion with soft tissue attenuation, usually irregular margins, and contrast enhancement, ± calcifications and cystic changes. *Ultrasound:* Tumors can have irregular shapes and borders, internal echoes, and hypervascularity. *MRI:* Tumors have low-intermediate signal on T1-weighted imaging, intermediate to slightly high signal on T2-weighted imaging, ± cystic changes. Tumors often show heterogeneous gadolinium contrast enhancement. MRI is useful in the evaluation of tumor spread beyond the thyroid capsule. *Radionuclide scintigraphy:* These neoplasms do not concentrate iodine. Therefore, iodine 123, iodine 131, or technetium 99m pertechnetate are not useful. Other radionuclides that are specific for neuroendocrine tissue (I-131 metaiodobenzylguanidine [MIBG] and somatostatin) can be used to evaluate for residual/recurrent tumor and metastatic disease. *PET/CT:* Tumors often show increased uptake of F-18 FDG.	Malignant primary thyroid tumors derived from neuroendocrine C cells that secrete calcitonin. Account for 4% of primary malignant thyroid tumors. Most tumors are solitary. Up to 80% are sporadic neoplasms, and the remaining 20% are related to inherited syndromes, such as autosomal dominant multiple endocrine neoplasia (MEN types 2a and 2b). Other lesions associated with MEN include parathyroid gland hyperplasia and pheochromocytoma. Medullary thyroid carcinomas do not concentrate iodine and iodine 131 ablation is not appropriate. The tumors are locally invasive and can spread to regional lymph nodes or metastasize to lungs, bone, and/or liver. Treatment is total thyroidectomy. The 10-year survival rate is 75%. Because these neoplasms derive from parafollicular cells, which secrete calcitonin, serum levels of calcitonin can be used for postoperative tumor assessment.
Poorly differentiated thyroid carcinoma (PDTC) (**Fig. 5.68**)	*CT:* Solitary lesion with soft tissue attenuation and irregular margins, typically showing contrast enhancement, ± calcifications and cystic changes. *Ultrasound:* Tumors can have irregular shapes and borders, internal echoes, and hypervascularity. *MRI:* Tumors have low-intermediate signal on T1-weighted imaging, intermediate to slightly high signal on T2-weighted imaging, + irregular margins, ± cystic changes. Tumors often show heterogeneous gadolinium contrast enhancement. MRI is useful in the evaluation of tumor spread beyond the thyroid capsule. *Radionuclide scintigraphy:* Postoperative evaluation with iodine 131 is used to assess for recurrent or metastatic tumor. *PET/CT:* Tumors often show increased uptake of F-18 FDG.	PDTCs are intermediate-grade malignant tumors of the thyroid gland, between more differentiated thyroid cancer (papillary thyroid carcinoma, follicular thyroid carcinoma) and undifferentiated/anaplastic thyroid carcinoma. PDTC tumor cells are not arranged into papillary structures. Most PDTCs can concentrate iodine and can be evaluated with, and treated with, radioactive Iodine.

(continued on page 546)

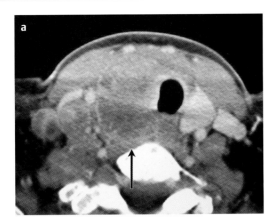
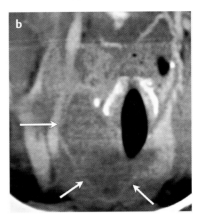

Fig. 5.66 **(a)** Axial and **(b)** coronal CT images of a 49-year-old woman show a large medullary carcinoma (*arrows*) involving the entire right thyroid lobe, isthmus, and anterior inferior portion of the left thyroid lobe. The neoplasm has ill-defined margins and invades the adjacent soft tissues. The tumor has mixed intermediate and low attenuation.

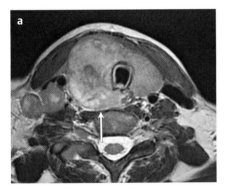
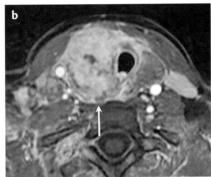
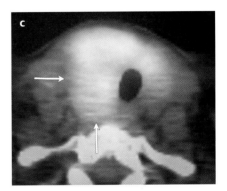

Fig. 5.67 **(a)** Axial T2-weighted imaging of a 59-year-old woman shows a medullary carcinoma in the right thyroid lobe, isthmus and anterior portion of the left thyroid lobe and that has ill-defined margins and heterogeneous signal with zones of intermediate, slightly high, and high signal (*arrow*). **(b)** The neoplasm (*arrow*) has heterogeneous gadolinium contrast enhancement on axial T1-weighted imaging. Metastatic right level IIIb and level V lymph nodes are seen. **(c)** Axial PET/CT shows abnormal increased uptake of F-18 FDG by the tumor (*arrows*).

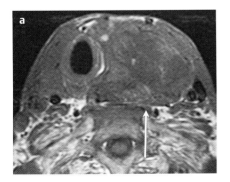
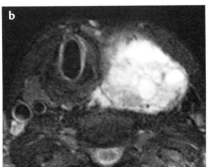
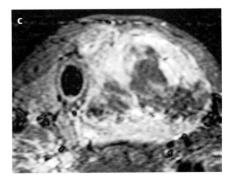

Fig. 5.68 **(a)** Axial T1-weighted imaging of a 73-year-old man shows a large poorly differentiated thyroid carcinoma (*arrow*) in the left thyroid lobe that has ill-defined margins and heterogeneous signal with zones of low and intermediate signal. **(b)** Axial fat-suppressed T2-weighted imaging shows the tumor to have mixed high and intermediate signal. **(c)** The large neoplasm has heterogeneous gadolinium contrast enhancement on axial fat-suppressed T1-weighted imaging and invades the adjacent soft tissues.

Table 5.3 *(cont.)* Visceral space: Lesions of the thyroid and parathyroid glands

Lesions	Imaging Findings	Comments
Anaplastic (undifferentiated) thyroid carcinoma (ATC) **(Fig. 5.69)**	*CT:* Diffuse large thyroid lesion with soft tissue attenuation, irregular margins, and extraglandular extension, measuring > 5 cm. Lesions can have necrotic/hemorrhagic zones (75%) and calcifications (60%) and can show heterogeneous contrast enhancement, ± cervical lymphadenopathy. *Ultrasound:* Tumors can have irregular shapes and borders and can be hypoechoic, with internal echoes. Hypervascularity is common. *MRI:* Tumors have heterogeneous low, intermediate, or high signal on T1- and T2-weighted imaging secondary to zones of necrosis and/or hemorrhage. Tumors often show heterogeneous gadolinium contrast enhancement. MRI is useful in the evaluation of tumor spread beyond the thyroid capsule. *Radionuclide scintigraphy:* These neoplasms do not usually concentrate iodine. Therefore, iodine 123, iodine 131, or technetium 99m pertechnetate are not useful. *PET/CT:* Tumors often show increased uptake of F-18 FDG.	ATCs are rare, malignant thyroid neoplasms that account for 2% of thyroid gland malignancies and account for up to 40% of deaths from thyroid cancer. These rapidly growing tumors usually occur in older patients (mean age = 71 years). Can occur in patients with long-standing goiter or arise from less-aggressive tumors, such as papillary thyroid carcinoma (PTC), follicular cell carcinoma (FCTC), or Hürthle cell carcinoma (HCTC). As a result, neoplastic cell types of PTC, FCTC, and HCTC can be seen along with the anaplastic tumor cells. At diagnosis, over 90% of tumors extend beyond the capsule, 40% have cervical lymphadenopathy, and 40% have metastatic disease. Lymphatic metastases are often necrotic. Prognosis is typically very poor, with a 1-year survival rate of 20%.
Thyroid lymphoma **(Fig. 5.70** and **Fig. 5.71)**	*CT:* Can present as a solitary lesion (80%) or as multiple (20%) lesions with low-intermediate attenuation. Ultrasound: Lesions are usually hypoechoic. *MRI:* Tumors have low-intermediate signal on T1-weighted imaging and slightly high signal on T2-weighted imaging, and can show gadolinium contrast enhancement. *Radionuclide scintigraphy:* These neoplasms do not concentrate iodine. Therefore, iodine 123, iodine 131, or technetium 99m pertechnetate are not useful. *PET/CT:* Tumors often show increased uptake of F-18 FDG.	Clonal proliferation of malignant lymphocytes accounts for ~ 3% of primary malignant thyroid neoplasms. Most common types are extranodal marginal zone B-cell lymphoma (mucosa-associated lymphoid tissue lymphoma [MALToma]) and diffuse large B-cell lymphoma. There is a slightly increased incidence of non-Hodgkin lymphoma in patients with history of Hashimoto's thyroiditis or long-standing goiter. Treatment is chemotherapy. Prognosis is poor for diffuse large B-cell lymphoma but is more favorable for MALToma.
Metastatic tumor	*CT:* Can present as one or multiple lesions with low-intermediate attenuation. *Ultrasound:* Lesions can be hypoechoic. *MRI:* Tumors have low-intermediate signal on T1-weighted imaging and slightly high signal on T2-weighted imaging, and often show gadolinium contrast enhancement. *Radionuclide scintigraphy:* These neoplasms do not concentrate iodine. Therefore, iodine 123, iodine 131, or technetium 99m pertechnetate are not useful. *PET/CT:* Tumors often show increased uptake of F-18 FDG.	Metastases can result from distant malignant neoplasms or by direct extension from adjacent tumors. Account for 5% of biopsied malignant thyroid tumors. Most common metastases are from primary malignant tumors of the lung, breast, or kidney.

(continued on page 548)

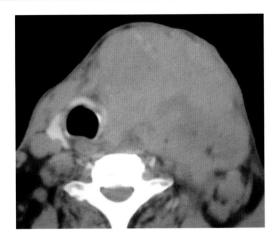

Fig. 5.69 Axial CT of an 83-year-old man with a large anaplastic thyroid carcinoma in the left thyroid lobe that has ill-defined margins and invades the adjacent soft tissues.

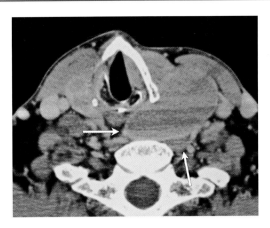

Fig. 5.70 Axial CT of a 60-year-old man shows a large lesion of primary lymphoma involving the left thyroid lobe (*arrows*). The tumor has relatively well-circumscribed margins.

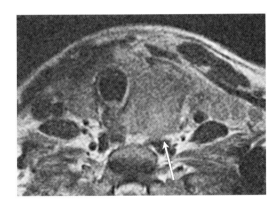

Fig. 5.71 Axial T2-weighted imaging of a 64-year-old man with B-cell non-Hodgkin lymphoma shows a large lesion involving the left thyroid lobe and isthmus (*arrow*) that has ill-defined margins and intermediate signal. Neoplastic adenopathy is also seen in the left neck anterior and lateral to the left carotid space.

Table 5.3 *(cont.)*   Visceral space: Lesions of the thyroid and parathyroid glands

Lesions	Imaging Findings	Comments
Infections involving the Thyroid		
Acute suppurative thyroiditis **(Fig. 5.72)**	*CT:* Diffuse enlargement of thyroid gland with ill-defined margins, heterogeneous attenuation, and contrast enhancement, ± abscess, ± underlying lesion in thyroid gland. *MRI:* Diffuse enlargement of gland with ill-defined margins, low-intermediate signal on T1-weighted imaging, slightly high to high signal on T2-weighted imaging, and heterogeneous gadolinium contrast enhancement of thyroid gland and adjacent soft tissue, ± abscess. *Ultrasound:* Diffuse decreased echogenicity, with hyperechoic trabeculae and mild increased vascularity, ± abscess.	Infection of the normal thyroid gland is uncommon because of its high iodine content (which limits bacterial growth), fibrous capsule, and rich lymphatic system. Infection of the thyroid gland can result from hematogenous dissemination, lymphatic spread, trauma, or spread from adjacent sites. Suppurative thyroiditis usually occurs in thyroid glands that have adenomas, goiters, carcinomas, lymphoma, or developmental anomalies, such as thyroglossal duct cysts, 3rd and 4th branchial cleft cysts, and piriform sinus fistulas, as well as in patients with a history of autoimmune thyroiditis. Infections are usually from gram-positive bacteria, such as staphylococci and streptococci. Less common organisms include *Salmonella* and fungi, such as *Actinomyces, Coccidioides,* or *Cryptococcus.* Clinical presentation includes tender, warm, firm, mobile mass that develops over days to weeks. Thyroid function tests are usually normal, although short-term hyper- or hypothyroidism can occur. Treatment is with antibiotics.
Subacute (de Quervain) thyroiditis	*CT:* Enlargement of one or both thyroid lobes with decreased attenuation and mild-moderate contrast enhancement. *MRI:* Enlargement of one or both thyroid lobes, ± irregular margins; intermediate signal on T1WI, high signal on T2WI, and heterogeneous Gd-contrast enhancement. *Ultrasound:* Decreased echogenicity. *Radionuclide scintigraphy:* Low uptake of iodine 123 or technetium 99m pertechnetate.	Self-limited transient granulomatous disorder involving the thyroid gland caused by viral infection (measles, mumps, adenovirus, influenza, Epstein-Barr virus, Coxsackie virus). Most common cause of a painful, rapid-onset thyroid lesion, which usually occurs in women between the ages of 20 and 50 years. Most patients are HLA-Bw positive. Patients have leukocytosis and elevated ESR, as well as transient early thyrotoxicity caused by release of T_3 and T_4 hormones from damaged thyroid tissue. Patients can become hypothyroid 6 months afterward, but this often eventually resolves.
Tuberculous thyroiditis	*CT:* Round or ovoid lesion with low attenuation centrally, surrounded by a contrast-enhancing rim, ± contrast enhancement of adjacent soft tissue from inflammation. *MRI:* Round or ovoid lesion, ± irregular margins, with low-intermediate signal on T1-weighted imaging, slightly high to high signal on T2-weighted imaging, and heterogeneous peripheral gadolinium contrast enhancement, ± enhancement in adjacent soft tissue. *Ultrasound:* Round or ovoid hypoechoic lesion with irregular borders, ± internal echoes. *Radionuclide scintigraphy:* Low uptake of iodine 123 or technetium 99m pertechnetate.	Rare type of infection of thyroid gland, most common in young and middle-aged females. Most commonly presents as a thyroid nodule without evidence of other sites of disease. Other presentations include: multiple lesions within the thyroid gland, acute or cold abscess, or goiter with caseation. Thyroid function is usually within normal limits. Patients can present with palsy/paresis of the recurrent laryngeal nerve.

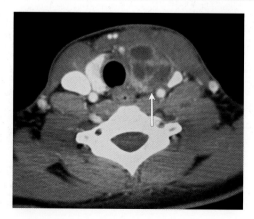

Fig. 5.72 Axial postcontrast CT of a 22-year-old woman with acute suppurative thyroiditis involving the left thyroid lobe (*arrow*), with multiple abscesses seen with peripheral contrast enhancement.

Lesions	Imaging Findings	Comments
Autoimmune Thyroid Diseases		
Graves disease	*CT:* Enlargement of the thyroid gland, which has slightly decreased attenuation and moderate contrast enhancement. *MRI:* Enlargement of the thyroid gland, with intermediate signal on T1-weighted imaging, slightly high to high signal on T2-weighted imaging, and heterogeneous gadolinium contrast enhancement. *Ultrasound:* Enlargement of thyroid gland, which often has decreased echogenicity, prominent increased vascularity on Doppler color flow imaging (referred to as "thyroid inferno"), and increased peak systolic velocities in thyroid vessels, ± multiple, small, 2–3 mm hypoechoic foci. *Radionuclide scintigraphy:* Prominent increased uptake of radiotracer (sodium-iodine 123, technetium 99m pertechnetate) in diffusely enlarged thyroid gland.	Graves disease is the most common cause of hyperthyroidism in developed countries. It occurs in 0.4% of the population in the United States, usually in females (female:male ratio is 8:1), at peak ages between the third and fourth decades. Results from the production of autoantibodies to the receptor for thyrotropin (also referred to as thyroid stimulating hormone or TSH) on the surface of thyroid epithelial cells. These autoantibodies (TRAbs) that bind to thyrotopin (TSH) receptors in the thyroid gland can result in growth of the thyroid gland, with increased thyroid hormone production and hyperthyroidism. These autoantibodies to thyrotropin receptor are also referred to as thryoid stimulating immunoglobulins. The abnormally enlarged thyroid gland has follicular cell hyperplasia and, prominent stromal vessels with adjacent lymphocytic infiltration. More than 50% of patients also have antithyroid peroxidase antibodies (anti-TPO). Patients may require hyperthyroidism medication, as well as requiring β-blockers for tachycardia. Treatment also includes radioiodine ablation or subtotal thyroidectomy.
Hashimoto thyroiditis (**Fig. 5.73** and **Fig. 5.74**)	*CT:* Enlargement of the thyroid gland, with heterogeneous decreased attenuation, as well as decreased contrast enhancement relative to normal thyroid tissue. *MRI:* Enlarged thyroid gland with low-intermediate signal on T1- and T2-weighted imaging (T2WI), heterogeneous intermediate to slightly high signal on fat-suppressed T2WI, and minimal-mild heterogeneous gadolinium contrast enhancement. *Ultrasound:* The thyroid gland can be enlarged and can contain poorly defined heterogeneous hypoechoic zones separated by fibrous strands, an appearance somewhat similar to that of multinodular goiter. *Radionuclide scintigraphy:* Uptake of technetium 99m pertechnetate is often heterogeneous and can be increased or decreased.	An autoimmune disease with diffuse thyroid enlargement, Hashimoto thyroiditis is the most common cause of hypothyroidism in the United States in patients > 6 years old. Hashimoto thyroiditis can be divided into two subtypes: IgG4 thyroiditis and non-IgG4 thyroiditis. IgG4-related disease is a systemic disease with diffuse lymphoplasmacytic infiltration of tissue, including IgG4-positive plasma cells, in combination with irregular fibrosis, eosinophils, and obliterative vasculitis. Thyroid peroxidase antibodies can be detected in most patients with Hashimoto thyroiditis. Antibodies to thyroglobulin also occur in more than half of these patients. Involves the thyroid gland as well as salivary glands, lacrimal glands, orbits, lymph nodes, pituitary stalk, and sinonasal cavity. Hashimoto thyroiditis occurs predominantly in women, with peak ages in the fourth to fifth decades. Associated with an increased incidence of lymphoma, leukemia, and Hürthle cell tumors.

(continued on page 550)

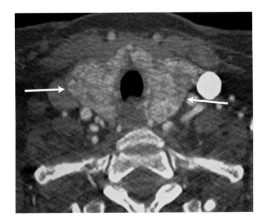

Fig. 5.73 Axial postcontrast CT of a 58-year-old woman with Hashimoto thyroiditis shows enlargement of the thyroid gland (*arrows*) with heterogeneous slightly decreased attenuation and contrast enhancement relative to normal thyroid tissue.

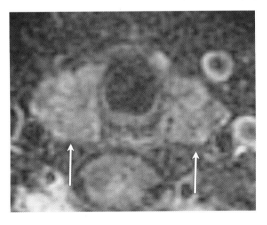

Fig. 5.74 Axial fat-suppressed T2-weighted imaging of a 33-year-old woman with Hashimoto thyroiditis shows slight enlargement of the thyroid gland, which has heterogeneous intermediate to slightly high signal (*arrows*).

Table 5.3 *(cont.)*   Visceral space: Lesions of the thyroid and parathyroid glands

Lesions	Imaging Findings	Comments
Riedel's thyroiditis	*CT:* Enlargement of thyroid gland with heterogeneous decreased attenuation, ± fibrous zones and irregular, ill-defined margins. Mild degree of irregular contrast enhancement, ± abnormality extending to involve adjacent soft tissues. *MRI:* Enlarged thyroid gland with low-intermediate signal on T1- and T2-weighted imaging related to fibrosis and minimal heterogeneous gadolinium contrast enhancement, ± irregular margins of thyroid gland. Abnormality can extend to involve adjacent soft tissues. *Ultrasound:* The thyroid gland can be enlarged and diffusely hypoechoic. *Radionuclide scintigraphy:* Uptake of technetium 99m pertechnetate is usually decreased.	Rarest form of autoimmune thyroiditis that is characterized by fibrosis of the thyroid gland, destruction of the normal thyroid follicular pattern, obliterative phlebitis, and infiltration of lymphocytes, eosinophils, and plasma cells that can be IgG4+. The fibrosis can extend beyond the thyroid gland into adjacent tissues. Usually occurs in females between the ages of 30 and 60 years. Results in hypothyroidism in 33% and hypoparathyroidism requiring medical management. Treatments also include surgical debulking or resection, tamoxifen, and/or steroids.
Granulomatous thyroiditis	*CT:* Can be a circumscribed nodular lesion with decreased attenuation relative to the normal thyroid gland. *Ultrasound:* Nodular hypoechoic lesion. *MRI:* Nodular lesion with low-intermediate signal on T1-weighted imaging and intermediate to slightly high signal on T2-weighted imaging, ± gadolinium contrast enhancement. *Radionuclide scintigraphy:* Uptake of technetium 99m pertechnetate is low— "cold nodule."	Granulomatous reaction that can result from fungal and mycobacterial infections, foreign body reaction, sarcoidosis, granulomatosis with polyangiitis (Wegener's granulomatosis), and Langerhans' cell histiocytosis.

Lesions	Imaging Findings	Comments
Benign Parathyroid Tumors		
Parathyroid adenoma (**Fig. 5.75**)	*Ultrasound:* Lesions are most commonly located dorsal to the thyroid gland or in ectopic locations, such as the anterosuperior mediastinum, posterosuperior mediastinum, or retropharynx. Lesions are round or ovoid, with circumscribed margins, and have homogeneous hypoechogenicity relative to the thyroid gland, ± cystic changes. On Doppler, a prominent extrathyroidal feeding artery can be seen at one pole ("polar artery") of the parathyroid adenoma. *CT:* Round or ovoid lesions with circumscribed margins, usually having soft tissue attenuation < 80 HU, + contrast enhancement. With dynamic contrast enhancement techniques, parathyroid adenomas show peak opacification of 130 HU at 45 seconds, followed by a decrease of > 20 HU on delayed images. *MRI:* Lesions have low-intermediate signal on T1-weighted imaging and slightly high to high signal on T2-weighted imaging (T2WI) and FS T2WI, ± cystic and/or hemorrhagic zones. Lesions show prominent gadolinium contrast enhancement. *Radionuclide scintigraphy:* Both the thyroid gland and parathyroid adenomas accumulate technetium 99m sestamibi. Technetium 99m sestamibi, however, washes out of the thyroid gland more rapidly than from parathyroid adenomas, and delayed imaging can demonstrate the parathyroid abnormality for localization. A dual isotope technique using iodine 123 and technetium 99m sestamibi can show discordant uptake of these agents in parathyroid lesions versus the normal pattern of concordant uptake. *SPECT/CT* can be used instead of planar imaging techniques, with improved results and increased sensitivity for detection of lesions. *PET/CT:* C-11 methionine uptake by hyperfunctioning parathyroid tissue has also been shown to be useful for preoperative localization of parathyroid adenomas.	Solitary parathyroid adenoma is the most common lesion of the parathyroid glands and is the cause of primary hyperparathyroidism (abnormally high serum levels of PTH) in up to 89% of patients. Other cases of hyperparathyroidism result from parathyroid hyperplasia (10%) and parathyroid carcinoma (1%). The prevalence of hyperparathyroidism is 1 per 500 women and 1 per 2,000 men more than 40 years old. Most adenomas contain chief cells or mitochondria-rich oxyphilic cells that take up technetium 99m sestamibi. Parathyroid adenomas are located dorsal to the thyroid gland in 80–85% of cases. The remainder can occur in ectopic locations, such as the mediastinum. Localization of the adenoma is important prior to surgical resection.

(continued on page 552)

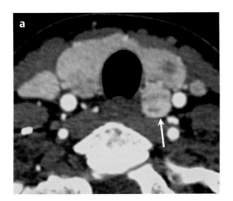 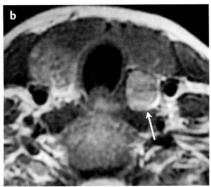 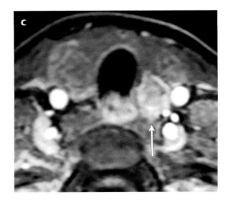

Fig. 5.75   **(a)** Axial CT of a 42-year-old woman shows a contrast-enhancing parathyroid adenoma (*arrow*) posterior to the left thyroid lobe. **(b)** The adenoma has slightly high signal (*arrow*) on axial T2-weighted imaging, and **(c)** shows gadolinium contrast enhancement (*arrow*) on axial fat-suppressed T1-weighted imaging.

Table 5.3 *(cont.)* Visceral space: Lesions of the thyroid and parathyroid glands

Lesions	Imaging Findings	Comments
Parathyroid hyperplasia	*CT:* Diffuse enlargement of the parathyroid glands, which have intermediate attenuation on nonenhanced CT, + prominent contrast enhancement. *MRI:* Parathyroid glands can be seen when they are enlarged more than the normal size of 5 mm. Hyperplastic glands have intermediate signal on T1-weighted imaging and slightly high signal on T2-weighted imaging. Usually show gadolinium contrast enhancement. *Radionuclide scintigraphy:* Both the thyroid gland and parathyroid hyperplasia accumulate technetium 99m sestamibi. Technetium 99m sestamibi, however, washes out of the thyroid gland more rapidly than from parathyroid hyperplasia, and delayed imaging can demonstrate the parathyroid abnormality. A dual isotope technique using iodine 123 and technetium 99m sestamibi can show discordant uptake of these agents in parathyroid lesions versus the normal pattern of concordant uptake. *SPECT/CT* can be used instead of planar imaging techniques, with improved results and increased sensitivity for detection of lesions. *PET/CT:* C-11 methionine uptake by hyperfunctioning parathyroid tissue has also been shown to be useful for preoperative localization of parathyroid hyperplasia.	Parathyroid gland hyperplasia accounts for 10% of cases of primary hyperparathyroidism. Usually involves more than one parathyroid gland.
Multiple parathyroid adenomas	*Ultrasound:* Lesions are round or ovoid, with circumscribed margins, and have homogeneous hypoechogenicity relative to the thyroid gland, ± cystic changes. On Doppler, a prominent extrathyroidal feeding artery can be seen at one pole ("polar artery") of the parathyroid adenoma. *CT:* Round or ovoid lesions with circumscribed margins, usually having soft tissue attenuation < 80 HU, + contrast enhancement. With dynamic contrast enhancement techniques, parathyroid adenomas show peak opacification of 130 HU at 45 seconds, followed by a decrease of > 20 HU on delayed images. *MRI:* Lesions have low-intermediate signal on T1-weighted imaging and slightly high to high signal on T2-weighted imaging (T2WI) and fat-suppressed T2WI, ± cystic and/or hemorrhagic zones. Lesions show prominent gadolinium contrast enhancement. Radionuclide scintigraphy: Both the thyroid gland and parathyroid adenomas accumulate technetium 99m sestamibi. Technetium 99m sestamibi, however, washes out of the thyroid gland more rapidly than from parathyroid adenomas, and delayed imaging can demonstrate the parathyroid abnormality for localization. A dual isotope technique using iodine 123 and technetium 99m sestamibi can show discordant uptake of these agents in parathyroid lesions versus the normal pattern of concordant uptake. *SPECT*/CT can be used instead of planar imaging techniques, with improved results. *PET/CT:* C-11 methionine uptake by hyperfunctioning parathyroid tissue has also been shown to be useful for preoperative localization of parathyroid adenomas.	Patients with multiple endocrine neoplasia (MEN) can have hyperplastic or neoplastic proliferation of one or more endocrine glands, including the pituitary gland, parathyroid glands (hyperplasia, adenoma, adenocarcinoma), adrenal glands (pheochromocytoma), and thyroid gland (medullary thyroid carcinoma). MEN type 1 is commonly associated with parathyroid, pituitary, and paraneoplastic neuroendocrine tumors. MEN type 2 is associated with a > 95% risk of developing medullary thyroid cancer. Up to 90% of patients with MEN type 1 have hyperparathyroidism. Hyperparathyroidism occurs in up to 30% of patients with MEN type 2.

Lesions	Imaging Findings	Comments
Malignant Parathyroid Tumors		
Parathyroid carcinoma	*Ultrasound:* Lesions are round or ovoid, with irregular margins, and can be hypoechoic or have heterogeneous echogenicity. Tumors range in size from 2 to 7 cm (average = 3.3 cm). Findings can overlap those for parathyroid adenoma. *CT:* Round or ovoid lesions with irregular margins, usually having soft tissue attenuation, ± cystic zones, + contrast enhancement. *MRI:* Lesions have low-intermediate signal on T1-weighted imaging and slightly high to high signal on T2-weighted imaging (T2WI) and fat-suppressed T2WI, ± cystic and/or hemorrhagic zones. Lesions show prominent gadolinium contrast enhancement. *Radionuclide scintigraphy:* Both the thyroid gland and parathyroid adenomas accumulate technetium 99m sestamibi. Technetium 99m sestamibi, however, washes out of the thyroid gland more rapidly than from parathyroid carcinomas, and delayed imaging can demonstrate the parathyroid abnormality for localization. A dual isotope technique using iodine 123 and technetium 99m sestamibi can show discordant uptake of these agents in parathyroid lesions versus the normal pattern of concordant uptake. *SPECT/CT* can be used instead of planar imaging techniques, with improved results. *PET/CT:* C-11 methionine uptake by hyperfunctioning parathyroid tissue has also been shown to be useful for preoperative localization of parathyroid carcinomas. F-18 FDG has also been shown to be useful for evaluation for metastatic tumor from parathyroid carcinoma.	A rare malignancy, parathyroid carcinoma accounts for less than 1% of primary parathyroid tumors. Patients can present with high serum calcium and elevated PTH levels, as well as a palpable neck mass, ± palsy of the recurrent laryngeal nerve. Most tumors occur in adults between 45 and 60 years old. Can occur in association with familial hyperparathyroidism or multiple endocrine neoplasia (MEN). Associated with mutations of the *HRPT2* gene. Histologically, tumors commonly have cellular atypia and pleomorphism, atypical mitoses and high mitotic rates, capsular, vascular, or perineural invasion, ± lymphadenopathy. Treatment is en bloc surgical resection with negative margins. Tumors tend to infiltrate adjacent tissue. Tumor size has not been shown to affect prognosis. Residual and recurrent disease occurs in over 50% of patients. Chemotherapy and external beam radiation are not effective. Five-year survival rates range from 40 to 85%.

Table 5.4 Visceral space: lesions of the pharynx, esophagus, and trachea

- Pharyngeal Lesions
  - Zenker's diverticulum
  - Pharyngocele (Lateral pharyngeal diverticulum)
  - Squamous cell carcinoma
- Esophageal Lesions
  - Esophageal duplication cyst
  - Neurenteric cyst
  - Esophageal carcinoma
- Tracheal Lesions
  - Tracheal carcinoma
  - Nonmalignant tracheal lesions
  - Paratracheal air cyst
  - Tracheal stenosis

Table 5.4 Visceral space: lesions of the pharynx, esophagus, and trachea

Lesions	Imaging Findings	Comments
Pharyngeal Lesions		
Zenker's diverticulum (**Fig. 5.76**)	*CT:* Circumscribed, unilocular, thin-walled expansion of the posterior hypopharynx at the junction of the pharynx and esophagus. The diverticulum can contain air, fluid, and/or solid food, ± air–fluid level.	Pulsion-type herniation of mucosa and submucosal tissue involving the hypopharynx just superior to the cricopharyngeus muscle, secondary to dysfunction of the muscle. The diverticulum commonly extends inferiorly and often contains liquid and food, resulting in halitosis, regurgitation, and dysphagia. Complications include aspiration pneumonia, bleeding, and increased risk for squamous cell carcinoma. Treatment can be by surgical resection or endoscopic methods.
Pharyngocele (lateral pharyngeal diverticulum) (**Fig. 5.77**)	*CT:* Circumscribed air-filled zone located lateral to the pharynx, usually unilateral but can be bilateral, typically measuring from 1 to 2.5 cm. Can increase in size with Valsalva maneuver.	Pulsion-type mucosal herniation involving the pharynx, typically at junctional sites between the superior and inferior constrictor muscles (level of the vallecula) or between the middle and inferior constrictor muscles (through the thyrohyoid membrane at the level of the lower piriform sinus). Usually occurs in older adults, and in men more than in women. Occurs in musicians playing wind instruments or in glass blowers. Considered to occur from weakening of the lateral pharyngeal wall from age-related loss of muscle elasticity and/or episodes of increased intrapharyngeal air pressure. Patients can present with dysphagia, neck swelling, food retention, or regurgitation. Treatment may require surgery or endoscopic repair.
Squamous cell carcinoma	*CT and MRI:* Soft tissue tumor with intermediate attenuation on CT and intermediate signal on T1-weighted imaging and intermediate to slightly high signal on T2-weighted imaging, + contrast enhancement, ± asymmetric thickening of the posterior pharyngeal wall, ± invasion of prevertebral space structures. *PET/CT:* Abnormal increased accumulation of F-18 FDG.	Most common malignant tumor of the pharynx. Tumor from the tongue base can extend into the hypopharynx.

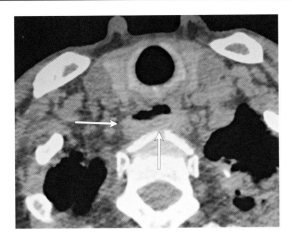

Fig. 5.76 Axial CT shows a Zenker's diverticulum (*arrows*) containing an air–fluid level.

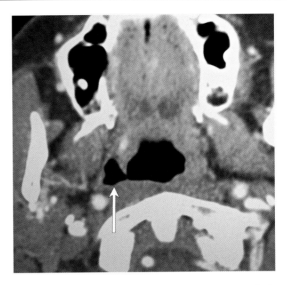

Fig. 5.77 Axial CT of a 53-year-old man with an air-filled right pharyngocele (*arrow*).

Lesions	Imaging Findings	Comments
Esophageal Lesions		
Esophageal duplication cyst	*MRI:* Well-circumscribed spheroid lesions, with low, intermediate, or high signal on T1- and T2-weighted imaging, and usually no gadolinium contrast enhancement. Can displace the trachea and/or esophagus. *CT:* Circumscribed structures with low-intermediate attenuation. Usually no contrast enhancement.	Type of foregut duplication cyst that also includes bronchogenic and neurenteric cysts. Esophageal duplication cysts result from foregut budding errors that occur in the third to sixth weeks of gestation. During gestation, the laryngotracheal groove forms separating the two structures that will become the dorsally positioned esophagus from the more ventrally located trachea. Esophageal duplication cysts result from abnormal formation of the esophageal channel. Can be asymptomatic or associated with dysphagia, respiratory distress, and epigastric or retrosternal pain. Symptomatic patients can be treated with surgery or endoscopic procedures.
Neurenteric cyst	*MRI:* Well-circumscribed spheroid lesions, with low, intermediate, or high signal on T1- and T2-weighted imaging, and usually no gadolinium contrast enhancement. Can occur between the dorsal margin of the esophagus and spinal canal. *CT:* Circumscribed structures with low-intermediate attenuation. Usually no contrast enhancement.	Neurenteric cysts are congenital foregut duplication cysts that extend into the spinal canal. This malformation results from persistent communication between the ventrally located endoderm and the dorsally located ectoderm secondary to developmental failure of separation of the notochord and foregut. Obliteration of portions of a dorsal enteric sinus can result in cysts lined by endothelium, fibrous cords, or sinuses. Observed in patients < 40 years old. Associated with anomalies of the adjacent vertebrae and clivus.

(continued on page 556)

Table 5.4 *(cont.)* Visceral space: lesions of the pharynx, esophagus, and trachea

Lesions	Imaging Findings	Comments
Esophageal carcinoma (**Fig. 5.78**)	*CT and MRI:* Soft tissue tumor with intermediate attenuation on CT and intermediate signal on T1-weighted imaging and intermediate to slightly high signal on T2-weighted imaging, + contrast enhancement, ± asymmetric thickening of the esophagus, ± tumor invasion beyond the visceral space into the carotid, retropharyngeal, and/or prevertebral spaces. Cervical lymph nodes commonly involved: levels VI, IV, and/or V. *PET/CT:* Abnormal increased accumulation of F-18 FDG.	Most esophageal squamous cell carcinomas occur at the gastroesophageal junction. Only 20% of these tumors occur in the cervical esophagus. Tumors typically occur in adults, at peak ages between 55 and 65 years, and in men more than in women (4:1 ratio). Associated with chronic tobacco and alcohol use, achalasia, prior radiation exposure, and Plummer-Vinson syndrome. Using the TNM classification system: T1: tumor invades the lamina propria T2: tumor invades the muscularis mucosa T3: tumor invades adventitia T4: tumor invades adjacent structures N0: no spread to nearby lymph nodes N1: spread to 1-2 nearby lymph nodes N2: spread to 3-6 nearby lymph nodes N3: spread to 7 or more lymph nodes M0: no distant metastases M1: spread to distant lymph nodes and/or other organs
Tracheal Lesions		
Tracheal carcinoma (**Fig. 5.79**)	*CT and MRI:* Soft tissue tumor within the tracheal lumen that has intermediate attenuation on CT and intermediate signal on T1-weighted imaging and intermediate to slightly high signal on T2-weighted imaging, + contrast enhancement, ± tracheal cartilage destruction, ± tumor invasion into the carotid, retropharyngeal, and/or prevertebral spaces. Cervical lymph nodes commonly involved: levels VI, IV, and/or V. *PET/CT:* Abnormal increased accumulation of F-18 FDG.	Squamous cell carcinomas are rare primary malignant tumors of the cervical trachea. More frequently, malignant tracheal tumors are caused by invasion from primary neoplasms of the larynx, thyroid, lung, and esophagus.
Nonmalignant tracheal lesions	*CT and MRI:* Soft tissue lesion within the tracheal lumen that can have intermediate attenuation on CT, intermediate signal on T1-weighted imaging, and intermediate to slightly high signal on T2-weighted imaging, + contrast enhancement. No evidence of cartilage destruction or lymphadenopathy.	Nonmalignant primary tumors of the trachea are very rare, and they include chondroma, hemangioma, nerve sheath tumor, leiomyoma, lipoma, papilloma, and pleomorphic adenoma.
Paratracheal air cyst (**Fig. 5.80**)	*CT:* Circumscribed, unilocular, thin-walled collection of air, usually located in the right posterior paratracheal region near the thoracic outlet.	Air-filled benign diverticulum of the trachea that occurs in up to 3% of patients, and it usually is asymptomatic.
Tracheal stenosis (**Fig. 5.81** and **Fig. 5.82**)	*CT:* Irregular narrowing of the tracheal airway from luminal soft tissue thickening, ± collapse and inward displacement of tracheal cartilage.	Narrowing of the trachea which can result from intubation, tracheostomy, relapsing polychondritis, granulomatosis with polyangiitis, sarcoidosis, amyloidosis, tracheobronchopathia osteochondroplastica, etc.

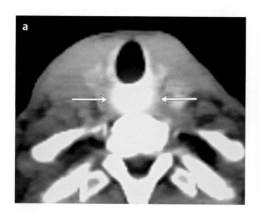

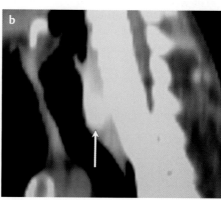

Fig. 5.78 **(a)** Axial and **(b)** sagittal PET/CT of a 67-year-old man shows an esophageal carcinoma with increased uptake of F-18 FDG (*arrows*).

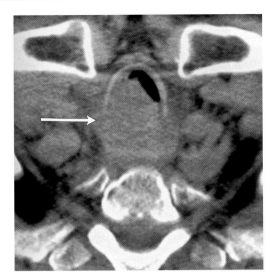

Fig. 5.79 Axial CT shows a squamous cell carcinoma with soft tissue attenuation filling most of the tracheal lumen (*arrow*) and extending into the adjacent soft tissues posteriorly.

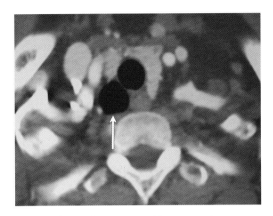

Fig. 5.80 Axial CT of a 68-year-old woman shows a posterior right paratracheal air cyst (*arrow*).

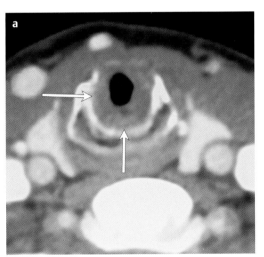
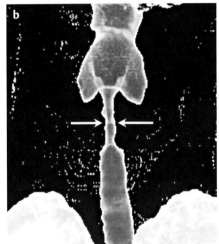

Fig. 5.81 **(a)** Axial CT shows luminal soft tissue thickening causing narrowing of the tracheal airway (*arrows*). **(b)** Coronal volume-rendered CT shows a segmental tracheal stenosis (*arrows*).

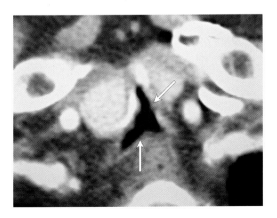

Fig. 5.82 Axial CT shows narrowing of the trachea (*arrows*) as a complication from prior endotracheal intubation.

5.5 Lesions of the Infrahyoid Carotid Space

The carotid space contains the internal carotid artery, internal jugular vein, cranial nerves IX, X, XI, and XII, sympathetic plexus, and deep cervical chain lymph nodes. The carotid space is anterior to the prevertebral space and posteromedial to the sternocleidomastoid muscle (SCM) (**Fig. 5.83**). The carotid space is enclosed by the carotid sheath, which is composed of the three layers (superficial, middle, and deep) of the deep cervical fascia. The suprahyoid portion of the carotid space is continuous with the retrostyloid parapharyngeal space.

Within the carotid sheath, the carotid artery (CA) is located medial to the internal jugular vein (IJV), and CN X (the vagus nerve) is located dorsal to both the CA and IJV. The cervical sympathetic plexus is located in the posterior portion of the carotid sheath. The ansa cervicalis is a loop of nerves of the cervical plexus arising from the ventral rami of the first three to four cervical nerves that innervate the infrahyoid, sternothyroid, sternohyoid, and omohyoid muscles. The ansa cervicalis is located in the anterior portion of the carotid sheath.

Cranial nerves IX, X, and XI exit the skull base within the jugular foramen. CN IX is located within the pars nervosa of the jugular foramen, along with its superior and inferior ganglia. CN X and CN XI are located within the pars vascularis portion of the jugular foramen. CN XII exits the medulla and passes through the skull base in the hypoglossal canal. Below the skull base, CN XII joins CN X and CN XI in the carotid space until it exits the carotid sheath lateral to the carotid bifurcation at the level of the posterior bellies of the digastric muscles.

Cranial nerve IX (the glossopharyngeal nerve) has its nuclei in the upper and middle medulla, and it has many functions: innervation of the stylopharyngeus muscle; taste sensation via sensory fibers from the posterior third of the tongue; sensation via sensory fibers from the tympanic membrane (Jacobson's nerve), pharynx, soft palate, and tongue base; parasympathetic innervation of the parotid glands; and parasympathetic supply to the carotid body, which is at its most inferior extent within the carotid sheath.

Cranial nerve X (the vagus nerve) is the longest cranial nerve and has parasympathetic nerve functions involving the head, neck, and thoracic and abdominal viscera, as well as conducting sensory information from the tympanic membrane (via Arnold's nerve), larynx, trachea, esophagus, and thoracic and abdominal viscera. Motor functions

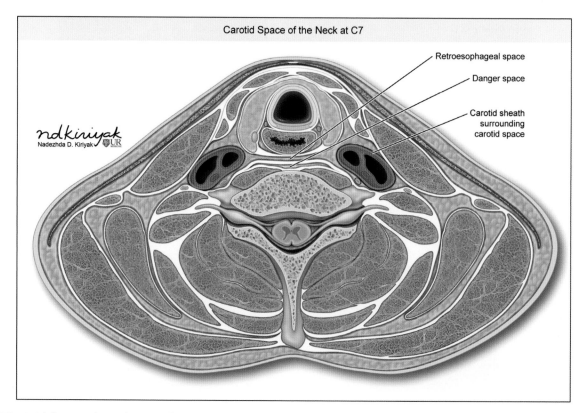

Carotid Space of the Neck at C7

Retroesophageal space

Danger space

Carotid sheath surrounding carotid space

Nadezhda D. Kiriyak

Fig. 5.83 Axial diagram shows the carotid spaces in color.

of CN X include innervation of the laryngeal muscles via the recurrent laryngeal nerves, of pharyngeal constrictor muscles, and of muscles involving the palate. Within the jugular foramen, the vagus neve has a superior jugular ganglion and an inferior ganglion (nodose ganglion). These ganglia communicate with the superior cervical sympathetic ganglia, CNs IX, XI, XII, and VII. Within the neck, CN X is located within the carotid sheath posterior to the carotid artery and anterior to the internal jugular vein.

CN XII is a motor nerve that innervates the intrinsic and extrinsic muscles of the tongue. The nucleus of CN XII is located in the lower medulla dorsally, which results in a bulge into the fourth ventricle (hypoglossal eminence). CN XII exits the brainstem between the medullary pyramid and olivary nucleus on each side, extends into the subarachnoid space, and exits the skull base via the hypoglossal canal below the jugular foramen.

Table 5.5 Lesions of the infrahyoid carotid space

- Benign Neoplasms
  - Paraganglioma
  - Schwannoma
  - Neurofibromas
  - Lipoma
  - Hemangioma
- Malignant Tumors
  - Direct extension from laryngeal squamous cell carcinoma or thyroid cancer
  - Rhabdomyosarcoma
  - Metastatic neoplasm
  - Non-Hodgkin lymphoma (NHL)
  - Hemangioendothelioma

- Tumorlike Lesions
  - Branchial cleft cyst
- Inflammatory Lesions
  - Spread of infection from neck phlegmon and/or abscess
- Vascular Abnormality
  - Ectasia and tortuosity of the carotid artery
  - Aneurysm of the carotid artery
  - Arterial dissection
  - Vasculitis
  - Idiopathic carotidynia ("Carotid pain syndrome")
  - Thrombosis and/or thrombophlebitis of the internal jugular vein (IJV)
  - Venolymphatic malformation

Table 5.5 Lesions of the infrahyoid carotid space

Lesions	Imaging Findings	Comments
Benign Neoplasms		
Paraganglioma (See **Fig. 4.41**, **Fig. 4.42**, and **Fig. 4.43**)	Ovoid or fusiform lesions with low-intermediate attenuation. *CT:* Lesions can show contrast enhancement. Can erode adjacent bone. *MRI:* Spheroid or lobulated lesion with intermediate signal on T1-weighted imaging (T1WI), intermediate-high signal on T2-weighted imaging (T2WI) and fat-suppressed T2WI, ± tubular zones of flow voids, usually prominent gadolinium contrast enhancement, ± foci of high signal on T1WI from mucin or hemorrhage, ± peripheral rim of low signal (hemosiderin) on T2WI.	Benign encapsulated neuroendocrine tumors that arise from neural crest cells associated with autonomic ganglia (paraganglia) throughout the body. Lesions, also referred to as chemodectomas, are named according to location (e.g., carotid body tumor, glomus jugulare, glomus tympanicum, glomus vagale). Paragangliomas represent 0.6% of tumors involving the head and neck, and 0.03% of all neoplasms.

(continued on page 560)

Table 5.5 *(cont.)* Lesions of the infrahyoid carotid space

Lesions	Imaging Findings	Comments
Schwannoma (**Fig. 5.84** and **Fig. 5.85**)	*MRI:* Circumscribed spheroid or ovoid lesions with low-intermediate signal on T1-weighted imaging, high signal on T2-weighted imaging (T2WI) and fat-suppressed T2WI, and usually prominent gadolinium (Gd) contrast enhancement. High signal on T2WI and Gd contrast enhancement can be heterogeneous in large lesions due to cystic degeneration and/or hemorrhage. *CT:* Circumscribed ovoid or spheroid lesions, intermediate attenuation, + contrast enhancement. Large lesions can have cystic degeneration and/or hemorrhage.	Schwannomas are benign encapsulated tumors that contain differentiated neoplastic Schwann cells. Most commonly occur as solitary, sporadic lesions. Multiple schwannomas are often associated with neurofibromatosis type 2 (NF2), which is an autosomal dominant disease involving a gene mutation at chromosome 22q12. In addition to schwannomas, patients with NF2 can also have multiple meningiomas and ependymomas. The incidence of NF2 is 1/37,000 to 1/50,000 newborns. Age at presentation = 22 to 72 years (mean age = 46 years). Peak incidence is in the fourth to sixth decades. Many patients with NF2 present in the third decade with bilateral vestibular schwannomas.
Neurofibromas (**Fig. 5.86**)	*MRI:* *Solitary neurofibromas* are circumscribed spheroid, ovoid, or lobulated lesions with low-intermediate signal on T1-weighted imaging (T1WI), intermediate-high signal on T2-weighted imaging (T2WI), + prominent gadolinium (Gd) contrast enhancement. High signal on T2WI and Gd contrast enhancement can be heterogeneous in large lesions. *Plexiform neurofibromas* appear as curvilinear and multinodular lesions involving multiple nerve branches, and have low to intermediate signal on T1WI and intermediate, slightly high to high signal on T2WI and fat-suppressed T2WI, with or without bands or strands of low signal. Lesions usually show Gd contrast enhancement. *CT:* Ovoid, spheroid, or fusiform lesions with low-intermediate attenuation. Lesions can show contrast enhancement. Often erode adjacent bone.	Benign nerve sheath tumors that contain mixtures of Schwann cells, perineural-like cells, and interlacing fascicles of fibroblasts associated with abundant collagen. Unlike schwannomas, neurofibromas lack Antoni A and B regions and cannot be separated pathologically from the underlying nerve. Most frequently occur as sporadic, localized, solitary lesions, less frequently as diffuse or plexiform lesions. Multiple neurofibromas are typically seen with neurofibromatosis type 1, which is an autosomal dominant disorder (1/2,500 births) due to mutations in the neurofibromin gene on chromosome 17q11.2. NF1 represents the most common type of neurocutaneous syndrome, and it is associated with neoplasms of the central and peripheral nervous system (optic gliomas, astrocytomas, plexiform and solitary neurofibromas) and skin (café-au-lait spots, axillary and inguinal freckling). It is also associated with meningeal and skull dysplasias, as well as hamartomas of the iris (Lisch nodules).
Lipoma (**Fig. 5.87**)	*MRI:* Lipomas have MRI signal isointense to subcutaneous fat on T1-weighted imaging (high signal), and on T2-weighted imaging, signal suppression occurs with frequency-selective fat saturation techniques or with a short time to inversion recovery (STIR) method. Typically there is no gadolinium contrast enhancement or peripheral edema. *CT:* Lipomas have CT attenuation similar to subcutaneous fat, and typically no contrast enhancement or peripheral edema.	Common benign hamartomas composed of mature white adipose tissue without cellular atypia. Most common soft tissue tumor, representing 16% of all soft tissue tumors. May contain calcifications and/or traversing blood vessels.

(continued on page 562)

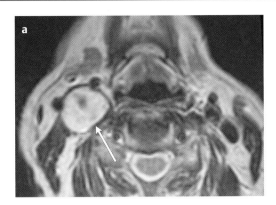
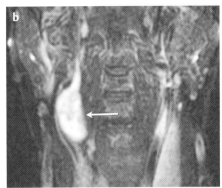

Fig. 5.84 **(a)** Axial T2-weighted image and **(b)** coronal fat-suppressed T2-weighted image show a schwannoma (*arrows*) with high signal in the right carotid space, which displaces the carotid arteries anteriorly.

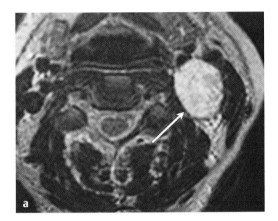
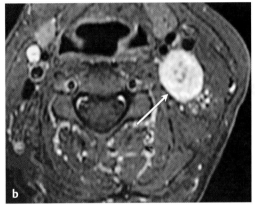

Fig. 5.85 **(a)** Axial T2-weighted imaging of a 46-year-old woman with a schwannoma (*arrow*) with high signal in the left carotid space that displaces the left carotid arteries anteriorly. **(b)** The schwannoma shows gadolinium contrast enhancement (*arrow*) on axial fat-suppressed T1-weighted imaging.

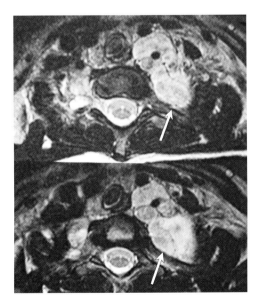

Fig. 5.86 Axial T2-weighted imaging of an 8-year-old male with neurofibromatosis type 1 shows multiple neurofibromas with high signal in the neck (*arrows*), including both carotid spaces, with anterior displacement of the carotid arteries.

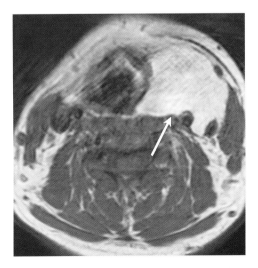

Fig. 5.87 Axial T1-weighted imaging shows a lipoma with high signal in the left neck, including the left carotid space (*arrow*).

Table 5.5 *(cont.)* Lesions of the infrahyoid carotid space

Lesions	Imaging Findings	Comments
Hemangioma **(Fig. 5.88)**	*MRI:* Circumscribed or poorly marginated structures (< 4 cm in diameter) in soft tissue or bone marrow with intermediate-high signal on T1-weighted imaging (often with portions that can be isointense to marrow fat), high signal on T2-weighted imaging (T2WI) and fat-suppressed T2WI, and typically gadolinium contrast enhancement, ± expansion of bone. *CT:* Hemangiomas in soft tissue have mostly intermediate attenuation, ± zones of fat attenuation.	Benign lesion of bone or soft tissue composed of capillary, cavernous, and/or venous malformations. Considered to be a hamartomatous disorder. Occurs in patients 1 to 84 years old (median age = 33 years).
Malignant Tumors		
Direct extension from laryngeal squamous cell carcinoma or thyroid cancer **(Fig. 5.89)**	*MRI:* Tumors often have intermediate signal on T1-weighted imaging, intermediate-slightly high signal on T2-weighted imaging, and mild gadolinium contrast enhancement. Can be large lesions (± necrosis and/or hemorrhage). *CT:* Tumors have intermediate attenuation and mild contrast enhancement. Can be large lesions (± necrosis and/or hemorrhage).	Malignant tumors from the hypopharynx, larynx, or thyroid gland can directly invade the carotid space.
Rhabdomyosarcoma (See **Fig. 4.52**)	*MRI:* Tumors can have circumscribed and/or poorly defined margins, and typically have low-intermediate signal on T1-weighted imaging and heterogeneous signal (various combinations of intermediate, slightly high, and/or high signal) on T2-weighted imaging (T2WI) and fat-suppressed T2WI. Tumors show variable degrees of gadolinium contrast enhancement, ± bone destruction and invasion. *CT:* Soft tissue lesions usually can have circumscribed or irregular margins. Calcifications are uncommon. Tumors can have mixed CT attenuation, with solid zones of soft tissue attenuation, cystic-appearing and/or necrotic zones, and occasional foci of hemorrhage, ± bone invasion and destruction.	Malignant mesenchymal tumors with rhabdomyoblastic differentiation that occur primarily in soft tissue, and only very rarely in bone. There are three subgroups of rhabdomyosarcoma: embryonal (50–70%), alveolar (18–45%), and pleomorphic (5–10%). Embryonal and alveolar rhabdomyosarcomas occur primarily in children < 10 years old, and pleomorphic rhabdomyosarcomas occur mostly in adults (median age in the sixth decade). Alveolar and pleomorphic rhabdomyosarcomas occur frequently in the extremities. Embryonal rhabdomyosarcomas occur mostly in the head and neck.
Metastatic neoplasm **(Fig. 5.90)**	*MRI:* Circumscribed spheroid lesions that often have low-intermediate signal on T1-weighted imaging and intermediate-high signal on T2-weighted imaging, ± hemorrhage, calcifications, and cysts, and variable gadolinium contrast enhancement. *CT:* Lesions usually have low-intermediate attenuation; ± hemorrhage, calcifications, and cysts; variable contrast enhancement; ± bone destruction; ± compression of neural tissue or vessels.	Metastatic tumor may cause variable destructive or infiltrative changes in single or multiple sites.

(continued on page 564)

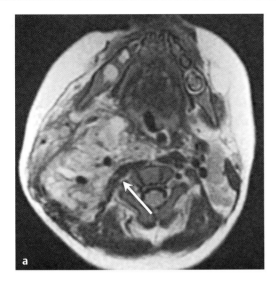
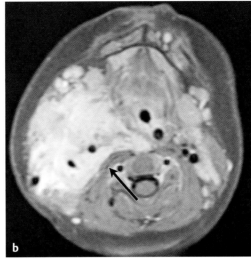

Fig. 5.88 **(a)** Axial T2-weighted imaging of an 8-month-old female shows a hemangioma in the right neck that has heterogeneous slightly high and high signal (*arrow*) and **(b)** shows prominent gadolinium contrast enhancement on axial fat-suppressed T1-weighted imaging (*arrow*). The hemangioma extends into the right carotid space (*arrows*).

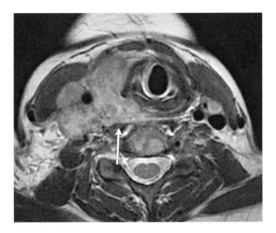

Fig. 5.89 Axial T2-weighted imaging of a 59-year-old woman shows a medullary carcinoma (*arrow*) in the right thyroid lobe that has heterogeneous signal with zones of intermediate, slightly high, and high signal. The neoplasm extends laterally to involve the right carotid space.

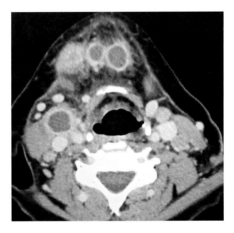

Fig. 5.90 Axial postcontrast CT shows multiple enlarged cervical lymph nodes, including involvement of the right carotid space, from metastatic squamous cell carcinoma. The nodes have low signal centrally surrounded by rims of contrast enhancement.

Table 5.5 *(cont.)* Lesions of the infrahyoid carotid space

Lesions	Imaging Findings	Comments
Non-Hodgkin lymphoma (NHL) (**Fig. 5.91**)	*CT:* Lesions have low-intermediate attenuation and may show contrast enhancement, ± bone destruction. *MRI:* Lesions have low-intermediate signal on T1-weighted imaging, intermediate to slightly high signal on T2-weighted imaging, + gadolinium contrast enhancement. Can be locally invasive and associated with bone erosion/destruction. B-cell NHL often occurs in the maxillary sinuses, whereas T-cell NHL frequently occurs in the midline, including the septum.	Lymphomas are a group of lymphoid tumors whose neoplastic cells typically arise within lymphoid tissue (lymph nodes and reticuloendothelial organs). Most lymphomas in the nasopharynx, nasal cavity, and paranasal sinuses are NHL (B-cell types more common than T-cell types).
Hemangioendothelioma (See **Fig. 4.54**)	*MRI:* Tumors have irregular or well-defined margins and often have intermediate signal on T1-weighted imaging and heterogeneous predominantly high signal on T2-weighted imaging, with or without internal low signal septations. Flow voids may be seen with the lesions. Tumors show heterogeneous gadolinium contrast enhancement. *CT:* Lesions have low-intermediate attenuation and usually show contrast enhancement, ± contrast-enhancing intralesional vessels.	Low-grade malignant neoplasms composed of vasoformative/endothelial elements that occur in soft tissues and bone. These tumors are locally aggressive and rarely metastasize, compared with high-grade endothelial tumors like angiosarcoma. Account for < 1% of malignant and all soft tissue tumors. Patients range in age from 17 to 60 years (mean age = 40 years).
Tumorlike Lesions		
Branchial cleft cyst (**Fig. 5.92**)	*CT:* Circumscribed, cystic lesion with low to intermediate attenuation depending on the proportions of protein and water. First branchial cleft cysts can be located adjacent to the external auditory canal (type 1 first branchial cleft cyst) or superficial portion of the parotid gland, ± extension into the parapharyngeal space, posterior to the submandibular gland, and/or up to the external auditory canal (type 2). Second branchial cleft cysts are often anterior or anteromedial to the sternocleidomatoid muscle (SCM) and medial to the carotid arteries, ± extension to the parapharyngeal space, and between the internal and external carotid arteries. Third branchial cleft cysts are located at the lower anterior margin of the SCM at the level of the upper thyroid lobe, ± extension of sinus tract posterior to the carotid artery and glossopharyngeal nerve, passing through the thyroid membrane above the level of the internal branch of the superior laryngeal nerve into the base of the piriform sinus. Fourth branchial cleft cysts occur in the lower third of the neck laterally, and anterior to the lower SCM and level of the aortic arch, ± visible connecting sinus tract on the right below the subclavian artery or on the left below the aortic arch that extend superiorly and dorsal to the carotid artery up to the level of the hypoglossal nerve and then downward along the SCM to the piriform sinus. *MRI:* Circumscribed lesions that often have low-intermediate signal on T1-weighted imaging and high signal on T2-weighted imaging. Usually there is no gadolinium contrast enhancement unless there is superimposed infection.	Branchial cleft cysts represent developmental anomalies of the branchial apparatus. The branchial apparatus consists of four major and two rudimentary arches of mesoderm lined by ectoderm externally and endoderm internally within pouches that form at the end of the fourth week of gestation. The mesoderm contains a dominant artery, nerve, cartilage, and muscle. The four major arches are separated by clefts. Each arch develops into a defined neck structure, with eventual obliteration of the branchial clefts. The first arch forms the external auditory canal, eustachian tube, middle ear, and mastoid air cells. The second arch develops into the hyoid bone and tonsillar and supratonsillar fossae. The third and fourth arches develop into the pharynx below the hyoid bone. Branchial anomalies include cysts, sinuses, and fistulas. Second branchial cleft cysts account for up to 90% of all branchial cleft malformations. Cysts are lined by squamous epithelium (90%), ciliated columnar epithelium (8%), or both types (2%). Sebaceous glands, salivary tissue, lymphoid tissue, and cholesterol crystals in mucoid fluid can also occur. There are four types of second branchial cleft cysts. Type 1 is located anterior to the SCM and deep to the platysma muscle; type 2 (the most common type) is located at the anteromedial surface of the SCM, lateral to the carotid space and posterior to the submandibular gland; type 3 is located lateral to the pharyngeal wall and medial to the carotid arteries, ± extension between the external and internal carotid arteries ("beak sign"); type 4 is located between the medial aspect of the carotid sheath and pharynx at the level of the tonsillar fossa, and can extend superiorly to the skull base. Typically, branchial cleft cysts are asymptomatic unless complicated by infection.

(continued on page 566)

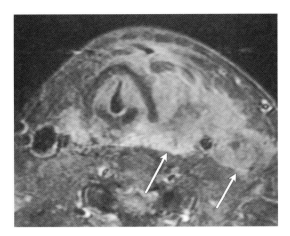

Fig. 5.91 Axial postcontrast fat-suppressed T1-weighted imaging of a 64-year-old man shows a large contrast-enhancing lesion in the left neck from B-cell non-Hodgkin lymphoma (*arrows*) that extends into the left anterior cervical, carotid, and visceral spaces, as well as extending into the left paraglottic space and left vocal cord.

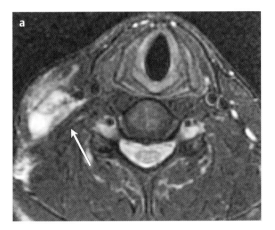
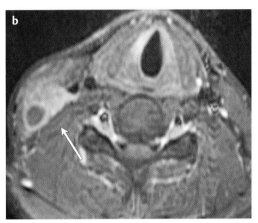

Fig. 5.92 **(a)** Axial fat-suppressed T2-weighted imaging shows an infected third branchial cleft cyst on the right (*arrow*) located posterior to the right sternocleidomastoid (SCM) muscle as well as involving the right SCM muscle and posterolateral portion of the right carotid space. The lesion has mixed slightly high and high signal with ill-defined margins. **(b)** Corresponding heterogeneous gadolinium contrast enhancement with ill-defined margins is seen on axial fat-suppressed T1-weighted imaging (*arrow*).

Table 5.5 *(cont.)*   Lesions of the infrahyoid carotid space

Lesions	Imaging Findings	Comments
Inflammatory Lesions		
Spread of infection from neck phlegmon and/or abscess (**Fig. 5.93** and **Fig. 5.94**)	*CT:* Irregular soft tissue thickening, ± adjacent lateral rim-enhancing fluid collection. Abnormal soft tissue thickening is seen surrounding the carotid space, ± thrombosis of the jugular vein. *MRI:* Irregular soft tissue thickening with poorly defined slightly high signal on T2-weighted imaging (T2WI) and fat-suppressed T2WI. Abscesses are collections with high signal on T2WI surrounded by a peripheral rim of gadolinium contrast enhancement. Soft tissue thickening with slightly high to high signal on T2WI without a rim-enhancing collection can represent a phlegmon.	Infection of the carotid space of the neck can result from hematogenous dissemination, lymphatic spread, trauma, or spread from adjacent sites, such as the oropharynx, hypopharynx, thyroid gland, and parapharyngeal, sublingual, and submandibular spaces. Clinical findings include: fever, pain, trismus, torticollis, Horner's sign, and palsies of cranial nerves IX, X, XI, and XII. Complications include thrombophlebitis of the jugular vein and/or septic embolization. Treatment is surgical drainage and antibiotics.
Vascular Abnormality		
Ectasia and tortuosity of the carotid artery (**Fig. 5.95**)	*CTA and MRA* show medial deviation of the course of the common and/or internal carotid arteries in the upper neck.	The internal and upper carotid arteries can be ectatic and tortuous. They may course medially, resulting in a pulsatile retropharyngeal or retrotonsillar mass. Identification of this arterial position is important for surgical planning and avoiding unnecessary biopsies.

(continued on page 568)

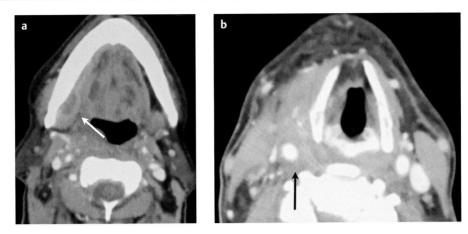

Fig. 5.93 **(a)** Axial postcontrast CT of a 74-year-old man with a phlegmon and pyogenic abscess (*arrow*) adjacent to the medial margin of the right mandible secondary to a dental infection. **(b)** Axial CT shows inferior extension of the infection along the outer margin of the right thyroid cartilage, with involvement of the right carotid space (*arrow*).

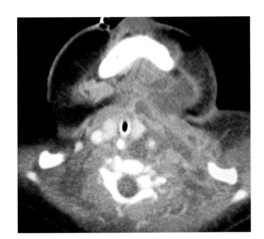

Fig. 5.94 Axial postcontrast CT of an endotracheally intubated patient with a left neck infection and abscess formation causing narrowing of the airway as well as thrombophlebitis, resulting in occlusion of the left internal jugular vein with lack of contrast enhancement (Lemierre syndrome).

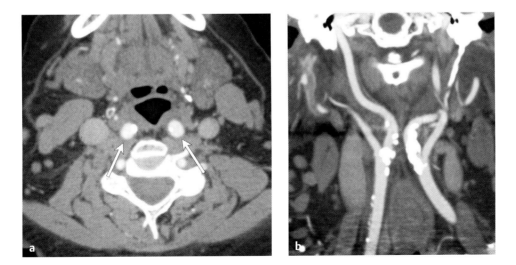

Fig. 5.95 **(a)** Axial and **(b)** coronal postcontrast CT images show tortuous carotid arteries that extend medially (*arrows* in **a**).

Table 5.5 *(cont.)* Lesions of the infrahyoid carotid space

Lesions	Imaging Findings	Comments
Aneurysm of the carotid artery **(Fig. 5.96)**	*Saccular aneurysm:* Focal well-circumscribed zone of contrast enhancement seen on conventional arteriography, CTA, and MRA. Can also be seen on noncontrast MRI and CT. *Fusiform aneurysm:* Tubular dilatation of involved artery. *Dissecting aneurysms (intramural hematoma):* Initially, the involved arterial wall is thickened in a circumferential or semilunar configuration and has intermediate attenuation with luminal narrowing. Evolution of the intramural hematoma can lead to focal dilatation of the arterial wall hematoma. *Giant aneurysm:* Saccular aneuryms that are more than 2.5 cm in diameter. Often contain mural thrombus, which has layers with intermediate to high attenuation on nonenhanced CT, and intermediate to high signal on T1- and T2-weighted imaging. The patent portion of the aneurysm shows contrast enhancement on CT, CTA, MRI, and MRA.	Abnormal fusiform or focal saccular dilatation of artery secondary to: acquired/degenerative etiology, polycystic disease, connective tissue disease, atherosclerosis, trauma, infection (mycotic), oncotic disorders, arteriovenous malformation, vasculitis, and drugs. Focal aneurysms, which are also referred to as saccular aneurysms, typically occur at arterial bifurcations and are multiple in 20% of cases. The chance of rupture of a saccular aneurysm causing subarachnoid hemorrhage is related to the size of the aneurysm. Saccular aneurysms > 2.5 cm in diameter are referred to as giant aneurysms. Fusiform aneurysms are often related to atherosclerosis or collagen vascular disease (Marfan syndrome, Ehlers-Danlos syndrome, etc.). In dissecting aneurysms, hemorrhage occurs in the arterial wall from incidental or significant trauma.
Arterial dissection **(Fig. 5.97)**	*MRI:* Crescentic zone with high signal on proton density-weighted imaging and fat-suppressed T1-weighted imaging involving the wall of a cervical carotid artery, resulting in narrowing of the intraluminal flow void. The intramural hematoma can progress and fill to occlude the lumen, obliterating the flow void of the artery. *CT:* The involved arterial wall is thickened in a circumferential or semilunar configuration and has intermediate attenuation. Lumen may be narrowed or occluded.	Arterial dissections can be related to trauma, collagen vascular disease (Marfan syndrome, Ehlers-Danlos syndrome, etc.), and fibromuscular dysplasia or they can be idiopathic. Hemorrhage occurs in the arterial wall and can cause stenosis, occlusion, and stroke.
Vasculitis **(Fig. 5.98)**	*MRI/MRA:* Zones of arterial occlusion, and/or foci of stenosis and poststenotic dilatation, can be seen involving small or medium-sized intracranial and extracranial arteries. Gadolinium contrast enhancement may be seen at the arterial walls related to acute/subacute inflammation. *CTA:* Zones of arterial occlusion, and/or foci of stenosis and poststenotic dilatation, can be seen involving small or medium-sized intracranial and extracranial arteries. *Conventional arteriography* shows zones of arterial occlusion, and/or foci of stenosis and poststenotic dilatation. May involve large, medium, or small intracranial and extracranial arteries.	Uncommon mixed group of inflammatory diseases/disorders involving the walls of blood vessels. Can involve small arteries (CNS vasculitis), small and medium-sized arteries (polyarteritis nodosa, Kawasaki disease), or large arteries with diameters of 7 to 35 mm, such as the aorta and its main branches (Takayasu arteritis, giant cell arteritis). Vasculitis can be a primary disease in which biopsies of meninges and brain show transmural vascular inflammation of vessels in the leptomeninges and brain parenchyma. Vasculitis can also occur secondary to other disorders, such as systemic disease (polyarteritis nodosa, granulomatosis with polyangiitis, giant cell arteritis, Takayasu arteritis, sarcoid, Behçet's disease, systemic lupus erythematosus, Sjögren's syndrome, dermatomyositis, mixed connective tissue disease), drugs (amphetamine, ephedrine, phenylpropylene, cocaine), or infections (virusal, bacterial, fungal, or parasitic).

(continued on page 570)

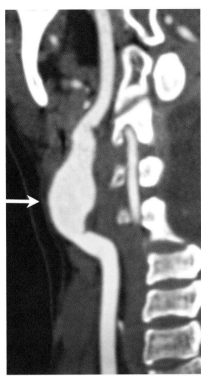

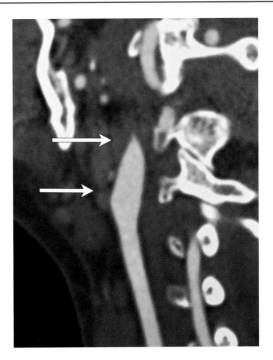

Fig. 5.96   Oblique sagittal CTA of a 27-year-old woman shows an aneurysm of the carotid artery (*arrow*).

Fig. 5.97   Oblique sagittal CTA of a 44-year-old man shows abrupt tapering and occlusion of the proximal internal carotid artery (*arrows*) from an intramural hematoma/arterial dissection.

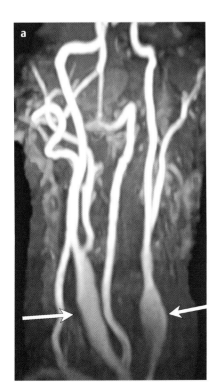

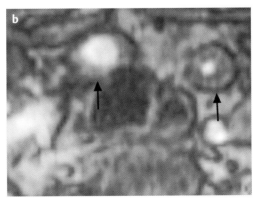

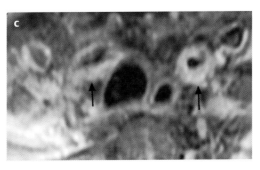

Fig. 5.98   (a) Coronal MRA of a 32-year-old woman with Takayasu arteritis shows abnormally dilated bilateral carotid arteries (*arrows*) as well as zones of distal stenosis. **(b)** Axial GRE shows thickening of the wall of a stenotic portion of the left carotid artery (*left arrow*) as well as a dilated right common carotid artery (*right arrow*), with **(c)** associated contrast enhancement of the wall of the left carotid artery (*left arrow*), which is not seen at the right carotid artery at this time (*right arrow*) on axial fat-suppressed T1-weighted imaging.

Table 5.5 (*cont.*)   Lesions of the infrahyoid carotid space

Lesions	Imaging Findings	Comments
Idiopathic carotidynia ("carotid pain syndrome") (**Fig. 5.99**)	*Ultrasound:* Hypoechoic arterial wall thickening at the carotid artery bifurcation in the neck, ± involvement of the proximal internal and external carotid arteries. Thickening of the arterial wall can be circumferential or involve a portion of the wall. Follow-up examinations can show regression of findings. *MRI:* Thickening of the carotid artery wall, which can have slightly high signal on fat-suppressed T2-weighted imaging. The arterial wall can show gadolinium (Gd) contrast enhancement, as well as poorly defined Gd contrast enhancement in the adjacent soft tissue. Minimal or no luminal narrowing. *CT:* Thickening of the carotid artery wall, which can show contrast enhancement, as well as poorly defined contrast enhancement in the adjacent soft tissue. Minimal or no luminal narrowing. *PET/CT:* Symptomatic site can show increased uptake of F-18 FDG.	Idiopathic self-limited syndrome of neck pain and tenderness at the carotid artery, in which there is arterial wall thickening and/or perivascular enhancement at or near the carotid bifurcation. Histologic findings include low-grade chronic inflammatory cells, fibroblasts, and vascular proliferation involving the adventitia surrounding the proximal carotid arteries. Patients are afebrile and do not have leukocytosis. Erythrocyte sedimentation rates are often within normal limits or minimally elevated. Carotidynia has a relatively benign clinical course, and typically resolves after 2 weeks. Treatment includes NSAIDs, ± steroids and benzodiazepines.
Thrombosis and/or thrombophlebitis of the internal jugular vein (IJV) (**Fig. 5.100** and **Fig. 5.101**)	*Contrast-enhanced CT and CTA:* Tubular intraluminal zone with low-intermediate attenuation, with reduced or absent contrast enhancement, ± peripheral contrast enhancement of the vaso vasorum of the vessel wall. *MRI:* Acute thrombus can have high signal on T2-weighted imaging (T2WI), whereas subacute thrombus can have low signal on T2WI. With Lemierre syndrome, poorly defined zones with high signal on T2WI and gadolinium contrast enhancement are seen in the adjacent soft tissues of the retrostyloid (RPPS), retropharyngeal space (RPS), and infrahyoid carotid space. *Ultrasound:* Dilated and incompressible vein, lack of blood flow on Doppler.	IJV thrombosis can result from surgical or procedural complications, trauma, polycythemia, coagulopathies, malignancies, IV drug abuse, and compression from adjacent lymphadenopathy. IJV thrombosis can also result from adjacent inflammation and/or infection. Extension of odontogenic and/or oropharyngeal infections can cause IJV thrombophlebitis (Lemierre syndrome). Lemierre syndrome often occurs in healthy young adults from oropharyngeal spread of infection by the usually commensal bacteria *Fusobacterium necrophorum* secondary to an altered host-defense mechanism with damage to the mucosa (trauma and bacterial or viral pharyngitis). Complications include septic embolization and bacteremia. Treatment of Lemierre syndrome is with broad-spectrum antibiotics, ± anticoagulation.
Venolymphatic malformation (**Fig. 5.102**)	Can be circumscribed lesions or occur in infiltrative pattern, with extension within soft tissue and between muscles. *MRI:* Often contain single or multiple cystic zones, which can be large (macrocystic type) or small (microcystic type), and which have predominantly low signal on T1-weighted imaging (T1WI) and high signal on T2-weighted imaging (T2WI) and fat-suppressed T2WI. Fluid–fluid levels and zones with high signal on T1WI and variable signal on T2WI may result from cysts containing hemorrhage, high protein concentration, and/or necrotic debris. Septa between the cystic zones can vary in thickness and gadolinium (Gd) contrast enhancement. Nodular zones within the lesions can have variable degrees of Gd contrast enhancement. Microcystic malformations typically show more Gd contrast enhancement than the macrocystic type. *CT:* Malformations of the macrocystic type are usually low-attenuation cystic lesions (10–25 HU) separated by thin walls, ± intermediate or high attenuation resulting from hemorrhage or infection, ± fluid–fluid levels.	Benign vascular anomalies (also referred to as lymphangioma or cystic hygroma) that primarily result from abnormal lymphangiogenesis. Up to 75% occur in the head and neck. Can be observed in utero with MRI or sonography, at birth (50–65%), or within the first 5 years. Approximately 85% are detected by age 2. Lesions are composed of endothelium-lined lymphatic ± venous channels interspersed within connective tissue stroma. Account for less than 1% of benign soft tissue tumors and 5.6% of all benign lesions of infancy and childhood. Can occur in association with Turner syndrome and Proteus syndrome.

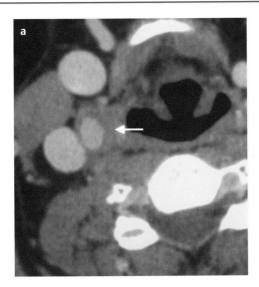
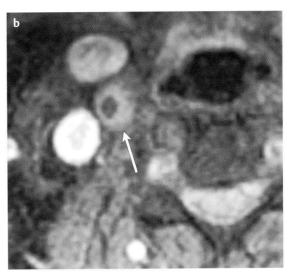

Fig. 5.99 **(a)** Axial postcontrast CT of a patient with carotidynia shows thickening of the carotid artery wall without luminal narrowing (*arrow*), as well as **(b)** poorly defined contrast enhancement in the adjacent soft tissue (*arrow*) on axial fat-suppressed T1-weighted imaging.

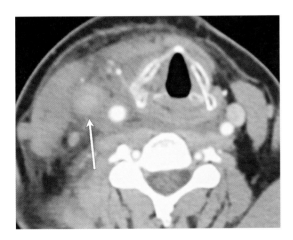

Fig. 5.100 Thrombophlebitis of the right internal jugular vein is seen on axial CT as an irregular, poorly defined zone of inflammatory soft tissue attenuation in the right neck, including the carotid space, with reduced contrast enhancement of the right internal jugular vein (*arrow*).

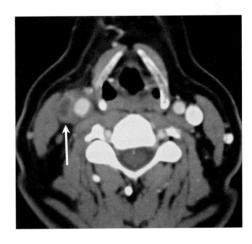

Fig. 5.101 Thrombosis of the right internal jugular vein is seen as low attenuation within the right internal jugular vein lacking contrast enhancement (*arrow*) on axial CT.

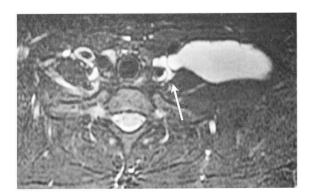

Fig. 5.102 Axial fat-suppressed T2-weighted imaging of a 15-year-old male with a macrocystic type of venolymphatic malformation (*arrow*), which has high signal in the left carotid space with lateral extension.

5.6 Abnormalities of the Anterior Cervical Space

The anterior cervical space (ACS) is a small fat-containing zone within the anterolateral portions of the neck. The ACS is located lateral to the visceral space, anterior to the carotid space, and medial to the sternocleidomastoid muscle (**Fig. 5.103**). The ACS is not enclosed by fascia and extends superiorly from the submandibular space down to the level of the clavicles. The posterior border of the ACS is the fascial layer covering the thyroid gland, and the posterolateral margin is the fascia surrounding the carotid sheath.

Table 5.6 Abnormalities of the anterior cervical space

- Congenital and Developmental
  - Thyroglossal duct cyst
  - Ectopic thyroid tissue
  - Venolymphatic malformation
  - Epidermoid
  - Dermoid
  - Dilated anterior jugular vein(s)
- Benign Tumors
  - Lipoma
  - Hemangioma
  - Schwannoma
  - Neurofibromas
- Malignant Neoplasms
  - Extension of tumors from adjacent locations
  - Sarcoma
  - Lymphoma
- Inflammation/Infection
  - Cellulitis/Abscess
- Trauma
  - Hematoma

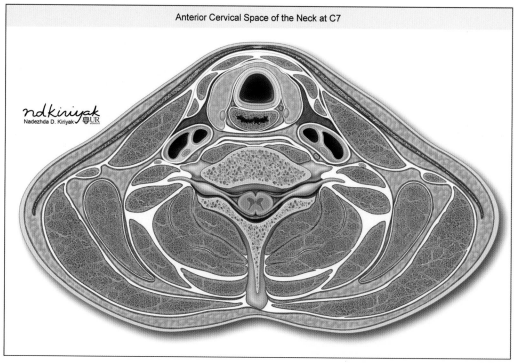

Anterior Cervical Space of the Neck at C7

Fig. 5.103 Axial view diagram shows the anterior cervical space in color.

Table 5.6   Abnormalities of the anterior cervical space

Abnormalities	Imaging Findings	Comments
Congenital and Developmental		
Thyroglossal duct cyst (See **Fig. 5.2** and **Fig. 5.3**)	*MRI:* Well-circumscribed spheroid or ovoid lesion at the tongue base or along the pathway of the thyroglossal duct that usually has low signal on T1-weighted imaging (T1WI) and diffusion-weighted imaging and high signal on T2-weighted imaging (T2WI). The wall of the thyroglossal duct cyst is typically thin, without gadolinium (Gd) contrast enhancement. Thyroglossal duct cysts complicated by hemorrhage and current or prior infection can have elevated protein with intermediate to slightly high signal on T1WI and T2WI. The walls of such cysts can be thick and show Gd contrast enhancement. Nodular Gd contrast enhancement involving the wall of a thyroglossal duct cyst can be seen with a potentially malignant lesion. *CT:* Well-circumscribed lesion with low (mucoid) attenuation ranging from 10 to 25 HU, surrounded by a thin wall. Occasionally contain thin septations. Thyroglossal duct cysts complicated by infection can have increased attenuation, thick walls, and loss/indistinctness of adjacent tissue planes. *Ultrasound:* Can be well-circumscribed anechoic cysts with through transmission or can have a pseudosolid appearance related to elevated protein concentration.	Thyroglossal duct cyst is the most common congenital mass in the neck and is related to altered development of the thyroid gland. The follicular cells of the thyroid gland develop from endodermal cells (median thyroid anlage) located between the first and second pharyngeal arches in the first 3 weeks of gestation. At 24 days of gestation, a small pit (thyroid bud) forms within the thyroid anlage that progressively forms a bilobed diverticulum that extends inferiorly along the midline adjacent to the aortic primordium. A small channel (thyroglossal duct) temporarily exists between the dorsal portion of the tongue (foramen cecum) and the inferiorly descending thyroid primordium. The thyroglossal duct normally involutes by the tenth week of gestation. The descending thyroid primordium and thyroglossal duct course anterior to the hyoid bone and loop slightly posterior to the inferior margin of the hyoid bone before descending anterior to the thyrohyoid membrane, thyroid cartilage, and trachea. The thyroglossal duct extends between the sternohyoid and sternothyroid strap muscles. The descending thyroid primordium reaches its normal position in the lower neck at 7 weeks of gestation. The parafollicular cells (C cells) of the thyroid develop from endodermal cells (lateral thyroid anlage) at the fourth pharyngeal pouch and migrate to join and merge with the descending thyroid primordium from the median thyroid anlage. Up to two-thirds of thyroglossal duct cysts occur in the infrahyoid neck and can be midline or extend laterally within, or deep to, the strap muscles. Nearly 50% present in patients < 20 years old as a progressively enlarging neck lesion.
Ectopic thyroid tissue (See **Fig. 5.4, Fig. 5.5,** and **Fig. 5.6**)	*CT:* Circumscribed ovoid or spheroid lesion at the dorsal portion (base) of the tongue that shows slightly increased attenuation (~ 70 HU), prominent contrast enhancement, ± low attenuation thyroid nodules, ± calcifications. *MRI:* Circumscribed lesions with low-intermediate signal on T1-weighted imaging and low, intermediate, or slightly high signal on T2-weighted imaging. Variable degrees of gadolinium contrast enhancement. *Nuclear medicine:* Iodine 123, iodine 131, or technetium 99m pertechnetate uptake in ectopic thyroid tissue in the tongue and lack of normal uptake in normal orthotopic location of thyroid bed.	The normal thyroid gland is located below the larynx, posterior to the strap muscles, medial to the carotid arteries, and anterolateral to the trachea. Ectopic thyroid tissue results from lack of normal embryologic descent of the primitive thyroid gland along the thyroglossal duct from the foramen cecum at the tongue base down to the lower neck. Lingual thyroid represents up to 90% of cases of ectopic thyroid. Other locations include: adjacent to the hyoid bone, midline infrahyoid neck, and lateral neck. Can be asymptomatic, or can occur in association with dysphagia, dysphonia, and/or stridor.

(continued on page 574)

Table 5.6 *(cont.)*   Abnormalities of the anterior cervical space

Abnormalities	Imaging Findings	Comments
Venolymphatic malformation (See **Fig. 5.11** and **Fig. 5.102**)	Can be circumscribed lesions or occur in an infiltrative pattern with extension within soft tissue and between muscles. *MRI:* Often contain single or multiple cystic zones, which can be large (macrocystic type) or small (microcystic type), and which have predominantly low signal on T1-weighted imaging (T1WI) and high signal on T2-weighted imaging (T2WI) and fat-suppressed T2WI. Fluid–fluid levels and zones with high signal on T1WI and variable signal on T2WI may result from cysts containing hemorrhage, high protein concentration, and/or necrotic debris. Septa between the cystic zones can vary in thickness and gadolinium (Gd) contrast enhancement. Nodular zones within the lesions can have variable degrees of Gd contrast enhancement. Microcystic malformations typically show more Gd contrast enhancement than the macrocystic type. *CT:* Malformations of the macrocystic type are usually low-attenuation cystic lesions (10–25 HU) separated by thin walls, ± intermediate or high attenuation from hemorrhage or infection, ± fluid–fluid levels.	Benign vascular anomalies (also referred to as lymphangioma or cystic hygroma) that primarily result from abnormal lymphangiogenesis. Up to 75% occur in the head and neck. Can be observed in utero with MRI or sonography, at birth (50–65%), or within the first 5 years. Approximately 85% are detected by age 2. Lesions are composed of endothelium-lined lymphatic ± venous channels interspersed within connective tissue stroma. Account for less than 1% of benign soft tissue tumors and 5.6% of all benign lesions of infancy and childhood. Can occur in association with Turner syndrome and Proteus syndrome.
Epidermoid	*MRI:* Well-circumscribed spheroid or multilobulated ectodermal-inclusion cystic lesions with low-intermediate signal on T1-weighted imaging, high signal on T2-weighted imaging and diffusion-weighted imaging, mixed low, intermediate, or high signal on FLAIR images, and no gadolinium contrast enhancement. *CT:* Well-circumscribed spheroid or multilobulated extra-axial ectodermal-inclusion cystic lesions with low-intermediate attenuation.	Nonneoplastic congenital or acquired lesions filled with desquamated cells and keratinaceous debris surrounded by a wall lined by simple squamous epithelium. Lesions result from congenital inclusion of epidermal elements during embryonic development of the first and second branchial arches, or from trauma. Often occur in patients between 5 and 50 years old (mean age = 30 years).
Dermoid	*MRI:* Well-circumscribed spheroid or multilobulated lesions, usually with high signal on T1-weighted imaging, and variable low, intermediate, and/or high signal on T2-weighted imaging, no Gd-contrast enhancement. *CT:* Well-circumscribed spheroid or multilobulated lesions, usually with low attenuation, ± fat–fluid or fluid–debris levels.	Nonneoplastic congenital or acquired ectodermal-inclusion cystic lesions filled with lipid material, cholesterol, desquamated cells, and keratinaceous debris surrounded by a wall lined by keratinizing squamous epithelium, ± related clinical symptoms. Lesions result from congenital inclusion of dermal elements during embryonic development or from trauma. Occur in males slightly more often than in females. Can cause chemical inflammation if dermoid cyst ruptures.
Dilated anterior jugular vein(s)	*MRI, CT, and Ultrasound:* Unilateral or bilateral enlargement of the anterior jugular veins.	Incidental finding on MRI and CT, with no clinical significance.

Abnormalities	Imaging Findings	Comments
Benign Tumors		
Lipoma (**Fig. 5.104**)	*MRI:* Lipomas have MRI signal isointense to subcutaneous fat on T1-weighted imaging (high signal), and on T2-weighted imaging, signal suppression occurs with frequency-selective fat saturation techniques or with a short time to inversion recovery (STIR) method. Typically there is no gadolinium contrast enhancement or peripheral edema. *CT:* Lipomas have attenuation similar to subcutaneous fat, and typically no contrast enhancement or peripheral edema.	Common benign hamartomas composed of mature white adipose tissue without cellular atypia. Most common soft tissue tumor, representing 16% of all soft tissue tumors.
Hemangioma (See **Fig. 5.13**)	*MRI:* Circumscribed or poorly marginated structures (< 4 cm in diameter) in bone marrow or soft tissue with intermediate-high signal on T1-weighted imaging (often with portions that are isointense to marrow fat), high signal on T2-weighted imaging (T2WI) and fat-suppressed T2WI, and typically gadolinium contrast enhancement, ± expansion of bone. *CT:* Expansile bone lesions with a radiating pattern of bony trabeculae oriented toward the center. Hemangiomas in soft tissue have mostly intermediate attenuation, ± zones of fat attenuation.	Benign lesions of bone or soft tissue composed of capillary, cavernous, and/or venous malformations. Considered to be a hamartomatous disorder. Occurs in patients 1 to 84 years old (median age = 33 years).
Schwannoma (See **Fig. 5.84** and **Fig. 5.85**)	*MRI:* Circumscribed spheroid or ovoid lesions with low-intermediate signal on T1-weighted imaging, high signal on T2-weighted imaging (T2WI) and fat-suppressed T2WI, and usually prominent gadolinium (Gd) contrast enhancement. High signal on T2WI and Gd contrast enhancement can be heterogeneous in large lesions due to cystic degeneration and/or hemorrhage. *CT:* Circumscribed or lobulated lesions with intermediate attenuation, + contrast enhancement. Large lesions can have cystic degeneration and/or hemorrhage.	Schwannomas are benign encapsulated tumors that contain differentiated neoplastic Schwann cells. Most commonly occur as solitary, sporadic lesions. Schwannomas rarely occur in the larynx, and account for less than 1.5% of benign laryngeal tumors. Most occur in the submucosal space and up to 80% involve the aryepiglottic fold. Multiple schwannomas are often associated with neurofibromatosis type 2 (NF2), which is an autosomal dominant disease involving a gene mutation at chromosome 22q12. In addition to schwannomas, patients with NF2 can also have multiple meningiomas and ependymomas. The incidence of NF2 is 1/37,000 to 1/50,000 newborns. Age at presentation = 22 to 72 years (mean age = 46 years). Peak incidence is in the fourth to sixth decades. Many patients with NF2 present in the third decade with bilateral vestibular schwannomas.

(continued on page 576)

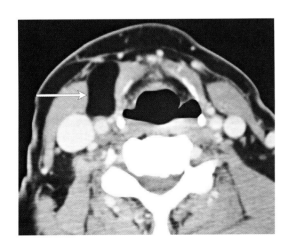

Fig. 5.104 Axial CT shows a lipoma (*arrow*) in the right anterior cervical space that has attenuation similar to subcutaneous fat.

Table 5.6 *(cont.)*　Abnormalities of the anterior cervical space

Abnormalities	Imaging Findings	Comments
Neurofibromas (See **Fig. 5.86**)	*MRI:* *Solitary neurofibromas* are circumscribed spheroid, ovoid, or lobulated lesions with low-intermediate signal on T1-weighted imaging (T1WI), intermediate-high signal on T2-weighted imaging (T2WI), + prominent gadolinium (Gd) contrast enhancement. High signal on T2WI and Gd contrast enhancement can be heterogeneous in large lesions. *Plexiform neurofibromas* appear as curvilinear and multinodular lesions involving multiple nerve branches and have low to intermediate signal on T1WI and intermediate, slightly high to high signal on T2WI and fat-suppressed T2WI, with or without bands or strands of low signal. Lesions usually show Gd contrast enhancement. *CT:* Ovoid, spheroid, or fusiform lesions with low-intermediate attenuation. Lesions can show contrast enhancement. Often erode adjacent bone.	Benign nerve sheath tumors that contain mixtures of Schwann cells, perineural-like cells, and interlacing fascicles of fibroblasts associated with abundant collagen. Unlike schwannomas, neurofibromas lack Antoni A and B regions and cannot be separated pathologically from the underlying nerve. Most frequently occur as sporadic, localized, solitary lesions, less frequently as diffuse or plexiform lesions. Multiple neurofibromas are typically seen with neurofibromatosis type 1, which is an autosomal dominant disorder (1/2,500 births) from mutations involving the neurofibromin gene on chromosome 17q11.2.
Malignant Neoplasms		
Extension of tumors from adjacent locations (**Fig. 5.105**)	*MRI:* Tumors often have intermediate signal on T1-weighted imaging, intermediate-slightly high signal on T2-weighted imaging, and mild gadolinium contrast enhancement. Can be large lesions (± necrosis and/or hemorrhage). *CT:* Tumors have intermediate attenuation and mild contrast enhancement. Can be large lesions (± necrosis and/or hemorrhage).	Malignant tumors from the hypopharynx, larynx, and thyroid gland can directly invade the anterior cervical space.
Sarcoma (**Fig. 5.106**)	*MRI:* Tumors can have circumscribed and/or poorly defined margins, and typically have low-intermediate signal on T1-weighted imaging and heterogeneous signal (various combinations of intermediate, slightly high, and/or high signal) on T2-weighted imaging (T2WI) and fat-suppressed T2WI. Tumors show variable degrees of gadolinium contrast enhancement, ± bone destruction and invasion. *CT:* Soft tissue lesions usually can have circumscribed or irregular margins. Calcifications are uncommon. Tumors can have mixed CT attenuation with solid zones of soft tissue attenuation, cystic-appearing and/or necrotic zones, and occasional foci of hemorrhage, ± bone invasion and destruction.	Primary sarcomas rarely occur in the neck.
Lymphoma (**Fig. 5.107**)	*CT:* Lesions have low-intermediate attenuation, and may show contrast enhancement, ± bone destruction. *MRI:* Lesions have low-intermediate signal on T1-weighted imaging, intermediate to slightly high signal on T2-weighted imaging, + gadolinium contrast enhancement. Can be locally invasive and associated with bone erosion/destruction.	Lymphomas are a group of lymphoid tumors whose neoplastic cells typically arise within lymphoid tissue (lymph nodes and reticuloendothelial organs). Most lymphomas involving the neck are non-Hodgkin lymphomas (B-cell types more common than T-cell types).

(continued on page 578)

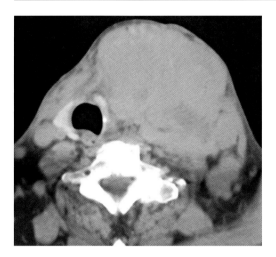

Fig. 5.105 Axial CT of an 83-year-old man with a large anaplastic thyroid carcinoma involving the left thyroid lobe that has ill-defined margins and invades the adjacent soft tissues, including the left anterior cervical space.

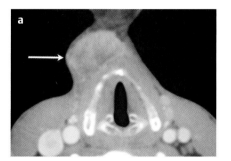
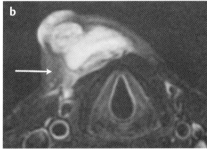
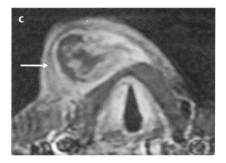

Fig. 5.106 **(a)** A 35-year-old woman with a myxoid liposarcoma in the superficial soft tissues of the neck, including the anterior cervical space, that has ill-defined margins and mixed intermediate and low signal on axial postcontrast CT (*arrow*). **(b)** The tumor has heterogeneous mostly high signal on axial fat-suppressed T2-weighted imaging (*arrow*) and **(c)** irregular gadolinium contrast enhancement on axial fat-suppressed T1-weighted imaging (*arrow*).

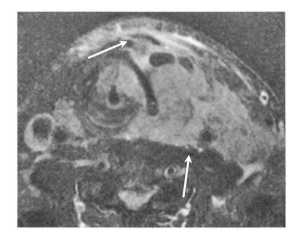

Fig. 5.107 Axial fat-suppressed T2-weighted imaging of a 64-year-old man with B-cell non-Hodgkin lymphoma shows a large lesion (*arrows*) in the left neck with ill-defined margins and slightly high signal that extends into the left anterior cervical, carotid, and visceral spaces, as well as extending into the left paraglottic space and left vocal cord.

Table 5.6 *(cont.)* Abnormalities of the anterior cervical space

Abnormalities	Imaging Findings	Comments
Inflammation/Infection		
Cellulitis/Abscess (**Fig. 5.108**)	*CT:* Irregular soft tissue thickening ± adjacent lateral rim-enhancing fluid collection (abscess). *MRI:* Irregular soft tissue thickening with poorly defined slightly high signal on T2-weighted imaging (T2WI) and fat-suppressed T2WI. Abscesses are collections with high signal on T2WI surrounded by a peripheral rim of gadolinium contrast enhancement. Soft tissue thickening with slightly high to high signal on T2WI without a rim-enhancing collection can represent a phlegmon.	Can result from trauma, infected thyroglossal or branchial cleft cysts, or extension of infection from the submandibular space (odontogenic osteomyelitis), hypopharynx, or thyroid gland. Treatment is surgical drainage and/or antibiotics.
Trauma		
Hematoma (**Fig. 5.109**)	*CT:* Nodular lesion with intermediate to slightly high attenuation, irregular margins, ± osseous or cartilage fracture.	Extravasated blood from trauma can be an isolated finding or associated with other injuries, including osseous or laryngeal cartilage fractures.

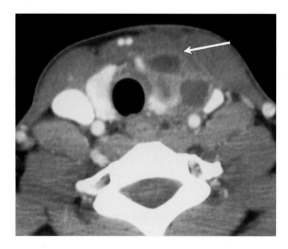

Fig. 5.108 Axial postcontrast CT of a 22-year-old woman shows acute suppurative thyroiditis in the left thyroid lobe. There are multiple abscesses seen with peripheral contrast enhancement and extension of the infection into the anterior cervical space (*arrow*).

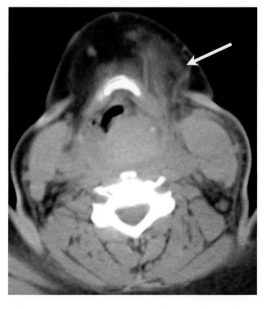

Fig. 5.109 Axial CT of a patient with history of blunt neck trauma shows a hematoma in the posterior larynx that has slightly high attenuation. Hematoma and edematous changes are seen in the left anterior cervical space (*arrow*).

5.7 Abnormalities of the Posterior Cervical Space

The posterior cervical space (PCS) corresponds to the posterior triangle of the neck. The PCS is located posterolateral to the carotid space, medial to the sternocleidomatoid muscle, anterior to the trapezius muscle, and lateral to the perispinal space (**Fig. 5.110**). The PCS extends from the skull base down to the clavicles. The PCS contains fat, CN XI, the spinal accessory chain of deep cervical lymph nodes, and the pre-axillary brachial plexus. The omohyoid muscle traverses the lower portion of the PCS.

Table 5.7   Abnormalities of the posterior cervical space

- Congenital and Developmental
  - Third branchial cleft cyst
  - Venolymphatic malformation
- Benign Tumors
  - Lipoma
  - Hemangioma
  - Schwannoma
  - Neurofibromas
- Malignant Neoplasms
  - Nodal metastases
  - Non-Hodgkin lymphoma (NHL) and Hodgkin disease (HD)
  - Sarcoma
- Inflammation/Infection
  - Lymphadenitis (Reactive adenopathy; Presuppurative and suppurative adenopathy; Granulomatous adenopathy)
  - Sarcoidosis
  - Cellulitis/Abscess

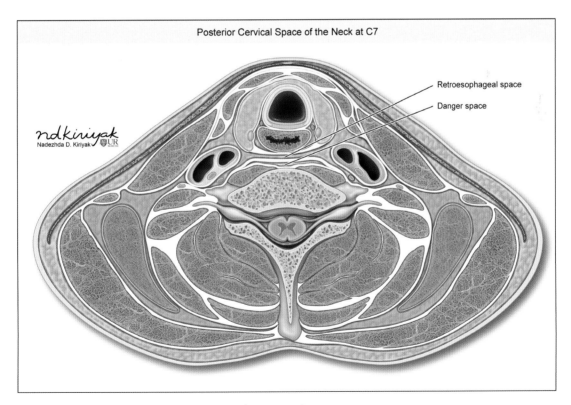

Fig. 5.110   Axial view diagram shows the posterior cervical space in color.

Table 5.7 Abnormalities of the posterior cervical space

Abnormalities	Imaging Findings	Comments
Congenital and Developmental		
Third branchial cleft cyst (**Fig. 5.111**)	*CT:* Circumscribed, cystic lesion with low to intermediate attenuation depending on the proportions of protein and water. Third branchial cleft cysts are located at the lower anterior margin of the sternocleidomastoid muscle at the level of the upper thyroid lobe, ± extension of sinus tract (± cyst) posterior to the carotid artery and glossopharyngeal nerve, passing through the thyroid membrane above the level of the internal branch of the superior laryngeal nerve into the base of the piriform sinus. *MRI:* Circumscribed lesion that often has low-intermediate signal on T1-weighted imaging and high signal on T2-weighted imaging. Usually there is no gadolinium contrast enhancement unless there is superimposed infection.	Branchial cleft cysts represent developmental anomalies of the branchial apparatus. The branchial apparatus consists of four major and two rudimentary arches of mesoderm lined by ectoderm externally and endoderm internally within pouches that form at the end of the fourth week of gestation. The mesoderm contains a dominant artery, nerve, cartilage, and muscle. The third and fourth arches develop into the pharynx below the hyoid bone. Branchial anomalies include cysts, sinuses, and fistulas. Second branchial cleft cysts account for up to 90% of all branchial cleft malformations. Cysts are lined by squamous epithelium (90%), ciliated columnar epithelium (8%), or both types (2%). Sebaceous glands, salivary tissue, lymphoid tissue, and cholesterol crystals in mucoid fluid can also occur. Typically, branchial cleft cysts are asymptomatic unless complicated by infection.
Venolymphatic malformation (See **Fig. 5.11** and **Fig. 5.102**)	Can be circumscribed lesions or occur in an infiltrative pattern with extension within soft tissue and between muscles. *MRI:* Often contain single or multiple cystic zones that can be large (macrocystic type) or small (microcystic type), and that have predominantly low signal on T1-weighted imaging (T1WI) and high signal on T2-weighted imaging (T2WI) and fat-suppressed T2WI. Fluid–fluid levels and zones with high signal on T1WI and variable signal on T2WI may result from cysts containing hemorrhage, high protein concentration, and/or necrotic debris. Septa between the cystic zones can vary in thickness and gadolinium (Gd) contrast enhancement. Nodular zones within the lesions can have variable degrees of Gd contrast enhancement. Microcystic malformations typically show more Gd contrast enhancement than the macrocystic type. *CT:* Macrocystic malformations are usually low-attenuation cystic lesions (10–25 HU) separated by thin walls, ± intermediate or high attenuation that can result from hemorrhage or infection, ± fluid–fluid levels.	Benign vascular anomalies (also referred to as lymphangioma or cystic hygroma) that primarily result from abnormal lymphangiogenesis. Up to 75% occur in the head and neck. Can be observed in utero with MRI or sonography, at birth (50–65%), or within the first 5 years. Approximately 85% are detected by age 2. Lesions are composed of endothelium-lined lymphatic ± venous channels interspersed within connective tissue stroma. Account for less than 1% of benign soft tissue tumors and 5.6% of all benign lesions of infancy and childhood. Can occur in association with Turner syndrome and Proteus syndrome.

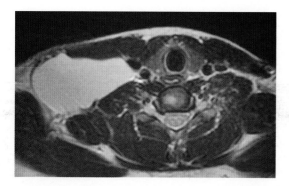

Fig. 5.111 Axial T2-weighted imaging shows a third branchial cleft cyst with high signal located dorsal to the right sternocleidomastoid muscle and posterolateral to the right carotid space.

Abnormalities	Imaging Findings	Comments
Benign Tumors		
Lipoma (See **Fig. 5.87**)	*MRI:* Lipomas have MRI signal isointense to subcutaneous fat on T1-weighted imaging (high signal), and on T2-weighted imaging, signal suppression occurs with frequency-selective fat saturation techniques or with a short time to inversion recovery (STIR) method. Typically there is no gadolinium contrast enhancement or peripheral edema. *CT:* Lipomas have CT attenuation similar to subcutaneous fat. Typically there is no contrast enhancement or peripheral edema.	Common benign hamartomas composed of mature white adipose tissue without cellular atypia. Most common soft tissue tumor, representing 16% of all soft tissue tumors. May contain calcifications and/or traversing blood vessels.
Hemangioma (**Fig. 5.112**)	*MRI:* Circumscribed or poorly marginated structures (< 4 cm in diameter) in soft tissue or bone marrow with intermediate-high signal on T1-weighted imaging (often isointense to marrow fat), high signal on T2-weighted imaging (T2WI) and fat-suppressed T2WI, and typically gadolinium contrast enhancement, ± expansion of bone. *CT:* Hemangiomas in soft tissue have mostly intermediate attenuation, ± zones of fat attenuation.	Benign lesions of soft tissue or bone composed of capillary, cavernous, and/or venous malformations. Considered to be a hamartomatous disorder. Occurs in patients 1 to 84 years old (median age = 33 years).
Schwannoma (See **Fig. 5.84** and **Fig. 5.85**)	*MRI:* Circumscribed spheroid or ovoid lesions with low-intermediate signal on T1-weighted imaging, high signal on T2-weighted imaging (T2WI) and fat-suppressed T2WI, and usually prominent gadolinium (Gd) contrast enhancement. High signal on T2WI and Gd contrast enhancement can be heterogeneous in large lesions due to cystic degeneration and/or hemorrhage. *CT:* Circumscribed spheroid or ovoid lesions with intermediate attenuation, + contrast enhancement. Large lesions can have cystic degeneration and/or hemorrhage.	Schwannomas are benign encapsulated tumors that contain differentiated neoplastic Schwann cells. Most commonly occur as solitary, sporadic lesions. Multiple schwannomas are often associated with neurofibromatosis type 2 (NF2), which is an autosomal dominant disease involving a gene mutation at chromosome 22q12. In addition to schwannomas, patients with NF2 can also have multiple meningiomas and ependymomas. The incidence of NF2 is 1/37,000 to 1/50,000 newborns. Age at presentation = 22 to 72 years (mean age = 46 years). Peak incidence is in the fourth to sixth decades. Many patients with NF2 present in the third decade with bilateral vestibular schwannomas.

(continued on page 582)

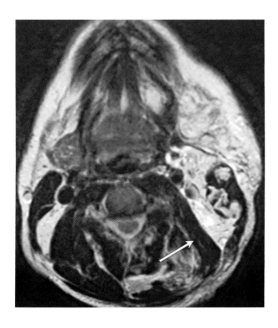

Fig. 5.112 Axial T2-weighted imaging shows an infiltrating hemangioma with high signal in the left neck, including the left submandibular, carotid, and posterior cervical spaces (*arrow*).

Table 5.7 *(cont.)* Abnormalities of the posterior cervical space

Abnormalities	Imaging Findings	Comments
Neurofibromas (**Fig. 5.113**)	*MRI:* Solitary neurofibromas are circumscribed spheroid, ovoid, or lobulated lesions, low-intermediate signal on T1-weighted imaging (T1WI), intermediate-high signal on T2-weighted imaging (T2WI), + prominent Gd-contrast enhancement. High signal on T2WI and Gd-contrast enhancement can be heterogeneous in large lesions. *Plexiform neurofibromas* appear as curvilinear and multinodular lesions involving multiple nerve branches, and have low to intermediate signal on T1WI; and intermediate, slightly high to high signal on T2WI and FS T2WI with or without bands or strands of low signal. Lesions usually show Gd-contrast enhancement. *CT:* Ovoid, spheroid, or fusiform lesions with low-intermediate attenuation. Lesions can show contrast enhancement. Often erode adjacent bone.	Benign nerve sheath tumors that contain mixtures of Schwann cells, perineural-like cells, and interlacing fascicles of fibroblasts associated with abundant collagen. Unlike schwannomas, neurofibromas lack Antoni A and B regions and cannot be separated pathologically from the underlying nerve. Most frequently occur as sporadic, localized, solitary lesions, less frequently as diffuse or plexiform lesions. Multiple neurofibromas are typically seen with neurofibromatosis type 1 (NF1), which is an autosomal dominant disorder (1/2,500 births) caused by mutations of the neurofibromin on chromosome 17q11.2. NF1 is the most common type of neurocutaneous syndrome, and is associated with neoplasms of central and peripheral nervous system (optic gliomas, astrocytomas, plexiform and solitary neurofibromas) and skin (café-au-lait spots, axillary and inguinal freckling). Also associated with meningeal and skull dysplasias, as well as hamartomas of the iris (Lisch nodules).
Malignant Neoplasms		
Nodal metastases (**Fig. 5.114**)	*MRI:* Enlarged spheroid or ovoid nodes that often have low-intermediate signal on T1-weighted imaging and intermediate-high signal on T2-weighted imaging (T2WI), ± high signal zones on T2WI (necrosis), ± irregular margins (capsule invasion), ± decreased ADC values on diffusion-weighted imaging (< 1.4 × 10^{-3} mm^2/sec). There is variable gadolinium contrast enhancement. *CT:* Involved nodes usually have low-intermediate attenuation, ± irregular margins (capsule invasion), ± low-attenuation zones (necrosis), and variable contrast enhancement. Nodes usually measure more than 8 mm in short axis. *Ultrasound:* Enlarged hypoechoic nodes, ± cystic-necrotic zones, ± irregular margins (capsule invasion). Color Doppler often shows hypervascularity.	Metastatic tumor in cervical lymph nodes can be caused by primary neck neoplasms, such as squamous cell carcinoma or thyroid cancer, or by spread from primary extracranial tumor source: lung > breast > GI > GU > melanoma. Can occur as single or multiple well-circumscribed or poorly defined lesions. Metastatic tumor may cause variable destructive or infiltrative changes in single or multiple sites.
Non-Hodgkin lymphoma (NHL) and Hodgkin disease (HD) (**Fig. 5.115**)	*CT:* Enlarged lymph nodes with soft tissue attenuation, ± contrast enhancement. *MRI:* Enlarged lymph nodes with intermediate signal on T1-weighted imaging and slightly high signal on T2-weighted imaging, ± gadolinium contrast enhancement. Necrosis and cystic changes rarely occur. *Ultrasound:* Enlarged hypoechoic nodes with circumscribed margins. Color Doppler often shows hypervascularity.	Both NHL and HD involve cervical lymph nodes.

(continued on page 584)

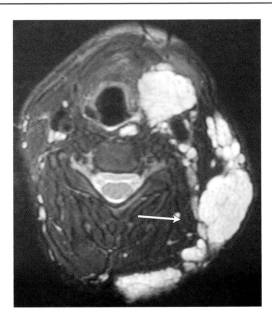

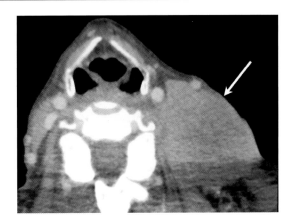

Fig. 5.114 Axial CT of a 65-year-old man with prostate carcinoma shows large nodal metastases (*arrow*) in the left posterior cervical space.

Fig. 5.113 Axial fat-suppressed T2-weighted imaging of a 15-year-old male with neurofibromatosis type 1 who has multiple neurofibromas with high signal in the neck, including the left posterior cervical space (*arrow*).

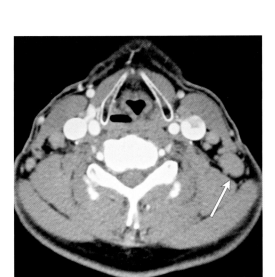

Fig. 5.115 Axial CT of a 63-year-old man with non-Hodgkin lymphoma shows an abnormally enlarged posterior cervical lymph node (*arrow*) on the left.

Table 5.7 *(cont.)* Abnormalities of the posterior cervical space

Abnormalities	Imaging Findings	Comments
Sarcoma	*MRI:* Tumors can have circumscribed and/or poorly defined margins, and typically have low-intermediate signal on T1-weighted imaging and heterogeneous signal (various combinations of intermediate, slightly high, and/or high signal) on T2-weighted imaging (T2WI) and fat-suppressed T2WI. Sarcomas with high cellularity can show low ADC values on diffusion-weighted imaging. Tumors show variable degrees of gadolinium contrast enhancement, ± bone destruction and invasion. *CT:* Soft tissue lesions can have circumscribed or irregular margins. Calcifications are uncommon. Tumors can have mixed CT attenuation with solid zones of soft tissue attenuation, cystic-appearing and/or necrotic zones, and occasional foci of hemorrhage, ± bone invasion and destruction. *PET/CT:* F-18 FDG is useful in grading primary tumors; high-grade tumors have higher standardized uptake value (2.6) than low-grade sarcomas (1.8) and benign tumors (< 1.4). PET/CT is also useful in the evaluation for metastatic disease.	Primary sarcomas rarely occur in the neck. The annual incidence of soft tissue sarcomas is 3 per 100,000. Sarcomas in the neck account for 15% of soft tissue sarcomas in adults and up to 35% of soft tissue sarcomas in children. The WHO categorizes sarcomas based on their predominant histologic findings, in concert with immunohistochemistry profiles, and genetic data if available. The subtypes of sarcomas include adipocytic tumors, fibroblastic tumors, myofibroblastic tumors, fibrohistiocytic tumors, smooth or skeletal muscle tumors, vascular tumors, nerve sheath tumors, chondro-osseous tumors, and undifferentiated tumors. Treatments and prognosis can vary based on the type of sarcoma, tumor grade, and stage.
Inflammation/Infection		
Lymphadenitis (reactive adenopathy; presuppurative and suppurative adenopathy; granulomatous adenopathy) (**Fig. 5.116** and **Fig. 5.117**)	*CT:* *Reactive adenopathy:* Enlarged lymph nodes measure less than 12 mm, with preservation of nodal architecture, ± prominent single hilar vessel or branching vascular pattern. In *presuppurative adenopathy,* enlarged lymph nodes are associated with loss of the fatty hilum, slightly decreased attenuation, increased contrast enhancement, and reticulation of adjacent fat. *Suppurative* lymph nodes are typically enlarged and can have zones with low attenuation centrally surrounded by a rim of contrast enhancement. *MRI:* Enlarged *presuppurative* nodes have intermediate signal on T1-weighted imaging (T1WI) and slightly high signal on T2-weighted imaging (T2WI), and show gadolinium (Gd) contrast enhancement. *Suppurative* nodes have low-intermediate signal on T1WI and slightly high to high signal on T2WI, and show rim Gd contrast enhancement. Irregular increased signal on T2WI and Gd contrast enhancement are typically seen in the adjacent soft tissue. *Ultrasound: Reactive nodes* are usually enlarged and hypoechoic and have circumscribed margins. *Suppurative nodes* range from enlarged, hypoechoic, hyperemic nodes to lobulated, anechoic/septated lesions with mild acoustic enhancement.	Enlarged lymph nodes that usually measure less than 12 mm, with preservation of nodal architecture, can result from infections of the oral cavity, oropharynx, and hypopharynx, and are referred to as reactive adenopathy or presuppurative lymphadenitis. In children, lymphadenitis can result from upper respiratory viral infections or bacteria, such as *Staphylococcus aureus* and *Streptococcus pyogenes*. Infection by the gram-negative bacillus *Bartonella henselae* can result in a self-limited regional granulomatous adenitis. This infection usually occurs in patients < 30 years old and is often related to contact with cats (cat-scratch disease). Other infectious granulomatous diseases that cause lymphadenopathy are caused by mycobacteria, such as *Mycobacterium tuberculosis, M. avium intracellulare, M. bovis,* and *M. kansasii*. Enlarged lymph nodes can undergo liquefactive necrosis (suppurative adenitis)—purulent lymph nodes. Purulent lymph nodes measure up to 4.5 cm. Treatment with IV antibiotics is usually effective when the suppurative low-attenuation nodes measures less than 2 cm. Larger suppurative lymph nodes usually require surgical drainage, especially with airway compromise. In adults, suppurative adenitis often results from trauma and procedural or surgical complications. Gram-positive cocci are common pathogens in suppurative adenitis in adults.
Sarcoidosis (**Fig. 5.118**)	*MRI:* Single or multiple enlarged cervical lymph nodes with low to intermediate signal on T1-weighted imaging and slightly high signal on T2-weighted imaging (T2WI) and fat-suppressed T2WI. After gadolinium (Gd) contrast administration, involved nodes can show Gd contrast enhancement. *CT:* Single or multiple enlarged lymph nodes with soft tissue attenuation. *Nuclear medicine:* Increased uptake of gallium 67 citrate and F-18 FDG-glucose.	Sarcoidosis is a multisystem noncaseating granulomatous disease of uncertain cause that can involve the CNS in 5–15% of cases. If untreated, it is associated with severe neurologic deficits, such as encephalopathy, cranial neuropathies, and myelopathy. Sarcoid can involve the major salivary glands and can be associated with cervical lymphadenopathy. Treatment includes oral corticosteroids and surgical debulking.

(continued on page 586)

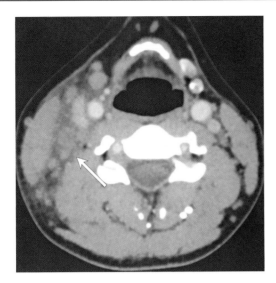

Fig. 5.116 Axial CT of a 32-year-old woman with a dental infection shows a presuppurative level IIb lymph node (*arrow*) with loss of the fatty hilum, slightly decreased attenuation, and reticulation of adjacent fat with extension into the posterior cervical space.

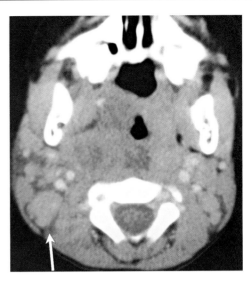

Fig. 5.117 Axial CT of a 5-year-old male shows a retropharyngeal abscess and reactive lymphadenopathy (*arrow*) in the right posterior cervical space.

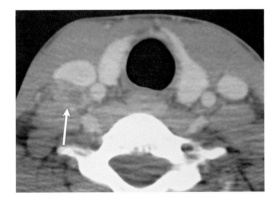

Fig. 5.118 Axial CT of a 30-year-old man with sarcoidosis shows an abnormally enlarged lymph node (*arrow*) with mixed intermediate and low attenuation located posterior to the right carotid space.

Table 5.7 *(cont.)*   Abnormalities of the posterior cervical space

Abnormalities	Imaging Findings	Comments
Cellulitis/Abscess (**Fig. 5.119**)	*CT:* Irregular soft tissue thickening ± adjacent lateral rim-enhancing fluid collection. *MRI:* Irregular soft tissue thickening with poorly defined slightly high signal on T2-weighted imaging (T2WI) and fat-suppressed T2WI. Abscesses are collections with high signal on T2WI surrounded by a peripheral rim of gadolinium contrast enhancement. Soft tissue thickening with slightly high to high signal on T2WI without a rim-enhancing collection can represent a phlegmon.	Cellulitis/abscess can result from trauma, infected branchial cleft cysts, suppurative lymphadenitis, or extension of infection from adjacent structures. Treatment is surgical drainage and/or antibiotics.

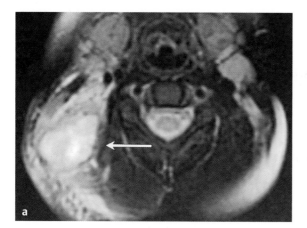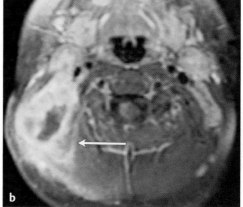

Fig. 5.119   **(a)** Axial fat-suppressed T2-weighted imaging of a 2-year-old male shows an abscess in the right posterior cervical space (*arrow*) with high signal centrally surrounded by ill-defined slightly high signal in the adjacent soft tissue. **(b)** Corresponding heterogeneous gadolinium contrast enhancement (*arrow*) is seen at the margins of the abscess and in the adjacent soft tissues on axial fat-suppressed T1-weighted imaging.

References

Ansa Cervicalis

1. Banneheka S. Anatomy of the ansa cervicalis: nerve fiber analysis. Anat Sci Int 2008;83(2):61–67

2. Khaki AA, Shokouhi G, Shoja MM, et al. Ansa cervicalis as a variant of spinal accessory nerve plexus: a case report. Clin Anat 2006;19(6):540–543

Anterior Cervical Space Lesions

3. Ojiri H, Tada S, Ujita M, et al. Infrahyoid spread of deep neck abscess: anatomical consideration. Eur Radiol 1998;8(6):955–959

4. Warshafsky D, Goldenberg D, Kanekar SG. Imaging anatomy of deep neck spaces. Otolaryngol Clin North Am 2012;45(6):1203–1221

5. Williams DW III. An imager's guide to normal neck anatomy. Semin Ultrasound CT MR 1997;18(3):157–181

Branchial Cleft Cyst

6. Acierno SP, Waldhausen JHT. Congenital cervical cysts, sinuses and fistulae. Otolaryngol Clin North Am 2007;40(1):161–176, vii–viii

7. Ahn JY, Kang SY, Lee CH, Yoon PH, Lee KS. Parapharyngeal branchial cleft cyst extending to the skull base: a lateral transzygomatic-transtemporal approach to the parapharyngeal space. Neurosurg Rev 2005;28(1):73–76

8. Dallan I, Seccia V, Bruschini L, Ciancia E, Franceschini SS. Parapharyngeal cyst: considerations on embryology, clinical evaluation, and surgical management. J Craniofac Surg 2008;19(6):1487–1490

9. Gaddikeri S, Vattoth S, Gaddikeri RS, et al. Congenital cystic neck masses: embryology and imaging appearances, with clinicopathological correlation. Curr Probl Diagn Radiol 2014;43(2):55–67

10. Gupta M, Gupta M. A rare parapharyngeal space branchial cleft cyst. BMJ Case Rep 2013;2013:6

12. Joshi MJ, Provenzano MJ, Smith RJH, Sato Y, Smoker WRK. The rare third branchial cleft cyst. AJNR Am J Neuroradiol 2009;30(9):1804–1806

13. Koeller KK, Alamo L, Adair CF, Smirniotopoulos JG. Congenital cystic masses of the neck: radiologic-pathologic correlation. Radiographics 1999;19(1):121–146, quiz 152–153

14. Panchbhai AS, Choudhary MS. Branchial cleft cyst at an unusual location: a rare case with a brief review. Dentomaxillofac Radiol 2012;41(8):696–702

15. Shin JH, Lee HK, Kim SY, et al. Parapharyngeal second branchial cyst manifesting as cranial nerve palsies: MR findings. AJNR Am J Neuroradiol 2001;22(3):510–512

Carotid Space Anatomy

16. Kuwada C, Mannion K, Aulino JM, Kanekar SG. Imaging of the carotid space. Otolaryngol Clin North Am 2012;45(6):1273–1292

17. Warshafsky D, Goldenberg D, Kanekar SG. Imaging anatomy of deep neck spaces. Otolaryngol Clin North Am 2012;45(6):1203–1221

Carotidynia

18. Inatomi Y, Nakajima M, Yonehara T, Hirano T. Contralateral recurrence of carotidynia during steroid therapy. J Stroke Cerebrovasc Dis 2014;23(1):184–186

19. Stanbro M, Gray BH, Kellicut DC. Carotidynia: revisiting an unfamiliar entity. Ann Vasc Surg 2011;25(8):1144–1153

20. van der Bogt KEA, Palm WM, Hamming JF. Carotidynia: a rare diagnosis in vascular surgery practice. EJVES Extra 2012;23:e18–e19

Esophageal Anomalies

21. Achildi O, Grewal H. Congenital anomalies of the esophagus. Otolaryngol Clin North Am 2007;40(1):219–244, viii

22. Fitoz S, Atasoy C, Yagmurlu A, Akyar S, Erden A, Dindar H. Three-dimensional CT of congenital esophageal atresia and distal tracheoesophageal fistula in neonates: preliminary results. AJR Am J Roentgenol 2000;175(5):1403–1407

23. Garge S, Rao KLN, Bawa M. The role of preoperative CT scan in patients with tracheoesophageal fistula: a review. J Pediatr Surg 2013;48(9):1966–1971

Gastrointestinal Duplication Cyst

24. Lee SY, Kim HY, Kim SH, Jung SE, Park KW. Thoracoscopic resection of a cervical esophageal duplication cyst in a 3-month-old infant: a case report. J Pediatr Surg 2013;48(4):873–875

25. Nayan S, Nguyen LHP, Nguyen VH, Daniel SJ, Emil S. Cervical esophageal duplication cyst: case report and review of the literature. J Pediatr Surg 2010;45(9):e1–e5

Hypopharyngeal and Laryngeal Infection

26. Bakir S, Tanriverdi MH, Gün R, et al. Deep neck space infections: a retrospective review of 173 cases. Am J Otolaryngol 2012;33(1):56–63

27. Capps EF, Kinsella JJ, Gupta M, Bhatki AM, Opatowsky MJ. Emergency imaging assessment of acute, nontraumatic conditions of the head and neck. Radiographics 2010;30(5):1335–1352

28. Maroldi R, Farina D, Ravanelli M, Lombardi D, Nicolai P. Emergency imaging assessment of deep neck space infections. Semin Ultrasound CT MR 2012;33(5):432–442

Kaposiform Hemangioendothelioma

29. Cooper JG, Edwards SL, Holmes JD. Kaposiform haemangioendothelioma: case report and review of the literature. Br J Plast Surg 2002;55(2):163–165

30. Lyons LL, North PE, Mac-Moune Lai F, Stoler MH, Folpe AL, Weiss SW. Kaposiform hemangioendothelioma: a study of 33 cases emphasizing its pathologic, immunophenotypic, and biologic uniqueness from juvenile hemangioma. Am J Surg Pathol 2004;28(5):559–568

31. Mukerji SS, Osborn AJ, Roberts J, Valdez TA. Kaposiform hemangioendothelioma (with Kasabach Merritt syndrome) of the head and neck: case report and review of the literature. Int J Pediatr Otorhinolaryngol 2009;73(10):1474–1476

32. Tsang WYW. Kaposiform haemangioendothelioma. In: Fletcher CDM, Unni KK, Mertens F, eds. World Health Organization Classification of Tumours. Pathology and Genetics of Tumours of Soft Tissue and Bone. Geneva: IARC Press; 2002:163–164

Klippel-Trenaunay Syndrome

33. Holak EJ, Pagel PS. Successful use of spinal anesthesia in a patient with severe Klippel-Trénaunay syndrome associated with upper airway abnormalities and chronic Kasabach-Merritt coagulopathy. J Anesth 2010;24(1):134–138

34. Oduber CEU, van der Horst CMAM, Hennekam RCM. Klippel-Trenaunay syndrome: diagnostic criteria and hypothesis on etiology. Ann Plast Surg 2008;60(2):217–223

Laryngeal Amyloidosis

35. Cankaya H, Egeli E, Unal O, Kiris M. Laryngeal amyloidosis: a rare cause of laryngocele. Clin Imaging 2002;26(2):86–88

36. Gallivan GJ, Gallivan HK. Laryngeal amyloidosis causing hoarseness and airway obstruction. J Voice 2010;24(2):235–239

Laryngeal Carcinoma

37. Beitler JJ, Muller S, Grist WJ, et al. Prognostic accuracy of computed tomography findings for patients with laryngeal cancer undergoing laryngectomy. J Clin Oncol 2010;28(14):2318–2322

38. Driessen JP, Caldas-Magalhaes J, Janssen LM, et al. Diffusion-weighted MR imaging in laryngeal and hypopharyngeal carcinoma: association between apparent diffusion coefficient and histologic findings. Radiology 2014;272(2):456–463

39. Kats SS, Muller S, Aiken A, et al. Laryngeal tumor volume as a predictor for thyroid cartilage penetration. Head Neck 2013;35(3):426–430

40. Kuno H, Onaya H, Fujii S, Ojiri H, Otani K, Satake M. Primary staging of laryngeal and hypopharyngeal cancer: CT, MR imaging and dual-energy CT. Eur J Radiol 2014;83(1):e23–e35

41. Maroldi R, Ravanelli M, Farina D. Magnetic resonance for laryngeal cancer. Curr Opin Otolaryngol Head Neck Surg 2014;22(2):131–139

Laryngeal Chondronecrosis

42. Beswick DM, Collins J, Nekhendzy V, Damrose EJ. Chondronecrosis of the larynx following the use of the laryngeal mask. Laryngoscope 2014; 10.1002/lary.24967

43. Takiguchi Y, Okamura HO, Kitamura K, Kishimoto S. Late laryngotracheal cartilage necrosis with external fistula 44 years after radiotherapy. J Laryngol Otol 2003;117(8):658–659

Laryngeal Chondrosarcoma

44. Sakai O, Curtin HD, Faquin WC, Fabian RL. Dedifferentiated chondrosarcoma of the larynx. AJNR Am J Neuroradiol 2000;21(3):584–586

Laryngeal Development

45. Som PM, Curtin HD. An updated and illustrated review of the complex embryology of the larynx and how laryngeal wens, atresias, and stenosis develop. Neurographics 2014;4:189–203

Laryngeal Myeloma

46. Sosna J, Slasky BS, Paltiel O, Pizov G, Libson E. Multiple myeloma involving the thyroid cartilage: case report. AJNR Am J Neuroradiol 2002;23(2):316–318

Laryngeal Schwannoma

47. Ebmeyer J, Reineke U, Gehl HB, et al. Schwannoma of the larynx. Head Neck Oncol 2009;1:24

Laryngeal Trauma

48. Becker M, Duboé PO, Platon A, et al. MDCT in the assessment of laryngeal trauma: value of 2D multiplanar and 3D reconstructions. AJR Am J Roentgenol 2013;201(4):W639–47

49. Becker M, Leuchter I, Platon A, Becker CD, Dulguerov P, Varoquaux A. Imaging of laryngeal trauma. Eur J Radiol 2014;83(1):142–154

Laryngocele

50. Alvi A, Weissman J, Myssiorek D, Narula S, Myers EN. Computed tomographic and magnetic resonance imaging characteristics of laryngocele and its variants. Am J Otolaryngol 1998;19(4):251–256

51. Dursun G, Ozgursoy OB, Beton S, Batikhan H. Current diagnosis and treatment of laryngocele in adults. Otolaryngol Head Neck Surg 2007;136(2):211–215

Larynx

52. Becker M, Burkhardt K, Dulguerov P, Allal A. Imaging of the larynx and hypopharynx. Eur J Radiol 2008;66(3):460–479

53. Huang BY, Solle M, Weissler MC. Larynx: anatomic imaging for diagnosis and management. Otolaryngol Clin North Am 2012; 45(6):1325–1361

Lemierre Syndrome

54. Hile LM, Gibbons MD, Hile DC. Lemierre syndrome complicating otitis externa: case report and literature review. J Emerg Med 2012;42(4):e77–e80

55. Ridgway JM, Parikh DA, Wright R, et al. Lemierre syndrome: a pediatric case series and review of literature. Am J Otolaryngol 2010;31(1):38–45

56. Righini CA, Karkas A, Tourniaire R, et al. Lemierre syndrome: study of 11 cases and literature review. Head Neck 2014;36(7):1044–1051

57. Syed MI, Baring D, Addidle M, Murray C, Adams C. Lemierre syndrome: two cases and a review. Laryngoscope 2007;117(9):1605–1610

Neck Teratoma

58. Gezer HO, Oğuzkurt P, Temiz A, Bolat FA, Hiçsönmez A. Huge neck masses causing respiratory distress in neonates: two cases of congenital cervical teratoma. Pediatr Neonatol 2014; doi: 10.1016/j.pedneo.2014.02.009

Parathyroid Adenomas

59. Beland MD, Mayo-Smith WW, Grand DJ, Machan JT, Monchik JM. Dynamic MDCT for localization of occult parathyroid adenomas in 26 patients with primary hyperparathyroidism. AJR Am J Roentgenol 2011;196(1):61–65

60. Carlson D. Parathyroid pathology: hyperparathyroidism and parathyroid tumors. Arch Pathol Lab Med 2010;134(11):1639–1644

61. Kunstman JW, Kirsch JD, Mahajan A, Udelsman R. Clinical review: Parathyroid localization and implications for clinical management. J Clin Endocrinol Metab 2013;98(3):902–912

62. Mariani G, Gulec SA, Rubello D, et al. Preoperative localization and radioguided parathyroid surgery. J Nucl Med 2003;44(9):1443–1458

63. Pasquali D, Di Matteo FM, Renzullo A, et al. Multiple endocrine neoplasia, the old and the new: a mini review. G Chir 2012;33(11-12):370–373

64. Patel CN, Salahudeen HM, Lansdown M, Scarsbrook AF. Clinical utility of ultrasound and 99mTc sestamibi SPECT/CT for preoperative localization of parathyroid adenoma in patients with primary hyperparathyroidism. Clin Radiol 2010;65(4):278–287

65. van Raalte DH, Vlot MC, Zwijnenburg A, Ten Kate RW. F18-choline PET/CT: a novel tool to localize parathyroid adenoma? Clin Endocrinol (Oxf) 2014; 10.1111/cen.12681

66. Weber T, Maier-Funk C, Ohlhauser D, et al. Accurate preoperative localization of parathyroid adenomas with C-11 methionine PET/CT. Ann Surg 2013;257(6):1124–1128

Parathyroid Carcinoma

67. Evangelista L, Sorgato N, Torresan F, et al. FDG-PET/CT and parathyroid carcinoma: Review of literature and illustrative case series. World J Clin Oncol 2011;2(10):348–354

68. Halenka M, Karasek D, Frysak Z. Four ultrasound and clinical pictures of parathyroid carcinoma. Case Rep Endocrinol 2012;2012:363690

69. Kassahun WT, Jonas S. Focus on parathyroid carcinoma. Int J Surg 2011;9(1):13–19

70. Schoretsanitis G, Daskalakis M, Melissas J, Tsiftsis DD. Parathyroid carcinoma: clinical presentation and management. Am J Otolaryngol 2009;30(4):277–280

71. Wei CH, Harari A. Parathyroid carcinoma: update and guidelines for management. Curr Treat Options Oncol 2012;13(1):11–23

Parathyroid Gland Hyperplasia

72. Oksüz MO, Dittmann H, Wicke C, et al. Accuracy of parathyroid imaging: a comparison of planar scintigraphy, SPECT, SPECT-CT, and C-11 methionine PET for the detection of parathyroid adenomas and glandular hyperplasia. Diagn Interv Radiol 2011;17(4):297–307

73. Welling RD, Olson JA Jr, Kranz PG, Eastwood JD, Hoang JK. Bilateral retropharyngeal parathyroid hyperplasia detected with 4D multidetector row CT. AJNR Am J Neuroradiol 2011;32(5):E80–E82

Parathyroid Gland Imaging

74. Kettle AG, O'Doherty MJ. Parathyroid imaging: how good is it and how should it be done? Semin Nucl Med 2006;36(3):206–211

75. Phillips CD, Shatzkes DR. Imaging of the parathyroid glands. Semin Ultrasound CT MR 2012;33(2):123–129

76. Phillips CD, Shatzkes DR. Imaging of the parathyroid glands. Semin Ultrasound CT MR 2012;33(2):123–129

Pharyngocele

77. Lee SW, Lee JY. Lateral pharyngeal diverticulum. Otolaryngol Head Neck Surg 2010;143(2):309–310

78. Naunheim M, Langerman A. Pharyngoceles: a photo-anatomic study and novel management. Laryngoscope 2013;123(7):1632–1638

79. Porcaro-Salles JM, Arantes Soares JM, Sousa AA, Meyer G, Sá Santos MH. Lateral pharyngeal diverticulum: a report of 3 cases. Ear Nose Throat J 2011;90(10):489–492

Postradiation Treatment Changes in Larynx

80. Mukherji SK, Weadock WJ. Imaging of the post-treatment larynx. Eur J Radiol 2002;44(2):108–119

Reinke's Edema

81. Díaz-Flores L, Gutiérrez R, del Pino García M, Álvarez-Argüelles H, Díaz-Flores L Jr, López-Campos D. CD34-positive fibroblasts in Reinke's edema. Laryngoscope 2014;124(3):E73–E80

82. Powell J, Cocks HC. Mucosal changes in laryngopharyngeal reflux—prevalence, sensitivity, specificity and assessment. Laryngoscope 2013;123(4):985–991

Relapsing Polychondritis

83. Cantarini L, Vitale A, Brizi MG, et al. Diagnosis and classification of relapsing polychondritis. J Autoimmun 2014;48-49:53–59

84. Childs LF, Rickert S, Wengerman OC, Lebovics R, Blitzer A. Laryngeal manifestations of relapsing polychondritis and a novel treatment option. J Voice 2012;26(5):587–589

85. Faix LE, Branstetter BF IV. Uncommon CT findings in relapsing polychondritis. AJNR Am J Neuroradiol 2005;26(8):2134–2136

86. Puéchal X, Terrier B, Mouthon L, Costedoat-Chalumeau N, Guillevin L, Le Jeunne C. Relapsing polychondritis. Joint Bone Spine 2014;81(2):118–124

87. Yamashita H, Takahashi H, Kubota K, et al. Utility of fluorodeoxyglucose positron emission tomography/computed tomography for early diagnosis and evaluation of disease activity of relapsing polychondritis: a case series and literature review. Rheumatology (Oxford) 2014;53(8):1482–1490

Retrostyloid Parapharyngeal Space Neoplasms

88. Varoquaux A, Fakhry N, Gabriel S, et al. Retrostyloid parapharyngeal space tumors: a clinician and imaging perspective. Eur J Radiol 2013;82(5):773–782

Rheumatoid Arthritis involving the Larynx

89. Berjawi G, Uthman I, Mahfoud L, et al. Cricothyroid joint abnormalities in patients with rheumatoid arthritis. J Voice 2010;24(6):732–737
90. Greco A, Fusconi M, Macri GF, et al. Cricoarytenoid joint involvement in rheumatoid arthritis: radiologic evaluation. Am J Otolaryngol 2012;33(6):753–755

Sarcomas in the Neck

91. Razek AA, Huang BY. Soft tissue tumors of the head and neck: imaging-based review of the WHO classification. Radiographics 2011;31(7):1923–1954

Thrombosis of the Internal Jugular Vein

92. Gallanos M, Hafner JW. Posttraumatic internal jugular vein thrombosis presenting as a painful neck mass in a child. Pediatr Emerg Care 2008;24(8):542–545
93. Ohba K, Matsushita A, Yamashita M, et al. The importance of imaging procedures in evaluating painful neck masses: two patients with a painful internal jugular vein thrombosis. Thyroid 2012;22(5):556–557

Thyroglossal Duct Cyst

94. Ahuja AT, Wong KT, King AD, Yuen EHY. Imaging for thyroglossal duct cyst: the bare essentials. Clin Radiol 2005;60(2):141–148
95. Gaddikeri S, Vattoth S, Gaddikeri RS, et al. Congenital cystic neck masses: embryology and imaging appearances, with clinicopathological correlation. Curr Probl Diagn Radiol 2014;43(2):55–67
96. Sameer KSM, Mohanty S, Correa MMA, Das K. Lingual thyroglossal duct cysts—a review. Int J Pediatr Otorhinolaryngol 2012;76(2):165–168

Thyroid Gland Cancer

97. Aiken AH. Imaging of thyroid cancer. Semin Ultrasound CT MR 2012;33(2):138–149
98. Gupta N, Norbu C, Goswami B, et al. Role of dynamic MRI in differentiating benign from malignant follicular thyroid nodule. Auris Nasus Larynx 2011;38(6):718–723
99. Loevner LA. Imaging of the thyroid gland. Semin Ultrasound CT MR 1996;17(6):539–562

100. Nachiappan AC, Metwalli ZA, Hailey BS, Patel RA, Ostrowski ML, Wynne DM. The thyroid: review of imaging features and biopsy techniques with radiologic-pathologic correlation. Radiographics 2014;34(2):276–293
101. Yuan Y, Yue XH, Tao XF. The diagnostic value of dynamic contrast-enhanced MRI for thyroid tumors. Eur J Radiol 2012;81(11):3313–3318

Thyroid Gland Development

102. Lu WH, Feng L, Sang JZ, et al. Various presentations of fourth branchial pouch sinus tract during surgery. Acta Otolaryngol 2012;132(5):540–545
103. Nicoucar K, Giger R, Pope HG Jr, Jaecklin T, Dulguerov P. Management of congenital fourth branchial arch anomalies: a review and analysis of published cases. J Pediatr Surg 2009;44(7):1432–1439
104. Policeni BA, Smoker WRK, Reede DL. Anatomy and embryology of the thyroid and parathyroid glands. Semin Ultrasound CT MR 2012;33(2):104–114
105. Shrime M, Kacker A, Bent J, Ward RF. Fourth branchial complex anomalies: a case series. Int J Pediatr Otorhinolaryngol 2003;67(11):1227–1233
106. Thomas B, Shroff M, Forte V, Blaser S, James A. Revisiting imaging features and the embryologic basis of third and fourth branchial anomalies. AJNR Am J Neuroradiol 2010;31(4):755–760

Thyroid Gland: Inflammatory Disease

107. Fujita A, Sakai O, Chapman MN, Sugimoto H. IgG4-related disease of the head and neck: CT and MR imaging manifestations. Radiographics 2012;32(7):1945–1958
108. Juliano AFY, Cunnane MB. Benign conditions of the thyroid gland. Semin Ultrasound CT MR 2012;33(2):130–137
109. Masuoka H, Miyauchi A, Tomoda C, et al. Imaging studies in sixty patients with acute suppurative thyroiditis. Thyroid 2011;21(10):1075–1080

Thyroid Gland Nodules

110. Hoang JK, Raduazo P, Yousem DM, Eastwood JD. What to do with incidental thyroid nodules on imaging? An approach for the radiologist. Semin Ultrasound CT MR 2012;33(2):150–157
111. Schueller-Weidekamm C, Schueller G, Kaserer K, et al. Diagnostic value of sonography, ultrasound-guided fine-needle aspiration cytology, and diffusion-weighted MRI in the characterization of cold thyroid nodules. Eur J Radiol 2010;73(3):538–544

Zenker's Diverticulum

112. Ferreira LE, Simmons DT, Baron TH. Zenker's diverticula: pathophysiology, clinical presentation, and flexible endoscopic management. Dis Esophagus 2008;21(1):1–8
113. Grant PD, Morgan DE, Scholz FJ, Canon CL. Pharyngeal dysphagia: what the radiologist needs to know. Curr Probl Diagn Radiol 2009;38(1):17–32

Chapter 6

Lesions That Can Involve Both Suprahyoid and Infrahyoid Neck

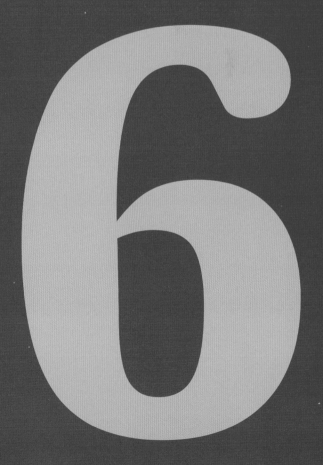

6 Lesions That Can Involve Both Suprahyoid and Infrahyoid Neck

Table 6.1	Cervical lymphadenopathy
Table 6.2	Prevertebral (perivertebral) space abnormalities

Introduction

Cervical Lymphadenopathy

Up to 40% of the lymph nodes in the body are located in the head and neck (**Fig. 6.1**). Malignant tumor cells commonly enter lymph nodes via invasion of the lymphatic system, although invasion can occur via a hematogenous pathway.

Once within nodes, tumor cells secrete extracellular proteases and plasminogen activators, which enable neoplastic spread through the lymph nodes to involve the lymphatic system, often in specific pathways. Based on the primary tumor location, neoplastic cells often follow the drainage patterns of the involved portions of the lymphatic system (**Box 6.1** and **Box 6.2**). Identification of pathologic lymph nodes is important for appropriate staging of tumors and treatment planning.

Box 6.1 Classification and Location of Lymph Nodes in the Head and Neck

Level	Location
Ia	Submental nodes: Below mylohyoid muscle between anterior bellies of digastric muscles above hyoid bone, posterior margin of submandibular gland
Ib	Submandibular nodes: Below mylohyoid muscle, lateral to digastric muscles
II	Anterior cervical/upper jugular nodes: From skull base to hyoid bone, posterior to submandibular gland, and medial to the sternocleidomastoid muscle (SCM)
IIa	Level II nodes located anterior to the jugular vein
IIb	Level II nodes located posterior to the jugular vein
III	Middle jugular nodes: From hyoid bone to cricoid, medial to SCM
IV	Lower jugular nodes: From cricoid to level of clavicles, lateral to carotid arteries
V	Posterior compartment/spinal accessory: Posterior to SCM from skull base to level of clavicles
Va	Level V nodes from skull base to cricoid
Vb	Level V nodes from cricoid to level of clavicles
VI	Visceral compartment: Medial to carotid arteries from hyoid bone to top of manubrium
VII	Superior mediastinal nodes: Between carotid arteries from the level of the manubrium to the level of the innominate vein

Box 6.2   Lymphatic Drainage Pathways

Level	Drainage Site
Retropharyngeal Nodes	Nasopharynx, sinonasal region, oral cavity
I	Sinonasal region, lip, oral cavity
II	Posterior oral cavity, oropharynx, parotid gland, supraglottic larynx
III	Hypopharynx, glottic and subglottic regions
IV	Subglottic region, esophagus, thyroid gland
V	Nasopharynx, superficial soft tissue of posterior scalp and neck
VI	Subglottic region, esophagus, thyroid gland
VII	Subglottic region, esophagus, thyroid gland
Supraclavicular Nodes	Thorax

Lymph Node Imaging Features

Normal lymph nodes are typically small, measuring 1 to 3 mm, have reniform shapes with a fatty hilum, and have circumscribed margins.

Enlarged nonmalignant nodes can occur when an immune response is initiated, causing follicular hyperplasia within the challenged lymph nodes. These reactive nodes have intermediate attenuation and sharp margins on CT, and on MRI they have homogeneous low-intermediate signal on T1-weighted imaging (T1WI) and slightly high signal on T2-weighted imaging (T2WI). Reactive lymph nodes usually have an oblong or "lima-bean" shape with a longitudinal to axial dimension ratio of > 2. Reactive nodes can retain the normal fatty appearance of the nodal hila.

Malignant lymph nodes have features associated with neoplastic nodal disease, including: changes in nodal size and shape, nodal necrosis, calcifications, heterogeneous nodal appearance on CT and MRI reflecting tumor cell characteristics, extracapsular tumor spread, and invasion of adjacent structures.

Nodal size alone is not a reliable marker for neoplastic disease. Lymph nodes can become enlarged from a hyperplastic response to inflammation. Using various size thresholds for neoplastic disease can alter the sensitivity and specificity of differential diagnosis. Using a minimal axial dimension threshold of 1 cm for neoplastic disease resulted in 88% sensitivity and 39% specificity (1). Using a minimum of 1.5 cm resulted in decreased sensitivity (56%) but increased specificity of 84%.[1] Measurements commonly used include minimal axial diameters of > 1.5 cm for nodes at levels I and II, and > 1 cm for the rest of the neck, although smaller lymph nodes can still be malignant.

As for nodal shape, malignant lymph nodes tend to be rounded or spheroid and often have a longitudinal to axial dimension ratio of < 2. Tumor infiltration typically replaces the normal fatty hila of lymph nodes.

Nodal necrosis is the most reliable imaging finding for neoplastic disease, with a specificity of over 90%. The occurrence of nodal necrosis increases with nodal size, although it can be seen with nodes of < 1 cm. On CT, nodal necrosis is seen as a zone of low attenuation surrounded by enhancing tissue at the involved node. On MRI, malignant nodes with necrosis have low-intermediate signal on T1WI, slightly high to high signal on T2WI and fat-suppressed (FS) T2WI, and peripheral solid gadolinium (Gd) contrast enhancement. Human papillomavirus-associated squamous cell carcinoma and thyroid carcinomas can have metastatic nodes that are mostly cystic.

Unlike calcified mediastinal lymph nodes, which are mostly caused by nonmalignant disease, calcified cervical lymph nodes are commonly associated with malignancy. Nodal calcifications can be seen with metastatic medullary or papillary thyroid carcinomas, as well as with mucinous adenocarcinomas, treated lymphoma or squamous cell carcinoma, and tuberculosis.

Extracapsular spread of tumor from involved lymph nodes is an important histologic finding affecting the patient's prognosis and treatment options. Findings of extracapsular spread on CT and MRI include irregular nodal margins and irregular contrast enhancement that extends into the adjacent tissue.

Invasion of adjacent structures can be evidenced, for example, as enlarged malignant nodes that coalesce and invade adjacent structures, including the carotid space. Invasion of the carotid artery can contraindicate surgery. If circumferential involvement by neoplastic nodes is less than 180 degrees, then direct vascular invasion is unlikely. Circumferential involvement by more than 270 degrees is usually indicative of vascular invasion. Deformation of the arterial wall is a marker of invasion of the carotid artery.

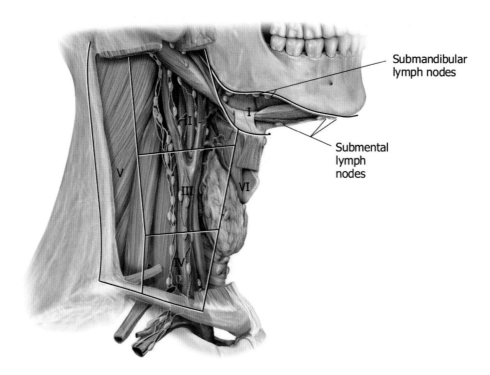

Fig. 6.1 Locations of cervical lymph node stations. From THIEME Atlas of Anatomy: Head and Neuroanatomy, © Thieme 2007, Illustration by Karl Wesker.

Table 6.1 Cervical lymphadenopathy

- Neoplastic Adenopathy
  - Metastatic disease
  - Non-Hodgkin lymphoma (NHL) and Hodgkin disease (HD)
  - Leukemia
- Infection
  - Reactive and presuppurative nodes
  - Suppurative nodes
  - Cat-scratch disease
  - Mycobacterial adenopathy (Tuberculous adenopathy)
  - Epstein-Barr viral lymphadenopathy—Mononucleosis
- Inflammatory Disease
  - Sarcoidosis
  - Langerhans' cell histiocytosis
  - Sinus histiocytosis (Rosai-Dorfman disease)
  - Castleman's disease
  - Kimura disease

Table 6.1   Cervical lymphadenopathy

Lymphadenopathy	Imaging Findings	Comments
Neoplastic Adenopathy		
Metastatic disease (**Fig. 6.2**, **Fig. 6.3**, **Fig. 6.4**, and **Fig. 6.5**)	*MRI:* Enlarged spheroid or ovoid nodes that often have low-intermediate signal on T1-weighted imaging, intermediate-high signal on T2-weighted imaging (T2WI), ± high signal zones on T2WI (necrosis), ± irregular margins (capsule invasion), ± decreased ADC values on diffusion-weighted imaging ($< 1.4 \times 10^{-3}$ mm^2/sec), and variable gadolinium contrast enhancement. Intranodal cystic changes are commonly seen with metastases from oropharyngeal squamous cell cancers caused by human papillomavirus (HPV) infection. *CT:* Involved nodes usually have low-intermediate attenuation, ± irregular margins (capsule invasion), ± low-attenuation zones (necrosis), and variable contrast enhancement. Usually measure more than 8 mm in short axis. *Ultrasound:* Enlarged hypoechoic nodes, ± cystic-necrotic zones, ± irregular margins (capsule invasion). Color Doppler often shows hypervascularity. *PET/CT:* Increased nodal uptake of F-18 FDG.	Metastatic tumor involving cervical lymph nodes can result from primary neck neoplasms, such as squamous cell carcinoma or thyroid cancer. Can result from spread from primary extracranial tumor source: lung > breast > GI > GU > melanoma. Can occur as single or multiple well-circumscribed or poorly defined lesions. Metastatic tumor may have variable destructive or infiltrative changes involving single or multiple sites of involvement.

(continued on page 597)

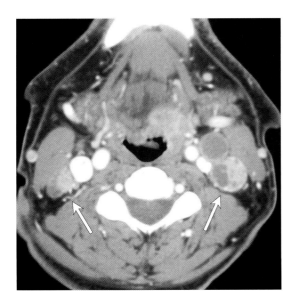

Fig. 6.2   Axial postcontrast CT of a 62-year-old man with squamous cell carcinoma involving the left side of the tongue shows level II metastatic lymphadenopathy (*arrows*) with heterogeneous contrast enhancement.

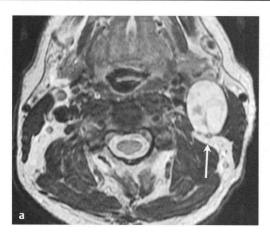
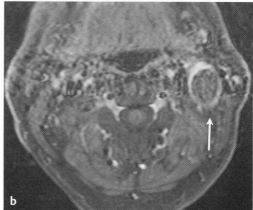

Fig. 6.3 **(a)** Axial T2-weighted imaging of a patient with an HPV-related oropharyngeal squamous cell carcinoma shows a cystic metastatic lymph node (*arrow*) with heterogeneous high signal. **(b)** Fat-suppressed T1-weighted imaging shows low signal centrally surrounded by a thin gadolinium-enhancing rim (*arrow*).

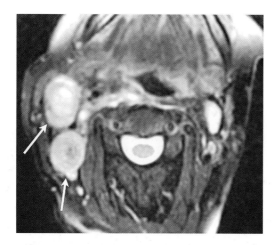

Fig. 6.4 Axial fat-suppressed T2-weighted imaging of a patient with nasopharyngeal carcinoma shows abnormally enlarged metastatic lymph nodes, which have heterogeneous slightly high and high signal (*arrows*).

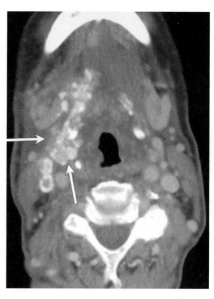

Fig. 6.5 Postcontrast CT of a patient with oropharyngeal squamous cell carcinoma treated with radiation shows conglomerate metastatic lymph nodes on the right containing dystrophic calcifications (*arrows*).

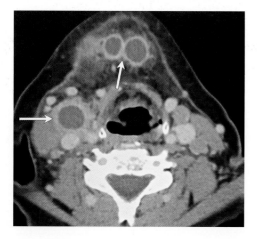

Fig. 6.6 Axial postcontrast CT of a patient with T-cell non-Hodgkin lymphoma shows abnormally enlarged lymph nodes that have low attenuation centrally surrounded by peripheral rims of enhancement (*arrows*).

Table 6.1 *(cont.)* Cervical lymphadenopathy

Lymphadenopathy	Imaging Findings	Comments
Non-Hodgkin lymphoma (NHL) and Hodgkin disease (HD) (**Fig. 6.6**)	*CT:* Enlarged lymph nodes with soft tissue attenuation, ± contrast enhancement. *MRI:* Enlarged lymph nodes with intermediate signal on T1-weighted imaging and slightly high signal on T2-weighted imaging, ± gadolinium contrast enhancement. Necrosis and cystic changes rarely occur. *Ultrasound:* Enlarged hypoechoic nodes with circumscribed margins. Color Doppler often shows hypervascularity. *PET/CT:* Increased nodal uptake of F-18 FDG.	Both NHL and HD involve cervical lymph nodes.
Leukemia (**Fig. 6.7** and **Fig. 6.8**)	*CT:* Enlarged lymph nodes with soft tissue attenuation, ± contrast enhancement. *MRI:* Enlarged lymph nodes with intermediate signal on T1-weighted imaging and slightly high signal on T2-weighted imaging, ± gadolinium contrast enhancement. Necrosis and cystic changes rarely occur. *Ultrasound:* Enlarged hypoechoic nodes with circumscribed margins. *PET/CT:* Increased nodal uptake of F-18 FDG.	Adenopathy can be a presentation with acute lymphocytic leukemia (ALL) in children or with chronic lymphocytic leukemia (CLL) in adults.

(continued on page 598)

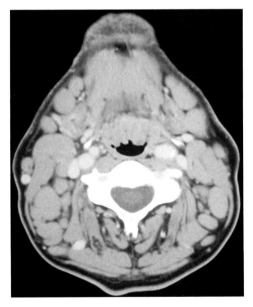

Fig. 6.7 Axial CT of a 61-year-old man with multiple enlarged cervical lymph nodes. The patient had a history of chronic lymphocytic leukemia (CLL) and development of aggressive B-cell lymphoma (Richter's transformation).

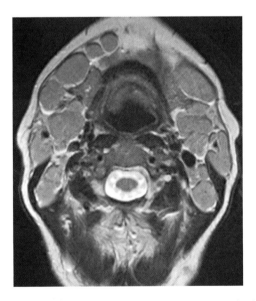

Fig. 6.8 Axial T2-weighted imaging of a patient with chronic lymphocytic leukemia (CLL) shows multiple abnormally enlarged cervical lymph nodes, which have intermediate signal.

Table 6.1 *(cont.)* Cervical lymphadenopathy

Lymphadenopathy	Imaging Findings	Comments
Infection		
Reactive and presuppurative nodes (**Fig. 6.9** and **Fig. 6.10**)	*CT:* *Reactive adenopathy* can have enlarged lymph nodes that measure < 12 mm, with preservation of nodal architecture, ± prominent single hilar vessel or branching vascular pattern. *Presuppurative nodes* can be enlarged lymph and are associated with loss of the fatty hilum, slightly decreased attenuation, increased contrast enhancement, and reticulation of adjacent fat. *MRI:* Enlarged *presuppurative* nodes have intermediate signal on T1-weighted imaging and slightly high signal on T2-weighted imaging, and show gadolinium contrast enhancement. *Ultrasound: Reactive nodes* are usually enlarged and hypoechoic and have circumscribed margins. *PET/CT:* Increased nodal uptake of F-18 FDG.	Enlarged lymph nodes, which usually measure < 12 mm, with preservation of nodal architecture, can result from infections of the oral cavity, oropharynx, and hypopharynx, and are referred to as reactive adenopathy or presuppurative lymphadenitis. In children, lymphadenitis can result from upper respiratory viral infections or bacterial infections, such as those caused by *Staphyloccous aureus* and *Streptococcus pyogenes*.
Suppurative nodes	*CT:* Suppurative lymph nodes are typically enlarged, and can have zones with low attenuation centrally surrounded by a rim of contrast enhancement. *MRI:* Suppurative nodes have low-intermediate signal on T1-weighted imaging and slightly high to high signal on T2-weighted imaging (T2WI), and show rim gadolinium (Gd) contrast enhancement. Irregular increased signal on T2WI and Gd contrast enhancement are typically seen in the adjacent soft tissue. *Ultrasound:* Suppurative nodes range from enlarged, hypoechoic, hyperemic nodes to lobulated anechoic/septated lesions with mild acoustic enhancement. *PET/CT:* Increased nodal uptake of F-18 FDG.	Enlarged lymph nodes from bacterial infection can undergo liquefactive necrosis (suppurative adenitis)—purulent lymph nodes. Purulent lymph nodes measure up to 4.5 cm. Treatment with IV antibiotics is usually effective when the suppurative low-attenuation nodes measure less than 2–3 cm. Larger suppurative lymph nodes usually require surgical drainage, especially when they cause airway compromise. In adults, suppurative adenitis often results from trauma or procedural or surgical complications. Gram-positive cocci are common pathogens for suppurative adenitis in adults.
Cat-scratch disease (**Fig. 6.11**)	*CT:* Enlarged lymph nodes associated with loss of the fatty hilum, slightly decreased attenuation, increased contrast enhancement, and reticulation of adjacent fat. *MRI:* Enlarged nodes have low-intermediate signal on T1-weighted imaging and slightly high to high signal on T2-weighted imaging (T2WI), + gadolinium (Gd) contrast enhancement. Irregular increased signal on T2WI and Gd contrast enhancement are typically seen in the adjacent soft tissue. *Ultrasound:* Findings range from enlarged, hypoechoic, hyperemic nodes to lobulated anechoic/septated lesions with mild acoustic enhancement.	Infection by the gram-negative bacillus *Bartonella henselae* can result in a self-limited regional granulomatous adenitis. This infection usually occurs in patients < 30 years old and is often related to contact with cats (cat-scratch disease).

(continued on page 600)

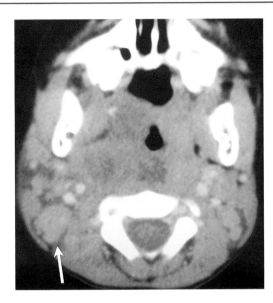

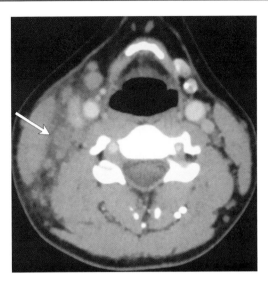

Fig. 6.9 Axial CT of a 5-year-old male with a retropharyngeal abscess and reactive lymphadenopathy (*arrow*) in the right posterior cervical space.

Fig. 6.10 Axial CT of a 32-year-old woman with a dental infection shows a presuppurative lymph node (*arrow*) on the right, with loss of the fatty hilum, slightly decreased attenuation, and reticulation of adjacent fat.

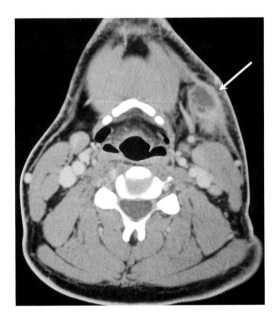

Fig. 6.11 Axial CT shows an abnormally enlarged lymph node (*arrow*) with low attenuation centrally surrounded by an irregular rim with ill-defined margin secondary to infection by the gram-negative bacillus *Bartonella henselae*—cat-scratch disease.

(continued on page 602)

Table 6.1 *(cont.)* Cervical lymphadenopathy

Lymphadenopathy	Imaging Findings	Comments
Mycobacterial adenopathy (Tuberculous adenopathy) (**Fig. 6.12**)	*CT:* Enlarged lymph nodes are associated with loss of the fatty hilum, slightly decreased attenuation centrally, peripheral contrast enhancement, and reticulation of adjacent fat, ± central necrosis, ± conglomeration/matting of lymph nodes, ± adjacent skin thickening, ± draining sinus tracts, ± nodal calcifications. *MRI:* Enlarged nodes have intermediate signal on T1-weighted imaging and slightly high signal on T2-weighted imaging, and show gadolinium contrast enhancement. *Ultrasound:* Nodes are usually enlarged and hypoechoic and can have circumscribed and/or slightly irregular margins. Hilar vascularity can be seen. *PET/CT:* Increased nodal uptake of F-18 FDG with active disease.	Granulomatous disease causing lymphadenopathy is caused by *Mycobacterium tuberculosis* and the atypical mycobacteria, *M. avium intracellulare, M. bovis,* and *M. kansasii.*
Epstein-Barr viral lymphadenopathy— Mononucleosis (**Fig. 6.13**)	*CT and MRI:* Multiple enlarged lymph nodes in the neck, + contrast enhancement. Often associated with enlargement of adenoids and palatine tonsils, ± enlargement of parotid and submandibular glands. *Ultrasound:* Enlarged rounded nodes. On Doppler, enlarged nodes often have a symmetric radial pattern of vessels.	In young adults, generalized lymphadenopathy can result from the Epstein-Barr virus infection (mononucleosis). Mononucleosis is a self-limited disease that is often associated with fever, malaise, pharyngotonsillitis, lymphadenopathy, and/or hepatosplenomegaly. Can involve major salivary glands. Other causes of viral lymphadenopathy include cytomegalovirus infection, mumps paramyxovirus, and infection by human T-cell lymphotropic virus type III (HIV), which can cause AIDS.
Inflammatory Disease		
Sarcoidosis (**Fig. 6.14**)	*MRI:* Single or multiple enlarged cervical lymph nodes with low to intermediate signal on T1-weighted imaging and slightly high signal on T2-weighted imaging (T2WI) and fat-suppressed T2WI. After gadolinium (Gd) contrast administration, involved nodes can show Gd contrast enhancement. Nodes can have circumscribed or slightly irregular margins. *CT:* Single or multiple enlarged lymph nodes with soft tissue attenuation. *Nuclear medicine:* Increased uptake of gallium 67 citrate. *PET/CT:* Increased uptake of F-18 FDG.	Sarcoidosis is a multisystem, noncaseating, granulomatous disease of uncertain etiology that can cause lymphadenopathy in 10–20% of cases. Treatment includes oral corticosteroids and surgical debulking.

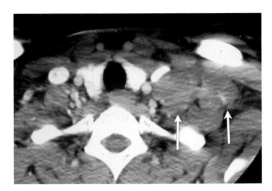

Fig. 6.12   Axial postcontrast CT of a 29-year-old woman with left supraclavicular tuberculous adenopathy (*arrows*).

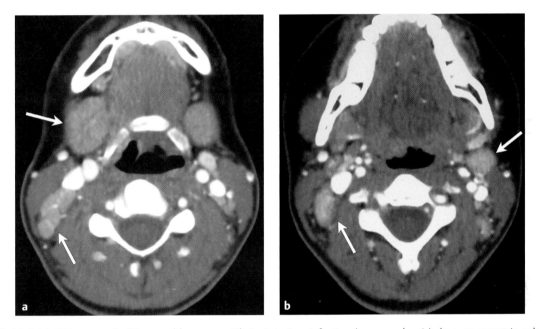

Fig. 6.13   **(a,b)** Axial CT images of a 22-year-old woman with Epstein-Barr infection (mononucleosis) show asymmetric enlargement of the right submandibular gland (*upper arrow* in **a**) and multiple enlarged contrast-enhancing cervical lymph nodes (*lower arrow* in **a**, and *both arrows* in **b**).

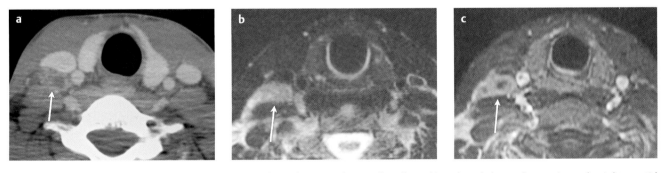

Fig. 6.14   **(a)** Axial CT of a 30-year-old man with sarcoidosis shows an abnormally enlarged lymph node located posterior to the right carotid space that has mixed intermediate and low attenuation (*arrow*). **(b)** On MRI, there is slightly high signal on axial fat-suppressed T2-weighted imaging (*arrow*) and **(c)** heterogeneous gadolinium contrast enhancement on axial fat-suppressed T1-weighted imaging (*arrow*).

Table 6.1 *(cont.)* Cervical lymphadenopathy

Lymphadenopathy	Imaging Findings	Comments
Langerhans' cell histiocytosis (**Fig. 6.15**)	*MRI:* Single or multiple enlarged cervical lymph nodes with low to intermediate signal on T1-weighted imaging and slightly high signal on T2-weighted imaging (T2WI) and fat-suppressed T2WI. After gadolinium (Gd) contrast administration, involved nodes can show Gd contrast enhancement. *CT:* Single or multiple enlarged lymph nodes with soft tissue attenuation. *PET/CT:* Increased uptake of F-18 FDG-glucose with active disease.	Disorder of reticuloendothelial system in which bone marrow-derived macrophages and dendritic Langerhans' cells infiltrate various organs as focal lesions or in diffuse patterns. Langerhans' cells have eccentrically located ovoid or convoluted nuclei within pale to eosinophilic cytoplasm. Lesions often consist of Langerhans' cells, macrophages, plasma cells, and eosinophils. Lesions are immunoreactive to S-100, CD1a, CD207, HLA-DR, and β_2-microglobulin. Prevalence of 2 per 100,000 in children < 15 years old; only a third of lesions occur in adults. Localized lesions (eosinophilic granuloma) can be single or multiple in bone. Intradural lesions occur at pituitary stalk/hypothalamus and can present with diabetes insipidus. Lesions rarely occur in brain tissue (< 4% of patients with Langerhans' cell histiocytosis). Involvement of lymph nodes occurs in 20% of cases. Occurs in patients with median age = 10 years (average age = 13.5 years), and peak incidence is between 5 and 10 years (80–85% of cases occur in patients < 30 years old).
Sinus histiocytosis (Rosai-Dorfman disease)	*MRI:* Single or multiple enlarged cervical lymph nodes with low to intermediate signal on T1-weighted imaging and slightly high signal on T2-weighted imaging (T2WI) and fat-suppressed T2WI. After gadolinium (Gd) contrast administration, involved nodes can show Gd contrast enhancement. *CT:* Single or multiple enlarged lymph nodes with soft tissue attenuation. *PET/CT:* Increased uptake of F-18 FDG-glucose with active disease.	Rare benign histiocytosis in which collections of lymphoplasmacytic cells and histiocytes occur in fibrous stroma within various tissues, such as lymph nodes, bone, orbits, nasal cavity, and intracranial dura. Immunoreactive to S-100 protein and CD68 (macrophages); no immunoreactivity to CD1a (Langerhans' cell marker). Occurs in children and young adults (peak age between 30 and 40 years).
Castleman's disease (**Fig. 6.16**)	*CT and MRI:* *Multicentric Castleman's disease:* Multiple enlarged lymph nodes with low-intermediate attenuation on CT, + contrast enhancement, and intermediate signal on T1-weighted imaging and intermediate to slightly high signal on T2-weighted imaging on MRI, + gadolinium (Gd) contrast enhancement in the thorax, abdomen, and/or neck, ± calcifications. *Unicentric Castleman's disease:* Solitary mass lesion, with intermediate attenuation on CT, + contrast enhancement. Intermediate signal on T1-weighted imaging and intermediate to slightly high signal on T2-weighted imaging, + gadolinium contrast enhancement. *Nuclear medicine:* Lymph node uptake of gallium 67. *PET/CT:* Increased uptake of F-18 FDG-glucose with active disease.	Castleman's disease is also known as angiofollicular lymph node hyperplasia or giant lymph node hyperplasia.. Adenopathy occurs in the thorax (70%), abdomen and pelvis (10–15%), and neck (10–15%). There are two types, multicentric and unicentric. The multicentric type consists of multiple enlarged lymph nodes with extensive accumulation of polyclonal plasma cells in the interfollicular regions. Patients with the multicentric type can also have hepatosplenomegaly and usually have a worse prognosis than those with the unicentric type. One variant of the multicentric type occurs in immunocompromised or HIV-positive patients and is related to infection by human herpesvirus type 8 (HHV-8). Treatment includes chemotherapy and rituximab. In the unicentric type, lymph nodes contain hyalinized vascular follicles with interfollicular capillary proliferations. Unicentric Castleman's can be treated with surgery and/or radiation, and it usually has a favorable prognosis.

Lymphadenopathy	Imaging Findings	Comments
Kimura disease	*MRI:* Enlarged lymph nodes with intermediate signal on T1-weighted imaging, slightly high to high signal on T2-weighted imaging, and gadolinium contrast enhancement. *CT:* Ill-defined lesions with intermediate attenuation. Lymphadenopathy occurs in up to 80% of cases, and enlarged lymph nodes usually show prominent contrast enhancement.	Kimura disease, also referred to as eosinophilic lymphogranuloma, is an immune-mediated inflammatory disease with multiple or solitary lesions in the head and neck (parotid gland, buccal space, lacrimal gland, submandibular gland, subcutaneous tissue) as well as enlarged lymph nodes. Lesions have a folliculoid configuration containing eosinophils, lymphocytes, plasma cells, and mast cells, in association with stromal fibrosis and vascular proliferation. May represent a self-limited autoimmune response with altered T-cell regulation and IgE-mediated type 1 hypersensitivity. Patients typically have > 10% hypereosinophilia and elevated IgE levels (800–35,000 IU/mL). Kimura disease usually occurs in Asian males (mean age = 32 years). Treatment includes surgery, systemic corticosteroids, cytotoxic medications, and/or cyclosporine.

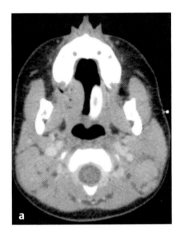 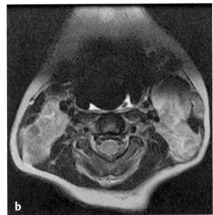 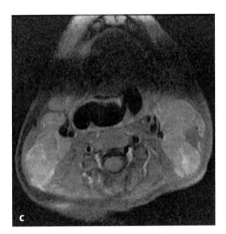

Fig. 6.15   **(a)** Axial CT of a patient with Langerhans' cell histiocytosis shows multiple abnormally enlarged cervical lymph nodes bilaterally that have **(b)** heterogeneous intermediate to slightly high signal on axial T2-weighted imaging, and **(c)** corresponding mild gadolinium contrast enhancement on axial fat-suppressed T1-weighted imaging.

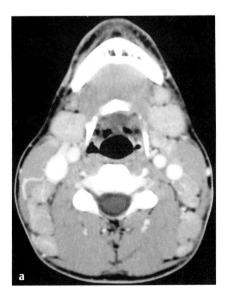 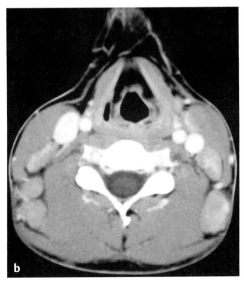

Fig. 6.16 **(a,b)** Axial postcontrast CT images of an 18-year-old man with Castleman's disease show multiple, abnormally enlarged, enhancing lymph nodes in both sides of the neck.

Prevertebral (Perivertebral) Space Abnormalities

The prevertebral (perivertebral) space is located posterior to the danger space and posteromedial to the carotid space (**Fig. 6.17**). The prevertebral space contains the prevertebral fascia (deep layer of the deep cervical fascia), longus colli and other paraspinal muscles, vertebrae, intervertebral disks, spinal canal, vertebral arteries and veins, phrenic nerve, and roots of the brachial plexus. Neoplastic or inflammatory involvement of the prevertebral space can occur by direct extension of vertebral lesions within the prevertebral space or by invasion by head and neck lesions.

The prevertebral space is enclosed by one of the deep layers of the deep cervical fascia (DCF). The deep layer of the DCF has a posterior major portion (also referred to as the prevertebral fascial layer) that encloses the pre-vertebral and paravertebral muscles and vertebral column and extends from the skull base down to the coccyx. This layer fuses with the anterior longitudinal ligament at the T3 level. The other layer of the DCF is the alar fascia, which is located anterior to the prevertebral fascial layer of the DCF, and extends from the skull base to the upper thoracic levels where it fuses with the visceral fascia (infrahyoid extension of the buccopharyngeal fascia/middle layer of the deep cervical fascia). In the suprahyoid neck, the alar fascial layer forms the posterior border of the retropharyngeal space. The inferior border of the retropharyngeal space is often at the C7–T1 level. Fusion of the visceral fascia with the alar fascia can, however, vary from the C6 to T4 levels. Between the alar fascia and the prevertebral fascia of the DCF is the potential danger space, which consists of loose areolar tissue. The inferior border of the danger space is at the level the diaphragm. Infections or neoplasms that extend into the retropharyngeal or danger spaces can spread between the skull base and mediastinum.

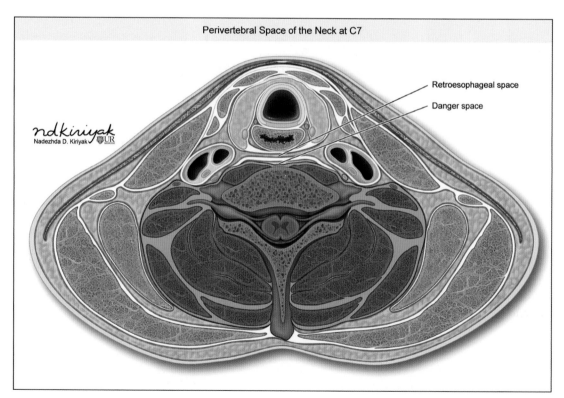

Fig. 6.17 Axial illustration shows the perivertebral space in color.

Table 6.2   Prevertebral (perivertebral) space abnormalities

- Malignant Vertebral Lesions
  - Metastatic osseous neoplasms
  - Myeloma/Plasmacytoma
  - Vertebral lymphoma
  - Leukemia
  - Chordoma
  - Chondrosarcoma
  - Osteosarcoma
- Spread from Malignant Neck Lesions
  - Squamous cell carcinoma
  - Nasopharyngeal carcinoma
  - Lymphoma
  - Thyroid cancer
  - Nodal metastases
  - Hemangioendothelioma
- Benign Tumors
  - Neurofibroma
  - Lipoma
  - Hemangioma

- Infection
  - Vertebral osteomyelitis
  - Tuberculous vertebral osteomyelitis
  - Perivertebral infection
  - Retropharyngeal and danger space phlegmon/abscess
- Inflammation
  - Calcium pyrophosphate dihydrate (CPPD) deposition disease
  - Acute calcific tendinitis of the longus colli muscle
  - Ankylosing spondylitis
  - Rheumatoid arthritis
  - Langerhans' cell histiocytosis
- Trauma
  - Vertebral fracture/hematoma
  - Traumatic and osteopenic vertebral fracture
  - Malignancy-related vertebral fracture
- Degenerative Lesions
  - Vertebral osteophytes
  - Paget disease
  - Melorheostosis

Table 6.2   Prevertebral (perivertebral) space abnormalities

Abnormalities	Imaging Findings	Comments
Malignant Vertebral Lesions		
Metastatic osseous neoplasms **(Fig. 6.18)**	Single or multiple well-circumscribed or poorly defined lesions involving vertebral marrow. *CT:* Lesions are usually radiolucent, may also be sclerotic, ± extraosseous tumor extension, usually + contrast enhancement, ± compression of neural tissue or vessels. *MRI:* Single or multiple well-circumscribed or poorly defined lesions involving the vertebrae, with low-intermediate signal on T1-weighted imaging, intermediate-high signal on T2-weighted imaging, and usually gadolinium contrast enhancement, ± bone destruction, ± pathologic fracture, ± compression of neural tissue or vessels, ± extraosseous tumor extension.	Metastatic lesions represent proliferating neoplastic cells that are located in sites or organs separated or distant from their origins. Metastatic carcinoma is the most frequent malignant tumor involving bone. In adults, metastatic lesions to bone occur most frequently from carcinomas of the lung, breast, prostate, kidney, and thyroid, as well as from sarcomas. Primary malignancies of the lung, breast, and prostate account for 80% of bone metastases. Metastatic tumor may cause variable destructive or infiltrative changes in single or multiple sites.
Myeloma/Plasmacytoma **(Fig. 6.19)**	Multiple (myeloma) or single (plasmacytoma) are well-circumscribed or poorly defined lesions involving vertebrae. *CT:* Lesions have low-intermediate attenuation, usually + contrast enhancement, + bone destruction. *MRI:* Well-circumscribed or poorly defined lesions involving vertebrae, with low-intermediate signal on T1-weighted imaging, intermediate-high signal on T2-weighted imaging, and usually gadolinium contrast enhancement, + bone destruction and pathologic vertebral fracture, ± extraosseous tumor extension, ± epidural tumor extension causing compression of neural tissue or vessels.	Multiple myeloma are malignant tumors composed of proliferating antibody-secreting plasma cells derived from single clones. Multiple myeloma primarily involves bone marrow. A solitary plasmacytoma is an infrequent variant in which a neoplastic mass of plasma cells occurs at a single site of bone or soft tissues. In the United States, 14,600 new cases occur each year. Multiple myeloma is the most common primary neoplasm of bone in adults. Median age at presentation = 60 years. Most patients are more than 40 years old. Tumors occur in the vertebrae > ribs > femur > iliac bone > humerus > craniofacial bones > sacrum > clavicle > sternum > pubic bone > tibia.

(continued on page 607)

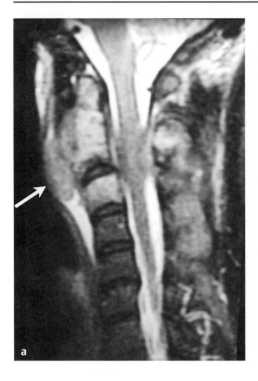

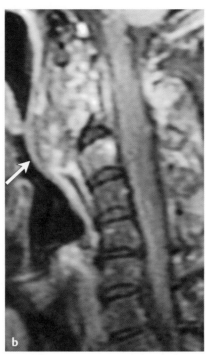

Fig. 6.18 **(a)** Sagittal fat-suppressed T2-weighted imaging of a 56-year-old woman with breast cancer shows destructive metastatic lesions involving the C2 and C3 vertebrae that have high signal (*arrow*) and **(b)** gadolinium contrast enhancement on sagittal fat-suppressed T1-weighted imaging (*arrow*). Intraosseous metastatic tumor extends anteriorly and posteriorly through destroyed bone cortex into the prevertebral space and spinal canal, respectively.

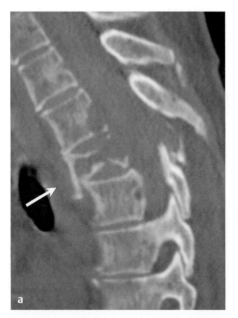

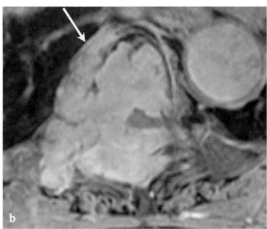

Fig. 6.19 **(a)** Sagittal CT of a 74-year-old man with myeloma shows osteolytic lesions of two adjacent vertebrae (*arrow*), including one with pathologic compression fractures. **(b)** The intraosseous tumor (*arrow*) shows gadolinium contrast enhancement on axial fat-suppressed T1-weighted imaging with extraosseous tumor extension through destroyed anterior bony cortex into the prevertebral space (*arrow*), as well as into the right paravertebral soft tissues and posteriorly into the spinal canal, causing spinal cord compression.

Table 6.2 *(cont.)*   Prevertebral (perivertebral) space abnormalities

Abnormalities	Imaging Findings	Comments
Vertebral lymphoma	Single or multiple well-circumscribed or poorly defined lesions. *CT:* Lesions have low-intermediate attenuation, may show contrast enhancement, ± bone destruction. Hodgkin disease may produce bony sclerosis as well as an "ivory vertebra" pattern that has diffuse high attenuation. *MRI:* Lesions have low-intermediate signal on T1-weighted imaging, intermediate to high signal on T2-weighted imaging, and gadolinium contrast enhancement. Can be locally invasive and may be associated with bone erosion/destruction and invasion of adjacent soft tissue.	Lymphomas are a group of lymphoid tumors whose neoplastic cells typically arise within lymphoid tissue (lymph nodes and reticuloendothelial organs). Unlike leukemia, lymphomas usually arise as discrete masses. Lymphomas are subdivided into Hodgkin disease (HD) and non-Hodgkin lymphoma (NHL). Distinction between HD and NHL is useful because of differences in clinical and histopathologic features, as well as treatment strategies. HD typically arises in lymph nodes and often spreads along nodal chains, whereas NHL frequently originates at extranodal sites and spreads in an unpredictable pattern. Almost all primary lymphomas of bone are B-cell NHL.
Leukemia	*MRI:* Diffuse abnormal signal in the marrow with low-intermediate signal on T1-weighted imaging, intermediate-high signal on T2-weighted imaging, ± gadolinium contrast enhancement, ± bone destruction, ± extraosseous extension into the adjacent soft tissues. *CT:* ± zones of bone destruction.	Leukemias are neoplastic proliferations of hematopoietic cells. Myeloid sarcomas (also referred to as chloromas or granulocytic sarcomas) are focal tumors composed of myeloblasts and neoplastic granulocyte precursor cells, and occur in 2% of patients with acute myelogenous leukemia. These lesions can involve the vertebral marrow, leptomeninges, and dura. Lesions can be solitary or multiple.
Chordoma (**Fig. 6.20**)	Well-circumscribed lobulated lesions along the dorsal surface of clivus, vertebral bodies, or sacrum, + localized bone destruction. *CT:* Lesions have low-intermediate attenuation, ± calcifications from destroyed bone carried away by tumor, + contrast enhancement. *MRI:* Lesions have low-intermediate signal on T1-weighted images, high signal on T2-weighted imaging, + gadolinium contrast enhancement (usually heterogeneous). Can be locally invasive and associated with bone erosion/destruction, encasement of vessels and nerves. Skull base-clivus is a common location, usually in the midline.	Chordomas are rare, locally aggressive, slow-growing, low to intermediate grade malignant tumors derived from ectopic notochordal remnants along the axial skeleton. Chondroid chondromas (5–15% of all chordomas) have both chordomatous and chondromatous differentiation. Chordomas that contain sarcomatous components are referred to as dedifferentiated or sarcomatoid chordomas (5% of all chordomas). Chordomas account for 2–4% of primary malignant bone tumors, 1–3% of all primary bone tumors, and less than 1% of intracranial tumors. The annual incidence has been reported to be 0.18–0.3 per million. With cranial chordomas, patients' mean age = 37 to 40 years.

(continued on page 608)

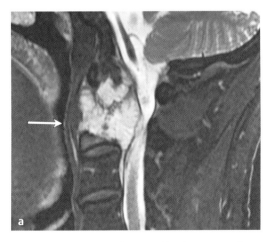 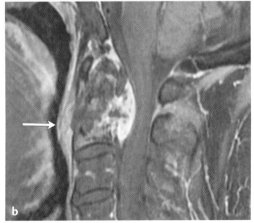

Fig. 6.20   (a) Sagittal fat-suppressed T2-weighted imaging of a 67-year-old man with a chordoma in the C2 vertebra that has heterogeneous high signal (*arrow*) and **(b)** heterogeneous gadolinium contrast enhancement (*arrow*) on sagittal fat-suppressed T1-weighted imaging. There is extraosseous tumor extension through destroyed anterior bony cortex into the prevertebral space as well as posteriorly into the spinal canal, causing spinal cord compression.

Table 6.2 *(cont.)*   Prevertebral (perivertebral) space abnormalities

Abnormalities	Imaging Findings	Comments
Chondrosarcoma (Fig. 6.21)	*CT:* Lesions have low-intermediate attenuation associated with localized bone destruction, ± chondroid matrix calcifications, + contrast enhancement. *MRI:* Lesions have low-intermediate signal on T1-weighted imaging, high signal on T2-weighted imaging (T2WI), ± matrix mineralization with low signal on T2WI, + gadolinium contrast enhancement (usually heterogeneous). Can be locally invasive and may be associated with bone erosion/destruction and encasement of vessels and nerves, and extraosseous tumor extension.	Chondrosarcomas are malignant tumors containing cartilage formed within sarcomatous stroma. Chondrosarcomas can contain areas of calcification/mineralization, myxoid material, and/or ossification, and they rarely arise within synovium. Chondrosarcomas represent 12–21% of malignant bone lesions, 21–26% of primary sarcomas of bone, 9–14% of all bone tumors, 6% of skull-base tumors, and 0.15% of all intracranial tumors.
Osteosarcoma	Destructive lesions involving vertebrae or skull base. *CT:* Tumors have low-intermediate attenuation, usually + matrix mineralization/ossification, and often show contrast enhancement (usually heterogeneous). *MRI:* Tumors often have poorly defined margins and commonly extend from the marrow through destroyed bone cortex into adjacent soft tissues. Tumors usually have low-intermediate signal on T1-weighted imaging. Zones of low signal often correspond to areas of tumor calcification/mineralization and/or necrosis. Zones of necrosis typically have high signal on T2-weighted imaging (T2WI), whereas mineralized zones usually have low signal on T2WI. Tumors can have variable signal on T2WI and fat-suppressed (FS) T2WI, depending on the relative amounts of calcified/mineralized osteoid, chondroid, fibroid, hemorrhagic, and necrotic components. Tumors may have low, low-intermediate, or intermediate to high signal on T2WI and FS T2WI. After gadolinium contrast administration, osteosarcomas typically show prominent enhancement in nonmineralized/calcified portions.	Osteosarcomas are malignant tumors comprised of proliferating neoplastic spindle cells that produce osteoid and/or immature tumoral bone. Occur in children as primary tumors and in adults are associated with Paget disease, irradiated bone, chronic osteomyelitis, osteoblastoma, giant cell tumor, and fibrous dysplasia.
Spread from Malignant Neck Lesions		
Squamous cell carcinoma (Fig. 6.22)	*MRI:* Invasive soft tissue tumors in the neck, ± bone destruction or perineural spread. Lesions have intermediate signal on T1-weighted imaging, intermediate-slightly high signal on T2-weighted imaging, and mild gadolinium contrast enhancement. Can be large lesions (± necrosis and/or hemorrhage), ± invasion of adjacent soft tissue. *CT:* Tumors have intermediate attenuation, and mild contrast enhancement. Can be large lesions (± necrosis and/or hemorrhage).	Malignant epithelial tumors originating from the mucosal epithelium. Include both keratinizing and nonkeratinizing types. Account for 3% of malignant tumors of the head and neck. Occur in adults (usually > 55 years old), and in males more than in females. Associated with occupational or other exposure to tobacco smoke, nickel, chlorophenols, chromium, mustard gas, radium, and material in the manufacture of wood products.

(continued on page 610)

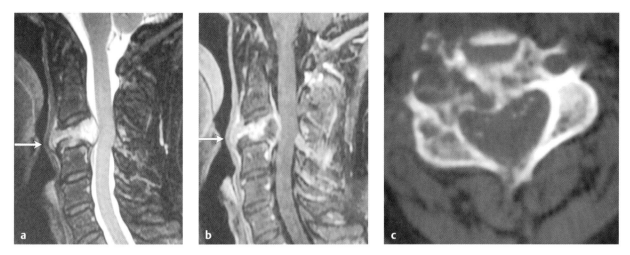

Fig. 6.21 **(a)** A 60-year-old woman with a chondrosarcoma causing pathologic compression fractures of the C3 vertebral body. The intraosseous tumor has high signal on sagittal fat-suppressed T2-weighted imaging (*arrow*). **(b)** The tumor shows heterogeneous gadolinium contrast enhancement on sagittal fat-suppressed T1-weighted imaging (*arrow*) and **(c)** contains chondroid matrix mineralization on axial CT. Intraosseous tumor extends through destroyed anterior bony cortex into the prevertebral space, as well as posteriorly into the spinal canal, causing spinal cord compression.

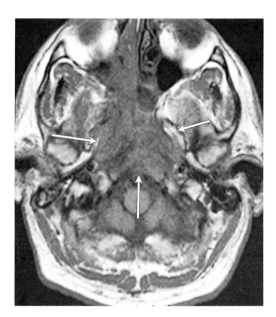

Fig. 6.22 Axial T1-weighted imaging of a patient with a squamous cell carcinoma (*arrows*) in the nasopharynx that posteriorly invades the prevertebral space and occipital portion of the lower clivus.

Table 6.2 *(cont.)* Prevertebral (perivertebral) space abnormalities

Abnormalities	Imaging Findings	Comments
Nasopharyngeal carcinoma (**Fig. 6.23**)	*CT:* Tumors have intermediate attenuation and mild contrast enhancement. Can be large lesions (± necrosis and/or hemorrhage). *MRI:* Invasive lesions in the nasopharynx (lateral wall/fossa of Rosenmüller and posterior upper wall), ± intracranial extension via bone destruction or perineural spread. Have intermediate signal on T1-weighted imaging, intermediate-slightly high signal on T2-weighted imaging, and often gadolinium contrast enhancement. Can be large lesions (± necrosis and/or hemorrhage), ± invasion of adjacent soft tissue, ± metastatic disease.	Carcinomas arising from the nasopharyngeal mucosa with varying degrees of squamous differentiation. Subtypes include squamous cell carcinoma, nonkeratinizing carcinoma (differentiated and undifferentiated), and basaloid squamous cell carcinoma. Nasopharyngeal carcinoma occurs at higher frequency in Southern Asia and Africa than in Europe and the Americas. Peak ages = 40–60 years. Occurs two to three times more frequently in men than in women. Associated with Epstein-Barr virus, diets containing nitrosamines, and chronic exposure to tobacco smoke, formaldehyde, chemical fumes, and dust. Invasion of the prevertebral space occurs in up to 40% of patients and is associated with a poor prognosis.
Lymphoma (**Fig. 6.24**)	*CT:* Enlarged lymph nodes with soft tissue attenuation, ± contrast enhancement. *MRI:* Enlarged lymph nodes with intermediate signal on T1-weighted imaging and slightly high signal on T2-weighted imaging, ± gadolinium contrast enhancement. Necrosis and cystic changes rarely occur. Extracapsular spread of tumor from lymph nodes can invade adjacent tissue, including the prevertebral space.	Both non-Hodgkin lymphoma and Hodgkin disease can invade adjacent tissue, including the prevertebral space.
Thyroid cancer (**Fig. 6.25**)	*CT:* Large thyroid lesions with soft tissue attenuation, irregular margins, and extraglandular extension, showing heterogeneous contrast enhancement, ± cervical lymphadenopathy. *MRI:* Tumors have heterogeneous low, intermediate, or high signal on T1- and T2-weighted imaging secondary to zones of necrosis and/or hemorrhage. Tumors often show heterogeneous gadolinium contrast enhancement.	High-grade malignant thyroid tumors (medullary, poorly differentiated, and undifferentiated types) commonly invade adjacent tissues, occasionally through the prevertbral fascia into the prevertebral space.
Nodal metastases	*MRI:* Enlarged spheroid or ovoid nodes that often have low-intermediate signal on T1-weighted imaging and intermediate-high signal on T2-weighted imaging (T2WI), ± high-signal zones on T2WI (necrosis), ± irregular margins (capsule invasion), ± decreased ADC values on diffusion-weighted imaging ($< 1.4 \times 10^{-3}$ mm^2/sec), and variable gadolinium contrast enhancement. Extracapsular spread of tumor from lymph nodes can invade adjacent tissue, including the prevertebral space. *CT:* Involved nodes usually have low-intermediate attenuation, ± irregular margins (capsule invasion), ± low-attenuation zones (necrosis) and variable contrast enhancement. Usually measure more than 8 mm in short axis. *PET/CT:* Increased nodal uptake of F-18 FDG.	Metastatic tumor involving cervical lymph nodes can result from primary neck neoplasms, such as squamous cell carcinoma or thyroid cancer. Can also result from spread from primary extracranial tumor source: Lung > breast > GI > GU > melanoma. Can occur as single or multiple well-circumscribed or poorly defined lesions. Metastatic tumor may cause variable destructive or infiltrative changes in single or multiple sites.

(continued on page 612)

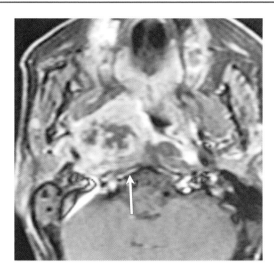

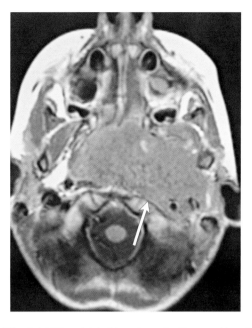

Fig. 6.23 Axial fat-suppressed T1-weighted imaging of a 60-year-old woman with a nasopharyngeal carcinoma in the right parapharyngeal space that shows heterogeneous irregular contrast enhancement. The tumor has irregular margins and invades the retropharyngeal and right prevertebral spaces (*arrow*).

Fig. 6.24 Axial T1-weighted imaging of a 6-year-old male with lymphoma in the nsaopharynx that has intermediate signal and invades the prevertebral space on the left (*arrow*).

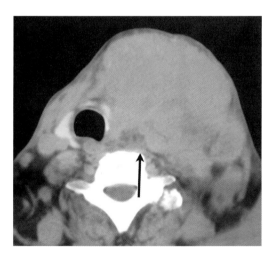

Fig. 6.25 Axial CT of an 83-year-old man with a large anaplastic thyroid carcinoma in the left thyroid lobe that has ill-defined margins and invades the adjacent soft tissues, including the prevertebral space on the left (*arrow*).

Table 6.2 *(cont.)* Prevertebral (perivertebral) space abnormalities

Abnormalities	Imaging Findings	Comments
Hemangioendothelioma (**Fig. 6.26**)	*MRI:* Tumors have lobulated well-defined or irregular margins, and have intermediate signal on T1-weighted imaging and heterogeneous predominantly high signal on T2-weighted imaging, with or without internal low-signal septations. Flow voids may be seen with the lesions. Tumors show heterogeneous gadolinium contrast enhancement. *CT:* Lesions have lobulated well-defined or irregular margins and mostly soft-tissue/intermediate attenuation. Usually show contrast enhancement, ± calcifications and prominent blood vessels.	Low-grade locally aggressive neoplasms with vascular differentiation. Tumors contain spindle-shaped and plump epithelioid endothelial cells as well as vascular spaces. Hemangioendotheliomas rarely metastasize. Frequently occur in patients from 2 weeks to 20 years old (mean age = 3.75 years), but also occur in adults as old as 64 years. Large lesions can be associated with anemia and consumptive coagulopathy (Kasabach-Meritt syndrome or phenomenon) due to clot activation within the neoplastic vasculature. The prognosis is poorer for large intraabdominal lesions associated with Kasabach-Merritt syndrome than for those located in the superficial soft tissues with easier surgical access. Tumors can occasionally spread to regional perinodal tissue, but typically do not metastasize to distant sites.
Benign Tumors		
Neurofibroma (**Fig. 6.27**)	*MRI:* *Solitary neurofibromas* are circumscribed or lobulated extra-axial lesions, with low-intermediate signal on T1-weighted imaging and intermediate-high signal on T2-weighted imaging (T2WI), + prominent gadolinium (Gd) contrast enhancement. High signal on T2WI and Gd contrast enhancement can be heterogeneous in large lesions. *Plexiform neurofibromas* appear as curvilinear and multinodular lesions involving multiple nerve branches, and have low to intermediate signal on T1WI and intermediate, slightly high to high signal on T2WI and fat-suppressed T2WI, with or without bands or strands of low signal. Lesions usually show gadolinium contrast enhancement. *CT:* Ovoid or fusiform lesions with low-intermediate attenuation. Lesions can show contrast enhancement. Often erode adjacent bone.	Benign nerve sheath tumors that contain mixtures of Schwann cells, perineural-like cells, and interlacing fascicles of fibroblasts associated with abundant collagen. Unlike schwannomas, neurofibromas lack Antoni A and B regions and cannot be separated pathologically from the underlying nerve. Most frequently occur as sporadic, localized, solitary lesions, less frequently as diffuse or plexiform lesions. Multiple neurofibromas are typically seen with neurofibromatosis type 1 (NF1), which is an autosomal dominant disorder (1/2,500 births) caused by mutations involving the neurofibromin gene on chromosome 17q11.2. NF1 is the most common type of neurocutaneous syndrome and is associated with neoplasms of the central and peripheral nervous systems (optic gliomas, astrocytomas, plexiform and solitary neurofibromas) and skin (café-au-lait spots, axillary and inguinal freckling). Also associated with meningeal and skull dysplasias, as well as hamartomas of the iris (Lisch nodules).
Lipoma	*MRI:* Lipomas have MRI signal isointense to subcutaneous fat on T1-weighted imaging (high signal), and on T2-weighted imaging, signal suppression occurs with frequency-selective fat saturation techniques or with a short time to inversion recovery (STIR) method. Typically there is no gadolinium contrast enhancement or peripheral edema. *CT:* Lipomas have CT attenuation similar to subcutaneous fat. Typically there is no contrast enhancement or peripheral edema.	Common benign hamartomas composed of mature white adipose tissue without cellular atypia. Most common soft tissue tumor, representing 16% of all soft tissue tumors. May contain calcifications and/or traversing blood vessels.
Hemangioma (**Fig. 6.28**)	*MRI:* Circumscribed or poorly marginated structures (< 4 cm in diameter) in soft tissue or bone marrow with intermediate-high signal on T1-weighted imaging (often with portions that are isointense to marrow fat), high signal on T2-weighted imaging (T2WI) and fat-suppressed T2WI, and typically gadolinium contrast enhancement, ± expansion of bone. *CT:* Hemangiomas in soft tissue have mostly intermediate attenuation, ± zones of fat attenuation. Intraosseous hemangiomas are expansile bone lesions with a radiating pattern of bony trabeculae oriented toward the center.	Benign lesions of soft tissue or bone composed of capillary, cavernous, and/or venous malformations. Considered to be a hamartomatous disorder. Occurs in patients 1 to 84 years old (median age = 33 years).

(continued on page 614)

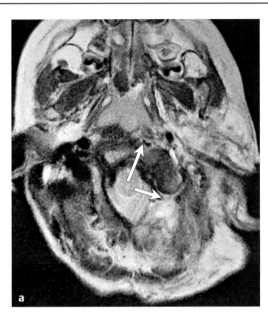
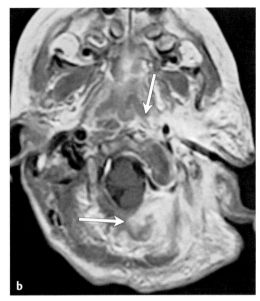

Fig. 6.26 **(a)** Axial T2-weighted imaging of a 5-year-old male with Kasabach-Merritt syndrome and a hemangioendothelioma with ill-defined margins in the left lower face and neck, including the left prevertebral space, that has heterogeneous mostly high signal (*arrows*). **(b)** The lesion shows heterogeneous gadolinium contrast enhancement on axial T1-weighted imaging (*arrows*).

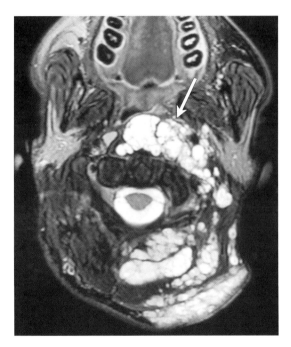

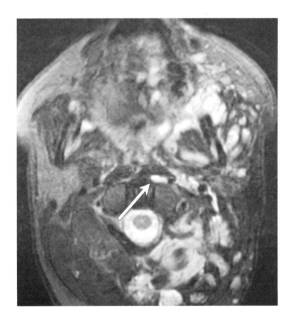

Fig. 6.28 Axial fat-suppressed T2-weighted imaging shows an infiltrating hemangioma with high signal in the left neck, including the left masticator, parapharyngeal, and prevertbral spaces (*arrow*).

Fig. 6.27 Axial fat-suppressed T2-weighted imaging of a 15-year-old male with neurofibromatosis type 1 shows multiple neurofibromas with high signal in the neck, including the left parapharyngeal, retropharyngeal, and prevertebral spaces (*arrow*).

Table 6.2 *(cont.)* Prevertebral (perivertebral) space abnormalities

Abnormalities	Imaging Findings	Comments
Infection		
Vertebral osteomyelitis (**Fig. 6.29**)	*CT:* Poorly defined radiolucent zones (bone destruction) involving the endplates and subchondral bone of two or more adjacent vertebral bodies, ± fluid collections in the adjacent paraspinal soft tissues. Complications include epidural abscess and meningitis. *MRI:* Zones with low-intermediate signal on T1-weighted imaging and high signal on T2-weighted imaging (T2WI) and fat-suppressed T2WI within marrow, with associated gadolinium contrast enhancement, + high signal on T2WI involving the disk, + erosion/destruction of vertebral endplates, ± epidural or paravertebral abscess. Also shows variable enhancement of disk (patchy zones within disk) and/or thin or thick peripheral enhancement, ± vertebral compression deformity, ± spinal cord or spinal canal compression.	Vertebral osteomyelitis represents 3% of osseous infections. Can have hematogenous source from distant infection (most common) or intravenous drug abuse. Can also be a complication of surgery, trauma, or diabetes, or can spread from contiguous soft tissue infection. Initially involves end-arterioles in marrow adjacent to endplates with eventual destruction and spread to the adjacent vertebrae through the disk. Occurs in children and in adults more than 50 years old. Gram-positive organisms (*Staphylococcus aureus, S. epidermidis, Streptococcus*, etc.) account for 70% of pyogenic osteomyelitis and gram-negative organisms (*Pseudomonas aeruginosa, Escherichia coli, Proteus*, etc.) represent 30%. Fungal osteomyelitis can appear similar to pyogenic infection of the spine.
Tuberculous vertebral osteomyelitis	*CT:* Poorly defined radiolucent zones (bone destruction) involving the bone of two or more adjacent vertebral bodies, ± fluid collections in the adjacent paraspinal soft tissues. Complications include epidural abscess and meningitis. *MRI:* Zones with low-intermediate signal on T1-weighted imaging and high signal on T2-weighted imaging (T2WI) and fat-suppressed T2WI within marrow, with associated gadolinium contrast enhancement, ± high signal on T2WI involving the disk, ± erosion/destruction of vertebral endplates, ± epidural or paravertebral abscess, ± vertebral compression deformity, ± spinal cord or spinal canal compression.	Osteomyelitis (bone infection) can result from surgery, trauma, hematogenous dissemination from another source of infection, or direct extension of infection from an adjacent site. Initially involves marrow in the anterior portion of the vertebral body, with spread to the adjacent vertebrae along the anterior longitudinal ligament, often sparing the disk until later in the disease process. Usually associated with paravertebral abscesses, which may be more prominent than the vertebral abnormalities.
Perivertebral infection (**Fig. 6.30**)	*MRI:* Irregular zones with low-intermediate signal on T1-weighted imaging and slightly high to high signal on T2-weighted imaging (T2WI), as well as rim gadolinium (Gd) contrast enhancement. Irregular increased signal on T2WI and Gd contrast enhancement are typically seen in the adjacent soft tissue. *CT:* Irregular soft tissue thickening, ± low-attenuation fluid collection (abscess) in the retropharyngeal space, with anterior expansion of the prevertebral space. Irregular contrast enhancement ± peripheral contrast enhancement around abscess.	Infection of the soft tissues adjacent to the spine can result from spread from adjacent tissues, surgery, biopsies, or hematogenous seeding of pathogens from distant sites. Common causative microorganisms include *Staphylococcus aureus, Mycobacterium tuberculosis, Escherichia coli*, and occasionally fungi in immunocompromised patients. Predisposing conditions include intravenous drug abuse, diabetes, renal insufficiency/failure, and alcoholism.
Retropharyngeal and danger space phlegmon/abscess (**Fig. 6.31**)	*CT:* Asymmetric abnormal soft tissue thickening (phlegmon) or low-attenuation fluid collection (abscess) in the retropharyngeal and danger spaces with anterior displacement of the posterior wall of the nasopharynx and/or oropharynx from the prevertebral space. Irregular, thin, and/or peripheral contrast enhancement with scalloped/lobulated margins can be seen, ± extension into the prevertebral space. *MRI:* Lesions with low-intermediate signal on T1-weighted imaging and slightly high to high signal on T2-weighted imaging, as well as rim gadolinium (Gd) contrast enhancement for abscess. Irregular increased signal on T2WI and Gd contrast enhancement are typically seen in the adjacent soft tissue, ± extension into the prevertebral space.	Retropharyngeal infection can result from inadequately treated suppurative lymphadenitis, trauma, foreign bodies, or extension of infection from adjacent structures. Can extend posteriorly to involve the danger and prevertebral spaces. A trial of IV antibiotics may be successful for a phlegmon or small abscesses, whereas larger abscesses (> 2 cm) associated with narrowing of the airway are usually treated with surgical drainage in addition to IV antibiotics.

(continued on page 616)

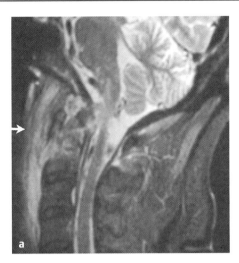

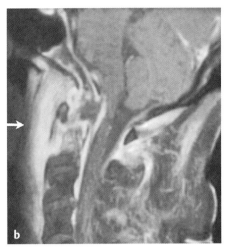

Fig. 6.29 **(a)** Sagittal fat-suppressed T2-weighted imaging of a 59-year-old man with vertebral osteomyelitis from oxacillin-resistant *Staphylococcus aureus* shows abnormal slightly high and high signal in the marrow of the C2 vertebra (*arrow*). **(b)** On sagittal fat-suppressed T1-weighted imaging, there is corresponding abnormal gadolinium contrast enhancement that extends through destroyed anterior bony cortex into the prevertebral space (*arrow*), as well as posteriorly into the spinal canal.

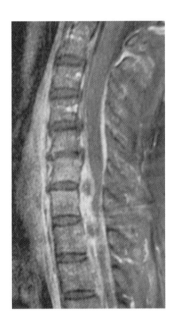

Fig. 6.30 Sagittal fat-suppressed T1-weighted imaging shows abnormal gadolinium contrast enhancement involving thickened soft tissue in the prevertebral space from infection extending from the C3 to the T2 level, as well as a peripherally enhancing epidural abscess at the C6 to T2 levels.

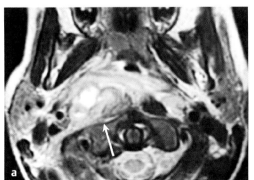

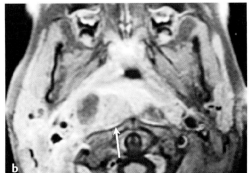

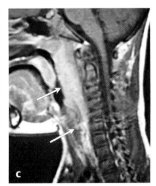

Fig. 6.31 **(a)** Axial T2-weighted imaging of a 6-year-old male shows poorly defined zones with abnormal high signal (*arrow*) and **(b)** corresponding gadolinium contrast enhancement on axial fat-suppressed T1-weighted imaging (*arrow*) from retropharyngeal phlegmon and abscess involving the right prestyloid and retrostyloid parapharyngeal spaces as well as the retropharyngeal, danger, and prevertebral spaces. **(c)** Sagittal T1-weighted imaging shows abnormal gadolinium contrast enhancement from the infection extending inferiorly within the danger space (*arrows*).

Table 6.2 *(cont.)* Prevertebral (perivertebral) space abnormalities

Abnormalities	Imaging Findings	Comments
Inflammation		
Calcium pyrophosphate dihydrate (CPPD) deposition disease (**Fig. 6.32**)	*CT:* Thickened synovium at C1–C2 containing multiple calcifications. *MRI:* At the C1–odontoid articulation, hypertrophy of synovium can be seen, with low-intermediate signal on T1- and T2-weighted imaging. Small zones of low signal may correspond to calcifications seen with CT. Minimal or no gadolinium contrast enhancement.	CPPD disease is a common disorder, usually in older adults, in which there is deposition of CPPD crystals, resulting in calcifications of hyaline and fibrocartilage. The disease is associated with cartilage degeneration, subchondral cysts, and osteophyte formation. Symptomatic CPPD disease is referred to as pseudogout because of clinical features overlapping those of gout. Usually occurs in the knee, hip, shoulder, elbow, and wrist, and rarely at the odontoid–C1 articulation.
Acute calcific tendinitis of the longus colli muscle (**Fig. 6.33**)	*CT:* Thickening of the cervical prevertebral soft tissues, + calcifications in the longus colli muscle, commonly at the C1–C3 levels. No contrast enhancement. No destruction of adjacent bone. *MRI:* Thickening of the cervical prevertebral soft tissues, with low-intermediate signal on T1-weighted imaging and high signal on T2-weighted imaging. No gadolinium contrast enhancement. No destruction of adjacent bone.	Rare, benign, aseptic inflammatory condition involving the cervical prevertebral space that results from deposition of calcium hydroxyapatite in the longus colli muscles and tendons. Occurs in patients from 21 to 65 years old. Clinical findings include acute or subacute onset of pain, odynophagia, limited range of neck motion, and neck stiffness. Usually a self-limited disorder. Can be treated with NSAIDs, steroids, and immobilization. Typically resolves 3 weeks after treatment.
Ankylosing spondylitis (**Fig. 6.34**)	Inflammation occurs at entheses (sites of attachment of ligaments, tendons, and joint capsules to bone). *MRI:* Zones with high signal on T2-weighted imaging and contrast enhancement can be seen in marrow at sites of active inflammation at corners of vertebral bodies, sacroiliac joints, and other bones. Progression of inflammation leads to squaring of vertebral bodies with mineralized syndesmophytes across disks, osteopenia, and erosions at sacroiliac joints, with eventual fusion across the joints and facets. The spine in these cases is referred to as "bamboo spine."	Chronic progressive autoimmune inflammatory disease involving the spine and sacroiliac joints. Associated with HLA-B27 in 90% of cases. Onset occurs in patients 20–30 years old, with a male:female ratio of 3:1. Fractures can occur in the horizontal plane through the osteopenic and fused "bamboo spine" at the level of the disks and/or vertebral bodies, as well as in the posterior elements.

(continued on page 618)

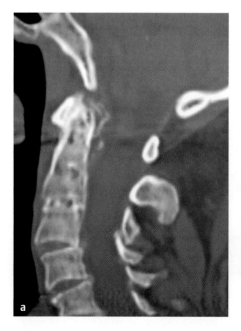
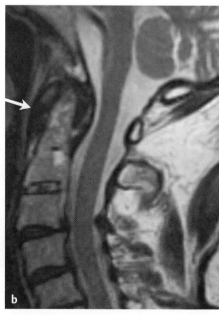

Fig. 6.32 (a) Sagittal CT of an 83-year-old man shows amorphous calcifications at C1–C2 from calcium pyrophosphate dihydrate deposition disease. **(b)** There is associated thickened synovium (*arrow*) that has low-intermediate signal on sagittal T2-weighted imaging.

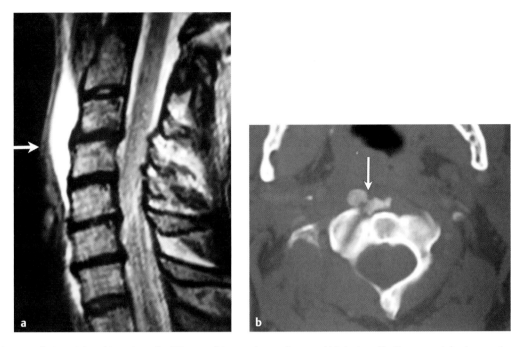

Fig. 6.33   **(a)** Sagittal T2-weighted imaging of a 67-year-old man shows abnormal high signal in the prevertebral space (*arrow*) from acute calcific tendinitis of the longus colli muscle. **(b)** Axial CT shows calcifications (*arrow*).

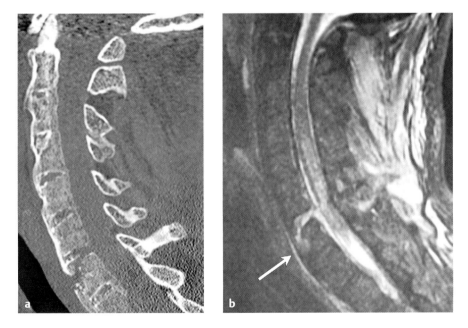

Fig. 6.34   **(a)** Sagittal CT of a 55-year-old man with ankylosing spondylitis shows a fracture through the anterior portion of the C7 vertebral body. **(b)** There is corresponding high signal on sagittal fat-suppressed T2-weighted imaging in the vertebral body as well as in the prevertebral space (*arrow*) and anterior epidural space from associated hematomas.

Table 6.2 *(cont.)*   Prevertebral (perivertebral) space abnormalities

Abnormalities	Imaging Findings	Comments
Rheumatoid arthritis (**Fig. 6.35**)	*MRI:* Hypertrophied synovium (pannus) can be diffuse, nodular, and/or villous, and usually has low to intermediate or intermediate signal on T1-weighted imaging (T1WI). On T2-weighted imaging (T2WI), pannus can have low to intermediate, intermediate, and/or slightly high to high signal. Signal heterogeneity of hypertrophied synovium on T2WI can result from variable amounts of fibrin, hemosiderin, and fibrosis. Chronic fibrotic nonvascular synovium usually has low signal on T1- and T2WI. Hypertrophied synovium can show prominent homogeneous or variable heterogeneous gadolinium contrast enhancement. Erosion of the dens and destruction of the transverse ligament can occur, as well as basilar impression. *CT:* Irregular enlarged enhancing synovium (pannus, with low-intermediate attenuation) at atlanto-dens articulation results in erosions of dens and transverse ligament, ± destruction of transverse ligament, with C1 on C2 subluxation and neural compromise, ± basilar impression. Also, erosions of vertebral endplates, spinous processes, and uncovertebral and apophyseal joints can occur.	Chronic multisystem disease of unknown etiology with persistent inflammatory synovitis involving peripheral joints in a symmetric distribution. Most common type of inflammatory arthropathy that results in synovitis causing destructive/erosive changes of cartilage, ligaments, and bone. Cervical spine involvement occurs in two-thirds of patients with both juvenile and adult types of rheumatoid arthritis. The disease affects ~ 1% of the world's population. Eighty percent of adult patients present between the ages of 35 and 50 years. In patients with juvenile idiopathic arthritis, patients range from 5 to 16 years old (mean age = 10.2 years).
Langerhans' cell histiocytosis (**Fig. 6.36**)	Single or multiple circumscribed soft-tissue lesions in vertebral marrow associated with focal bony destruction/erosion, with extension extra- or intracranially or both. *CT:* Single or multiple circumscribed radiolucent lesions in the vertebral body marrow, associated with focal bony destruction/erosion and extension into the adjacent soft tissues. Lesions usually have low-intermediate attenuation and involve the vertebral body and not the posterior elements, and can show with contrast enhancement, ± enhancement of the adjacent dura. Progression of lesion can lead to vertebra plana (collapsed, flattened vertebral body), with minimal or no kyphosis and relatively normal-size adjacent disks. *MRI:* Lesions typically have low-intermediate signal on T1-weighted imaging and heterogeneous slightly high to high signal on T2-weighted imaging (T2WI) and fat-suppressed (FS) T2WI. Poorly defined zones of high signal on T2WI and FS T2WI are usually seen in the marrow and soft tissues peripheral to the lesions secondary to inflammatory changes. Lesions typically show prominent gadolinium contrast enhancement in marrow and extraosseous soft tissue.	Disorder of reticuloendothelial system in which bone marrow-derived dendritic Langerhans' cells infiltrate various organs as focal lesions or in diffuse patterns. Langerhans' cells have eccentrically located ovoid or convoluted nuclei within pale to eosinophilic cytoplasm. Lesions often consist of Langerhans' cells, macrophages, plasma cells, and eosinophils. Lesions are immunoreactive to S-100, CD1a, CD207, HLA-DR, and β_2-microglobulin. Prevalence of 2 per 100,000 children < 15 years old; only a third of lesions occur in adults. Localized lesions (eosinophilic granuloma) can be single or multiple in the skull, usually at the skull base. Single lesions are commonly seen in males more than in females, and in patients < 20 years old. Proliferation of histiocytes in medullary bone results in localized destruction of cortical bone with extension into adjacent soft tissues. Multiple lesions are associated with Letterer-Siwe disease (lymphadenopathy and hepatosplenomegaly) in children < 2 years old and Hand-Schüller-Christian disease (lymphadenopathy, exophthalmos, and diabetes insipidus) in children 5–10 years old.

(continued on page 620)

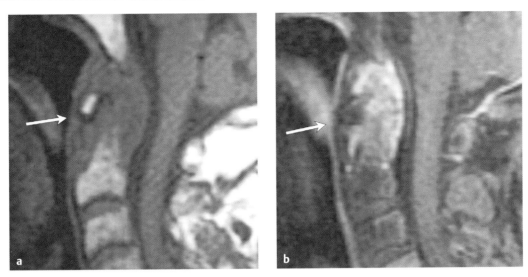

Fig. 6.35   **(a)** Sagittal T1-weighted imaging of a 72-year-old woman with rheumatoid arthritis shows pannus with intermediate signal and corresponding gadolinium contrast enhancement on **(b)** sagittal fat-suppressed T1-weighted imaging at the C1–C2 level (*arrows*) eroding the upper dens and extending into the prevertebral space.

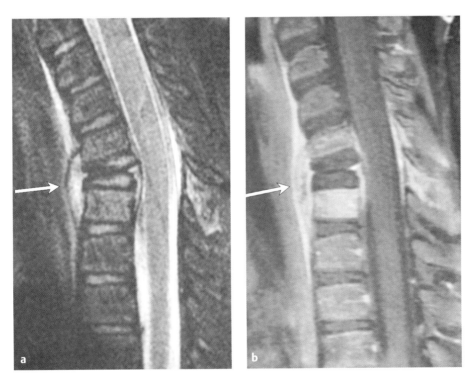

Fig. 6.36   **(a)** Sagittal fat-suppressed T2-weighted imaging of an 8-year-old female with Langerhans' cell histiocytosis shows collapse of a cervical vertebral body related to an intraosseous eosinophilic granuloma (*arrow*). **(b)** The lesion is associated with high signal and corresponding gadolinium contrast enhancement on sagittal fat-suppressed T1-weighted imaging in the prevertebral space (*arrow*) and anterior epidural space from associated hematomas. Abnormal increased signal on T2-weighted imaging and corresponding gadolinium contrast enhancement are also seen in the marrow of the vertebral bodies above and below the collapsed vertebral body.

Table 6.2 *(cont.)*   Prevertebral (perivertebral) space abnormalities

Abnormalities	Imaging Findings	Comments
Trauma		
Vertebral fracture/ hematoma (**Fig. 6.37**) Traumatic and osteopenic vertebral fracture Malignancy-related vertebral fracture	*Traumatic and osteopenic vertebral fracture* *CT:* Acute/subacute fractures have sharply angulated cortical margins, no destructive changes at cortical margins of fractured endplates, ± convex outward angulated configuration of compressed vertebral bodies, ± spinal cord and/or spinal canal compression related to fracture deformity, ± retropulsed bone fragments into spinal canal, ± subluxation, ± kyphosis, ± epidural hematoma. *MRI:* Poorly defined zones with low signal on T1-weighted imaging, high signal on T2-weighted imaging (T2WI) and fat-suppressed T2WI, and corresponding gadolinium contrast enhancement in the marrow, ± serpiginous curvilinear zones of low signal, ± hematoma adjacent to fracture. *Malignancy-related vertebral fracture* *CT:* Fractures related to radiolucent and/or sclerotic lesions, ± destructive changes at cortical margins of vertebrae, ± convex outward-bowed configuration of compressed vertebral bodies, ± paravertebral mass lesions, ± spheroid or poorly defined lesions in other noncompressed vertebral bodies. *MRI:* Intramedullary zones with low-intermediate signal on T1-weighted imaging (T1WI) and slightly high to high signal on T2-weighted imaging (T2WI) and fat-suppressed T2WI. Sclerotic lesions often have low signal on T1WI and mixed low, intermediate, and/ or high signal on T2WI. Metastatic spinal lesions may be focal or involve most of a vertebra. Metastatic skeletal lesions usually show varying degrees of gadolinium contrast enhancement, ± extraosseous or epidural tumor extension.	Vertebral fractures can result from trauma, primary bone tumors/lesions, metastatic disease, bone infarcts (steroids, chemotherapy, and radiation treatment), osteoporosis, osteomalacia, metabolic disorders (calcium/ phosphate imbalances), vitamin deficiencies, Paget disease, and genetic disorders (osteogenesis imperfecta, etc).
Degenerative Lesions		
Vertebral osteophytes (**Fig. 6.38** and **Fig. 6.39**)	*CT:* Bone spurs (osteophytes) occur along the margins of one or more vertebral bodies, typically in association with degenerative disk disease. *MRI:* Osteophytes have low peripheral signal on T1- and T2-weighted imaging overlying fatty marrow with or without edematous reaction. Smooth undulating zones of ossification involving the anterior longitudinal ligament can be seen along the anterior margins of the vertebral bodies and extending across the disks.	Bony outgrowths usually related to degenerative athropathy at synovial joints, or degenerative disk disease adjacent to the anterior and posterior longitudinal ligaments. At synovial joints, these bony protrusions may be a response to increase the articular surface to reduce load. At the spine, osteophytes occur as a metaplastic bone response related to degenerative disk bulges displacing the longitudinal ligaments. Flowing or bridging osteophytes at four or more adjacent vertebral bodies have been referred to as diffuse idiopathic skeletal hyperostosis (DISH).

(continued on page 622)

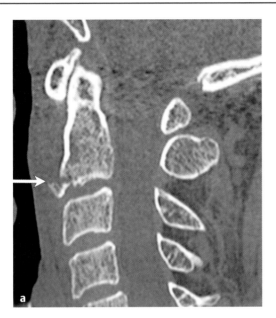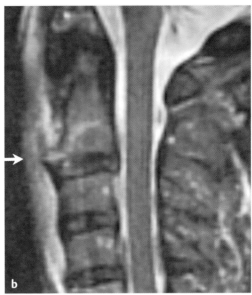

Fig. 6.37   **(a)** Sagittal CT shows a fracture at the anterior inferior portion of the C2 vertebral body (*arrow*), with **(b)** associated hematoma with high signal on sagittal fat-suppressed T2-weighted imaging in the prevertebral soft tissues (*arrow*).

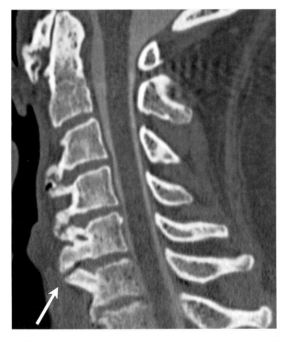

Fig. 6.38   Sagittal CT shows multiple prominent osteophytes (*arrow*) at the anterior margins of multiple cervical vertebral bodies.

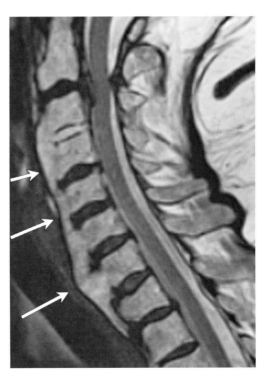

Fig. 6.39   Sagittal T2-weighted imaging shows anterior bridging osteophytes (*arrows*) at six adjacent vertebral bodies, representing diffuse idiopathic skeletal hyperostosis (DISH); the osteophytes protrude into the prevertebral space. Spinal canal narrowing is seen at the C2–C3 level from a posterior disk-bulge osteophyte complex that is likely related to lack of mobility of the spine from DISH at the adjacent lower cervical levels.

Table 6.2 *(cont.)*   Prevertebral (perivertebral) space abnormalities

Abnormalities	Imaging Findings	Comments
Paget disease (**Fig. 6.40**)	*CT:* Expansile sclerotic/lytic process involving a single vertebra or multiple vertebrae with mixed intermediate high attenuation and irregular/indistinct borders between marrow cortical bone. Can also result in diffuse sclerosis, "ivory vertebral pattern." *MRI:* Most cases involving vertebrae are the late or inactive phases. Findings include osseous expansion, cortical thickening with low signal on T1-weighted imaging (T1WI) and T2-weighted imaging (T2WI). The inner margins of the thickened cortex can be irregular and indistinct. Zones of low signal on T1WI and T2WI can be seen in the diploic marrow secondary to thickened bony trabeculae. Marrow in late or inactive phases of Paget disease can have signal similar to normal marrow, contain focal areas of fat signal, have low signal on T1WI and T2WI secondary to regions of sclerosis, and have areas of high signal on fat-suppressed T2WI from edema or persistent fibrovascular tissue.	Paget disease is a chronic skeletal disease in which there is disordered bone resorption and woven bone formation, resulting in osseous deformity. A paramyxovirus may be the etiologic agent. Paget disease is polyostotic in up to 66% of patients. Paget disease is associated with a risk of less than 1% for developing secondary sarcomatous changes. Occurs in 2.5 to 5% of Caucasians > 55 years old, and in 10% of those > 85 years old.
Melorheostosis (**Fig. 6.41**)	*CT:* Attenuation is based on the relative proportions of chondroid, mineralized osteoid, and soft tissue components in the lesions. Mineralized zones typically have high attenuation along sites of thickened cortical bone; typically no contrast enhancement is seen in bone lesions. Nonmineralized portions can have low-intermediate attenuation and can show contrast enhancement. *MRI:* Signal varies based on the relative proportions of, mineralized osteoid, chondroid and soft tissue components in the lesions. Mineralized osteoid zones involving bone cortex typically have low signal on T1-weighted imaging (T1WI) and T2-weighted imaging (T2WI), and no gadolinium contrast enhancement. Soft tissue lesions may also occur adjacent to the cortical lesions, and they have mixed signal on T1WI and T2WI.	Rare bone dysplasia with cortical thickening that has a "flowing candle wax" configuration. Associated soft tissue masses occur in ~ 25% of cases. The soft tissue lesions often contain mixtures of chondroid material, mineralized osteoid, and fibrovascular tissue. Surgery is usually performed only for lesions causing symptoms.

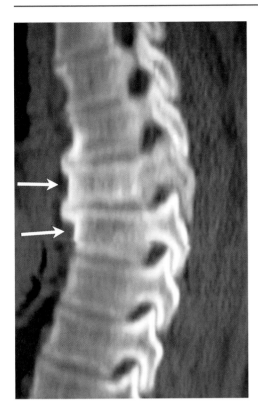

Fig. 6.40   Sagittal CT of a patient with Paget disease shows expansile sclerosis of two adjacent thoracic vertebral bodies (*arrows*), with irregular borders between marrow cortical bone, and anterior osteophytes that protrude into the prevertebral space.

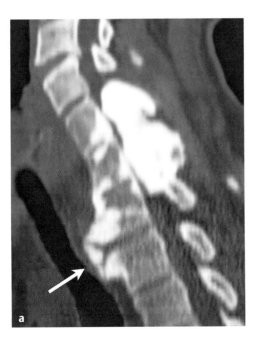
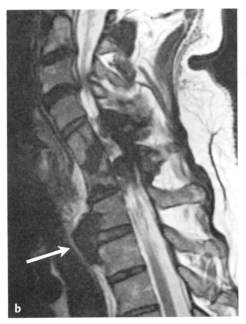

Fig. 6.41   (**a**) Sagittal CT of a 46-year-old man with melorheostosis shows thick zones of cortical hyperostosis involving the C5 through T1 vertebrae, with (**b**) corresponding low signal on sagittal T2-weighted imaging. Hyperostosis anteriorly at the C7–T1 level protrudes into the prevertebral space (*arrows*).

References

Cervical Lymphadenopathy

1. Bryson TC, Shah GV, Srinivasan A, Mukherji SK. Cervical lymph node evaluation and diagnosis. Otolaryngol Clin North Am 2012; 45(6):1363–1383

2. Curtin HD, Ishwaran H, Mancuso AA, Dalley RW, Caudry DJ, McNeil BJ. Comparison of CT and MR imaging in staging of neck metastases. Radiology 1998;207(1):123–130

3. Goldenberg D, Begum S, Westra WH, et al. Cystic lymph node metastasis in patients with head and neck cancer: An HPV-associated phenomenon. Head Neck 2008;30(7):898–903

4. Gupta P, Babyn P. Sinus histiocytosis with massive lymphadenopathy (Rosai-Dorfman disease): a clinicoradiological profile of three cases including two with skeletal disease. Pediatr Radiol 2008;38(7): 721–728, quiz 821–822

5. Hoang JK, Vanka J, Ludwig BJ, Glastonbury CM. Evaluation of cervical lymph nodes in head and neck cancer with CT and MRI: tips, traps, and a systematic approach. AJR Am J Roentgenol 2013;200(1):W17–W25

6. Hock ATE, Long MTM, Sittampalam K, Eng DNC. Rosai-Dorfman disease: FDG PET/CT findings in a patient presenting with pyrexia and cervical adenopathy. Clin Nucl Med 2010;35(8):576–578

7. Jiang XH, Song HM, Liu QY, Cao Y, Li GH, Zhang WD. Castleman disease of the neck: CT and MR imaging findings. Eur J Radiol 2014;83(11):2041–2050

8. Karunanithi S, Singh H, Sharma P, Naswa N, Kumar R. 18F-FDG PET/CT imaging features of Rosai Dorfman disease: a rare cause of massive generalized lymphadenopathy. Clin Nucl Med 2014;39(3):268–269

9. Krestan C, Herneth AM, Formanek M, Czerny C. Modern imaging lymph node staging of the head and neck region. Eur J Radiol 2006;58(3):360–366

10. Lee ES, Paeng JC, Park CM, et al. Metabolic characteristics of Castleman disease on 18F-FDG PET in relation to clinical implication. Clin Nucl Med 2013;38(5):339–342

11. Wen L, Zhang D, Zhang ZG. CT characteristics of cervical Castleman's disease. Clin Imaging 2005;29(2):141–143

12. Mack MG, Rieger J, Baghi M, Bisdas S, Vogl TJ. Cervical lymph nodes. Eur J Radiol 2008;66(3):493–500

13. Morani AC, Eisbruch A, Carey TE, Hauff SJ, Walline HM, Mukherji SK. Intranodal cystic changes: a potential radiologic signature/biomarker to assess the human papillomavirus status of cases with oropharyngeal malignancies. J Comput Assist Tomogr 2013;37(3):343–345

14. Restrepo R, Oneto J, Lopez K, Kukreja K. Head and neck lymph nodes in children: the spectrum from normal to abnormal. Pediatr Radiol 2009;39(8):836–846

15. Sathekge M, Maes A, Van de Wiele C. FDG-PET imaging in HIV infection and tuberculosis. Semin Nucl Med 2013;43(5):349–366

16. Saindane AM. Pitfalls in the staging of cervical lymph node metastasis. Neuroimaging Clin N Am 2013;23(1):147–166

17. Sobic-Saranovic D, Artiko V, Obradovic V. FDG PET imaging in sarcoidosis. Semin Nucl Med 2013;43(6):404–411

18. Treglia G, Annunziata S, Sobic-Saranovic D, et al. The role of 18F-FDG and PET/CT in patients with sarcoidosis. Acad Radiol 2014; 21:675–684

19. Valeyre D, Prasse A, Nunes H, Uzunhan Y, Brillet PY, Müller-Quernheim J. Sarcoidosis. Lancet 2014;383(9923):1155–1167

20. Vogl T, Bisdas S. Lymph node staging. Top Magn Reson Imaging 2007; 18(4):303–316

21. Windebank K, Nanduri V. Langerhans cell histiocytosis. Arch Dis Child 2009;94(11):904–908

22. Yasui T, Morii E, Yamamoto Y, et al. Human papillomavirus and cystic node metastasis in oropharyngeal cancer and cancer of unknown primary origin. PLoS ONE 2014;9(4):e95364

23. Zaveri J, La Q, Yarmish G, Neuman J. More than just Langerhans cell histiocytosis: a radiologic review of histiocytic disorders. Radiographics 2014;34(7):2008–2024

Prevertebral Space

24. Debnam JM, Guha-Thakurta N. Retropharyngeal and prevertebral spaces: anatomic imaging and diagnosis. Otolaryngol Clin North Am 2012;45(6):1293–1310

25. Hsu WC, Loevner LA, Karpati R, et al. Accuracy of magnetic resonance imaging in predicting absence of fixation of head and neck cancer to the prevertebral space. Head Neck 2005;27(2):95–100

26. Larawin V, Naipao J, Dubey SP. Head and neck space infections. Otolaryngol Head Neck Surg 2006;135(6):889–893

27. Lee CC, Chu ST, Chou P, Lee CC, Chen LF. The prognostic influence of prevertebral space involvement in nasopharyngeal carcinoma. Clin Otolaryngol 2008;33(5):442–449

28. Paik NC, Lim CS, Jang HS. Tendinitis of longus colli: computed tomography, magnetic resonance imaging, and clinical spectra of 9 cases. J Comput Assist Tomogr 2012;36(6):755–761

29. Park R, Halpert DE, Baer A, Kunar D, Holt PA. Retropharyngeal calcific tendinitis: case report and review of the literature. Semin Arthritis Rheum 2010;39(6):504–509

30. Zibis AH, Giannis D, Malizos KN, Kitsioulis P, Arvanitis DL. Acute calcific tendinitis of the longus colli muscle: case report and review of the literature. Eur Spine J 2013;22(Suppl 3):S434–S438

Chapter 7
Brachial Plexus

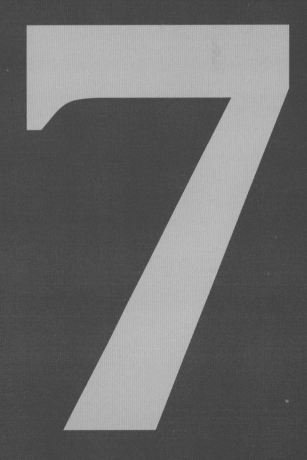

7 Brachial Plexus

Table 7.1 Brachial plexus abnormalities

Introduction

The brachial plexus is a network of nerves innervating the muscles of the shoulder, arm, forearm, and upper chest (**Fig. 7.1** and **Fig. 7.2**). A major function of the brachial plexus is sensorimotor innervation of the arm and forearm. The brachial plexus is supplied by the C5–C8 spinal nerves and the T1 spinal nerve. From medial to lateral, the brachial plexus is composed of roots and trunks (located above the clavicles), divisions (posterior to the clavicles), cords, and branches (below the clavicles).

Within the foramina, the anterior spinal rootlets (motor function) and posterior spinal rootlets (sensory function) merge into ganglia, and then separate into anterior and posterior rami that contain both motor and sensory fibers. The anterior rami (roots) continue to form the brachial plexus, whereas the posterior rami continue to innervate the paraspinal muscles and not the brachial plexus.

The nerve roots of the brachial plexus extend laterally beyond the neural foramina through a triangular space at the thoracic (interscalene) outlet, also referred to as the scalene triangle, between the anterior scalene muscle and the middle and posterior scalene muscles. Located below the nerve roots within the interscalene triangular space are the subclavian artery and lung apex. Within the interscalene outlet, spinal nerves C5 and C6 join to form the superior trunk, C7 forms the middle trunk, and the C8 and T1 nerves join to form the inferior trunk. Nerves that arise from the superior trunk include the suprascapular and subclavius nerves (C5 and C6). The phrenic nerve (C3–C5) also passes between the anterior and middle scalene muscles and extends inferiorly along the surface of the anterior scalene muscle. The three nerve trunks continue laterally and posterior to the clavicle and subclavian muscle, where each trunk separates into single anterior and posterior divisions.

Inferior to the clavicle and distal to the lateral margin of the first rib, the six divisions subsequently merge into three cords. The posterior cord is formed by the union of the three posterior divisions, the lateral cord from the union of the anterior divisions of the upper and middle trunks, and medial cord from the anterior division of the inferior trunk. The posterior cord branches into the radial and axillary nerves. The lateral cord branches into the lateral pectoral nerve (C5–C7 fibers), lateral root of the median nerve, and musculocutaneous nerve. The medial cord branches into the medial root of the median nerve, medial pectoral nerve (C8, T1), medial brachial cutaneous nerve of the upper arm (C8, T1), and median cutaneous nerve of the forearm (C8, T1).

MR imaging of the brachial plexus can be done with conventional techniques, or with high-resolution fat-suppressed three-dimensional (3D) T2-weighted imaging in combination with maximum intensity projections to generate images referred to as MR neurography. Diffusion-weighted imaging can be used to evaluate pathologic changes, measured as fractional anisotropy, in disorders involving the brachial plexus.

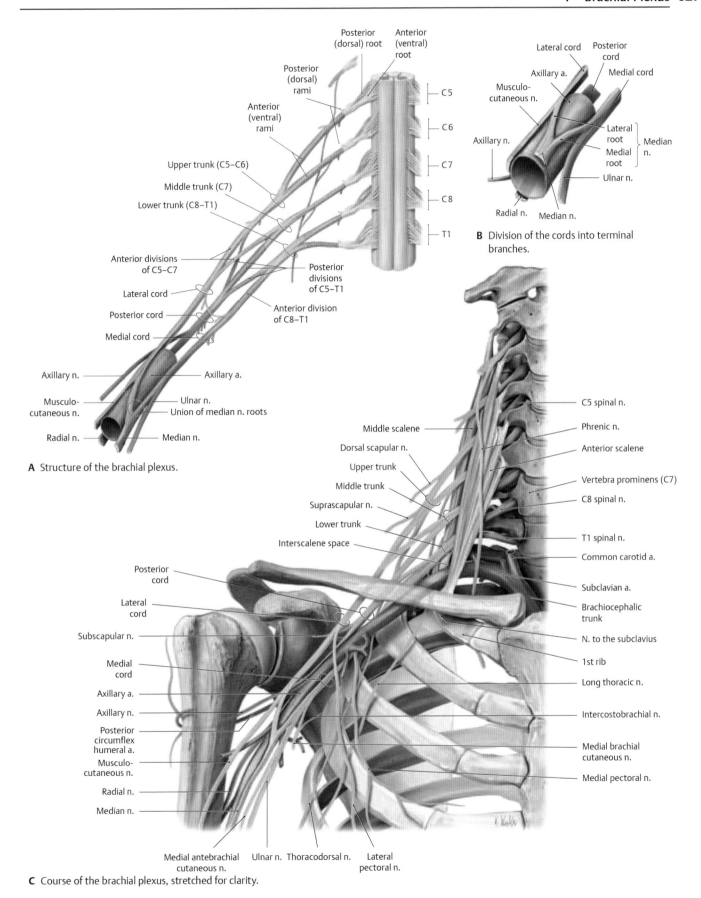

Posterior (dorsal) root
Anterior (ventral) root

Posterior (dorsal) rami

Anterior (ventral) rami

Upper trunk (C5–C6)

Middle trunk (C7)

Lower trunk (C8–T1)

Anterior divisions of C5–C7

Lateral cord

Posterior cord

Medial cord

Axillary n.

Musculo-cutaneous n.

Radial n.

Posterior divisions of C5–T1

Anterior division of C8–T1

Axillary a.

Ulnar n.

Union of median n. roots

Median n.

C5
C6
C7
C8
T1

A Structure of the brachial plexus.

Lateral cord
Posterior cord
Medial cord

Axillary a.

Musculo-cutaneous n.

Axillary n.

Radial n.
Median n.

Lateral root
Medial root
Median n.

Ulnar n.

B Division of the cords into terminal branches.

Middle scalene

Dorsal scapular n.

Upper trunk

Middle trunk

Suprascapular n.

Lower trunk

Interscalene space

Posterior cord

Lateral cord

Subscapular n.

Medial cord

Axillary a.

Axillary n.

Posterior circumflex humeral a.

Musculo-cutaneous n.

Radial n.

Median n.

Medial antebrachial cutaneous n.

Ulnar n.   Thoracodorsal n.

Lateral pectoral n.

C5 spinal n.

Phrenic n.

Anterior scalene

Vertebra prominens (C7)

C8 spinal n.

T1 spinal n.

Common carotid a.

Subclavian a.

Brachiocephalic trunk

N. to the subclavius

1st rib

Long thoracic n.

Intercostobrachial n.

Medial brachial cutaneous n.

Medial pectoral n.

C Course of the brachial plexus, stretched for clarity.

Fig. 7.1 Coronal view of the right brachial plexus and anatomic relationships to adjacent structures. From THIEME Atlas of Anatomy: Head and Neuroanatomy, © Thieme 2007, Illustration by Karl Wesker.

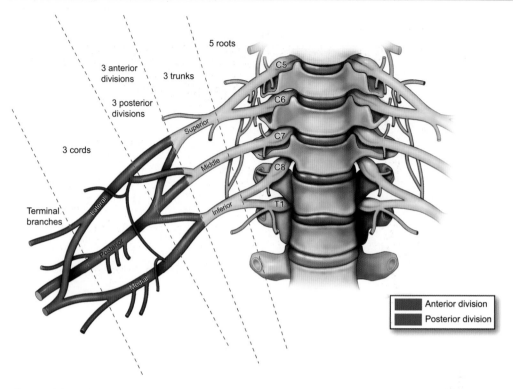

Fig. 7.2 Coronal view of the components of the right brachial plexus.

Table 7.1   Brachial plexus abnormalities

- Benign Neoplasms
  - Schwannoma
  - Neurofibroma
  - Hemangioma
  - Lipoma
- Malignant Neoplasms
  - Metastatic tumor
  - Metastatic lymphadenopathy
  - Lung carcinoma/Pancoast tumor
  - Lymphoma
  - Malignant peripheral nerve sheath tumors (MPNST)
  - Sarcoma
- Tumorlike Lesions
- Venolymphatic malformation

- Charcot-Marie-Tooth disease (Hereditary motor-sensory neuropathy)
- Inflammatory Disease
  - Parsonage-Turner syndrome (Neuralgic amyotrophy)
  - Chronic acquired immune-mediated multifocal demyelinating neuropathy (CIDP)
  - Multifocal motor neuropathy (MMN)
  - Radiation-induced plexopathy
  - Viral infection
  - Bacterial infection
- Traumatic Lesions
  - Erb-Duchenne palsy (Avulsion of nerve roots)
  - Stretch injuries of the brachial plexus
  - Fracture
- Congenital/Developmental
  - Thoracic outlet syndrome

Table 7.1 Brachial plexus abnormalities

Abnormalities	Imaging Findings	Comments
Benign Neoplasms		
Schwannoma **(Fig. 7.3)**	*MRI:* Circumscribed ovoid or spheroid lesions with low-intermediate signal on T1-weighted imaging, high signal on T2-weighted imaging (T2WI) and fat-suppressed T2WI, and usually prominent gadolinium (Gd) contrast enhancement. High signal on T2WI and Gd contrast enhancement can be heterogeneous in large lesions due to cystic degeneration and/or hemorrhage. *CT:* Circumscribed ovoid or spheroid lesions, with intermediate attenuation + contrast enhancement. Large lesions can have cystic degeneration and/or hemorrhage.	Schwannomas are benign encapsulated tumors that contain differentiated neoplastic Schwann cells. Most commonly occur as solitary, sporadic lesions. Schwannomas occur in neurofibromatosis type 2 (NF2), which is an autosomal dominant disease involving a gene mutation at chromosome 22q12. Patients with NF2 can also have multiple meningiomas and ependymomas. The incidence of NF2 is 1/37,000 to 1/50,000 newborns. Age at presentation = 22 to 72 years (mean age = 46 years). Peak incidence is in the fourth to sixth decades. Many patients with NF2 present in the third decade with bilateral vestibular schwannomas.

(continued on page 630)

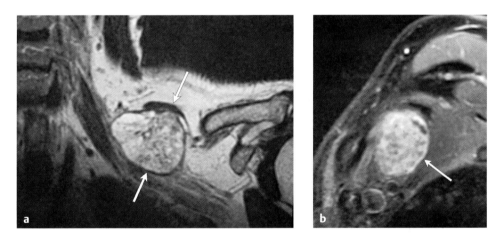

Fig. 7.3 **(a)** Coronal T2-weighted imaging of a 60-year-old man shows a schwannoma involving the left brachial plexus with circumscribed margins, mostly high signal, and irregular zones of low signal (*arrows*). **(b)** The lesion shows heterogeneous gadolinium contrast enhancement (*arrow*) on sagittal fat-suppressed T1-weighted imaging.

Table 7.1 *(cont.)*   Brachial plexus abnormalities

Abnormalities	Imaging Findings	Comments
Neurofibroma (**Fig. 7.4** and **Fig. 7.5**)	*MRI:* *Solitary neurofibromas* are circumscribed spheroid, ovoid, or lobulated extra-axial lesions with low-intermediate signal on T1-weighted imaging (T1WI), intermediate-high signal on T2-weighted imaging (T2WI), + prominent gadolinium (Gd) contrast enhancement. High signal on T2WI and Gd contrast enhancement can be heterogeneous in large lesions. A central zone of low signal on T2WI can be seen in a neurofibroma from collagen/fibrous deposits giving a "target sign." *Plexiform neurofibromas* appear as curvilinear and multinodular lesions involving multiple nerve branches and have low to intermediate signal on T1WI and intermediate, slightly high to high signal on T2WI and fat-suppressed T2WI, with or without bands or strands of low signal. Lesions usually show Gd contrast enhancement. *CT:* Ovoid, spheroid, or fusiform lesions with low-intermediate attenuation. Lesions can show contrast enhancement. Often erode adjacent bone.	Benign nerve sheath tumors that contain mixtures of Schwann cells, perineural-like cells, and interlacing fascicles of fibroblasts associated with abundant collagen. Unlike schwannomas, neurofibromas lack Antoni A and B regions and cannot be separated pathologically from the underlying nerve. Most frequently occur as sporadic, localized, solitary lesions, less frequently as diffuse or plexiform lesions. Multiple neurofibromas are typically seen in neurofibromatosis type 1 (NF1), which is an autosomal dominant disorder (1/2,500 births) caused by mutations in the neurofibromin gene on chromosome 17q11.2. NF1 is the most common type of neurocutaneous syndrome and is associated with neoplasms of the central and peripheral nervous system (optic gliomas, astrocytomas, plexiform and solitary neurofibromas) and skin (café-au-lait spots, axillary and inguinal freckling). Also associated with meningeal and skull dysplasias, as well as hamartomas of the iris (Lisch nodules).
Hemangioma	*MRI:* Circumscribed or poorly marginated structures (< 4 cm in diameter) in soft tissue or bone marrow with intermediate-high signal on T1-weighted imaging (often with portions that are isointense to marrow fat), high signal on T2-weighted imaging (T2WI) and fat-suppressed T2WI, and typically gadolinium contrast enhancement, ± expansion of bone. *CT:* Hemangiomas in soft tissue have mostly intermediate attenuation, ± zones of fat attenuation.	Benign lesions of soft tissue or bone composed of capillary, cavernous, and/or venous malformations. Considered to be a hamartomatous disorder. Occurs in patients 1 to 84 years old (median age = 33 years).
Lipoma (**Fig. 7.6**)	*MRI:* Lipomas have MRI signal isointense to subcutaneous fat on T1-weighted imaging (high signal), and on T2-weighted imaging, signal suppression occurs with frequency-selective fat saturation techniques or with a short time to inversion recovery (STIR) method. Typically there is no gadolinium contrast enhancement or peripheral edema. *CT:* Lipomas have CT attenuation similar to subcutaneous fat, and typically no contrast enhancement or peripheral edema.	Common benign hamartomas composed of mature white adipose tissue without cellular atypia. Most common soft tissue tumor, representing 16% of all soft tissue tumors. May contain calcifications and/or traversing blood vessels.

(continued on page 632)

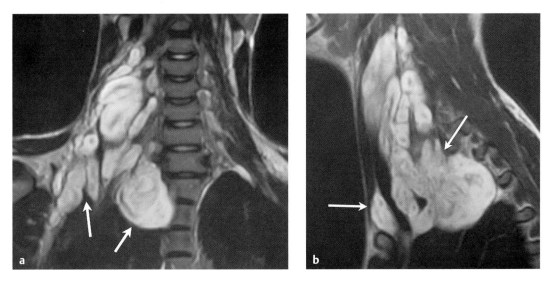

Fig. 7.4 **(a)** Coronal and **(b)** sagittal T2-weighted imaging of a 15-year-old male with neurofibromatosis type 1 shows multiple neurofibromas with high signal involving the left brachial plexus (*arrows*). Low signal foci in the central portions of the neurofibromas are seen. These findings are have been referred to as "target signs."

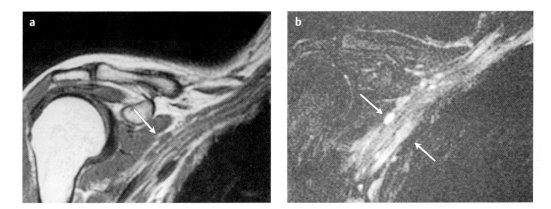

Fig. 7.5 **(a)** Coronal T1-weighted imaging of a 26-year-old woman with neurofibromatosis type 1 shows multiple small neurofibromas (*arrow*) involving the right brachial plexus. **(b)** The lesions have corresponding high signal on coronal fat-suppressed T2-weighted imaging (*arrows*).

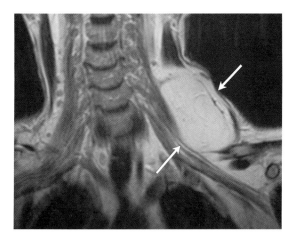

Fig. 7.6 Coronal T1-weighted imaging shows a lipoma with high signal (*arrows*) indenting the upper portions of the left brachial plexus.

Table 7.1 *(cont.)* Brachial plexus abnormalities

Abnormalities	Imaging Findings	Comments
Malignant Neoplasms		
Metastatic tumor **(Fig. 7.7)**	*MRI:* Circumscribed spheroid or diffusely infiltrating lesions that often have low-intermediate signal on T1-weighted imaging, intermediate-high signal on T2-weighted imaging, ± hemorrhage, calcifications, and cysts and variable gadolinium contrast enhancement. *CT:* Lesions usually have low-intermediate attenuation, ± hemorrhage, calcifications, and cysts, variable contrast enhancement, ± bone destruction, ± compression of neural tissue or vessels.	Metastatic tumor may cause variable destructive or infiltrative changes in single or multiple sites. Metastatic tumor involving the brachial plexus can result from direct spread from lung or breast carcinomas.
Metastatic lymphadenopathy	*MRI:* Enlarged spheroid or ovoid nodes that often have low-intermediate signal on T1-weighted imaging, intermediate-high signal on T2-weighted imaging (T2WI), ± high signal zones on T2WI (necrosis), ± irregular margins (capsule invasion), ± decreased ADC values on diffusion-weighted imaging ($< 1.4 \times 10^{-3}$ mm^2/sec), and variable gadolinium contrast enhancement. Extracapsular spread of tumor from lymph nodes can invade adjacent tissue. *CT:* Involved nodes usually have low-intermediate attenuation, ± irregular margins (capsule invasion), ± low-attenuation zones (necrosis), and variable contrast enhancement. Usually measure more than 8 mm in short axis. *PET/CT:* Increased nodal uptake of F-18 FDG.	Metastatic tumor involving cervical and supraclavicular lymph nodes can result from primary neck neoplasms, such as squamous cell carcinoma or thyroid cancer. Can also result from spread from primary extracranial tumor source: Lung > breast > GI > GU > melanoma. Can occur as single or multiple well-circumscribed or poorly defined lesions. Metastatic tumor may cause variable destructive or infiltrative changes in single or multiple sites. Clinical findings include neck and upper-extremity pain, muscle weakness, and/or paresthesias.
Lung carcinoma/ Pancoast tumor **(Fig. 7.8)**	*MRI:* Lesions often have intermediate signal on T1-weighted imaging and slightly high to high signal on T2-weighted imaging, + gadolinium contrast enhancement. Tumors often have irregular margins, with extension into the brachial plexus and neural foramina. Bone destruction is commonly seen. *CT:* Soft tissue lesions at the lung apex that often have irregular margins. Bone invasion and destruction are commonly seen.	Primary lung carcinomas (adenocarcinoma, squamous cell carcinoma, large cell carcinoma, small cell carcinoma) at the upper lung and lung apex (Pancoast tumor) can invade the brachial plexus, causing shoulder and arm pain from the tumor involving the C8 and T1 nerve roots, as well as Horner syndrome (20%) and head and neck pain. Radiation treatment followed by surgery can used.
Lymphoma **(Fig. 7.9)**	*CT:* Lesions have low-intermediate attenuation, may show contrast enhancement, ± bone destruction. *MRI:* Lesions have low-intermediate signal on T1-weighted imaging, intermediate to slightly high signal on T2-weighted imaging, + gadolinium contrast enhancement. Can be locally invasive and associated with bone erosion/destruction and intracranial extension with meningeal involvement (up to 5%).	Lymphomas are a group of lymphoid tumors whose neoplastic cells typically arise within lymphoid tissue (lymph nodes and reticuloendothelial organs). Unlike leukemia, lymphomas usually arise as discrete masses. Lymphomas are subdivided into Hodgkin disease (HD) and non-Hodgkin lymphoma (NHL). Distinction between HD and NHL is useful because of differences in clinical and histopathologic features, as well as treatment strategies. HD typically arises in lymph nodes and often spreads along nodal chains, whereas NHL frequently originates at extranodal sites and spreads in an unpredictable pattern. Almost all primary lymphomas of bone are B-cell NHL.
Malignant peripheral nerve sheath tumors (MPNST)	*MRI:* MPNST usually have heterogeneous signal on T1- and T2-weighted imaging, as well as heterogeneous gadolinium contrast enhancement because of necrosis and hemorrhage. Some MPNST are similar in appearance to benign nerve sheath tumors. *CT:* Soft tissue lesions that usually can have circumscribed or irregular margins. Calcifications are uncommon. Tumors can have mixed CT attenuation, with solid zones of soft tissue attenuation, cystic-appearing and/or necrotic zones, and occasional foci of hemorrhage, ± bone invasion and destruction.	MPNST are malignant tumors of the peripheral nerve sheath that contain mixtures of packed hyperchromatic spindle cells with elongated nuclei and slightly eosinophilic cytoplasm, mitotic figures, and zones of necrosis. Approximately 50% of MPNSTs occur in patients with neurofibromatosis type 1, followed by de novo evolution from peripheral nerves. MPNST infrequently arise from schwannomas, ganglioneuroblastomas/ganglioneuromas, and pheochromocytomas.

(continued on page 634)

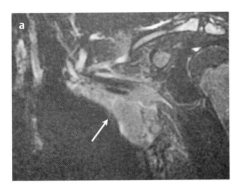
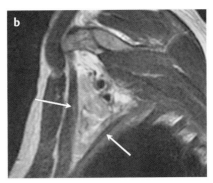
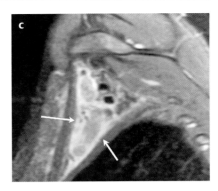

Fig. 7.7 **(a)** Coronal fat-suppressed T2-weighted imaging and **(b)** sagittal T2-weighted imaging of a 36-year-old woman with breast cancer show a metastatic lesion at the upper left hemithorax (*arrows*) with intermediate to high signal. **(c)** The lesion has corresponding gadolinium contrast enhancement on sagittal fat-suppressed T1-weighted imaging and extends into the left brachial plexus (*arrows*).

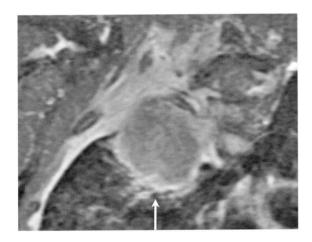

Fig. 7.8 Coronal fat-suppressed T1-weighted imaging of a 50-year-old woman shows a gadolinium-enhancing lung carcinoma at the upper right hemithorax (Pancoast tumor). The tumor (*arrow*) invades the right brachial plexus.

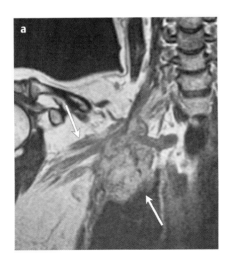
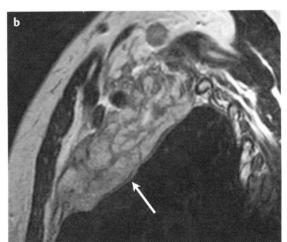

Fig. 7.9 **(a)** Coronal and **(b)** sagittal T2-weighted images of a 58-year-old woman with non-Hodgkin lymphoma show a mass lesion at the upper right hemithorax with heterogeneous intermediate to slightly high signal. The lesion invades the right brachial plexus (*arrows*).

Table 7.1 *(cont.)* Brachial plexus abnormalities

Abnormalities	Imaging Findings	Comments
Sarcoma (**Fig. 7.10** and **Fig. 7.11**)	*MRI:* Tumors can have circumscribed and/or poorly defined margins, and typically have low-intermediate signal on T1-weighted imaging and heterogeneous signal (various combinations of intermediate, slightly high, and/or high signal) on T2-weighted imaging (T2WI) and fat-suppressed T2WI. Tumors show variable degrees of gadolinium contrast enhancement, ± bone destruction and invasion. *CT:* Soft tissue lesions usually can have circumscribed or irregular margins. Calcifications are uncommon. Tumors can have mixed CT attenuation with solid zones of soft tissue attenuation, cystic-appearing and/or necrotic zones, and occasional foci of hemorrhage, ± bone invasion and destruction.	Primary sarcomas rarely occur in the neck.
Tumorlike Lesions		
Venolymphatic malformation (**Fig. 7.12**)	Can be circumscribed lesions or occur in an infiltrative pattern with extension within soft tissue and between muscles. *MRI:* Often contain single or multiple cystic zones that can be large (macrocystic type) or small (microcystic type), and that have predominantly low signal on T1-weighted imaging (T1WI) and high signal on T2-weighted imaging (T2WI) and fat-suppressed T2WI. Fluid–fluid levels and zones with high signal on T1WI and variable signal on T2WI may result from cysts containing hemorrhage, high protein concentration, and/or necrotic debris. Septa between the cystic zones can vary in thickness and gadolinium (Gd) contrast enhancement. Nodular zones within the lesions can have variable degrees of Gd contrast enhancement. Microcystic malformations typically show more Gd contrast enhancement than the macrocystic type. *CT:* Macrocystic malformations are usually low-attenuation cystic lesions (10–25 HU) separated by thin walls, ± intermediate or high attenuation resulting from hemorrhage or infection, ± fluid–fluid levels.	Benign vascular anomalies (also referred to as lymphangioma or cystic hygroma) that primarily result from abnormal lymphangiogenesis. Up to 75% occur in the head and neck. Can be observed in utero with MRI or sonography, at birth (50–65%), or within the first 5 years. Approximately 85% are detected by age 2. Lesions are composed of endothelium-lined lymphatic ± venous channels interspersed within connective tissue stroma. Account for less than 1% of benign soft tissue tumors and 5.6% of all benign lesions of infancy and childhood. Can occur in association with Turner syndrome and Proteus syndrome.
Charcot-Marie-Tooth disease (Hereditary motor-sensory neuropathy)	*MRI:* Focal or diffuse enlargement of one or more nerves, which have low-intermediate signal on T1-weighted imaging, slightly high to high signal on T2-weighted imaging (T2WI) and fat-suppressed T2WI, + diffuse gadolinium contrast enhancement of nerves, ± denervation of muscles, which have high signal on T2WI in the acute/subacute phases, followed by eventual fatty replacement.	Charcot-Marie-Tooth (CMT) disease is a heterogeneous group of genetic disorders (30 causative genes on chromosome 17, usually autosomal dominant) characterized clinically by slowly progressive muscle wasting, weakness > sensory loss, ± foot deformities (pes cavus, hammer toes). CMT disease is a relatively common inherited neurologic disorder, with a prevalence of 15/100,000. Frequently presents in children or young adults. Mutation makes a peripheral myelin protein unstable, which results in repetitive cycles of demyelination and remyelination, producing enlarged nerves with concentric myelin layers around the axon, giving it an "onion bulb" histologic appearance. Most frequently involves the peripheral nerves of the arms and legs, although can also involve the brachial plexus. Associated with acute or chronic muscle denervation. Conservative treatment includes injury prevention, physical therapy, and ankle/foot orthotics.

(continued on page 636)

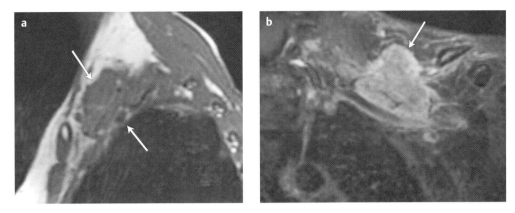

Fig. 7.10 **(a)** Sagittal T1-weighted imaging of a patient who has a pleomorphic sarcoma involving the left brachial plexus (*arrows*), which has intermediate signal and shows gadolinium contrast enhancement on **(b)** coronal fat-suppressed T1-weighted imaging (*arrow*).

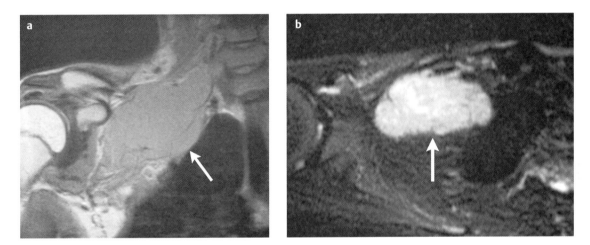

Fig. 7.11 An 11-year-old female with an extraosseous Ewing sarcoma involving the right brachial plexus. **(a)** The tumor has intermediate signal on coronal proton density-weighted imaging (*arrow*) and **(b)** high signal on axial fat-suppressed T2-weighted imaging (*arrow*).

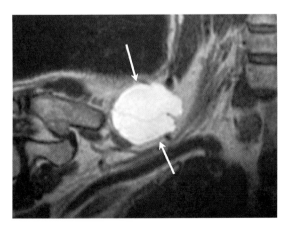

Fig. 7.12 Coronal T2-weighted imaging of a 53-year-old man shows a veno-lymphatic malformation with high signal (*arrows*) at the upper border of the right brachial plexus.

Table 7.1 *(cont.)*   Brachial plexus abnormalities

Abnormalities	Imaging Findings	Comments
Inflammatory Disease		
Parsonage-Turner syndrome (Neuralgic amyotrophy) (**Fig. 7.13**)	*MRI:* Abnormal thickening of nerve roots, which have slightly high to high signal on T2-weighted imaging (T2WI) and fat-suppressed T2WI. There is denervation of muscles, which have high signal on T2WI in the acute/subacute phases, followed by eventual fatty replacement.	Acute idiopathic inflammation of the brachial plexus associated with acute onset of muscle pain, followed by weakness and wasting of the shoulder muscles (serratus anterior, supraspinatus and infraspinatus muscles are the most frequently involved). Incidence is at least 3 per 100,000 per year, and usually occurs in patients between the third and seventh decades, with a male predominance. Most commonly involves the upper trunks of the brachial plexus, but can involve other nerves. Sporadic cases may occur after viral or bacterial infections, immunizations, drug reactions, burn injuries, stress, and/or episodes of vasculitis. Can also occur as a genetic syndrome of hereditary neuralgic amyotrophy (HNA), which results from mutations involving the septin 9 gene on chromosome 17q25. EMG shows acute and chronic denervation. Treatment includes long-acting NSAIDs and physical therapy. Symptoms often resolve after 4–12 weeks.
Chronic acquired immune-mediated multifocal demyelinating neuropathy (CIDP) (**Fig. 7.14**)	*MRI:* Most frequently involves the nerves of the lumbar plexus and cauda equina, and infrequently involves the brachial plexus. Diffuse enlargement of multiple nerves, with slightly high signal on T2-weighted imaging (T2WI) and fat-suppressed T2WI, with variable mild-moderate gadolinium contrast enhancement. Localized zones of nodular thickening may be seen within the enlarged nerves. Enlarged nerves can be bilateral and symmetric or asymmetric. Abnormally enlarged nerves can extend from the ventral rami to the lateral portions of the brachial plexus.	Acquired immune-mediated progressive/recurrent neuropathy that occurs more commonly in adults than in children. Prevalence of up to 7/100,000. Usually involves the spinal nerves, ± proximal nerve trunks of the brachial plexus. Patients present with relapsing or progressive, symmetric, proximal and distal muscle weakness without or with sensory loss. Diagnosis is based on biopsy and clinical and electrophysiologic examinations. EMGs show slowed conduction velocities from demyelination. Cycles of demyelination and remyelination produce enlarged nerves with inflammatory infiltrates (lymphocytes, macrophages). Can occur in association with IgG or IgA monoclonal gammopathy, inflammatory bowel disease, hepatitis C infection, HIV infection, diabetes, Sjögren's syndrome, and lymphoma. Immunosuppressive medications can be used for treatment.
Multifocal motor neuropathy (MMN)	*MRI:* Diffuse or multiple sites of enlargement of nerves (brachial plexus and median, ulnar, and/or radial nerves) that have increased signal on T2-weighted imaging and involve the nerves of the brachial plexus, including the ventral rami, ± gadolinium contrast enhancement. Imaging findings typically correlate with distribution of symptoms.	Immune-mediated progressive demyelinating disorder that results in a purely motor neuropathy without objective sensory loss. MMN occurs from an autoimmune response directed toward an antigen specific to the motor nerves, impairing function. Up to 50% of patients have IgM antibodies to the ganglioside GM_1 located in peripheral nerves. MMN has a prevalence of 0.6/100,000, usually occurs in adults 20 to 70 years old (mean age = 40 years), and occurs two to three times more often in males than in females. Clinical findings include slowly progressive asymmetric weakness and atrophy in the distribution of spinal segments rather than specific nerves. Asymmetric motor weakness more frequently involves the nerves of the distal > proximal upper extremities > lower extremities. Usually involves more than two separate motor nerve distributions. EMGs show motor conduction blocks. Can be treated with immunotherapy with intravenous immunoglobulins, rituximab, or cyclosporine.

(continued on page 638)

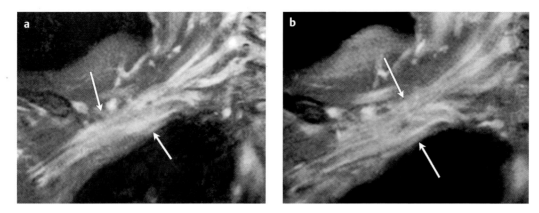

Fig. 7.13 **(a)** Coronal fat-suppressed T2-weighted imaging of a 65-year-old woman with Parsonage-Turner syndrome shows abnormal thickening of the right brachial plexus nerves (*arrows*), which have slightly high to high signal. **(b)** There is corresponding gadolinium contrast enhancement on coronal fat-suppressed T1-weighted imaging (*arrows*).

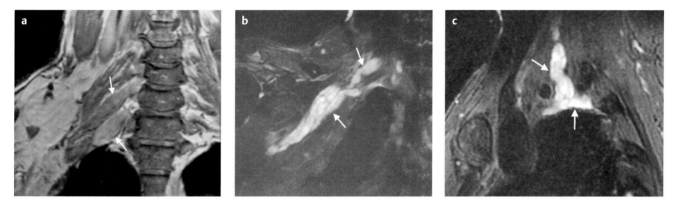

Fig. 7.14 **(a)** Coronal T1-weighted imaging of a 54-year-old man with chronic acquired immune-mediated multifocal demyelinating neuropathy (CIDP) shows abnormally thickened right C7 and C8 nerve roots and trunks, which have heterogeneous intermediate signal (*arrows*), and high signal on **(b)** coronal and **(c)** sagittal fat-suppressed T2-weighted imaging (*arrows*).

Table 7.1 *(cont.)*   Brachial plexus abnormalities

Abnormalities	Imaging Findings	Comments
Radiation-induced plexopathy (**Fig. 7.15**)	*MRI:* Diffuse thickening of the nerves at the treated site, ± indistinct margins. In the first few years, radiation-induced inflammatory changes often result in nerves with intermediate signal on T1-weighted imaging (T1WI), slightly high to high signal on T2-weighted imaging (T2WI), and gadolinium (Gd) contrast enhancement. In the late phases, when fibrotic changes predominate, nerves may have low-intermediate signal on both T1WI and T2WI, with minimal or no Gd contrast enhancement. *CT:* Thickening of nerve roots, poorly defined margins with adjacent adipose tissue, ± adjacent radiation-induced pleuritis and pneumonitis. *PET/CT:* Usually low uptake of F-18 FDG.	Radiation-induced fibrosis can occur within 6 months of radiation treatment, usually with doses more than 60 Gray. Radiation treatment results in a combination of inflammatory changes and progressive fibrosis. May be difficult to distinguish from recurrent tumor in some cases.
Viral infection	*MRI:* Enlarged nerves with slightly high signal on T2-weighted imaging (T2WI) and fat-suppressed T2WI, ± gadolinium contrast enhancement.	Primary viral infections (cytomegalovirus, Coxsackie, Epsein-Barr, HIV) can cause direct infection of the brachial plexus.
Bacterial infection	*MRI:* Enlarged nerves with poorly defined margins, slightly high signal on T2-weighted imaging (T2WI) and fat-suppressed T2WI, + gadolinium contrast enhancement of nerves and adjacent soft tissues, ± abscess.	Extension of pyogenic vertebral infections can involve the brachial plexus.
Traumatic Lesions		
Erb-Duchenne palsy (Avulsion of nerve roots) (**Fig. 7.16**, **Fig. 7.17**, and **Fig. 7.18**)	*MRI:* Nerve root avulsions may be seen as discontinuous nerves with bulbous ends within dura or extradural fluid collections (pseudomeningoceles). A common finding is the presence of periscalene soft tissue with intermediate signal on T1-weighted imaging (T1WI) and slightly high signal on T2-weighted imaging (T2WI) adjacent to the anterior scalene muscle, which occurs in up to 95% of patients. Other findings include empty nerve root sleeves, posttraumatic nerve root pouch cysts. If avulsed nerve roots are not reattached, terminal neuromas can occur within the first year, which have low-intermediate signal on T1WI and mildly heterogeneous intermediate to high signal on T2WI and fat-suppressed T2WI, ± gadolinium contrast enhancement. *CT myelography:* Contrast can be seen within traumatic meningocele/pseudomeningocele, and/or epidural space through a dural tear.	Obstetric trauma can result in downward traction, causing stretch injuries of the brachial plexus involving the C5 and/or C6 nerves, resulting in a flaccid ipsilateral upper extremity. Accounts for up to 90% of obstetric-related injuries involving the brachial plexus. When nerve roots are stretched but not avulsed during obstetric delivery, clinical findings often resolve within weeks to months after birth. Avulsion of the nerve roots, however, results in an *Erb palsy* (shoulder and arm in adducted and internally rotated position, elbow extension and forearm pronation). Injuries to the brachial plexus also occur in young adults due to blunt trauma from motor vehicle collisions or falls, as well as gunshots. These injuries usually occur in association with significant traumatic head and/or spine injuries. *Klumpke-Dejerine syndrome* is an uncommon type of injury involving the brachial plexus that occurs from upward traction, resulting in damage to the C8 and/or T1 nerve roots or lower trunks of the brachial plexus, causing paralysis of the intrinsic muscles of the hand, wrist, and finger flexor muscles. Damage to the proximal T1 nerve can be associated with injury to the sympathetic chain and concomitant Horner syndrome. For *postganglionic nerve injuries,* treatment includes surgical removal of mass effect on injured brachial plexus and nerve root grafting if nerve fascicles are not intact. For *preganglionic nerve injuries,* surgical grafting can be performed to the nerve stumps of C5 and C6 to restore biceps function and shoulder mobility. If not repaired, the proximal ends of the damaged or transected nerves undergo a benign proliferative process (terminal neuroma) that occurs 1 to 12 months after injury.

(continued on page 641)

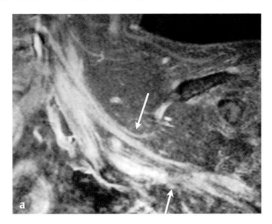 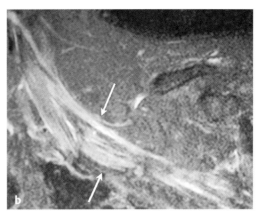

Fig. 7.15 **(a)** Coronal fat-suppressed T2-weighted imaging of a 70-year-old man with radiation-induced left brachial plexopathy shows abnormal thickening of the brachial plexus nerves (*arrows*), which have high signal and **(b)** corresponding gadolinium contrast enhancement on coronal fat-suppressed T1-weighted imaging (*arrows*).

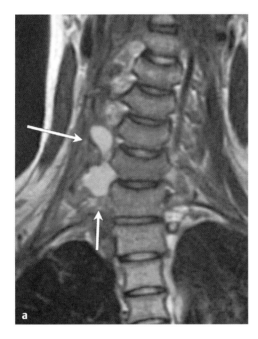 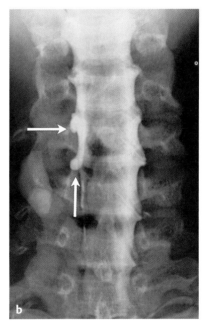

Fig. 7.16 **(a)** Coronal T2-weighted imaging of a 15-year-old male shows sites of nerve root avulsions, with extradural fluid collections (pseudomeningoceles) with high signal on T2-weighted imaging (*arrows*) and empty nerve root sleeves. **(b)** AP myelographic image shows contrast filling the traumatic pseudomeningoceles (*arrows*).

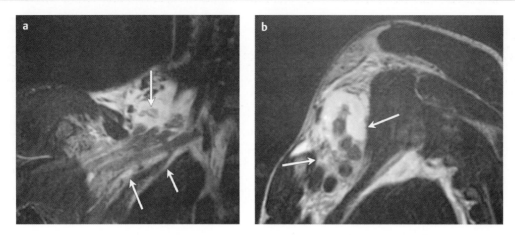

Fig. 7.17 **(a)** Coronal and **(b)** sagittal T2-weighted images of a 17-year-old male show multiple traumatic nerve root avulsions involving the right brachial plexus. The discontinuous distal portions of the nerves are thickened and retracted laterally, with associated high-signal edema and seromas in the adjacent soft tissue (*arrows*).

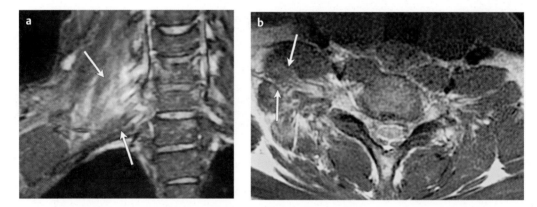

Fig. 7.18 **(a)** Coronal fat-suppressed T2-weighted imaging of a 40-year-old man shows traumatic tears of multiple nerve roots of the right brachial plexus, which are thickened and have ill-defined margins with high signal (*arrows*). **(b)** Axial T2-weighted imaging shows an ill-defined ovoid zone of periscalene soft tissue with slightly high signal on axial T2-weighted imaging adjacent to the anterior scalene muscle (*arrows*).

Table 7.1 *(cont.)*   Brachial plexus abnormalities

Abnormalities	Imaging Findings	Comments
Stretch injuries of the brachial plexus (**Fig. 7.19**)	*MRI:* Nerve roots can be thickened, with intermediate signal on T1-weighted imaging and high signal on T2-weighted imaging, + gadolinium contrast enhancement.	Stretch injuries to the brachial plexus can result in nerve damage without frank avulsion of nerve fibers (neuropraxia). Resolution of clinical findings and/or recovery can depend on the duration and severity of injury.
Fracture (**Fig. 7.20**)	*CT:* Shows clavicular fractures and location of displaced fragments. *MRI:* Can show the position of clavicular fracture in relation to the brachial plexus, as well as the presence of hematomas and seromas and disrupted nerves.	At the junction of the medial and mid portions of the clavicle, the subclavian artery, brachial plexus, and subclavian vein are located within 2 cm. Fractures of these portions of the clavicle are associated with increased risk of injuries to the nearby neurovascular structures.

(continued on page 642)

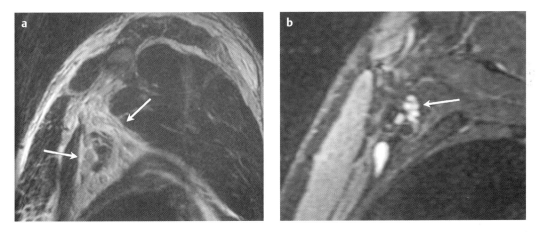

Fig. 7.19   **(a)** Sagittal T2-weighted imaging of a 47-year-old man with an acute traction stress injury involving the brachial plexus shows abnormally thickened edematous nerves with slightly high-to-high signal (*arrows*). **(b)** Sagittal fat-suppressed T2-weighted imaging 10 months later shows atrophied nerves with high signal (*arrow*).

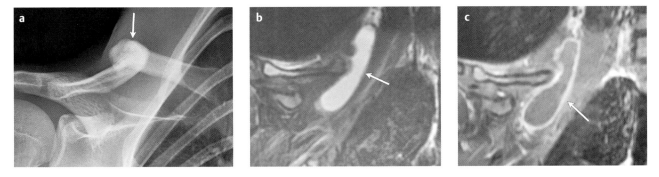

Fig. 7.20   **(a)** AP radiograph shows a fracture of the right clavicle (*arrow*) that is associated with a seroma at the upper margins of the right brachial plexus, which has **(b)** high signal on coronal fat-suppressed T2-weighted imaging (*arrow*) and shows **(c)** peripheral gadolinium contrast enhancement on coronal fat-suppressed T1-weighted imaging (*arrow*).

Table 7.1 *(cont.)*   Brachial plexus abnormalities

Abnormalities	Imaging Findings	Comments
Congenital/Developmental		
Thoracic outlet syndrome (**Fig. 7.21** and **Fig. 7.22**)	*CT or MRI:* Can show cervical ribs, enlarged C7 transverse processes, fibrous bands, or posttraumatic deformities adjacent to the subclavian artery, subclavian vein, and/or brachial plexus. *CTA:* With arms extended may demonstrate impingement on the nerves or vessels in the scalene triangle.	Signs and symptoms of thoracic outlet syndrome (TOS) occur from compression of the brachial plexus (neurogenic TOS), subclavian artery (arterial TOS), and/or subclavian vein (venous TOS). Neurogenic TOS accounts for ~ 90% of TOS cases. Compression of the thoracic outlet structures can be static or positional. Causes of compression include cervical ribs, fibrous bands, and hypertrophy or anomalies of the scalene muscles.

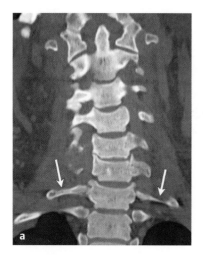
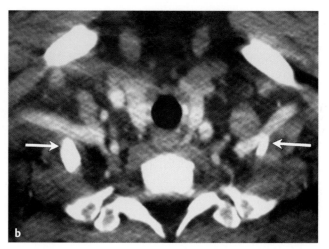

Fig. 7.21   **(a)** Coronal CT in thoracic outlet syndrome shows bilateral cervical ribs (*arrows*). **(b)** The ribs impress on the subclavian arteries (*arrows*), as seen on postcontrast axial CT.

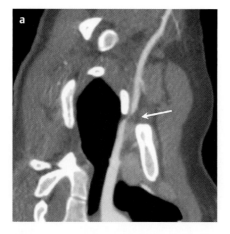
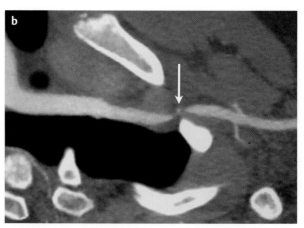

Fig. 7.22   **(a)** Oblique sagittal and **(b)** axial CTA acquired with the upper extremity elevated shows localized impingement and narrowing of the subclavian artery (*arrows*) in the scalene triangle resulting in thoracic outlet syndrome.

References

Brachial Neuritis

1. Jain S, Bhatt GC, Rai N, Bhan BD. Idiopathic brachial neuritis in a child: A case report and review of the literature. J Pediatr Neurosci 2014; 9(3):276–277

Brachial Plexus: Imaging

2. Castillo M. Imaging the anatomy of the brachial plexus: review and self-assessment module. AJR Am J Roentgenol 2005;185(6, Suppl): S196–S204
3. Chen WC, Tsai YH, Weng HH, et al. Value of enhancement technique in 3D-T2-STIR images of the brachial plexus. J Comput Assist Tomogr 2014;38(3):335–339
4. Chhabra A, Thawait GK, Soldatos T, et al. High-resolution 3T MR neurography of the brachial plexus and its branches, with emphasis on 3D imaging. AJNR Am J Neuroradiol 2013;34(3):486–497
5. Lutz AM, Gold G, Beaulieu C. MR imaging of the brachial plexus. Neuroimaging Clin N Am 2014;24(1):91–108
6. Posniak HV, Olson MC, Dudiak CM, Wisniewski R, O'Malley C. MR imaging of the brachial plexus. AJR Am J Roentgenol 1993;161(2):373–379
7. Todd M, Shah GV, Mukherji SK. MR imaging of brachial plexus. Top Magn Reson Imaging 2004;15(2):113–125

Brachial Plexus: Nontraumatic Lesions

8. Boulanger X, Ledoux JB, Brun AL, Beigelman C. Imaging of the non-traumatic brachial plexus. Diagn Interv Imaging 2013;94(10):945–956

Brachial Plexus: Traumatic Injuries

9. Buchanan EP, Richardson R, Tse R. Isolated lower brachial plexus (Klumpke) palsy with compound arm presentation: case report. J Hand Surg Am 2013;38(8):1567–1570
10. Robinson L, Persico F, Lorenz E, Seligson D. Clavicular caution: an anatomic study of neurovascular structures. Injury 2014; 45(12):1867–1869
11. Sakellariou VI, Badilas NK, Mazis GA, et al. Brachial plexus injuries in adults: evaluation and diagnostic approach. ISRN Orthop 2014;2014:726103
12. Silbermann-Hoffman O, Teboul F. Post-traumatic brachial plexus MRI in practice. Diagn Interv Imaging 2013;94(10):925–943
13. Wandler E, Lefton D, Babb J, Shatzkes D. Periscalene soft tissue: the new imaging hallmark in Erb palsy. AJNR Am J Neuroradiol 2010;31(5):882–885

Charcot-Marie-Tooth Disease

14. Reilly MM, Murphy SM, Laurá M. Charcot-Marie-Tooth disease. J Peripher Nerv Syst 2011;16(1):1–14

Chronic Inflammatory Demyelinating Polyradiculopathy

15. Bradley LJ, Wilhelm T, King RHM, Ginsberg L, Orrell RW. Brachial plexus hypertrophy in chronic inflammatory demyelinating polyradiculoneuropathy. Neuromuscul Disord 2006;16(2):126–131

Hypertrophic Mono- and Polyneuropathies

16. De Smet K, De Maeseneer M, Talebian Yazdi A, Stadnik T, De Mey J. MRI in hypertrophic mono- and polyneuropathies. Clin Radiol 2013;68(3):317–322
17. Lawson VH, Arnold WD. Multifocal motor neuropathy: a review of pathogenesis, diagnosis, and treatment. Neuropsychiatr Dis Treat 2014;10:567–576
18. Vlam L, van der Pol WL, Cats EA, et al. Multifocal motor neuropathy: diagnosis, pathogenesis and treatment strategies. Nat Rev Neurol 2012;8(1):48–58

Parsonage-Turner Syndrome (Neuralgic Amyotrophy)

19. Tjoumakaris FP, Anakwenze OA, Kancherla V, Pulos N. Neuralgic amyotrophy (Parsonage-Turner syndrome). J Am Acad Orthop Surg 2012;20(7):443–449
20. Park MS, Kim H, Sung DH. Magnetic resonance neurographic findings in classic idiopathic neuralgic amyotrophy in subacute stage: a report of four cases. Ann Rehabil Med 2014;38(2):286–291

Index